Clinical Interventional Oncology

First Edition

Stephen T. Kee, MD
Professor of Radiology
Chief, Interventional Radiology
UCLA Health Sciences
Los Angeles, California

Ravi Murthy, MD, FACP
Professor of Radiology
Interventional Radiology Section
Division of Diagnostic Imaging
University of Texas
M.D. Anderson Cancer Center
Houston, Texas

David C. Madoff, MD
Professor of Radiology
Chief, Division of Interventional Radiology
New York-Presbyterian Hospital/ Weill Cornell Medical Center
New York, New York

ELSEVIER
SAUNDERS

ELSEVIER
SAUNDERS

1600 John F. Kennedy Blvd.
Ste 1800
Philadelphia, PA 19103-2899

CLINICAL INTERVENTIONAL ONCOLOGY
First Edition

ISBN: 978-1-4557-1221-2

Notices

Knowledge and best practice in this field are constantly changing. As new research and experience broaden our understanding, changes in research methods, professional practices, or medical treatment may become necessary.

Practitioners and researchers must always rely on their own experience and knowledge in evaluating and using any information, methods, compounds, or experiments described herein. In using such information or methods they should be mindful of their own safety and the safety of others, including parties for whom they have a professional responsibility.

With respect to any drug or pharmaceutical products identified, readers are advised to check the most current information provided (i) on procedures featured or (ii) by the manufacturer of each product to be administered, to verify the recommended dose or formula, the method and duration of administration, and contraindications. It is the responsibility of practitioners, relying on their own experience and knowledge of their patients, to make diagnoses, to determine dosages and the best treatment for each individual patient, and to take all appropriate safety precautions.

To the fullest extent of the law, neither the Publisher nor the authors, contributors, or editors, assume any liability for any injury and/or damage to persons or property as a matter of products liability, negligence or otherwise, or from any use or operation of any methods, products, instructions, or ideas contained in the material herein.

ISBN: 978-1-4557-1221-2

Content Strategist: Helene T. Caprari
Content Development Strategist: Jacob Harte
Publishing Services Manager: Julie Eddy
Senior Project Manager: Marquita Parker
Design Direction: Steven Stave

Printed in China

Last digit is the print number: 9 8 7 6 5 4 3 2 1

Mohamed Abdelsalem, MD
Section of Interventional Radiology
Department of Diagnostic Radiology
The University of Texas M.D. Anderson Cancer Center
Houston, Texas
United States
Intra-Arterial Procedures for the Musculoskeletal System

Ghassan K. Abou-Alfa, MD
Memorial Sloan-Kettering Cancer Center
New York, New York
United States
Systemic Therapy in Advanced Hepatocellular Carcinoma

Fereidoun Abtin, MD
Associate Professor of Radiology
Thoracic Radiology, Department of Radiological Sciences
David Geffen School of Medicine at UCLA
Los Angeles, California
United States
Primary Lung Carcinoma

Andreas Adam, PhD, FRCR, FmedSci
Professor of Interventional Radiology
Department of Interventional Radiology
King's College
Honorary Consultant Radiologist
Department of Radiology
Guy's and St. Thomas' Hospital
London
United Kingdom
The Role of Interventional Oncology in Modern Cancer Care

Quazi Zubair Al-Tariq, MD
Resident Physician
Department of Radiology
University of California at Los Angeles
Los Angeles, California
United States
Metastatic Disease

Jordan Anaokar, MD
Resident Radiologist
Department of Radiology
University of California
Los Angeles, California
United States
Interventional Strategies in the Treatment of Gynecologic Cancers

Celina Ang, MD
Assistant Professor
Medicine, Hematology/Oncology
Tisch Cancer Institute, Mount Sinai School of Medicine
New York, New York
United States
Systemic Therapy in Advanced Hepatocellular Carcinoma

Rony Avritscher, MD
Section of Interventional Radiology
Department of Diagnostic Radiology
The University of Texas M.D. Anderson Cancer Center
Houston, Texas
United States
Intra-Arterial Procedures for the Musculoskeletal System

Matthew Callstrom, MD, PhD
Consultant
Department of Radiology
Mayo Clinic
Associate Professor of Radiology
Mayo Clinic College of Medicine
Rochester, Minnesota
United States
Ablation of Musculoskeletal Metastatic Lesions Including Cementoplasty

Daniel Cherqui, MD
Professor of Surgery
Weill Cornell Medical College
Attending Surgeon
New York-Presbyterian Hospital
Chief, Hepatobiliary Surgery and Liver Transplantation
New York-Presbyterian/Weill Cornell
New York, New York
United States
Surgical Management of Hepatocellular Carcinoma

Sophie Chheang, MD
Interventional Radiology Fellow
Department of Interventional Radiology
New York-Presbyterian Hospital/Weill Cornell
New York, New York
United States
Tumor Response for IGI - Assessment and Validation

Bruno Damascelli, MD
Department of Interventional Radiology GVM
Emocuore Columbus
Milan
Italy
Transcatheter Chemotherapy for Cancer in the Head and Neck Area

Benjamin M. Ellingson, PhD, MS
Assistant Professor
Department of Radiological Sciences
David Geffen School of Medicine at University of California at Los Angeles
Los Angeles, California
United States
Head: Intracranial - Gliomas, and Meningiomas and Extracranial - Orbits, Internal Auditory Canals, and Skull Base

Scott Genshaft, MD
Clinical Instructor
Department of Radiology
University of California at Los Angeles
Los Angeles, California
United States
Primary Lung Carcinoma
Metastatic Disease

Sanjay Gupta, MD
Section of Interventional Radiology
Department of Diagnostic Radiology
The University of Texas M.D. Anderson Cancer Center
Houston, Texas
United States
Gastroenteropancreatic Neuroendocrine Tumors
Interventional Oncology Management of Non-Colorectal and Non-Neuroendocrine Hepatic Metastatic Disease
Intra-Arterial Procedures for the Musculoskeletal System

Charbel Ishak, MD
Cardiovascular and Interventional Radiology Fellow
Department of Radiology
Weill Cornell Medical College
Cardiovascular and Interventional Radiology Fellow
Department of Radiology
Memorial Sloan Kettering Cancer Center
New York, New York
United States
Principles of Percutaneous Ablative Therapies

Alexis D. Kelekis, MD, PhD, EBIR
Assistant Professor of Interventional Radiology
2nd Radiology Department
Attikon University Hospital
University of Athens
Athens
Greece
Vertebroplasty/Kyphoplasty in Malignant Vertebral Fracture

Lizbeth Kenny, MD, FRANZCR, FACR (hon), FBIR (hon), FRCR (hon)
Senior Radiation Oncologist
Royal Brisbane and Women's Hospital
Medical Director
Central Integrated Regional Cancer Service, Queensland Health
Chair, Queensland Statewide Cancer Clinical Network
Queensland, Australia
The Role of Interventional Oncology in Modern Cancer Care

Sarah N. Khan, MD
Research Fellow
Department of Radiological Sciences
University of California Los Angeles
Los Angeles, California
United States
Head: Intracranial - Gliomas, and Meningiomas and Extracranial - Orbits, Internal Auditory Canals, and Skull Base

Pavan Khurana, MD
Fellow
Department of Vascular Interventional Radiology
New York-Presbyterian Hospital/Weill Cornell
New York, New York
United States
Principles of Embolization

Michael D. Kluger, MD
Assistant Attending Surgeon
New York Presbyterian Hospital
Assistant Professor of Surgery (Transplant Surgery)
Weill Cornell Medical College
New York, New York
United States
Surgical Management of Hepatocellular Carcinoma

Katsuhiro Kobayashi, MD, PhD
Physician
Michael E. DeBakey VA Medical Center
Assistant Professor
Department of Radiology
Baylor College of Medicine
Houston, Texas
United States
Intra-Arterial Procedures for the Musculoskeletal System

Anil Nicholas Kurup, MD
Assistant Professor of Radiology
Mayo Clinic College of Medicine
Consultant
Department of Radiology
Mayo Clinic
Rochester, Minnesota
United States
Ablation of Musculoskeletal Metastatic Lesions Including Cementoplasty

Edward W. Lee, MD, PhD, MSc
Assistant Professor-in-Residence
Department of Interventional Radiology/Radiology
University of California at Los Angeles Medical Center
Los Angeles, California
United States
Trends in Basic Science Research in Interventional Radiology: Nanotechnology, Stem Cell, RNAi and Radiogenomics

Ser Yee Lee, MBBS, M.Med(Surgery), M.Sc, FRCS, FAMS
Clinical Fellow
Hepatobiliary Surgery and Liver Transplantation
New York-Presbyterian Hospital/Weill Cornell
New York, New York
United States
Surgical Management of Hepatocellular Carcinoma

Mohamed Mansour, MD
Section of Interventional Radiology
Department of Diagnostic Radiology
The University of Texas M.D. Anderson Cancer Center
Houston, Texas
United States
Interventional Oncology Management of Non-Colorectal and Non-Neuroendocrine Hepatic Metastatic Disease

Daniel J. A. Margolis, MD
Assistant Professor
Department of Radiology
David Geffen School of Medicine at University of California at Los Angeles
Los Angeles, California
United States
Editor: Part 4. Genitourinary and Gynecologic Oncology
Prostate Cancer Intervention

Maurie Markman, MD
Senior Vice President of Clinical Affairs
National Director of Medical Oncology
Cancer Treatment Centers of America
Philadelphia, Pennsylvania
United States
Philosophy of Locoregional Therapies

Michael N. Mavros, MD
Department of Surgery
The Johns Hopkins Hospital
Baltimore, Maryland
United States
Cholangiocarcionma: Diagnosis, Management and Prognosis

Timothy D. McClure, MD
Resident Radiologist
Department of Radiology
University of California
Los Angeles, California
United States
Percutaneous Management of Renal Tumors

Sandy Mong, MD
Post-Doctoral Research Fellow
Department of Radiology
David Geffen School of Medicine at University of California at Los Angeles
Los Angeles, California
United States
Head: Intracranial - Gliomas, and Meningiomas and Extracranial - Orbits, Internal Auditory Canals, and Skull Base

Jamil Muasher, MD
Department of Radiology and Medical Imaging
Division of Vascular Interventional Radiology
University of Virginia Health System
Charlottesville, Virginia
United States
Percutaneous Management of Cholangiocarcinoma

Nita Nayak, MD
Resident Radiologist
Department of Radiology
University of California
Los Angeles, California
United States
Image Based Interventional Therapies for Benign Uterine Neoplasms

Dwight Owen, MB, BCh, BAO
Chief Medical Resident
Department of Medicine
Memorial Sloan-Kettering Cancer Center
New York, New York
United States
Systemic Therapy in Advanced Hepatocellular Carcinoma

Gianluigi Patelli, MD
Department of Interventional Radiology
Pesenti Fenaroli Hospital
Alzano Lombardo
Italy
Transcatheter Chemotherapy for Cancer in the Head and Neck Area

Timothy M. Pawlik, MD, MPH, PhD, FACS
Associate Professor of Surgery and Oncology
John L. Cameron M.D. Professor of Alimentary Tract Diseases
Chief, Division of Surgical Oncology
Director, Johns Hopkins Medicine Liver Tumor Center Multi-Disciplinary Clinic
Johns Hopkins Hospital
Baltimore, Maryland
United States
Cholangiocarcionma: Diagnosis, Management and Prognosis

Elena N. Petre, MD
Research Associate
Department of Interventional Radiology
Memorial Sloan-Kettering Cancer Center
New York, New York
United States
Interventional Radiology in the Management of Colorectal Cancer Liver Metastases

Alexandria T. Phan, MD
Associate Professor
Department of Gastrointestinal Medical Oncology
Division of Cancer Medicine
The University of Texas M.D. Anderson Cancer Center
Houston, Texas
United States
Gastroenteropancreatic Neuroendocrine Tumors

David E. Piccioni, MD, PhD
UCLA Neuro-Oncology Program
Neuro-Oncology Fellow, Adult Brain Tumors
The Ronald Reagan UCLA Medical Center
Los Angeles, California
United States
Head: Intracranial - Gliomas, and Meningiomas and Extracranial - Orbits, Internal Auditory Canals, and Skull Base

Whitney Pope, MD, PhD
Associate Professor
Department of Radiology
University of California Los Angeles
Los Angeles, California
United States
Editor: Part 5. Head and Neck Oncology
Head: Intracranial - Gliomas, and Meningiomas and Extracranial - Orbits, Internal Auditory Canals, and Skull Base
Imaging of Head and Neck Cancer

Bradley Pua, MD
Assistant Professor of Radiology
Division of Interventional Radiology
Weill Cornell Medical College
Assistant Attending Radiologist
Department of Vascular and Interventional Radiology
NewYork-Presbyterian Hospital
New York, New York
United States
Principles of Embolization
Tumor Response for IGI - Assessment and Validation

Steven S. Raman, MD
Diagnostic Radiology
Ronald Reagan Santa Monica UCLA Medical Center
Los Angeles, California
United States
Interventional Strategies in the Treatment of Gynecologic Cancers

Richard E. Royal, MD, FACS
Associate Professor
Department of Surgical Oncology and Melanoma Medical Oncology
M. D. Anderson Cancer Center, University of Texas
Houston, Texas
Principles of Isolated Regional Perfusion of the Extremity or Liver

Wael Saad, MD, FSIR
Professor of Radiology
University of Virginia Health System
Department of Radiology and Medical Imaging
Division of Vascular Interventional Radiology
Charlottesville, Virginia
United States
Percutaneous Management of Cholangiocarcinoma

Ali R. Sepahdari, MD
Assistant Professor
Department of Radiological Sciences
David Geffen School of Medicine at University of California at Los Angeles
Los Angeles, California
United States
Head: Intracranial - Gliomas, and Meningiomas and Extracranial - Orbits, Internal Auditory Canals, and Skull Base
Imaging of Head and Neck Cancer

Colette Shaw, MB, BCh, BAO
Assistant Professor
Department of Interventional Radiology
Thomas Jefferson University Hospital
Philadelphia, Pennsylvania
United States
Percutaneous Musculoskeletal Biopsy

Junichi Shindoh, MD, PhD
Department of Surgical Oncology
The University of Texas M.D. Anderson Cancer Center
Houston, Texas
United States
Surgical Management of Hepatic Metastases

Panagiotis A. Sideras, MD, PhD
Mount Sinai School of Medicine
Department of Radiology
New York, New York
United States
Interventional Radiology in the Management of Colorectal Cancer Liver Metastases

Akhilesh K. Sista, MD
Assistant Professor of Radiology
Division of Interventional Radiology
Weill Cornell Medical College
Assistant Attending Radiologist
Department of Vascular and Interventional Radiology
NewYork-Presbyterian Hospital
New York, New York
United States
Principles of Embolization
Interventional Management of Hepatocellular Carcinoma

Constantinos T. Sofocleous, MD, PhD, FSIR
Interventional Radiologist
Department of Radiology
Memorial Sloan-Kettering Cancer Center
New York, New York
United States
Interventional Radiology in the Management of Colorectal Cancer Liver Metastases

Stephen B. Solomon, MD
Chief, Interventional Radiology Service
Director, Center for Image-Guided Intervention
Memorial Sloan-Kettering Cancer Center
New York, New York
United States
Principles of Percutaneous Ablative Therapies

Alda L. Tam, MD, FRCPC, MBA
Section of Interventional Radiology
Department of Diagnostic Radiology
The University of Texas M.D. Anderson Cancer Center
Houston, Texas
United States
Editor: Part 7. MSK Oncology
Musculoskeletal Interventions for Benign Bone Lesions
Intra-Arterial Procedures for the Musculoskeletal System

Raymond H. Thornton, MD
Vice Chair for Quality, Safety, and Performance Improvement
Department of Radiology
Division of Interventional Radiology
Memorial Sloan-Kettering Cancer Center
New York, New York
United States
Principles of Percutaneous Ablative Therapies

Vladimira Tichà, MD
Department of Interventional Radiology GVM
Emocuore Columbus
Milan
Italy
Transcatheter Chemotherapy for Cancer in the Head and Neck Area

Sean Merrill Tutton, MD, FSIR
Professor of Radiology and Surgery
Department of Radiology
Medical College of Wisconsin
Froedtert Memorial Lutheran Hospital
Milwaukee, Wisconsin
Chief, Vascular and Interventional
Clement J. Zablocki Veteran's Hospital
United States
Musculoskeletal Interventions for Benign Bone Lesions

Jean-Nicolas Vauthey, MD
Professor
Chief, Liver Service
Department of Surgical Oncology
Division of Surgery
The University of Texas M.D. Anderson Cancer Center
Houston, Texas
United States
Surgical Management of Hepatic Metastases

Christopher Willett, MD
Professor and Chairman
Department of Radiation Oncology
Duke University Medical Center
Durham, North Carolina
United States
Principles of Radiotherapy

Minzhi Xing, MD
Division of Interventional Radiology
Department of Radiology
David Geffen School of Medicine at UCLA
Los Angeles, California
United States
Trends in Basic Science Research in Interventional Radiology: Nanotechnology, Stem Cell, RNAi and Radiogenomics

James C. Yao, MD
Associate Professor
Department of Gastrointestinal Medical Oncology
Division of Cancer Medicine
The University of Texas M.D. Anderson Cancer Center
Houston, Texas
United States
Gastroenteropancreatic Neuroendocrine Tumors

David Yoo, MD, PhD
Medical Instructor
Department of Radiation Oncology
Duke University Medical Center
Durham, North Carolina
United States
Principles of Radiotherapy

Jennifer Zhang, MD
Department of Surgery
The Johns Hopkins Hospital
Baltimore, Maryland
United States
Cholangiocarcionma: Diagnosis, Management and Prognosis

Giuseppe Zimmitti, MD
Department of Surgical Oncology
The University of Texas M.D. Anderson Cancer Center
Houston, Texas
United States
Surgical Management of Hepatic Metastases

Adam Zoga, MD
Section of Musculoskeletal Radiology
Department of Radiology
Thomas Jefferson University Hospital
Philadelphia, Pennsylvania
United States
Percutaneous Musculoskeletal Biopsy

Rodrick C. Zvavanjanja, MD
Section of Interventional Radiology
Department of Diagnostic Radiology
The University of Texas M.D. Anderson Cancer Center
Houston, Texas
United States
Musculoskeletal Interventions for Benign Bone Lesions

PREFACE

The first edition of *Clinical Interventional Oncology* is intended to educate practicing Interventionists on the state of the profession, while disseminating the specialty's artistry to referring Oncologists and primary care physicians. Far too often, we have heard patients or their loved ones express that they have little knowledge of the available treatment options. Many interventional oncologic practices have developed over the last 20 years and have few major publications in journals to which our referring physicians subscribe. Interventional oncologic practices are also less common due to poor understanding of techniques, even by members of our own discipline. As the field of Interventional Oncology matures, it is important that we resist the temptation to seek approval from our closest peers, but rather that we share the information, good or bad, with those doctors who deal with cancer patients at the point of initial contact.

Embolic and ablative therapies have historically been considered palliative therapies that are only sought out after all traditional methods have failed. As a result, we frequently receive patients for treatments that could clearly have been better served, and potentially even cured, had they come to our attention earlier in the course of their disease. The fault for this lies with us, the practitioners. We need to do a better and more comprehensive job of informing the medical profession, and even the public, of where we currently stand with interventional cancer therapies, and where we are exploring new horizons.

This book endeavors to address methods for treating most of the major cancers seen by Interventional Oncologists. Our approach is intended to give readers an understanding of what major therapeutic options are currently available; to teach how interventional techniques are being applied and how they work; and to prompt which patients may benefit from an Interventional Oncologist.

The practice of Radiology and Interventional Radiology, in particular, has evolved considerably over the last 20 years. It is now a routine part of most Interventional Oncologist's practices to establish out-patient clinics where the physician may evaluate patients and their imaging to determine if they could be appropriate candidates for alternative therapies. Once these treatments have been applied, it is common to follow patients in a longitudinal fashion, usually working in concert with a more traditional oncologist. Most, if not all, of these therapies are applied while patients continue their traditional course of oncologic regimen. Patients will have follow-up imaging coordinated in such a way that the full value of treatment can be evaluated.

The practice of Interventional Oncology continues to evolve rapidly. There are a number of advanced treatment regimens that have been studied in extensive double-blind trials and have demonstrated their worth. Many are currently in ongoing trials and it has become almost common for novel cancer treatment studies to include interventional techniques in their options. Practicing physicians, however, may not always know where to turn for a reference because this area of medicine is undergoing changes much more rapidly than most. The editorial team and I hope to position this volume at the top of physicians' reading lists for the understanding of what to perform, when, and in whom. We will endeavor to update the various options available as advances are made.

We would like to profusely thank all of the authors who dedicated their time and skills to assist us in the production of this first edition of *Clinical Interventional Oncology,* as well as the excellent team at Elsevier. We hope to provide you with many updates over the upcoming years in the ongoing battle against Cancer.

ACKNOWLEDGMENTS

I would like to express my thanks to all the authors, my co-editors and publishers for their tremendous work putting this book together. Also to my colleagues at UCLA for all their clinical support during this process. I owe much to my mentors and leaders who have provided me with guidance and support. Lastly to my friends and family, especially the Ponz, for their patience and understanding.

Stephen T. Kee

To my parents for their unconditional love and sacrifices, my wife and children for providing purpose and support, to my mentors for their guidance and selflessness. Finally to the trainees and patients whose presence provides the impetus for remaining focused, challenged and innovative.

Ravi Murthy

My sincerest gratitude to my wife, children and parents for their love and patience without which no endeavor would have been possible nor worthwhile. To my associates past and current for providing the environment for continuous learning and success. Lastly, to the patients I take pride in treating and to those who plan to practice Interventional Oncology today and in the future.

David C. Madoff

CONTENTS

THE ROLE OF INTERVENTIONAL ONCOLOGY IN MODERN CANCER CARE

LIZBETH KENNY | ANDREAS ADAM

Throughout recorded history, surgery has been the mainstay of potentially curative treatment for people with cancer. Its importance increased over the centuries as physicians gained progressively greater understanding of the natural history of cancers and the importance of defining the extent of the disease and as surgical techniques and anesthesia evolved. Surgery for many cancers has become increasingly less invasive.

Surgery continues to play a vital and central role in cancer management, spanning diagnosis, through curative resection and palliative intervention. Cross-sectional imaging has greatly reduced the need for surgical methods of staging malignant disease, and most biopsies are now performed percutaneously or endoscopically. Surgical debulking remains important for some tumors, such as ovarian carcinoma or tumors obstructing airways.

Since the last century, radiation therapy has played an increasingly important role in the treatment of cancer, and evidence would now support its use in more than half of all patients with cancer. A better understanding of radiobiology, the impact of computers and modern imaging, and more sophisticated methods of radiation treatment delivery have increased its effectiveness and reduced the complications associated with it. The ability to avoid or reduce the dose to sensitive structures using advanced techniques such as intensity-modulated radiotherapy (IMRT) and image guidance reduces short- and long-term morbidity and may allow for dose escalation to increase local cure. Radiosurgery is now commonplace for some tumors.

Chemotherapy is definitive treatment for some malignancies and can increase the cure rate in some cancers by either reducing local recurrence in combination with surgery and/or radiation treatment, or by reducing the risk of subsequent disseminated disease. Chemotherapy has a significant role in palliation.

In recent years, combinations of surgery, radiotherapy, and chemotherapy have been used with increasing frequency, and there has been better understanding of the benefits of integrating such treatments in a planned and sequenced manner. The role of multidisciplinary treatment teams has greatly enhanced care delivery and interdisciplinary cooperation. Chemotherapy may be used to downstage tumors prior to surgical excision and for adjuvant postoperative treatment; radiation may be used either pre- or postoperatively to reduce the risk of loco-regional recurrence, and radiation alone or chemoradiation may be used with curative intent. Often all three modalities are used with imaging guiding staging and assessing response to treatment. Modern imaging, collaboration by cancer specialists, particularly through multidisciplinary teams, evidence-based and consistent treatment decisions, and the use of multiple modalities of treatment have greatly improved outcomes for people with cancer in the past two decades.

Surgery, radiation treatment, and chemotherapy may produce significant short- and long-term consequences including effects on a patient's functional or physical anatomy, surrounding normal tissues, or significant systemic side effects, respectively.

Increasing the chance of cure, where cure is possible, and at the same time reducing short- and long-term morbidity is a critical focus of research and evolution of treatment for all oncologic disciplines. The benefits for people with cancer are obvious. These are also likely to translate into reductions not only in personal and possibly lifelong cost to our patients but also to the health system at large. The realization of the wealth of possibilities for truly minimally invasive cancer therapy has driven the interventional radiology community to develop such techniques. The clear aim is to destroy the tumor while minimizing the effect on the structure and function of the body.

The term *interventional oncology* has raised questions among some oncologists, who are concerned about interventional radiologists without extensive training in oncology assuming responsibility for the overall care of cancer patients. However, this term is intended to denote "a doctor who uses interventional radiologic techniques to treat patients with cancer." Interventional oncologists need to work in multidisciplinary teams that include specialists from all other modalities involved in cancer care. It is important that they have sufficient understanding of the basic principles of surgical, medical, and radiation oncology in order to be able to explain to the patient and their oncology colleagues the place of interventional radiologic techniques in the context of other methods of treatment, and to integrate their care with other modalities. It is very important, however, for the interventional oncologist to assume clinical responsibility for the care of the patient during treatment and to observe the patient both short- and long-term. We would strongly counsel against the interventionist acting as a technician, expecting all nontechnical aspects of patient care to be dealt with by someone else. This approach can lead to significant problems: the person carrying out a procedure is in the best position to prepare the patient appropriately for it, to anticipate interactions with chemotherapeutic or radiotherapeutic regimens, to deal with any complications, and to observe the patient appropriately. The assumption of a purely technical role can lead to misunderstandings and delays, as other specialists try to interpret what is done by the interventional radiologist and to deal with its results. Misinterpretation of follow-up imaging, and miscommunication among specialists not involved with the procedure, can have adverse consequences, which can be avoided if the interventional radiologist assumes a full clinical role. Important clinical data, including morbidity and outcomes, must be collected and analyzed.

Importantly, if interventional oncologists are not part of multidisciplinary teams, interventional oncology may not reach its full potential and its benefits may not reach people with cancer.

This excellent book covers all the important potentially curative interventional radiologic procedures used to treat patients with malignant tumors. It will not only serve to teach interventional radiologists involved in this field all important aspects of the techniques used to treat cancer but will also serve as a comprehensive source of information for surgeons, radiation oncologists, and medical oncologists who wish to refer patients for interventional oncological treatment.

Oncology is one of the most rapidly changing fields of medicine and imaging is one of the strongest forces responsible for the pace of change. The information available from structural and functional imaging regarding the extent, location, and, increasingly, the characteristics of malignant tumors is astonishing in its detail, and in many cases has outstripped our capacity to treat the disease. However, imaging is also being used to guide methods of treatment and to increase their effectiveness. This is particularly true of interventional radiologic and radiotherapeutic techniques. One of the most exciting developments in this field is the growing overlap and partial convergence of these disciplines. We believe that institutions involved in the organization of professional practice and education in radiology and radiation oncology have an exciting opportunity to consider how training and clinical practice in these intimately related fields can be enhanced by closer collaboration between its practitioners.

PHILOSOPHY OF LOCOREGIONAL THERAPIES

MAURIE MARKMAN

For the nononcologic physician the concept of local-regional antineoplastic therapy might appear to be really quite simple: *Treat the cancer where you know it is located.*

And this is, of course, the goal of curative local anticancer therapeutic strategies (e.g., surgery, external beam radiation). In theory, successful removal of all visible (macroscopic) tumor masses should eliminate the local cancer.

Unfortunately, decades of observation and extensive clinical trial experience have confirmed that this overly simplistic view of cancer management does not begin to adequately explain the remarkably complex biology of malignant disease, including the large number of factors, many of which surely remain unidentified, which determine how and when local invasion, lymphatic and hematogenous spread, and drug resistance occur. Further, it is now well established that micro-metastatic disease is commonly present in many clinical settings long before metastatic cancer is clinically evident, and extending the total size or volume of definitive local therapy will not "cure the cancer."

For example, the previous generally accepted oncologic concept of radical mastectomy in the routine management of breast cancer was rejected following the conduct of evidence-based trials that revealed this extensive and often morbid procedure failed to improve survival compared to less aggressive strategies (e.g., modified radical mastectomy; partial mastectomy with radiation) designed to achieve adequate control of local disease while not compromising the ultimate survival outcome.

In sharp contrast to the lack of utility for more extended local treatment, the routine use of *systemic therapy* in the adjuvant setting (following definitive local therapy) has been shown in breast cancer (and other solid tumors) to improve survival. This results from the ability of such treatment to effectively kill viable cancer that had spread beyond the confines of the local-regional area (micro-metastatic disease).

When macroscopic metastatic cancer (either at diagnosis or developing later in the clinical course) is documented to be present, systemic treatment is the "standard-of-care" as this approach will (at least in theory) permit malignant cells present throughout the body to be exposed to the cytotoxic or cytostatic properties of the antineoplastic.

Thus, considering the above discussion and existing clinical data, the question to be asked in this chapter is as follows: *What is the justification for employing antineoplastic drug therapy as a local-regional treatment approach rather than delivering the agent(s) systemically to maximize the opportunity to achieve the greatest exposure and optimize the therapeutic impact?*

Local-Regional Antineoplastic Drug Delivery

In fact, it can certainly be rationally argued that *if* the antineoplastic drugs to be delivered in a particular clinical setting were highly effective and *if* they produced minimal side effects, there would be very little (if any) justification for the time, effort, and potential morbidity (e.g., placement of catheters, risk of infection, etc.) associated with attempting to deliver such agents locally or regionally. Surely, the argument continues, exposing the entire systemic circulation to optimal concentrations of the antineoplastic must be far more effective than applying the agent only locally. Is this not a correct conclusion?

Unfortunately, this statement does not describe the general state of affairs in many oncologic settings.

Consider, for example, the observation that although 70%–80% of women with advanced ovarian cancer achieve a major, highly clinically relevant response to a primary platinum-taxane-based chemotherapy regimen, the large majority of patients in this setting will experience a recurrence of the disease process and ultimately die of complications of progressive cancer.[1] Thus, it is not difficult to justify efforts to improve the efficacy of the current systemic antineoplastic drug delivery paradigm in this patient population.

Another poignant example of a potential role for regional therapy is in the management of lymphomatous or carcinomatous meningitis, where it is recognized that limited blood supply (among other factors) from the systemic circulation to the central nervous tissue may profoundly negatively impact outcome, despite the fact that cancer present elsewhere in the body (including bone marrow) can be controlled or completely eradicated.[2–5] This outcome results at least in part from delivery of active drugs in *adequate concentrations* to the cancer in these other regions *by capillary flow*. Thus, at least conceptually, the idea of local drug delivery with sufficient biologically active concentrations of an antineoplastic agent to susceptible tissue within the central nervous system has considerable appeal (overcoming the "blood–brain barrier").

Regional Antineoplastic Drug Delivery is not a New Concept

The idea of delivering anticancer agents directly into the involved body compartment was proposed more than 50 years ago, initially principally as an approach to control malignant fluid accumulation.[6,7]

A more focused interest in this fundamental concept was stimulated following the success of peritoneal dialysis as a strategy to manage renal insufficiency.[8,9] Both preclinical and clinical studies revealed the capacity of drugs to enter and leave body compartments based on basic biological properties of cells and tissues as well as the specific agents themselves, with the potential for substantial increases in the exposure of the contents of the compartment to the drugs following local or regional delivery.

Both animal and early-phase clinical trials revealed an impressive pharmacokinetic advantage associated with the regional administration of certain agents (e.g., 1000-fold increased exposure of the peritoneal cavity to paclitaxel compared to the systemic compartment following instillation into the cavity)[10], as well as the potential toxicity observed with drugs when delivered in this manner (e.g., intense inflammation resulting from doxorubicin given via the intraperitoneal route).[11] Additional

TABLE 1 Theoretical and Pragmatic Considerations in the Use of Locoregional Antineoplastic Drug Therapy

1. Preclinical data (in vitro, in vivo) supporting the extent of a *pharmacokinetic advantage* (peak concentration or increased AUC [area-under-the-concentration-versus-time-curve], or both) associated with a particular locoregional administration strategy (e.g., intraperitoneal drug delivery) for a specific antineoplastic agent (e.g., cisplatin, paclitaxel)
2. Preclinical data (in vitro, in vivo) supporting the concept of *superior therapeutic efficacy* associated with either higher peak or AUC concentrations achieved following locoregional administration of the particular antineoplastic agents against a specific tumor type (e.g., ovarian cancer)
3. Preclinical data (in vivo) supporting the safety of a particular locoregional administration approach (e.g., intrahepatic arterial infusion) with a specific antineoplastic agent (e.g., floxuridine [FUDR])
4. Development of an approach to safely and effectively apply the locoregional strategy, initially within the clinical trials setting, but ultimately in routine clinical practice
5. Establishment of *sufficient evidence* (e.g., results of phase 3 randomized trials) to consider a particular locoregional approach to be a component of "standard of care" oncologic practice (by patients, the clinical community, regulatory bodies, and third-party payers of medical care), rather than merely an investigative strategy
6. Continuous refinement of the approach (e.g., modification of drugs, dosages, technical details) to optimize the chances that patients with particular clinical conditions documented to be benefitted by the use of locoregional therapy are able to safely complete the proposed management program

TABLE 2 Locoregional Antineoplastic Drug Delivery Strategies Currently Employed in Routine Oncologic Practice

Intravesical therapy of superficial bladder cancer
Intrathecal therapy (and prophylaxis) or meningeal leukemia (or lymphoma)
Intrathecal therapy of meningeal metastases from selected solid tumors (e.g., breast cancer)
Intraperitoneal chemotherapy of ovarian cancer
Hyperthermic intraperitoneal chemotherapy (HIPEC) of gastrointestinal malignancies and ovarian cancer
Intrahepatic arterial therapy of colon cancer (and other solid tumors) metastatic to the liver
Isolation-perfusion of arterial blood supply for localized treatment of solid tumors (e.g., isolated limb involvement with malignant melanoma)

studies documented wide variations in the duration of exposure of the body compartments associated with regional treatment employing specific agents and the actual limited direct depth of drug penetration into tumor tissue following this approach (Table 1).[12,13]

Subsequently conducted phase 2 studies employing multiple drugs (single agent or in combination regimens) and various routes of regional delivery have confirmed both impressive biological and therapeutic effects associated with this management strategy in a number of clinical settings (e.g., peritoneal cavity, bladder, pleura, pericardium, meninges, hepatic, and other arteries).[14,15] In a number of areas, phase 3 trials have been completed (e.g., cisplatin-based intraperitoneal chemotherapy in the management of small-volume residual advanced ovarian cancer) which have revealed the superiority (e.g., improved progression-free and overall survival) of this approach compared to systemic antineoplastic drug delivery.

Further, it is fair to conclude that regional antineoplastic drug delivery is currently considered to be *an acceptable* standard of care or *the established* standard of care in a number of clinical settings (Table 2).

Concerns with Local or Regional Antineoplastic Drug Delivery

Despite the documented utility of regional antineoplastic therapy, it is critical to acknowledge both the limitations of the available data supporting its use in certain settings as well as clinical experience demonstrating specific patient populations where such therapy should logically not be used.

For example, although a number of phase 3 trials have explored the clinical utility of direct hepatic arterial infusion of chemotherapy in the management of colon cancer metastatic to the liver, and high objective response rates have been documented, the impact of this strategy on overall survival in this setting remains unclear. One recognized explanation for this serious problem is that for ethical considerations, in many evidence-based randomized trials patients have been appropriately permitted to "cross over" to receive the regional treatment strategy at the time of progression if they were randomized to initially receive treatment with systemic therapy on the study's "control arm."[16] (Of course, this decision to permit cross-over to the investigative study arm assumes the patient remains an appropriate candidate to potentially benefit from the regional management strategy.)

Thus, failure to demonstrate an impact on overall survival in such a trial may simply have been due to the fact the majority of patients ultimately received the "experimental" regional therapeutic strategy and patients *on both study arms* may have benefited from utilization of the innovative approach.

A second issue in the examination of the impact on survival associated with regional antineoplastic treatment is the recognized fact that the therapy itself is objectively only directly influencing disease in the specific area treated. As a result, even if such therapy was highly effective in controlling both the signs and symptoms associated with the local disease process (e.g., malignant fluid accumulation; bleeding from a blood vessel invaded by a metastatic mass lesion) the cancer may progress elsewhere with the patient succumbing to the effects of cancer at a distant site. Further, in a randomized trial, survival may not have been improved even if truly favorable clinically relevant effects were observed.

Finally, it must be recognized that (in general) regional drug delivery is more complex and labor intensive and is potentially associated with greater morbidity than that resulting from systemic antineoplastic therapy. A recent example of this phenomenon is the use of hyperthermic intraperitoneal chemotherapy (HIPEC) in the management of gastrointestinal and ovarian cancers.[17] Although both retrospective case series and prospective phase 2 trials have suggested prolonged disease-free and overall survival following use of this approach, the strategy can be associated with considerable morbidity, which mandates very careful patient selection when considering this therapeutic option.

Unfortunately, further complicating the issue, the appropriate *clinical judgment* employed by a physician in the decision to deliver a novel regional management program leads to concern for *selection bias* in the interpretation of outcomes when attempting to directly compare the survival of an unselected population to those individuals treated with the innovative strategy. As a result, controversy continues as to the benefits of the treatment itself, versus the natural history of the disease process in a select patient population.

Conclusion

Existing data provide strong support for the conclusion that in specific clinical settings local or regional antineoplastic drug delivery plays a critically important role in routine cancer management (Table 2), whereas in other circumstances the approach remains under active investigation. It is also reasonable to conclude that local-regional drug administration may be a highly rational approach to deliver novel "targeted molecular-based" antineoplastic strategies, especially in a setting where there is concern for side effects resulting from the drug impacting the specific target on normal tissue outside the confines of the local area or where there is evidence for the potential of a serious "off-target" effect with the agent following exposure to the systemic compartment.

REFERENCES

1. Hennessy BT, Coleman RL, Markman M: Ovarian cancer, *Lancet* 374:1371–1382, 2009.
2. Stevens G, Peereboom DM: Principles of intrathecal chemotherapy. In Markman M, editor: *Regional chemotherapy: clinical research and practice*, Totowa, NJ, 2000, Humana Press, pp 305–318.
3. Overmoyer BA: Regional chemotherapy for meningeal involvement with breast cancer. In Markman M, editor: *Regional chemotherapy: clinical research and practice*, Totowa, NJ, 2000, Humana Press, pp 319–330.
4. Pohlman B: Regional chemotherapy for treatment and prophylaxis of meningeal lymphoma. In Markman M, editor: *Regional chemotherapy: clinical research and practice*, Totowa, NJ, 2000, Humana Press, pp 331–338.
5. Kalaycio ME: Regional chemotherapy for the treatment and prophylaxis of meningeal leukemia. In Markman M, editor: *Regional chemotherapy: clinical research and practice*, Totowa, NJ, 2000, Humana Press, pp 339–356.
6. Weisberger AS, Levine B, Storaasli JP: Use of nitrogen mustard in the treatment of serous effusions of neoplastic origin, *J Am Med Assoc* 159:1704–1707, 1955.
7. Suhrland LG, Weisberger AS: Intracavitary 5-fluorouracil in malignant effusions, *Arch Intern Med* 116:431–433, 1965.
8. Dedrick RL, Myers CE, Bungay PM, DeVita VT Jr: Pharmacokinetic rational for peritoneal drug administration in the treatment of ovarian cancer, *Cancer Treat Rep* 62:1–9, 1978.
9. Kraft AR, Tompkins RK, Jesseph JE: Peritoneal electrolyte absorption: analysis of portal, systemic venous and lymphatic transport, *Surgery* 64:148–153, 1968.
10. Markman M, Rowinsky E, Hakes T, et al: Phase 1 trial of intraperitoneal taxol: a Gynecologic Oncology Group study, *J Clin Oncol* 10:1485–1491, 1992.
11. Ozols RF, Young RC, Speyer JL, et al: Phase 1 and pharmacological studies of adriamycin administered intraperitoneally to patients with ovarian cancer, *Cancer Res* 42:4265–4269, 1982.
12. Los G, Mutsaers PHA, van der Vijgh WJF, et al: Direct diffusion of cis-diamminedichloroplatinum(II) in intraperitoneal rat tumors after intraperitoneal chemotherapy: a comparison with systemic chemotherapy, *Cancer Res* 49:3380–3384, 1989.
13. Ozols RF, Locker GY, Doroshow JH, et al: Pharmacokinetics of adriamycin and tissue penetration in murine ovarian cancer, *Cancer Res* 39:3209–3214, 1979.
14. Markman M: *Regional chemotherapy: clinical research and practice* Totowa, NJ, 2000, Humana Press.
15. Gasion JPB, Cruz JFJ: Improving efficacy of intravesical chemotherapy, *Eur Urol* 50:225–234, 2006.
16. Kemeny NE, Atiq OT: Intrahepatic chemotherapy for metastatic colorectal cancer. In Markman M, editor: *Regional chemotherapy: clinical research and practice*, Totowa, NJ, 2000, Humana Press, pp 5–20.
17. Chua TC, Yan TD, Saxena A, et al: Should the treatment of peritoneal carcinomatosis by cytoreductive surgery and hyperthermic intraperitoneal chemotherapy still be regarded as a highly morbid procedure? a systemic review of morbidity and mortality, *Ann Surg* 249: 900–907, 2009.

PART 1

Principles of Locoregional Therapy

BRADLEY B. PUA

1

Principles of Embolization

BRADLEY B. PUA | PAVAN KHURANA | AKHILESH K. SISTA

KEY POINTS

- Properly identify the indications and goals for the procedure to guide selection of embolic material.
- Become familiar with available embolic agents and common uses for each.
- A clear understanding of the relevant anatomy will allow for a safe and efficient embolization.

Introduction

Transcatheter and percutaneous embolization therapies are a large part of the Interventional Radiologists' armamentarium. Embolotherapy has a wide array of applications such as control of bleeding in a variety of settings, tumor therapy, and treatment of certain vascular abnormalities. In this chapter, we provide a brief overview of the different embolic agents currently available. The choice of agent must be made according to the appropriate clinical scenario, which can be varied. For example, compare the following two patients: the first being one who is involved in a motor vehicle accident sustaining solid organ injury with evidence of active arterial bleeding on imaging; the second, a consultation regarding nonsurgical treatment options for a liver tumor. Both can be treated with transcatheter embolization; however, because of the different clinical scenarios, the approach to each, risks of embolization, and the choice of embolic agent are all radically different. Some key factors that should be considered include the following:

1. What is the goal of the procedure? Is temporary or permanent occlusion required?
2. What is the desired level of occlusion?
3. What is the relevant anatomy? How does this influence the risks of nontarget embolization?
4. What is the appropriate delivery system?

In this chapter, we will provide an overview of the most commonly employed embolic agents and their typical uses. We divide embolic agents into two major categories: temporary versus permanent. The temporary agents are commonly used in the setting of trauma or times when a permanent occlusion may result in unacceptable end-organ damage. Gelfoam is the prototypical temporary agent and is versatile in both its uses and methods of deployment.

Among the permanent embolic agents, we first discuss particles such as polyvinyl alcohol (PVA) and acrylic spheres, which are available in a number of different size ranges and commonly used in tumor and solid organ embolization procedures. Coils are another commonly used embolic agent and are available in a variety of sizes to occlude small, medium, and large vessels. Some common uses for coils include treatment of pseudoaneurysms, blockage of collateral vessels during Y-90 treatments, and treatment of pulmonary arteriovenous malformations (AVMs). Finally, we will review some commonly employed sclerosants and glues, frequently used for the treatment of peripheral vascular malformations. Figure 1-1 provides a brief overview of the most commonly employed embolic agents.

Temporary Agents

GELFOAM

Gelfoam is a water-insoluble hemostatic gelatin sponge that expands on contact with fluid. A gelatin derived from purified porcine skin, gelfoam is a flow-directed embolic agent used for temporary vascular occlusion that induces hemostasis by promoting platelet aggregation, vessel wall inflammation, and thrombus formation.[1] As a temporary agent, it is most useful in the setting of trauma to control bleeding. Gelfoam is available as sterile sheets of varying thicknesses that can be cut into smaller pieces or as a fine powder, approximately 50 μm in size.[2] Care must be taken when used in the powder form as occlusion is often permanent because of the small size of the particles, and can result in tissue necrosis. Gelfoam sheets are versatile and can also be prepared in a slurry by cutting or shaving small strips of the gelfoam and loading them into a syringe mixed with contrast and/or saline.

It has been observed histologically that within 6 days of gelfoam embolization, an acute inflammatory and foreign body reaction occurs as characterized by giant cells followed by an inflammatory cascade resulting in thrombus formation.[3] Recanalization has been estimated to be anywhere from 3 weeks to 4 months in animal studies with vessel recanalization in two patients undergoing embolization for renal cell carcinoma occurring in 5 and 6 months.[4,5] It must be reiterated though that permanent gelfoam occlusion has also been demonstrated and is thought to be secondary to aggressive and densely packed gelfoam.[6]

AVITENE

Avitene (Davol Inc., Warwick RI) is a microfibrillar collagen preparation that comes in a variety of forms including powder, sheets, and sponges. The uses and preparation are similar to that described for gelfoam although it is not as commonly used. Although considered a temporary agent with vessel recanalization in a few weeks, this agent causes an intense inflammatory reaction with immediate thrombosis in large and small vessels, which may be permanent in some cases.

Permanent Agents

PARTICLES

Polyvinyl Alcohol

PVA particles are derived from shavings of blocks of inert plastic (polyvinyl alcohol) sponges. They are irregular in size and shape and come in a variety of differing size ranges from 50 to 2500 μm.

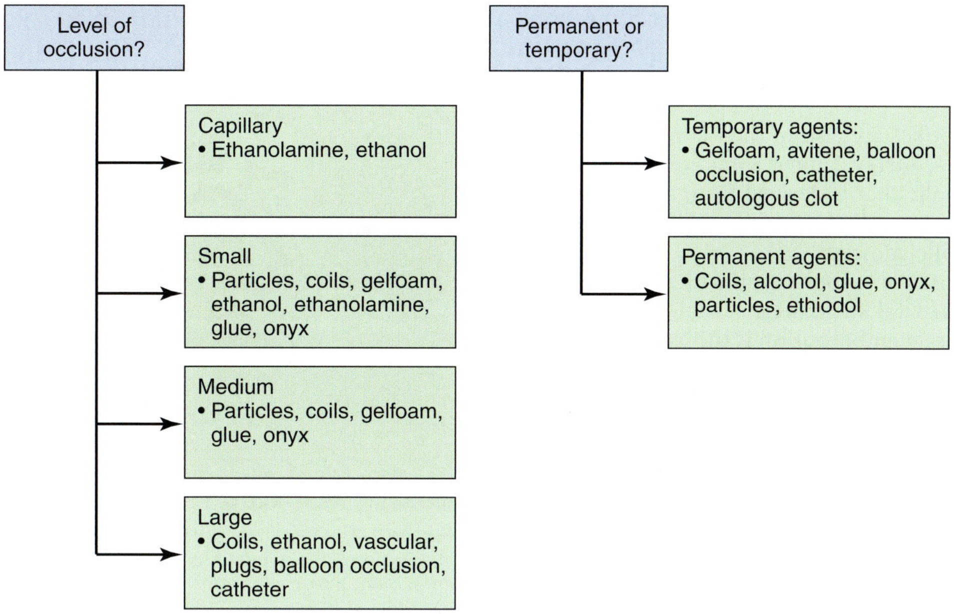

Figure 1-1 Agents for embolization.

PVA is injected via a catheter to occlude small arteries and arterioles by both a mechanical occlusion and creation of an inflammatory reaction in the vessel wall that leads to fibrosis, thrombosis, and occlusion.[7] Because the particles expand on contact with fluid and tend to clump together, there is a tendency for this embolic to produce a more proximal blockade in comparison to uniformly sized particles.[8] Albumin can be added to the suspension to help prevent clumping of these irregular particles.

As a permanent embolic agent that is available in a variety of different sizes, PVA is well suited for a variety of procedures, including tumor embolization. As with other particles, the operator must be aware of the risk of reflux and nontarget embolization. Also, very dense solutions of PVA can cause clumping of the particles, leading to catheter occlusion or proximal vessel occlusion. Angiographically, this may appear to be a successful embolization with cessation of flow to the target area. However, the particles that had clumped together may potentially break down later, leading to an incomplete embolization.[8,9]

Acrylic Spheres

Tris-acryl spheres are particles that are uniform in size and shape that can be cross-linked to gelatin. The spheres are hydrophilic and designed to be non-aggregating to deliver a more predictable distribution.[9] The soft, elastic nature of these spheres allows for compressibility of the particles by up to 33% in diameter. This reduces the problem of catheter clogging that can be found with PVA, and allows for more distal penetration in the vascular bed as compared to similarly sized PVA.[9,10] Once ejected from the delivery catheter, the particles are carried to their eventual point of occlusion via arterial blood flow around the delivery catheter. In this manner, hypervascular tumors are preferentially embolized. The compressibility and nonaggregating nature of the particles result in a more distal vessel occlusion compared to similarly sized particles of another material. Because the particles occlude a more distal vascular bed, there are higher rates of infarction. Knowledge of the appropriate-size particle to utilize for each tumor type is important because if incorrectly sized, there are risks of escape to the systemic circulation via arteriovenous shunts.[9,10,13] This agent is available from various manufacturers. Embosphere particles (BioSphere Medical, South Jordan, UT) are available in 1–2 mL aliquots suspended in sterile saline and in the following size distributions (Figure 1-2):

- 40–120 μm
- 100–300 μm
- 300–500 μm
- 500–700 μm
- 700–900 μm
- 900–1200 μm

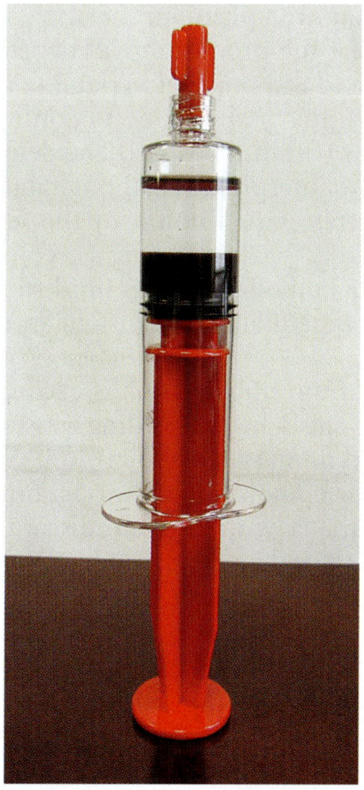

Figure 1-2 Embospheres (BioSphere Medical, South Jordan, UT) are typically supplied in prefilled syringes in ranges of sizes. Some varieties, as shown here, are color coded for size (100–300-μm particles).

Embozene® Microspheres (CeloNova BioSciences, San Antonio, TX) is another particle embolic that offers microspheres that are color-coded by individual particle size, which ranges from 40 to 1300 μm.

Other particle embolics are also in the market such as Bead Block (Biocompatibles, Surrey, United Kingdom), which represents a spherical embolic that is derived from a PVA hydrogel. There is tremendous interest in determining the relative efficacy of each of these embolic choices.[11,12,14]

One of the major risks of embolization with particles is nontarget embolization to vital structures. A tool for minimizing the risk of such nontarget embolization is the balloon occlusion catheter.[15,16] These catheters are designed to enhance the safety of the delivery of embolic agents to an intended target by minimizing or eliminating the risk of reflux around the catheter to nontarget sites.[17] This end-hole catheter, commonly designed with a balloon set 1 cm from its tip, can be inflated to temporarily occlude the vessel feeding the target. Once this vessel is occluded, the embolic material can be injected. One drawback with such a design is that total vessel occlusion does not allow for antegrade blood flow, which would limit the ability of controlling the amount of embolic agent reaching the intended target. Novel designs of some newer antireflux catheters are able to circumvent this issue (Surefire Medical, Inc., Westminster, CO). Such antireflux catheters make use of an expandable, thin-walled, funnel-shaped tip that is designed to expand and occlude the vessel during retrograde flow and prevent particle reflux. The funneled tip is designed to collapse during antegrade flow, thus allowing for delivery of the embolic agent to the intended target.[17]

When performing an embolization procedure using particles, there is a degree of variability among different operators in the exact details; however, the following steps are helpful to keep in mind. Many operators will allow the particles to settle in the syringe and decant most of the saline, replacing the decanted volume with 5–10 mL of contrast to allow maximal visualization during embolization.

The endpoint of the procedure will depend on the goal of the task at hand and is a point of variability among operators. In some instances, the goal may be to continue embolization until there is stasis within the vessel. The definition of stasis in the vessel is open to interpretation, though many consider stasis as persistent contrast visualization in the feeding vessel that persists for 5 cardiac beats. Another accepted endpoint is to continue instilling embolic particles until tumor vascularity is no longer seen, yet maintaining persistent antegrade flow in the parent vessel.[19]

The further out the embolization is carried, the greater will be the degree of stasis in the feeding vessel, thus increasing the risk reflux and nontarget embolization. When approaching the endpoint of the embolization, the operator should flush the volume of the catheter with saline to discard any unnecessary particles. Contrast can then be injected via the delivery catheter to assess the degree of progress.

Transarterial Embolization Versus Chemoembolization

Although a detailed discussion of the differences between transarterial "bland" embolization (TAE) and chemoembolization (TACE) is beyond the scope of this chapter, it is important to understand the basic differences between these techniques.

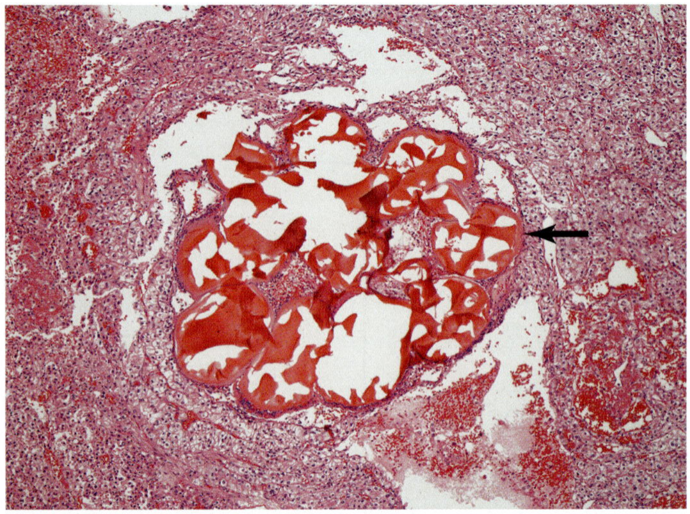

Figure 1-3 Hematoxylin and eosin stain at 10× magnification demonstrating embolic material (*arrow*) within a field of renal cell carcinoma in an explant after preoperative bland embolization.

Transarterial embolization, otherwise known as "bland" embolization, refers to the administration of embolic material without delivery of chemotherapeutic agents (Figure 1-3), whereas transarterial chemoembolization refers to the concomitant administration of an embolic agent and a chemotherapeutic drug. TACE can in turn be subdivided into conventional TACE (cTACE) and drug-eluting bead TACE (DEB-TACE). The former is formally defined as the delivery of an agent, most commonly doxorubicin, cisplatin, and/or mitomycin C with or without lipiodol, followed by or coadministered with an embolic agent (either gelfoam or particles).[20] DEB-TACE refers to the procedure by which beads loaded with doxorubicin are transarterially administered.

The premise of transarterial treatment of hepatocellular carcinoma (HCC), for example, is that hepatomas derive the majority of their blood supply from the arterial supply to the liver, whereas the rest of the liver derives most of its blood supply from the portal vein.[21] This unique property of HCC prompted the development of intraarterial chemotherapy and arterial embolization to (1) concentrate chemotherapeutic agents in the tumor and (2) cause selective ischemic necrosis of the arterially supplied tumor. Although these principles appear simple on initial examination, differing practice techniques over the past several decades have sparked a debate as to which of these mechanisms plays a more important role.

TAE works by causing occlusion of the terminal tumor arterioles, leading to ischemic necrosis and cell death. Although tumor necrosis has been demonstrated in several papers, some have argued that tumor hypoxia may actually stimulate angiogenesis and incite mechanisms to resist apoptosis, leading them to question the use of embolization alone in the treatment of HCC.[22,23] The counterargument is that more distal embolization is associated with less vascular recruitment and angiogenesis than proximal embolization.[24] This debate has been fueled by the lack of standardization of the size of embolic material used; agents have ranged from 40-μm microspheres to gelfoam cubes.

Conventional TACE aims to concentrate cytotoxic drugs within the tumor and prevent systemic toxicity by using a combination of lipiodol and embolic material. Lipiodol is iodinated poppy seed oil, and it has several unique properties that support its use such as selective uptake in target tumors; slowing the release of cytotoxic drugs it is mixed with; and when used in the liver, is thought to pass through hepatic sinusoids into portal venules, leading to dual embolization of the tumor.[25,26]

Once the combination of lipiodol and cytotoxic drugs is infused, embolic material (e.g., gelfoam, PVA, and tris-acryl microspheres) is administered into the same artery, with the goals of preventing washout of the lipiodol/chemotherapy infusion and causing ischemic necrosis.

DEB-TACE has evolved to improve the pharmacokinetic profile of chemoembolization. In spite of similar quantities of drug infused, drug-eluting beads result in lower systemic doses of doxorubicin compared with conventional TACE.[27] These beads lodge in the tumor microcirculation and elute the loaded drug into the tumor over time. In an animal model, 43% of the drug eluted off the beads after 28 days and ~90% after 90 days. Drug was detected as far as 600 μm from the bead, and there was a 30% decrease in doxorubicin tissue concentration from 1 to 3 months.[28]

The most commonly used beads are either made of PVA (DC beads, Biocompatibles) or a sodium acrylate–polyvinyl alcohol copolymer (Quadrasphere, Biosphere Medical). These beads range in size from 40 to 900 μm. It should be noted that as of this writing, the United States Food and Drug Administration (FDA) has not approved these beads for drug delivery.

Beads are loaded with doxorubicin in the pharmacy. In the case of DC beads, an ion-exchange mechanism loads oppositely charged doxorubicin onto the beads at a maximum of 45 mg doxorubicin per milliliter of beads, irrespective of bead size.[29] When smaller and larger beads were compared, higher plasma concentrations of doxorubicin were seen with the smaller beads, a finding that was attributed to a higher surface area–volume ratio of the smaller beads, leading to a more robust release of the drug.[30] Quadraspheres expand when hydrated, leading to a final diameter of 200–800 μm.[31] They can be loaded with either doxorubicin or cisplatin, and have CE Mark approval for the treatment of unresectable HCC when loaded with doxorubicin.

A preloaded microsphere (Precision Bead, Biocompatibles) has also been developed. This PVA polymer hydrogel with a sulfonic acid component has 37.5 mg of doxorubicin per milliliter of beads, and ranges in diameter from 100 to 900 μm.[32]

Coils

Coils are thin metal wires that are used for permanent vessel occlusion in a variety of vessels sizes, generally at the prearteriolar level. Coils are most often stainless steel or platinum, although platinum coils are preferred because of their increased radiopacity and thrombogenicity. Coils cause vascular occlusion in part by mechanical obstruction, but mainly by inducing thrombus in the vessel. It is important to allow sufficient time for thrombus to form in between coil deployment. Often, a gelfoam slurry can be used in addition to coils to hasten thrombus formation and provide a more complete embolization. Most coils are manufactured with tiny thrombogenic synthetic fibers that are attached to promote clot formation. Coils are available in a variety of shapes, and once deployed in the vessel will try to reassume this shape to help facilitate filling of the entire vessel volume. An example of one such embolic is shown in Figure 1-4.

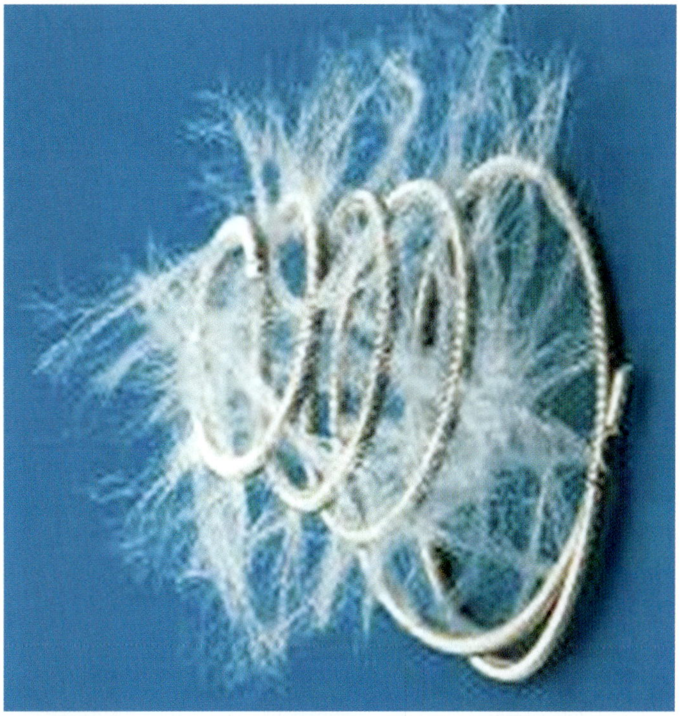

Figure 1-4 Tornado embolization coils with polyester fibers.

Once the delivery catheter is optimally positioned in the target vessel, ensure that it is in a secure location prior to deployment of coils. Test for catheter recoil by advancing the guidewire out of catheter before coil deployment. At this point, the coils are loaded and may be pushed through the catheter with an appropriately sized coil pusher. Alternatively, the catheter can be injected aggressively with a small amount of saline to "blow" the coil out the end of the catheter. The deployment of the first coil during an embolization, termed the "bookend," should be done in as precise a manner as possible. The first coil chosen is often stiffer than subsequent coils, with a higher radial force to allow for vessel occlusion. This is especially important in treating AVMs as an undersized coil may embolize to a nontarget area.[32]

Techniques such as the anchor technique is often utilized in these situations. The anchor technique refers to partially deploying the coil in a side branch of the target artery and subsequently deploying the remaining body of the coil into the main artery. This often allows this first coil extra support against the pressure from the high antegrade arterial flow (Figure 1-5).[33]

The Amplatz Occluder and the Amplatzer vascular plug (St Jude Medical, Plymouth, MN) are devices designed to provide a bookend upon which one can lay down additional coils. The Occluder is a cone-shaped plug with struts that fix it to the vessel wall. The design serves to provide a foundation against which the operator can lay down coils while minimizing the risk of downstream migration. The Amplatzer vascular plugs not only are designed to provide a scaffold for coils, but may obviate the need for or decrease the number of coils required to achieve a technically successful embolization (Figure 1-6).[34,35] Although techniques have been previously discussed to facilitate safe deployment of coils, certain scenarios may require very precise placement. Detachable coils have been developed to help in these instances. These coils are delivered while still

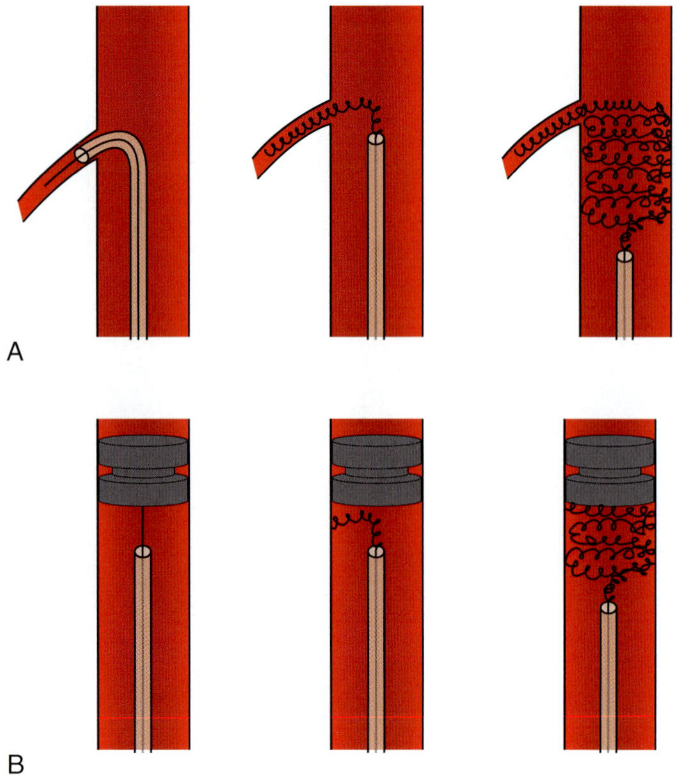

Figure 1-5 Graphic demonstrating anchor technique of initial coil deployment (A) and utilization of an Amplatz Occluder in a scaffold technique of coil deployment (B).

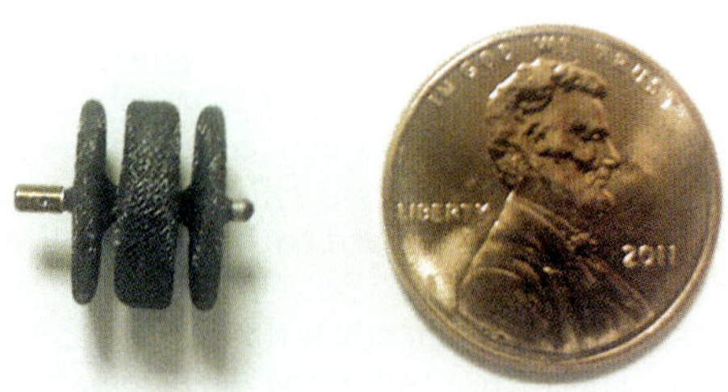

Figure 1-6 Image of an Amplatzer II Vascular Plug (10 mm), taken next to a penny for scale.

attached to the delivery wire so that they can be easily withdrawn and repositioned. Once proper coil positioning is achieved, these coils can be detached from the delivery system. As these coils are more costly, it may be prudent to use these devices to create a scaffolding to allow traditional coils to be used.

Other Embolic Agents

Ethanolamine Oleate

Ethanolamine oleate (Ethamolin 5%) is a mixture of 5% ethanolamine oleate and Ethiodol. It is a fatty acid–based sclerosing agent with thrombosing properties secondary to the ability of oleic acid to incite a mild inflammatory response in the vessel wall causing thrombosis, fibrosis, and occlusion. It is used primarily in venous sclerosis of gastroesophageal varices in portal hypertension and for venous malformations. Less commonly, this solution can be used as a sclerosing agent for cysts or varicose veins, though other agents are preferred for these uses.

Ethiodol, which is a radiopaque, inert, iodinated oil, is also used as a medium for delivery of chemotherapy in chemoembolization procedures. It is especially useful for treating HCC because of preferential uptake of Ethiodol by the tumor.

Alcohol

Absolute ethanol is an extremely potent liquid agent for embolization, the use of which is limited by its toxicity to normal tissue and the painful, intense inflammatory response it causes. Alcohol causes a complete, permanent vascular occlusion by denaturing proteins in the vessel wall, which leads to thrombosis and eventual fibrosis. It induces further thrombosis on contact with blood. This leads to a complete, permanent vascular occlusion. In addition to occluding blood flow, absolute ethanol ablates tissue as well. Ethanol can be injected intravascularly or by direct percutaneous puncture.

Although the potency of absolute alcohol makes it an excellent agent for embolization, its use is limited because of risks of damage to adjacent structures. The risk for systemic toxicity increases with doses above 1 mL/kg, or if the total volume exceeds 60 mL. Patients are also at risk for systemic toxicity from inadvertent vascular injection of the agent. The risks of systemic toxicity include intoxication, hypotension, and rarely cardiopulmonary collapse. Pulmonary hypertension can also be seen, leading to cardiopulmonary arrest requiring resuscitation. For this reason, some authors recommend pulmonary artery Swan-Ganz catheter and arterial pressure monitoring when using ethanol for arteriovenous malformations.[36,37] Ethanol ablation procedures are usually performed with general anesthesia because of the intense pain associated with its use.

Glue (Cyanoacrylate)

Cyanoacrylates are liquid adhesives that cause permanent occlusion and incite an acute inflammatory response.

Although an effective embolic agent, the use of cyanoacrylate glue is often limited as considerable experience is often required to effectively utilize it. The material rapidly polymerizes on contact with anionic substances such as plasma, blood cells, endothelium, or saline. In fact, the polymerization time is so rapid that a stabilization agent, ethiodized oil (Ethiodol, Lipiodol), is mixed with the glue, commonly in a 1:1 to 1:4 ratio in order to delay the solidification to about 1–4 seconds, to prevent solidification in the delivery catheter. As these agents are often not very radiopaque, tantalum can also be added in order to increase the radiopacity during injection. D5W is used to flush the catheter both before and after the injection of glue. Following injection of the solution and flush with D5W, the delivery catheter must immediately be withdrawn to avoid gluing the catheter tip to the vessel.

Appropriate solution preparation is of paramount importance because if the solution solidifies too early, the catheter may become glued in place. If the polymerization time is too long, the cyanoacrylate can pass into the venous circulation, resulting in pulmonary emboli.

Cyanoacrylate incites a very intense inflammatory reaction that involves the wall of the vessel and the adjacent interstitial areas. This inflammatory reaction ultimately leads to vessel necrosis, fibrous ingrowth, and permanent occlusion.

On account of its viscous, liquid nature, cyanoacrylates are well suited for embolizing AVMs. Ideally, the solution viscosity should be prepared to allow the glue to penetrate and fill the nidus without flowing through the venous end or occluding the feeding artery. Glue can also be used as a second- or third-line option in other situations, including aneurysms, pseudoaneurysms, varicocele treatment, and gastrointestinal bleeding.

Ethylene Vinyl Alcohol (Onyx)

Ethylene vinyl alcohol (EVOH), commonly known by the trade name Onyx (Covidien, Plymouth, MN), is FDA approved for the preoperative embolization of brain arteriovenous malformations. It is a solid copolymer that is dissolved in the organic solvent dimethyl sulfoxide (DMSO). In this form, it is used as a nonadhesive liquid embolic agent. Suspended tantalum powder provides the contrast for visibility under fluoroscopy (Figure 1-7).

The agent must be used with DMSO-compatible catheters to prevent catheter occlusion. DMSO-compatible syringes are also mandatory and are supplied with the delivery kit.

DMSO is injected into the microcatheter to fill the dead space, prior to the administration of the EVOH. The EVOH is mixed continuously for at least 20 minutes in a mixer prior to injection, in order to adequately suspend the tantalum. When the EVOH is initially injected, it remains in liquid form as it traverses the DMSO-coated catheter, and when the EVOH comes into contact with an ionic solution (such as saline, contrast, or blood), it immediately begins to solidify into a spongy, cohesive embolus. The DMSO solvent dissipates into the blood. It is imperative to watch the Onyx as it is delivered, if during the injection the operator does not see the solution exiting the catheter tip, the catheter may be occluded. If the solution is injected into an occluded catheter, with even a small degree of pressure, there is risk of catheter rupture and embolic delivery to unintended locations.[38]

In April 2007, the FDA approved the use of Onyx HD-500 (9.4% EVOH) to occlude certain types of cerebral aneurysms. This is a more viscous form of Onyx approved for intracranial, saccular, and sidewall aneurysms that have a wide neck ($\geq$4 mm) or with a dome-to-neck ratio $<$2 that are not amenable to treatment with surgical clipping. Prior to embolization with EVOH, a balloon occlusion catheter is used across the neck of the aneurysm to reduce the risk of the agent exiting the aneurysm and entering the systemic circulation.

One of the pitfalls that may arise during the delivery of Onyx involves entrapment of the catheter by the Onyx cast as it is deployed. Tips for removing an entrapped catheter, as mentioned in the instructions for use, include the following[39]:

- Pull gently on the catheter while visualizing the vasculature to assess the risk rupture. Apply 3–4 cm of traction on the catheter for a few seconds; release and repeat.
- If the above fails, another method of catheter removal is to use a quick wrist snapping motion from left to right. Again, assess the vasculature during attempted removal and do not apply more than 20 cm of traction to the catheter to minimize the risk of catheter fracture.

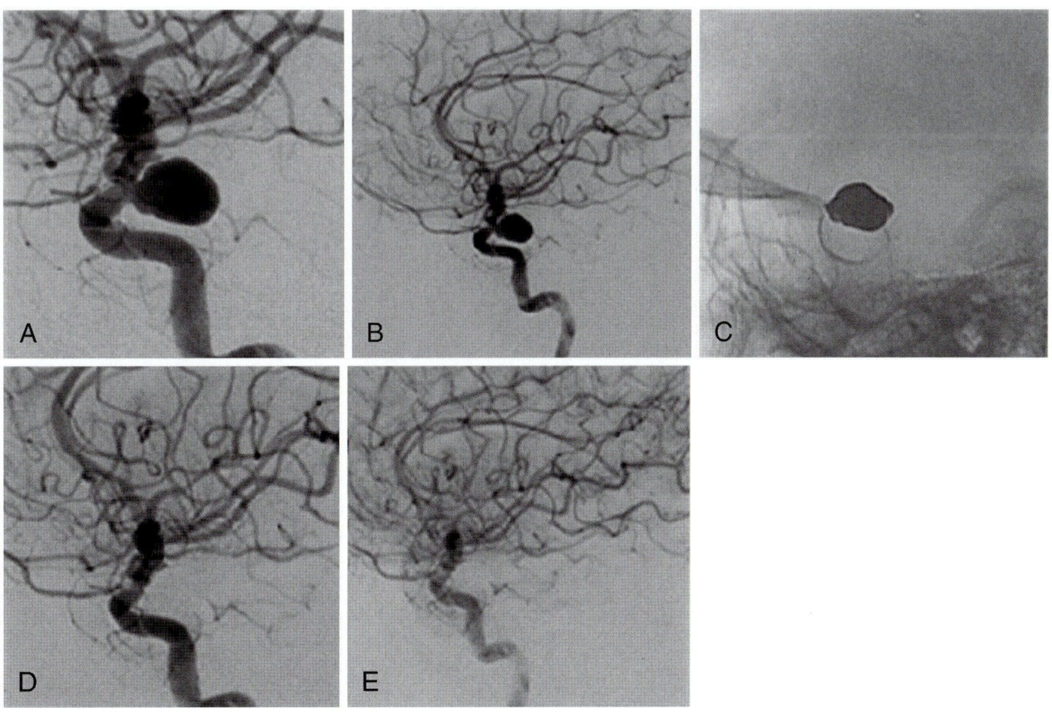

Figure 1-7 Ethylene vinyl alcohol (Onyx) selective left internal carotid artery (ICA) lateral angiogram. (A, B) Large aneurysm of the ICA–posterior communicating artery with a posterior orientation. (C) Unmasked fluoroscopic lateral view of radiopaque Onyx HD-500® filling the lumen of the aneurysm. (D, E) Postprocedural control angiography demonstrates total occlusion of the aneurysm. *(From Tevah J, Senf R, Cruz J, Fava M: Endovascular treatment of complex cerebral aneurysms with Onyx HD-500® in 38 patients,* J Neuroradiol *38:238–290, 2011, Figure 1.)*

- If all attempts to remove the catheter have failed, it may not be possible to safely remove the catheter without the risk of hemorrhagic complications. In this instance, it may be safer to leave the catheter in the vascular system. As a last resort measure, the catheter can be stretched and cut near the point of access. The catheter would then remain in the artery.

In this chapter, we have outlined the most commonly used embolic agents and provided an overview of their properties and uses. There are a wide variety of different embolic agents and each has unique characteristics that make it suitable for use in a given clinical scenario. The choice of agent must be tailored to the appropriate situation and a thorough understanding of the risks and benefits of each agent is imperative in order to make an appropriate selection.

REFERENCES

The complete reference list is available online at www.expertconsult.com.

2 Principles of Percutaneous Ablative Therapies

CHARBEL ISHAK | RAYMOND H. THORNTON | STEPHEN B. SOLOMON

KEY POINTS

- Percutaneous image-guided tumor ablation uses the cytotoxic properties of thermal energy or electric field strength to cause cell death.
- The thermal ablative effect due to coagulation necrosis is generated by the **Radiofrequency** probe, which acts as the cathode in an electrical circuit closed by attaching grounds pads to the patient.
- Cytotoxicity of **Cryoablation** results from denaturation of protein structures, and cellular membrane disruption caused by freezing and thawing.
- **Microwave** frequency causes rapid molecular friction and significant rise in water temperature, leading to cellular death and coagulation necrosis.
- **Irreversible Electroporation** mechanism is entirely electric and nonthermal, using pulses of high electrical current to disrupt the lipid cellular membrane with formation of multiple permanent nanopores leading to cell death.
- **Chemical ablation** uses acetic acid and ethanol to destroy tissues, leading to immediate cytoplasmic dehydration, vascular thrombosis, protein denaturation, and consequent coagulation and ischemic necrosis.

Percutaneous image-guided tumor ablation with both thermal and nonthermal techniques has gained growing attention for the treatment of many focal neoplasms with a parallel continuous advance in energy delivery and technical developments. Percutaneous ablative therapy, delivered by using needlelike applicators connected to a generator, uses the cytotoxic effects of thermal energy, electric field strength, or chemicals to cause cell death.

This chapter will review the principles of percutaneous ablative therapies currently used in the field of interventional oncology, including thermal techniques (radiofrequency ablation [RFA], cryoablation, microwave ablation) as well as nonthermal techniques (irreversible electroporation and chemical ablations). High-intensity focused ultrasound (HIFU) and laser ablative therapies are beyond the scope of this chapter. The clinical practice of these percutaneous ablative therapies will be discussed in different chapters.

Radiofrequency Ablation

MECHANISM OF ACTION

RFA is the most frequently used percutaneous ablative technique for many focal neoplasms, especially liver and lung tumors. Most RFA systems operate in a monopolar mode by using two different types of electrodes: interstitial electrodes inserted into the lesion and dispersive electrodes placed on the skin surface known as ground pads.[1,2] The interstitial electrode delivers energy to the tumor, creating a volume of high current density and localized heating around the electrode tip.[3] The ground pad closes the electrical current circuit with dispersing energy over a large surface area to reduce the likelihood of thermal injury to the skin (Figure 2-1).[4]

Radiofrequency (RF) waves range from 300 to 600 kHz in the electromagnetic spectrum, and it is followed in an increasing frequency by microwave, infrared, visible, ultraviolet, x-rays, and gamma rays (Figure 2-2). Molecules close to the active component of the RF electrode, especially dipolar molecules like water, respond with motion to the alternating current produced by the RF generator. The charged molecules move in order to constantly realign their electric poles with the continuously alternating current. This motion causes friction and results in the production of heat. Heat is locally conducted from hotter to cooler tissues, and heat can be drawn away from tissue on the basis of continuous transfer to flowing blood in vessels larger than 3 mm in diameter, a process called "heat sink." Tissues surrounding the electrode undergo coagulation necrosis because of a higher deposited energy flux in a small surface of the probe tip when compared to a lower energy flux in a large surface of the grounding pads.[4] This thermal ablative effect is generated by the RF probe, which acts as the cathode in an electrical circuit closed by attaching grounds pads to the patient.

Cellular death occurs within a few seconds at 55°C.[5] At 100°C, cell death is almost instantaneous, and it is accompanied by vaporization and microbubble formation. Nitrogen gas, released on cellular death at high temperatures, acts to insulate against the efficient conduction of heat to adjacent tissue. Clinically, this type of rapid tissue death caused by very high temperature is referred to as "charring." Therefore, a slow RF application, over many minutes, is more effective and efficient than a quick temperature rise. Slower transfer of heat results in less charring and tissue desiccation; otherwise, these undesirable factors act to further insulate the probe, limiting further extension of the ablation zone.[4,6] The physical properties involved in the production and transfer of heat energy away from the electrode into more distant tissue limits the size of the ablation achievable with a single probe. RFA appears to perform best when tumors have a diameter of 3 cm or less. In addition, an additional ablative margin of 1 cm is preferable to ensure complete tumor coverage, because the extent of coagulation necrosis is limited by the heat sink effect created by adjacent blood vessels.[6] Flowing blood, in vessels of 3 mm or larger, carries away heat on a continuous basis, preventing the sustained elevation of high temperature in adjacent tissue.

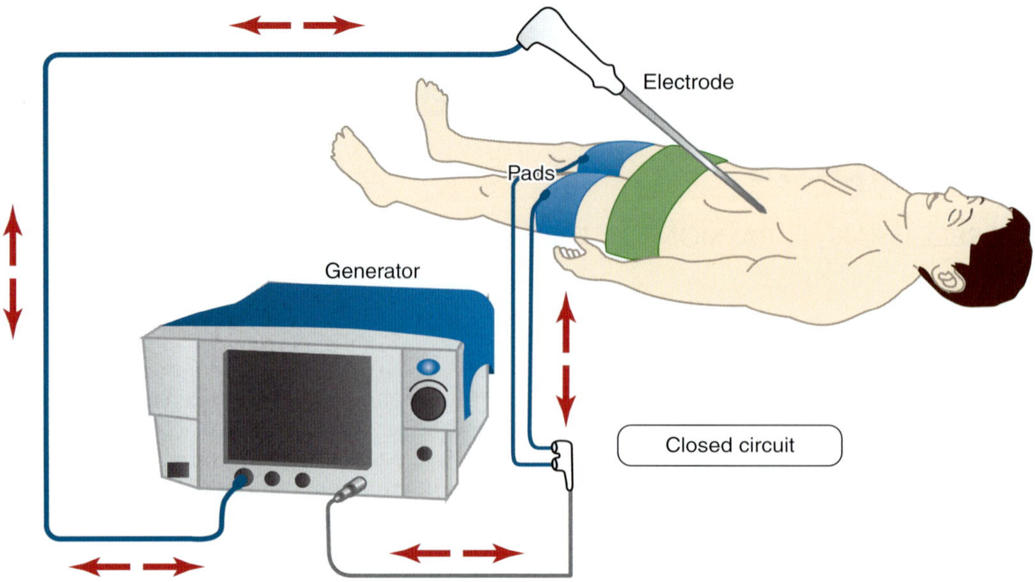

Figure 2-1 The thermal ablative effect is generated by the RF electrode, which acts as the cathode in an electrical circuit closed by attaching ground pads to the patient. *(Courtesy Covidien.)*

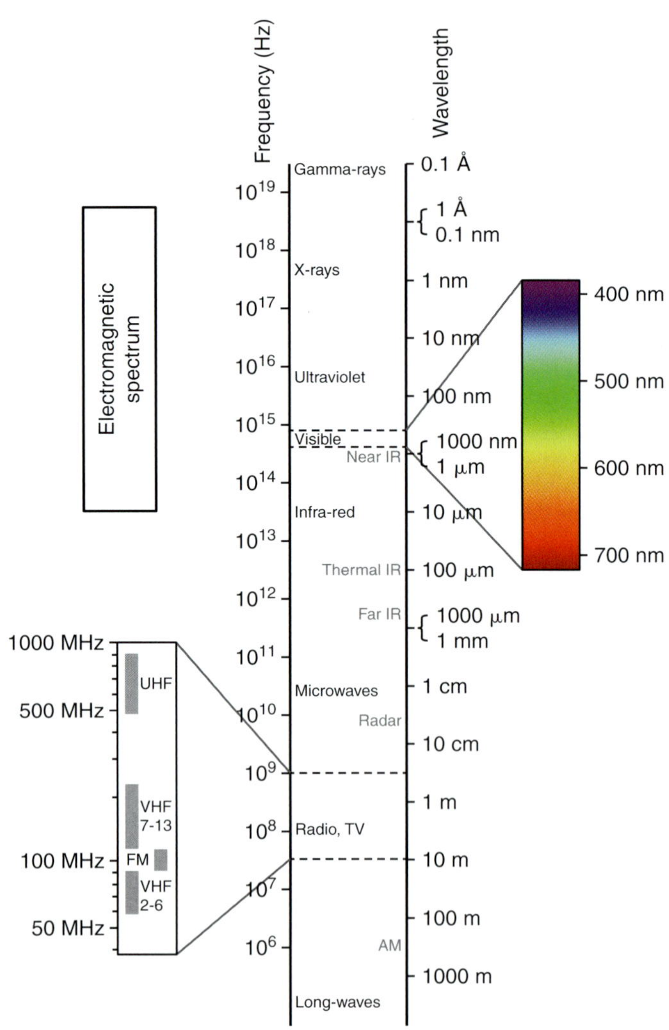

Figure 2-2 Electromagnetic spectrum is shown in an increasing frequency from radio waves followed by microwaves, infrared, visible, ultraviolet rays, x-rays, and gamma rays. *(Courtesy Microsulis.)*

This can limit effectiveness, leading to possible residual tumor and increasing the chance of tumor recurrence. The use of multiple electrodes can mitigate this problem and help in increasing the ablation area.

EQUIPMENT

Monopolar RFA

There are three major manufacturers of monopolar RFA devices on the market. Generators manufactured by the three major RFA companies provide maximum outputs of 150–200 W, delivering high-frequency (450–500 kHz) alternating current via RF electrodes in the size range of 14–17 gauge.

Boston Scientific RF System

The Boston Scientific RF system (Natick, MA), which includes the RF 3000 Generator that is an impedance-based direct feedback system designed to accurately monitor the extent of tissue desiccation, permits continued delivery of RF energy until desired ablation is achieved (Figure 2-3). There are a range of LeVeen RFA array probes, which include the SuperSlim, standard, co-access systems in addition to the Soloist straight-tip needle, single-needle electrode (Figure 2-4).

The SuperSlim RFA needle electrode (17-gauge) has size ranges from 2 to 3 cm and for each diameter size can be matched with cannula lengths of either 15 or 25 cm. The standard LeVeen needle electrode comes in diameters ranging from 2 cm (12 cm in length), 3 cm (12 cm in length), 3.5 cm (12 or 15 cm in length), 4 cm (15 cm in length), and 5 cm (15 cm in length). The needle electrodes for diameter sizes ranging from 2 to 3.5 cm, 4 cm, and 5 cm are 15, 14, and 13 gauge, respectively. The 15-gauge CoAccess electrode system has the ability to obtain a tissue biopsy by inserting an 18-gauge needle gun into the sheathed needle system before starting the ablation. The CoAccess probe has diameters ranging from 3, 3.5, and 4 cm with 15 cm length. The co-access RFA electrode shaft is not insulated and therefore cannot be used without the co-access sheath as this will cause skin burn (Figure 2-5).

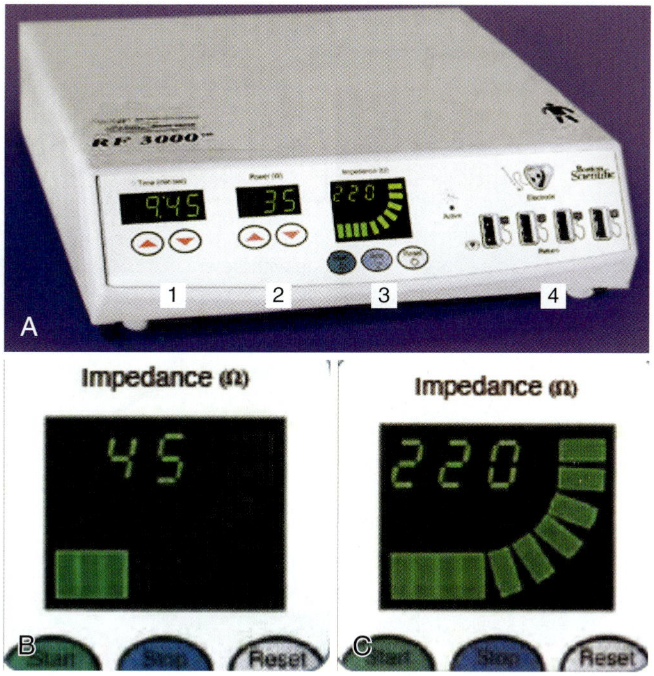

Figure 2-3 (A) Boston Scientific RF 3000 generator system: 1. Ablation time. 2. Power display. 3. Impedance display. 4. Pad-Guard current monitor for proper pad placement. (B) Initial tissue impedance is measured prior to application of RF energy and is typically within the range of 40–80 Ω, illuminating three bars on the front panel of the RF 3000 Generator. (C) Impedance rise is indicated by an increase in Ohms and a sequential illumination of the bars on the front panel, signaling cellular destruction and the completion of a thermal lesion. *(Courtesy Boston Scientific.)*

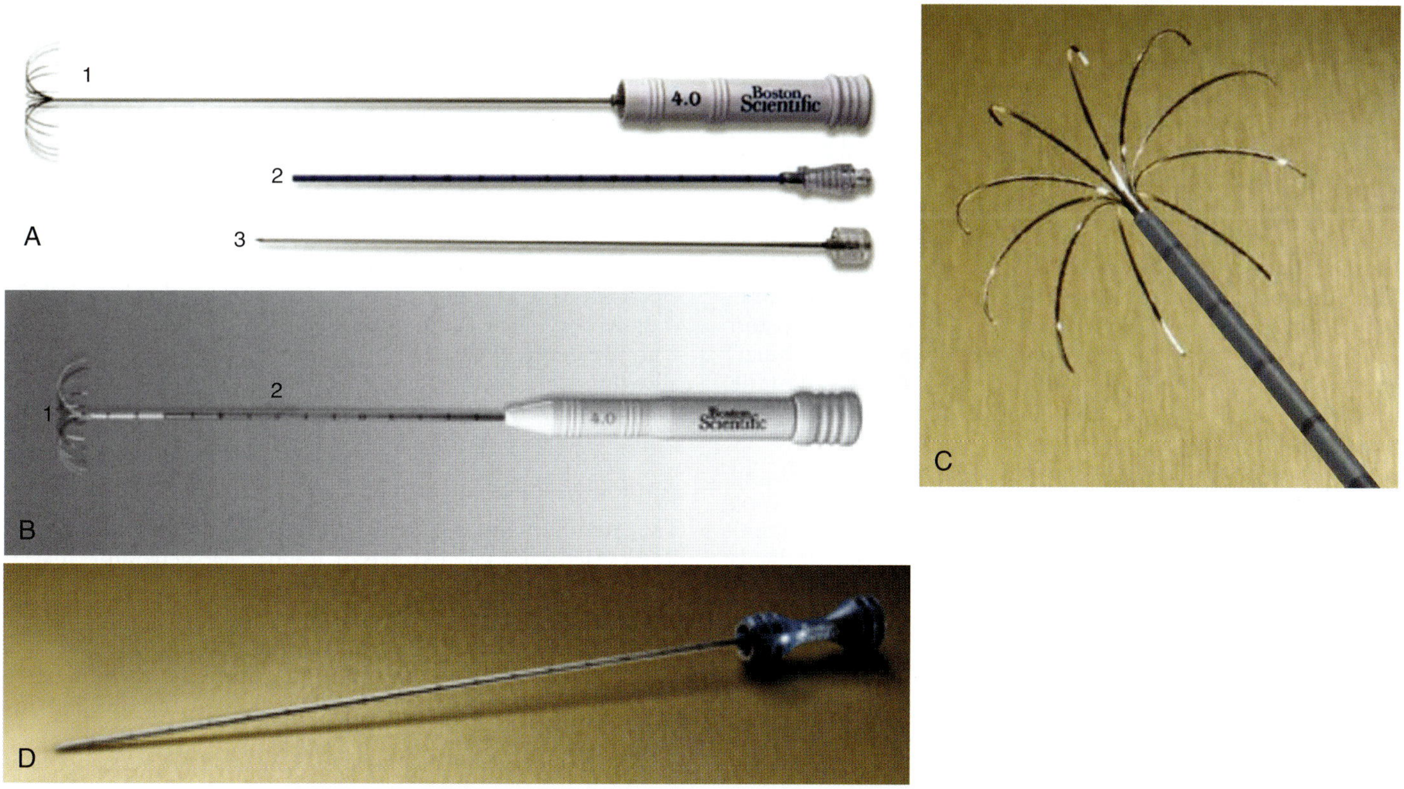

Figure 2-4 (A) 1. LeVeen CoAccess electrode with umbrella-shaped prongs. Introducer set consists of insulated cannula (2) and Stylet with Trocar tip (3). (B) 1. LeVeen Needle electrode. 2. Cannula marked at 1-cm intervals. (C) LeVeen device: 1 cm tine spacing is designed to facilitate the creation of a spherical thermal ablation zone. (D) Soloist straight-tip single-needle electrode (16.5-gauge) is useful for treating small tumors and can avoid any significant collateral damage. *(C and D: Courtesy Boston Scientific.)*

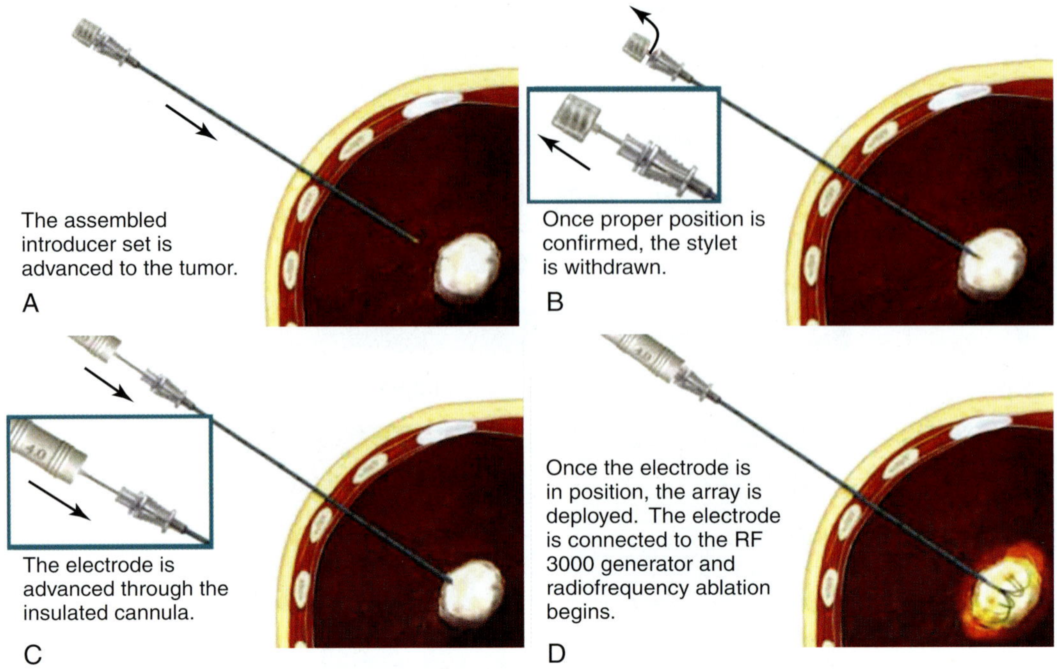

Figure 2-5 LeVeen CoAccess electrode system is a coaxial system. (A)–(D) show how to place the electrode. The electrode must be used in conjunction with the insulated cannula (C). *(Courtesy Boston Scientific.)*

The LeVeen probe consists of multiple curved prongs that deploy from the central needle and project a short distance beyond the needle before directing recurving in the opposite direction. Fully deployed, this creates the appearance of an umbrella (Figure 2-4, *C*). Each individual prong causes a separate area of coagulation necrosis that slowly increases in size by administering increasing amounts of RF energy in a stepwise fashion and creating a surrounding volume of necrosis (Figure 2-6). Electrode probe tips provide impedance feedback. The resulting increase in tissue resistance to current flow—impedance—is measured in Ohms and is displayed as a series of illuminated bars that progress to Roll-Off® Indication, an easy-to-read signal of the desired clinical endpoint. The end point of ablation with the LeVeen device is a dramatic increase in impedance, termed "roll-off" by Boston Scientific. The standard algorithm suggests a second "burn" starting at 70% of maximum Roll-Off power. At the end of the procedure, the probe tract can be ablated in order to reduce needle tract seeding.

There is also a straight-tip needle, the Soloist single-needle electrode (16.5 gauge), which is useful for treating small tumors and can avoid any significant collateral damage. The typical ablation zone with the Soloist needle is slightly oval in shape and measures ≈ 1 cm (diameter) × 1.5 cm (length).

Cool-tip™ Covidien RF System

The Cool-tip Covidien RF system (Boulder, CO, formerly known as Tyco Healthcare Valleylab) works on the basis of internally cooled electrodes, where chilled saline is pumped through the chamber of the needle, in order to reduce charring, to increase tumor volume ablation and to shorten ablation time (Figure 2-7). The internal electrode cooling mechanism keeps the temperature of the tissue around the electrode low, allowing the electrode to drive more energy into the tissue without the need to increase power.[6] The Covidien RF Ablation Generator, a 200-W power source, connected to the Cool-tip electrode features a feedback algorithm that continuously monitors tissue impedance. The generator senses maximum energy deposition into the lesion and uses pulsing to control the energy output (Figure 2-8). Impedance is adjusted to achieve the appropriate energy output for the electrode. Thermocouples at electrode tip also measure tissue temperature to help optimize energy deposition. Once the treatment cycle is complete, the electrode cooling can be stopped. The generator automatically shuts off at the end of the 12-minute ablation cycle. The Cool-tip electrode is a 17-gauge straight electrode with a beveled tip (Figure 2-9). There are multiple electrode lengths (10, 15, 25 cm) with five different electrode exposure lengths (1, 2, 2.5, 3, 4 cm), allowing control for varying lesion sizes. The entire electrode can be imaged with computed tomography (CT) or ultrasound guidance during the procedure.

AngioDynamics System

The AngioDynamics system (Latham, NY, formerly known as RITA Medical Systems) has a 1500X RF generator that is equipped with computer-driven protocols that automatically adjust wattage to maintain optimal temperatures during the ablation. The generator, with 250 W of power, combined with the IntelliFlow saline peristaltic infusion pump, is thought to allow for faster and larger ablations by reducing the charring effect (Figure 2-10).

The AngioDynamics StarBurst® family of probes consists of an attachable or preattached interface cable and an insulated primary trocar with needles and temperature sensors at the distal end. The temperature sensors determine the average temperature.

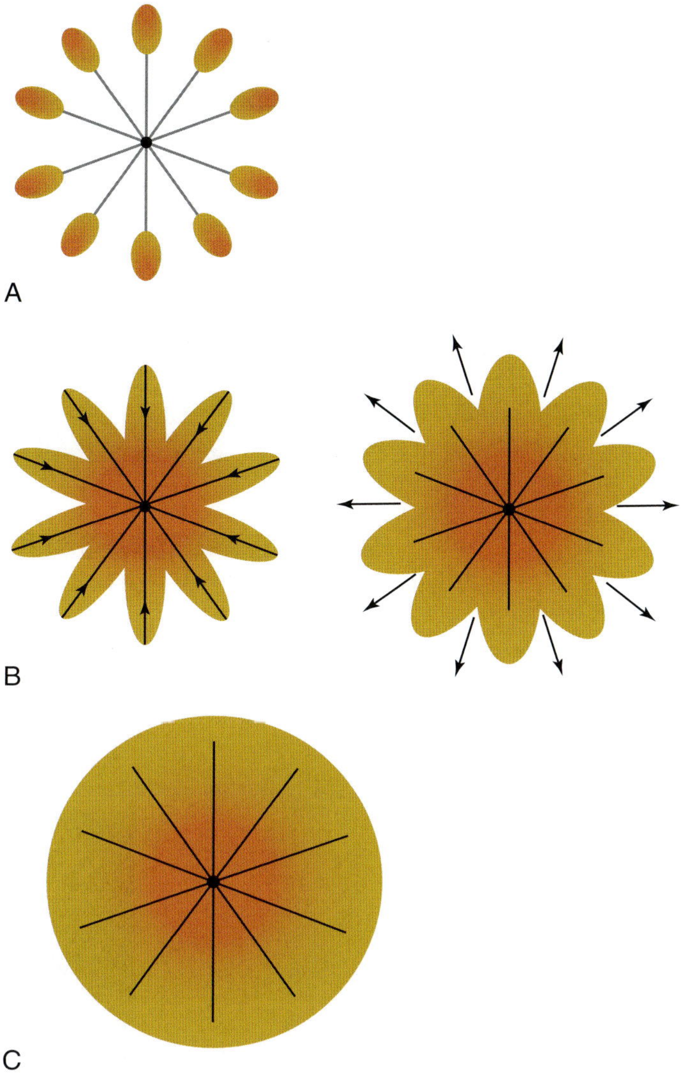

Figure 2-6 (A) The thermal lesion developed by the LeVeen Needle electrode begins at the tips of the array tines. The multiplicity of tines in the electrode allows the RF energy to shift away from any given tine as the adjacent tissue desiccates and increases in impedance. (B) As the tissue near the tips of the tines desiccates, the zone of ablation travels back along the tines toward the center of the array. The thermal lesion then moves outward and begins to fill in the gaps between the tines. (C) A complete thermal lesion is achieved once tissue desiccation has occurred throughout the target tissue. The RF 3000 Radiofrequency Generator is designed to receive feedback from the target tissue to reduce power and signal a complete thermal lesion. *(Courtesy Boston Scientific.)*

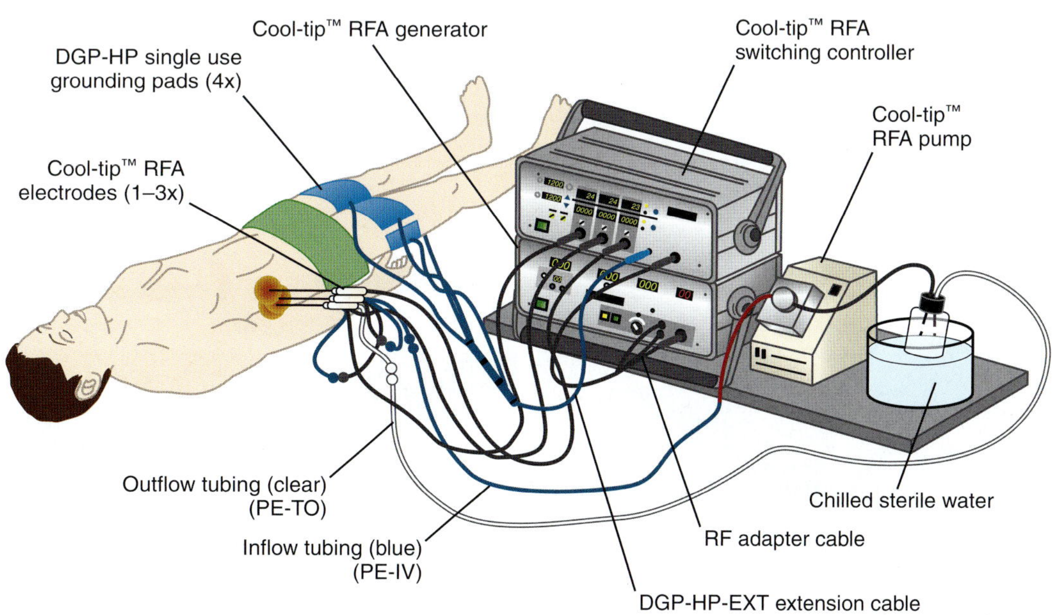

Figure 2-7 Covidien Cool-tip™ setup. Pads close the electrical current circuit. Chilled water pumped through electrodes. *(Courtesy Covidien.)*

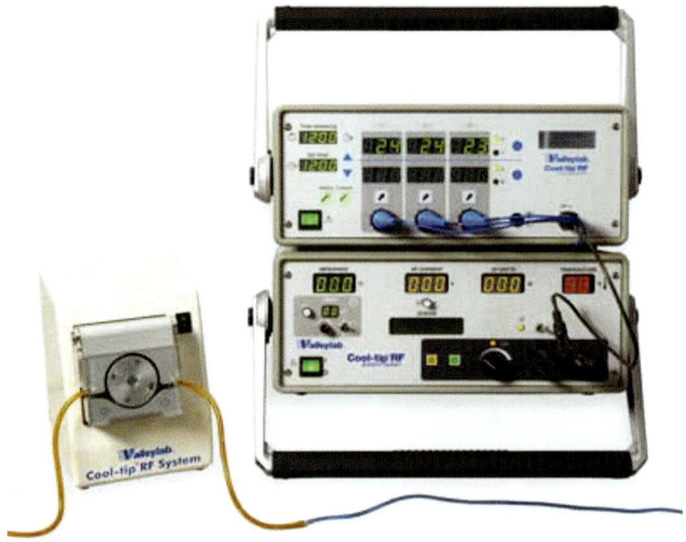

Figure 2-8 Cool-tip™ RF generator, switching controller: Output: 0–200 watts, 480 kHz. Display parameters: impedance, current, power, time, and temperature. *(Courtesy Covidien).*

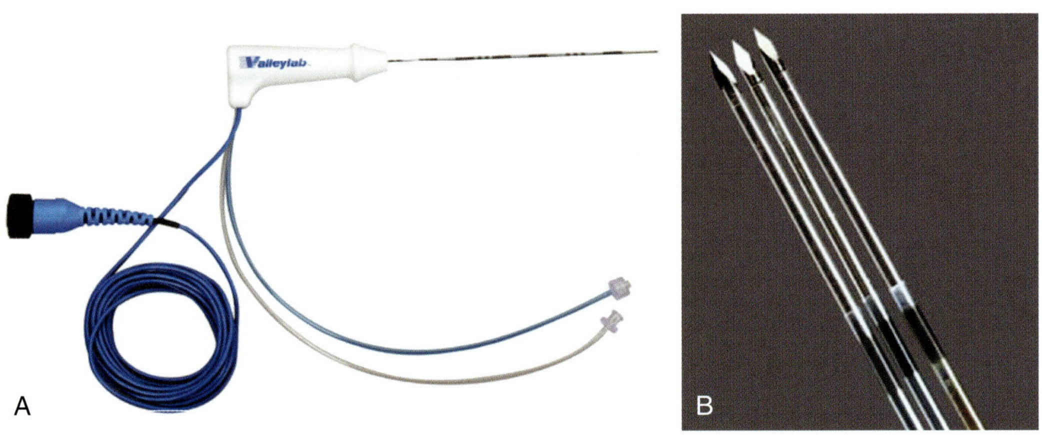

Figure 2-9 (A) 17-gauge straight Cool-tip™ electrodes with beveled tip (B) for easier insertion and reposition. There are multiple electrode lengths (10, 15, 25 cm) with five different electrode exposure lengths (1, 2, 2.5, 3, 4 cm) allowing for the control for varying lesion sizes. *(Courtesy Covidien.)*

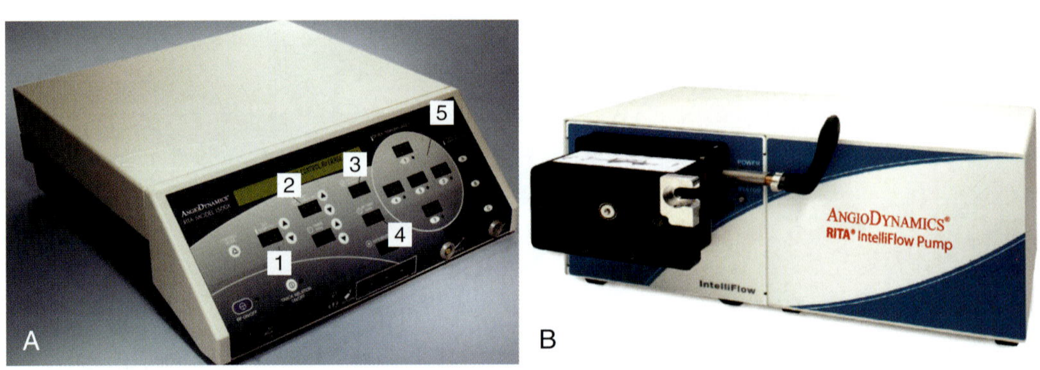

Figure 2-10 (A) AngioDynamics 500X RF generator: 1. Set temperature (°C). 2. Set power (W). 3. Delivered power (W). 4. RF time (minutes). 5. Device temperatures (°C) displaying the temperature readings of the probe thermocouples. (B) IntelliFlow saline peristaltic infusion pump without tubing set. *(Courtesy AngioDynamics.)*

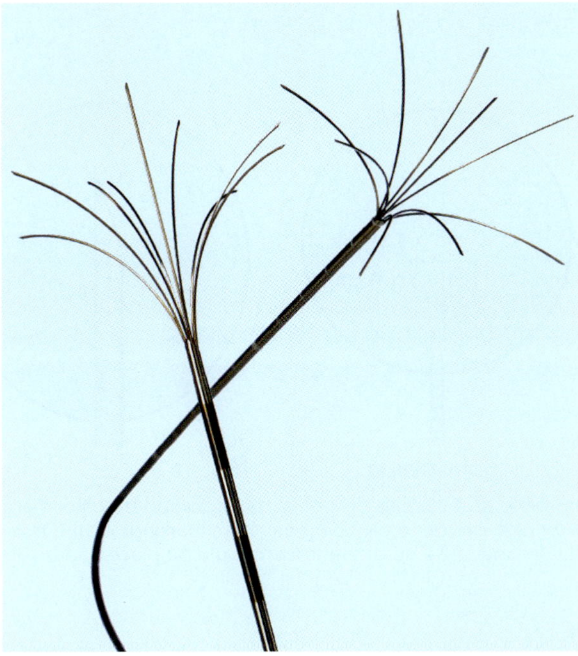

Figure 2-11 AngioDynamics StarBurst XL and Semi-Flex 14-gauge probes with nine deployable curved prongs oriented forward from the main needle shaft, capable of ablations from 3 to 5 cm. *(Courtesy AngioDynamics.)*

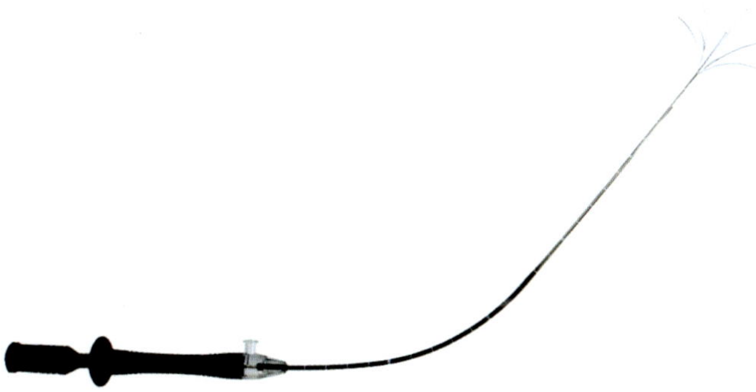

Figure 2-12 AngioDynamics flexible electrodes (StarBurst SemiFlex) with the ability to bend up to 90 degrees in all directions allowing for easy entry into the CT gantry. *(Courtesy AngioDynamics).*

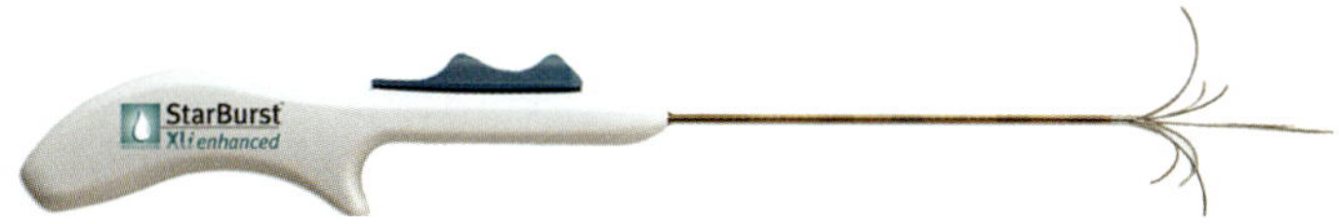

Figure 2-13 AngioDynamics system: StarBurst XLi-Enhanced probe as a perfusion electrode whereby saline or hypertonic saline is infused into the ablation tissue, to augment tissue electrical conductivity and ablation zone. *(Courtesy AngioDynamics.)*

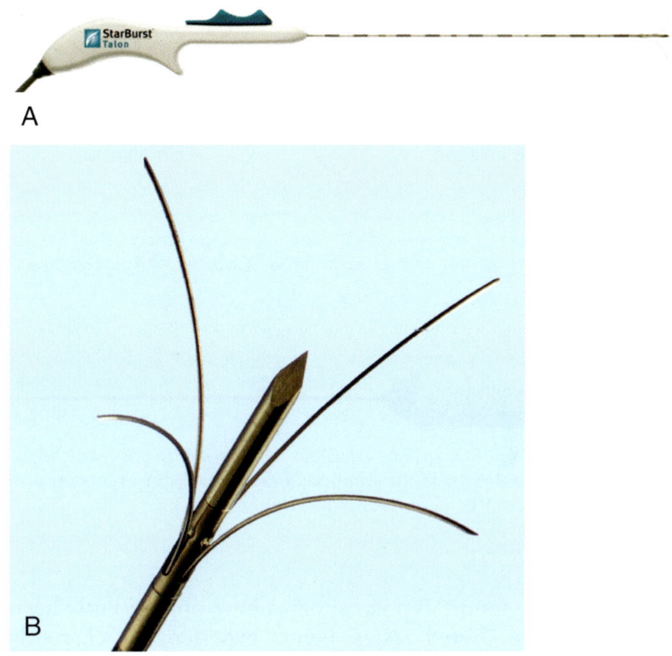

Figure 2-14 (A and B) AngioDynamics StarBurst Talon probe with four active arrays and trocar tip. Thermocouples exist in the tip of each active array. *(Courtesy AngioDynamics.)*

The AngioDynamics system has several electrodes, with the 14-gauge StarBurst XL as the basic probe capable of ablations from 3 to 5 cm (Figure 2-11). The probe contains nine deployable curved prongs oriented forward from the main needle shaft. The maximum diameter is 5 cm in a configuration of a Christmas tree when fully deployed. The tips of the AngioDynamics system hooks have thermocouples that monitor real-time temperature at the treatment volume margin. Real-time temperature readings are displayed on the generator console. Flexible electrodes are also available (StarBurst SemiFlex) (Figure 2-12) with the ability to bend up to 90 degrees in all directions, allowing for easy entry and navigation into the CT gantry. Similar to other systems, electrodes with perfusion capabilities are also offered, the StarBurst Xli Enhanced (Figure 2-13) and StarBurst Talon electrodes (Figure 2-14), whereby saline or hypertonic saline is infused into the ablation tissue, to augment tissue electrical conductivity with the aim of creating an ablation volume diameter up to 7 cm. The probe is placed at the proximal portion of the lesion, allowing the tine tips to be deployed forward (Figure 2-15, *A*). The one exception is the StarBurst Talon probe, which uses side deployment of the tines, and therefore requires insertion to the distal aspect of the lesion (Figure 2-15, *B*). The StarBurst Talon RFA electrode with side-deployment tines may be used in lesions adjacent to critical structures. AngioDynamics also manufactures a linear deployment "UniBlate" 17-gauge probe, which provides linear, scalable ablations from 1 to 3 cm in length and 1 to 2.5 cm in diameter. The UniBlate probe has a very low profile for CT gantry compatibility (Figure 2-16).

Bipolar RFA

Bipolar systems do not require attaching the patient to a grounding pad, thus minimizing risks of skin burns. The applied RF current is limited to between the two poles within the ablative electrode. The InCircle (RFA Medical, Fremont, CA) bipolar probes are placed on each side of the tumor without

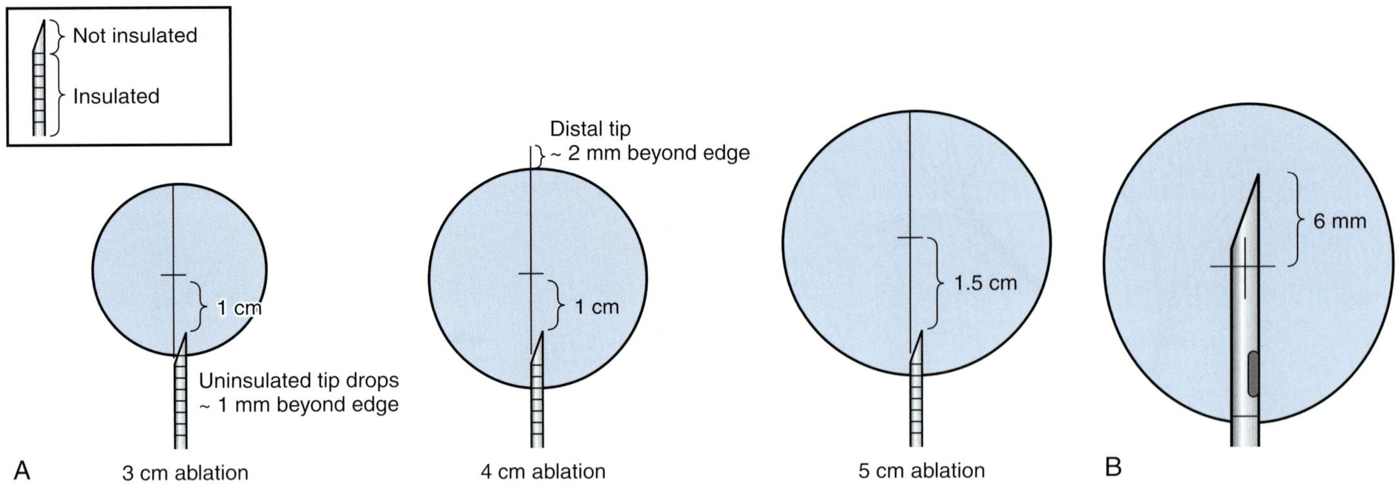

Figure 2-15 (A) Trocar position when using StarBurst XL, Semi-Flex, or MRI-compatible probes. The tip of the trocar should be placed approximately 1 cm (for a 3-cm ablation) to 1.5 cm (for a 5-cm ablation) proximal to the center of the target area. Using the 1-cm markings on the trocar can assist in placement of the device. (B) Trocar position when using StarBurst Talon, SDE probes. The tip of the trocar should be placed approximately 6 mm distal to the center of the target area. *(Courtesy AngioDynamics.)*

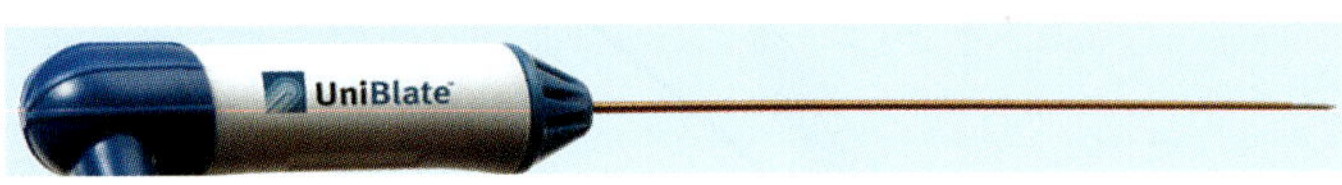

Figure 2-16 AngioDynamics "UniBlate" 17-gauge probe with linear deployment provides scalable ablations from 1 to 3 cm in length and 1 to 2.5 cm in diameter. *(Courtesy AngioDynamics.)*

penetrating the lesion. Bipolar systems have only recently been available in the United States; hence, experience is currently limited.

Cryoablation

MECHANISM OF ACTION

Image-guided percutaneous cryoablation is most commonly used for the treatment of small renal cancers, prostate cancer, soft tissue, and bone tumors. Renal cell carcinoma is the tumor most commonly treated with cryoablation. In addition, percutaneous cryoablation is used for the palliation of painful bone lesions and to a lesser extent for the treatment of liver and chest neoplasms, especially pleural-based lesions. More recently, cryoablation has been used for salvaging prostate applications and lung and breast tumors.

Cryoablation reduces the temperature of the target lesion to lethal levels (−20°C to −40°C). Additionally, cycling between cooling and thawing results in disruption of cell membranes, leading to a variety of cytotoxic effects. Cytotoxicity results from extracellular ice formation (producing dehydration, protein denaturation, lipid peroxidation, and increased free radicals), apoptosis (programmed cell death and mitochondrial damage), vascular stasis (creating hypoxia and lack of nutrients), and intracellular ice formation (shearing the cellular membrane caused by freezing and thawing).

The low thermal energy can be transferred from one tissue volume to another by conduction or convection. The direct physical contact and the molecular kinetic energy exchanges are seen in the conduction. However, flowing blood surrounding ablated tissue can transfer away the low thermal energy as seen in convection. Conduction constitutes stable energy transfer dependent on the temperature difference between ablated tissue and the cryoablation probe, whereas convection depends on the flow rate of the surrounding blood adjacent to the volume of interest. Therefore, large-diameter arteries will limit the extent of cryoablation.

The iceball created by cryoablation is visible under CT, ultrasonography, or magnetic resonance guidance, allowing visual monitoring throughout the procedure in most organs. The iceball margin demarcates a zone cooled to 0°C, which is not a lethal temperature. The zone starting 5 mm inside this 0°C isotherm zone will usually harbor the tissue at −20°C, which is considered a lethal temperature.[7] A cryoprobe tip should be placed beyond the distal margin of the tumor to provide 5–10 mm tumor margin as the ablation zone does not extend more than 2 mm past the probe tip.

Argon or helium are the two expanding gases used in commercial cryoablation systems. The inversion temperature is the critical temperature below which a gas that is expanded will experience a temperature decrease, and above which it will experience a temperature increase. According to the Joule-Thomson law,[8] an expanding gas cools if its inversion temperature is greater than the ambient temperature and warms if its inversion temperature is lower than the ambient temperature. Therefore, argon creates the cooling when expanding and circulating in the cryoprobe. The inversion temperature of helium is lower than room temperature; therefore, helium warms when it expands and circulates in the dual-chambered cryoprobe. Separate gas tanks are required to supply argon and helium to the probe via pressure regulators. Argon or helium, once expanding, cools or warms and exchanges thermal energy with the adjacent tissues before circulating back into the dual-chambered cryoprobe.

EQUIPMENT

Two cryoablation system manufacturers, Endocare and Galil Medical, distribute products in the U.S. market. Both companies use argon for freezing and helium for thawing.

Endocare

The Endocare (HealthTronics, Inc., Austin, TX) regulator is composed of gas inlet and outlet hookups for argon and helium, where up to eight cryoprobes and eight temperature sensors can be connected simultaneously (Figure 2-17). Three different cryoprobes (Perc-15, Perc-17, and Perc-24) exist, and selection depends on the size and shape of the target lesion (Figure 2-18). Endocare needles incorporate temperature sensors within the handle of the needle. The Endocare protocol generally consists of a 10-minute freeze, followed by an 8-minute active thaw and another 10-minute freeze (Figure 2-19). Cryoprobes should be started simultaneously to ensure proper coalescence of ice. Ideally, final iceball size should be 1 cm beyond edge of tumor and completely cover the mass (Figure 2-20).

Galil Medical

The Galil Medical (Arden Hills, MN) cryoablation systems (Visual-ICE® System, SeedNet® System, and Presice® System) are composed of gas inlet and outlet hookups for argon and helium (Figure 2-21). Different iceball sizes and shapes (IceBulb®, IceRod®, IceSphere®, IceSeed®, and IceEDGE®) can be generated depending on the operator's selection (Figure 2-22). Galil Medical cryoablation needles do not have incorporated thermocouples. Rather, the company offers 17-gauge multiple-point and single-point thermosensors that can be independently placed in tissue. These sensors can be placed between the target lesion and surrounding tissue to monitor the temperature, and therefore the safety and efficiency of the cryoablation.

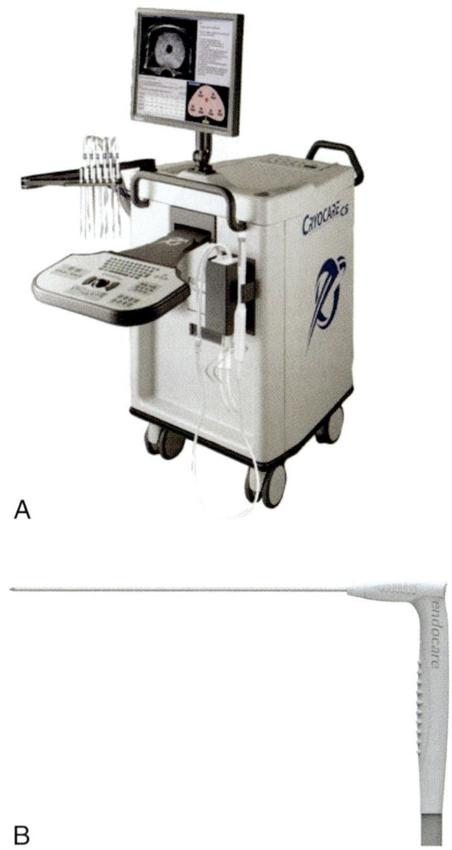

Figure 2-17 Endocare Cryoablation system (A) and PerCryo probe (B). *(Courtesy Endocare, Heathtronics.)*

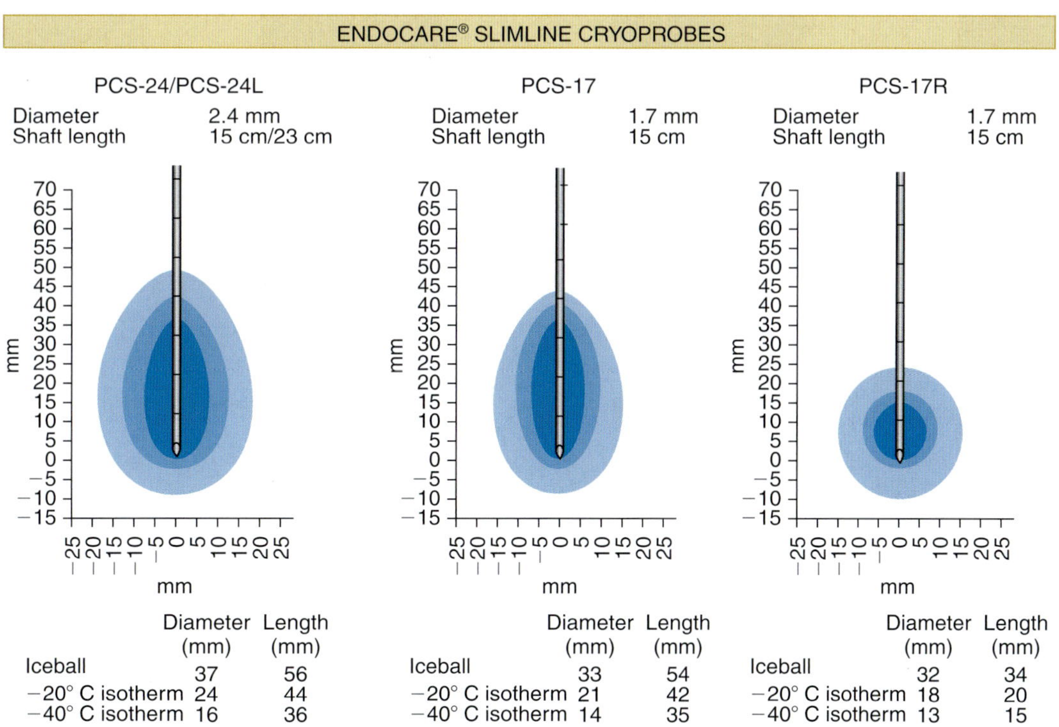

Figure 2-18 Different cryoprobes exist and selection depends on the size and shape of the target lesion. *(Courtesy Endocare, Heathtronics.)*

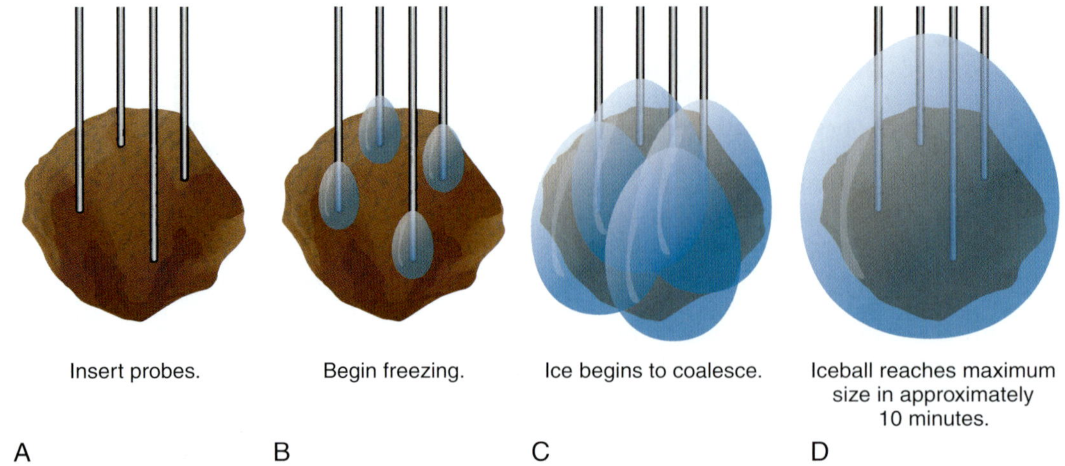

Figure 2-19 Tumor treated with four cryoprobes. (A) Insert probes. (B) Begin freezing. (C) Ice begins to coalesce. (D) Ice ball reaches maximum size in approximately 10 minutes. *(Courtesy Endocare, Heathtronics.)*

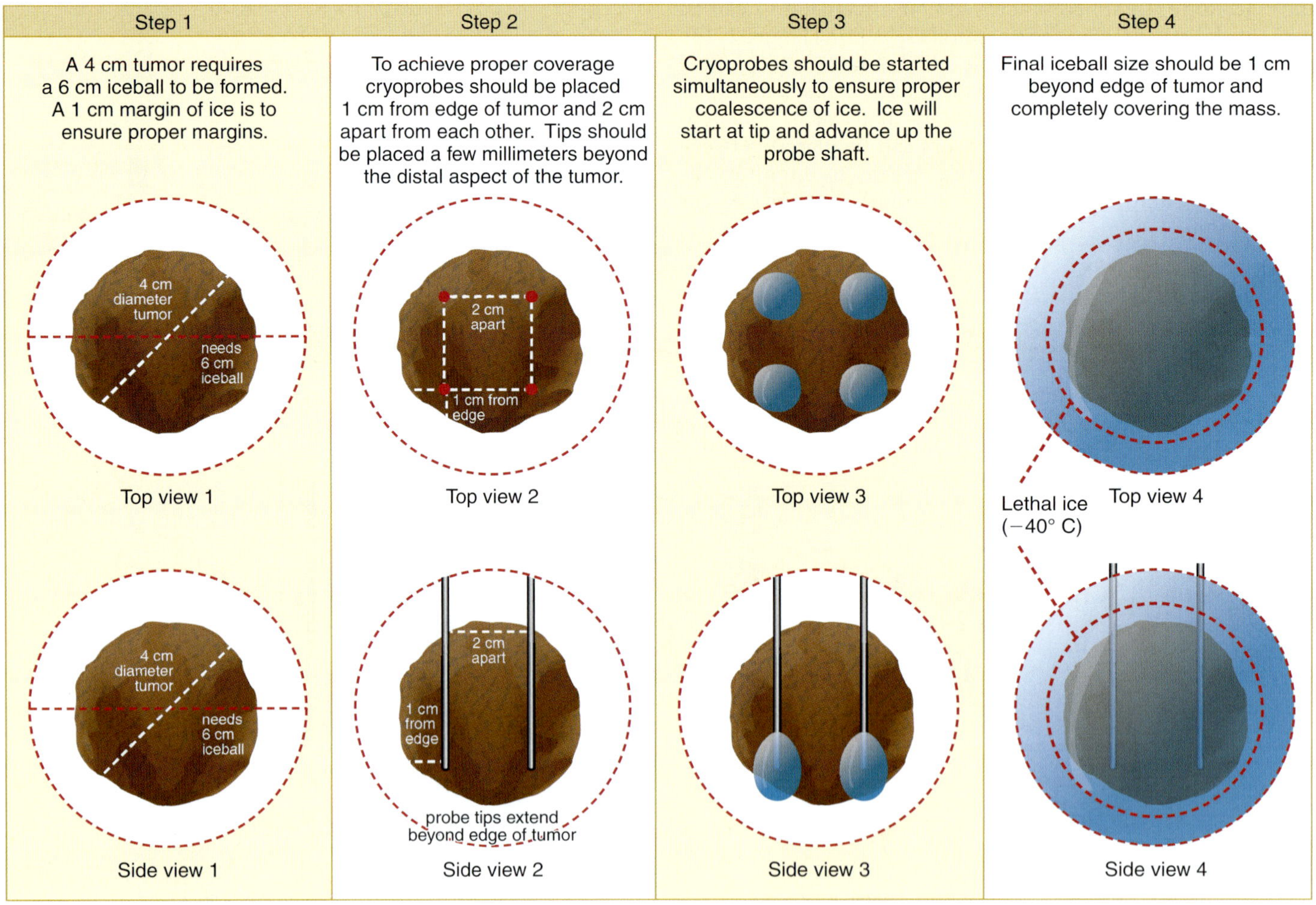

Figure 2-20 Endocare cryoprobes insertion. *(Courtesy Endocare, Heathtronics.)*

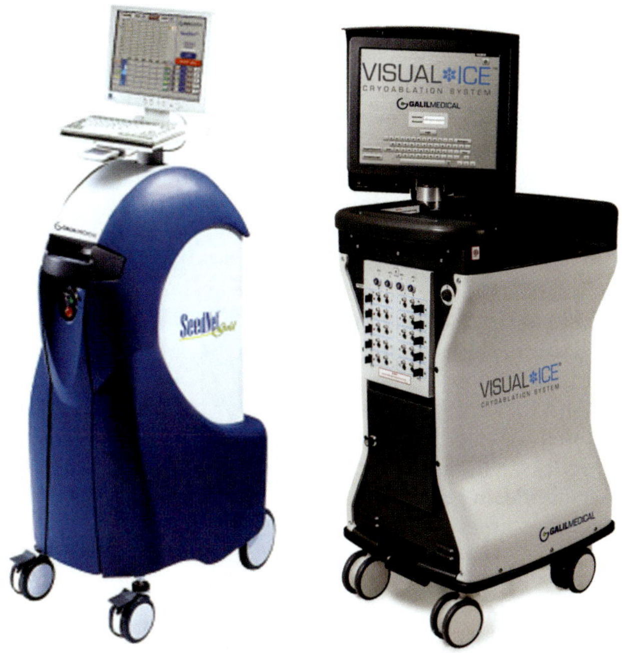

Figure 2-21 Galil Medical cryoablation systems (Visual-ICE® System, SeedNet® System) are composed of gas inlet and outlets hookups for argon and helium. *(Courtesy Galil Medical.)*

Isotherm data	IceSeed® 1.5 mm 17G	IceSphere® 1.5 mm 17G	IceRod® 1.5 mm 17G	IceRod®*PLUS* 1.5 mm 17G	IceBulb® 1.5 mm 17G	IceEDGE™ | 2.4 2.4 mm 13G
0°C	31 mm x 36 mm	37 mm x 45 mm	40 mm x 58 mm	43 mm x 60 mm	40 mm x 67 mm	49 mm x 63 mm
−20°C	19 mm x 26 mm	24 mm x 34 mm	27 mm x 50 mm	30 mm x 48 mm	28 mm x 55 mm	34 mm x 51 mm
−40°C	10 mm x 19 mm	15 mm x 25 mm	16 mm x 41 mm	18 mm x 42 mm	17 mm x 48 mm	22 mm x 43 mm

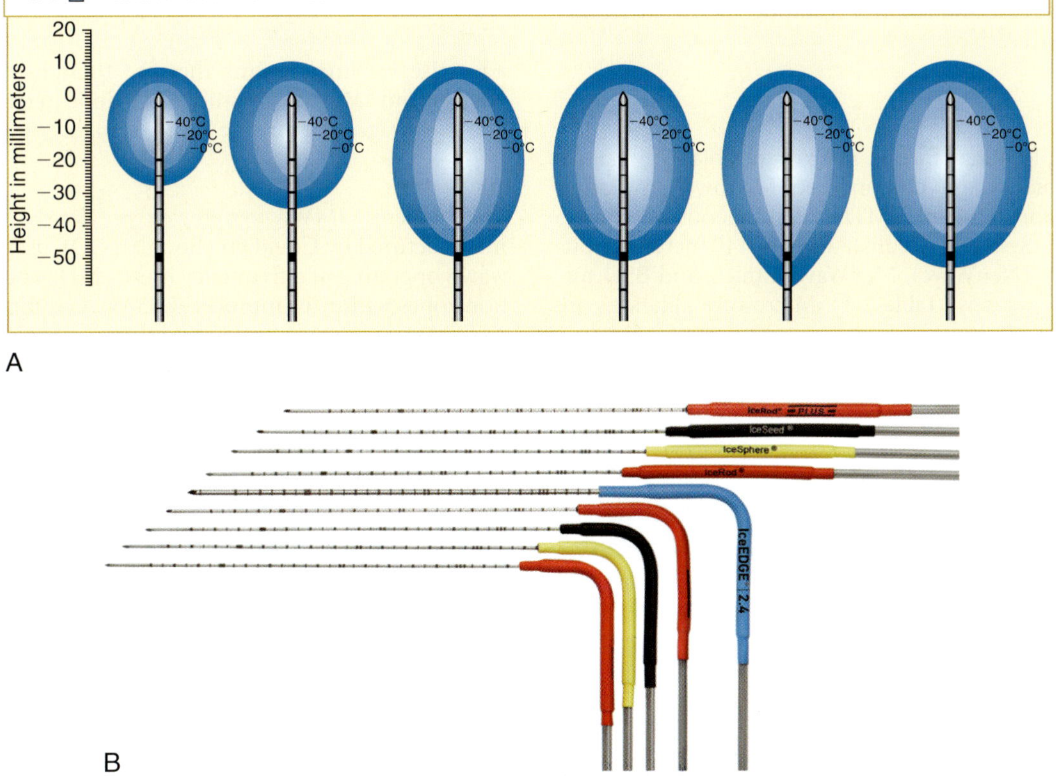

Figure 2-22 (A and B) Galil Medical Isotherms: Ice ball dimensions are provided to assist users in selecting the cryoablation needle(s) and needle placement to appropriately ablate the target area. Typically, in vivo dimensions are smaller than the dimensions generated in the laboratory. Measurements were made after two 10-minute Freeze cycles separated by a 5-minute passive Thaw cycle. In vivo ice ball dimensions and the resulting ablation zone are determined by the cryoablation needle type, number of needles placed, tissue and tumor characteristics, thermal heat sink from surrounding vasculature, and treatment duration. Monitoring ice ball formation provides direct control throughout the procedure and is crucial to cryotherapy success. *(Courtesy Galil Medical.)*

Microwave Ablation

MECHANISM OF ACTION

Microwave ablation is utilized in the treatment of hepatic, pulmonary, and renal malignancies and metastases.[9,10] Microwave ablation may be selected in most lesions where RFA can be used, and is thought to be more efficacious in lesions greater than 4 cm in size. Microwave is a promising thermal ablative technique even when targets are located adjacent to large vessels; this is due to minimal heat-sink effects seen with microwave when compared to other thermal ablation modalities.[11]

Microwave frequency, in the range of 300 MHz–300 GHz, follows RF waves in the electromagnetic spectrum. The asymmetric distribution of charges between the hydrogen and oxygen atoms causes water molecules to be polarized; thus, they carry electrical charges and interact with the oscillating electrical field transmitted from the antenna of the microwave probes.[12] Rapid molecular agitation causes friction, leading to a significant rise in water temperature and conductive heating of the target tissue surrounding the microwave probe (Figure 2-23). Cellular death and coagulation necrosis occur above 50°C–55°C because of protein and enzymatic degradation and DNA denaturation.[4,12]

A microwave probe generates a large zone of ablation extending up to 2–3 cm from the antenna. The operator should ensure that the radiating section is always fully inserted into tissue to prevent elongated waveform fields that can cause unintended thermal injury to the user and/or patient (Figure 2-24). The direct ablation zone for microwave, where the active molecular oscillation and frictional heating dwell, is approximately 2 cm from the probe. Microwave energy creates higher temperatures with larger ablation zones in a shorter period of time, without significant charring that increase impedance, resulting in the insulating effects seen with RFA.[14,15]

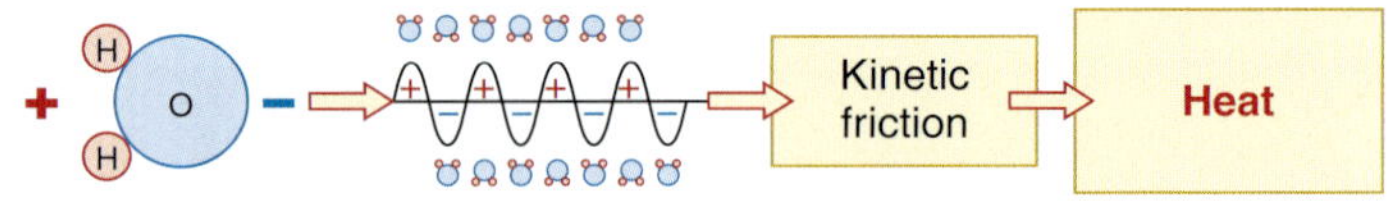

Figure 2-23 Dipole water molecule excitation from microwave antenna causes friction, leading to a significant rise in water temperature and conductive heating of the surrounding target tissue. *(Courtesy MedWaves Medical.)*

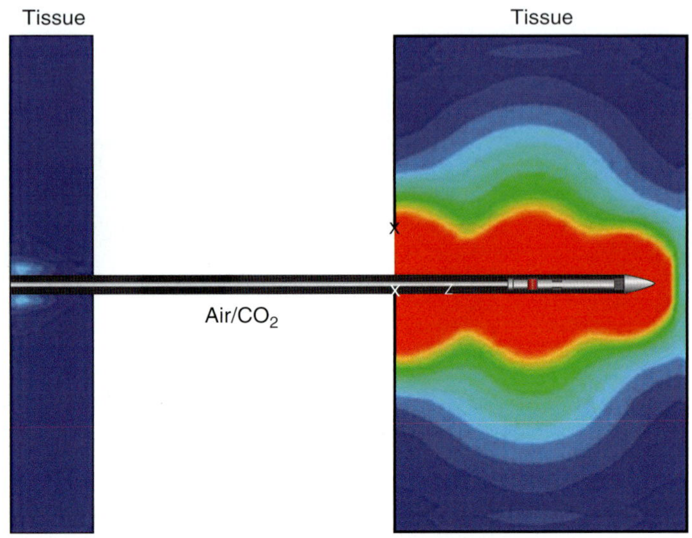

Figure 2-24 The radiating section of the antenna should be fully inserted into tissue to prevent elongated waveform fields that can cause unintended thermal injury to the user and/or patient's skin. *(Courtesy Covidien.)*

EQUIPMENT

There are multiple percutaneous microwave ablation systems currently available in the U.S. market: Microwave Ablation System (Valley Lab/Covidien), pMTA (percutaneous Microwave Tissue Ablation) System (Acculis), Certus 140 percutaneous microwave device (NeuWave), MedWave, Amica, and BSD microwave ablation systems (Table 2-1). Microwave ablations are generally performed under CT and/or ultrasound guidance. Microwave technology is in infancy when compared to RF technology. Therefore, as summarized herein, multiple manufacturers advertise varying designs that are thought to enhance both efficacy and safety. Until studies are done to determine the relative advantages of each, the choice is highly operator dependent.

Covidien

The Evident™ MWA system, or previously Valleylab system, manufactured by Covidien (Boulder, CO), uses electromagnetic waves operating at a frequency of 915 MHz and can create ablation zones within 10 minutes at 45 W. A continuous infusion of normal saline via a pump at 60 mL/min provides cooling to the outer shaft of each antenna in order to prevent thermal injury to the tissues along the length of the antenna shaft (Figure 2-25).

Table 2-1 Comparison of Currently Used Percutaneous Microwave Ablation Systems in the Market

Microwave systems	NeuWave Certus 140	Covidien Evident	MedWaves	Microsulis Acculis	BSD MicroThermX	HS Amica
Frequency	2.45 GHz	915 MHz	915 MHz	2.45 GHz	915 MHz	2.45 GHz
Probe sizes (gauge)	13 and 17	13	12 and 17	15	14	14 and 16
Max power, single probe (W)	140	45	32	180	60	70
Capacity, number of probes	3	1	1	1	3	1
Max power, all probes (W)	195	45	32	180	180	70
Cooling system	CO2	Water	None	Water	Water	Water
Synchronous	Yes	No	No	No	Yes	No

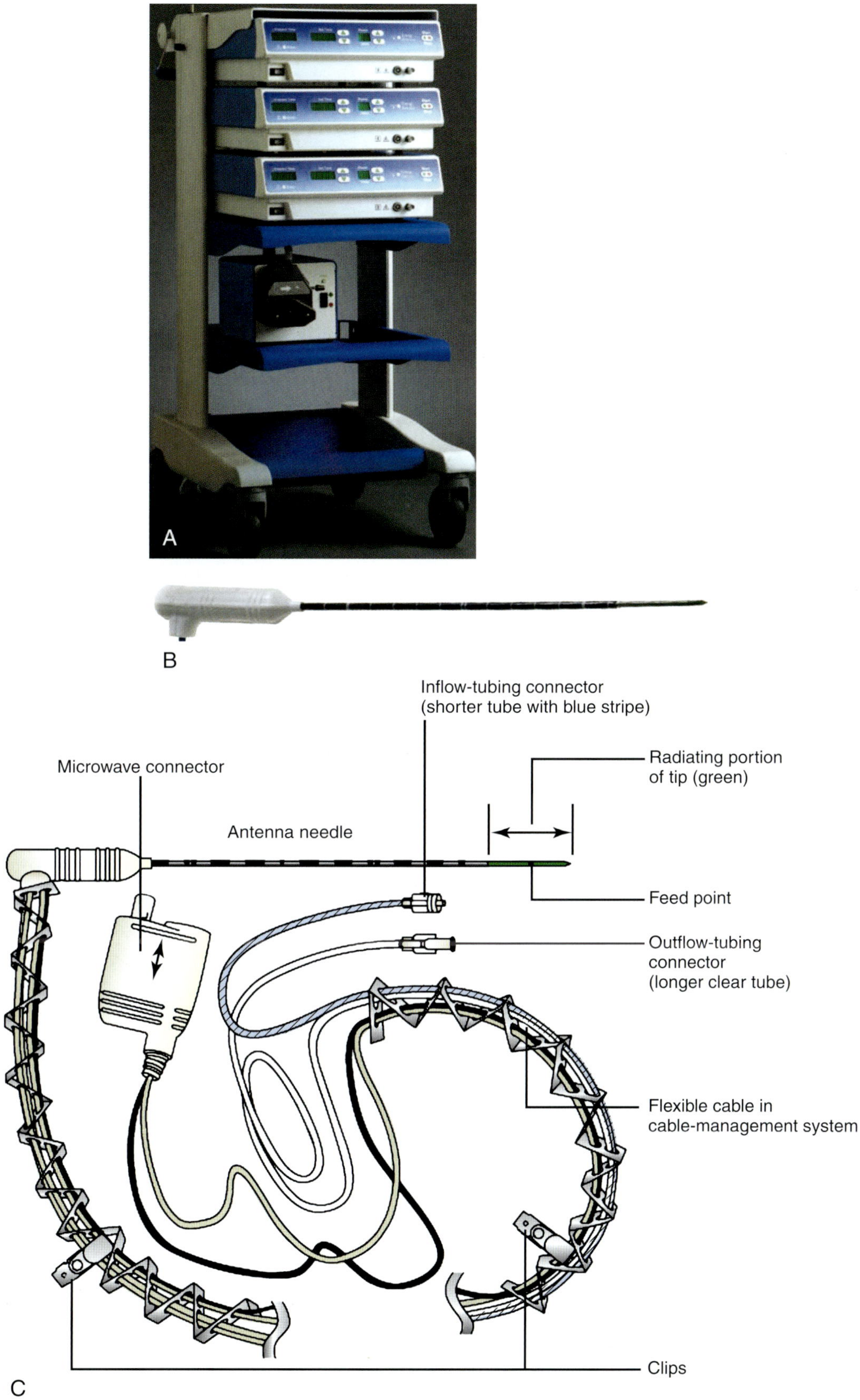

Figure 2-25 (A) MWA generator and pump. (B and C) Evident percutaneous antenna. *(Courtesy Covidien.)*

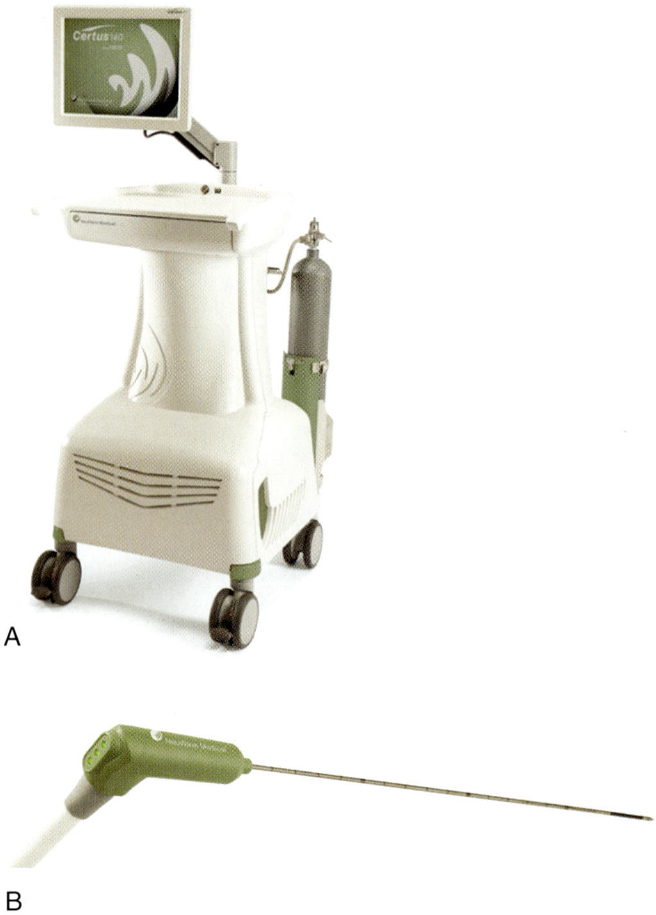

Figure 2-26 (A) NeuWave generator. (B) NeuWave antenna. *(Courtesy NeuWave.)*

Multiple microwave antennae (up to six) may be used per treatment. Using multiple microwave antennae allows for creation of larger ablation zones. It is important to ensure that antennae are spaced 2 cm apart to minimize excessive overheating that can occur because of overlapping ablation zones. There is no need to use grounding pads when using microwave. To minimize the risk of local skin burn injury, antennae are equipped with sensors that monitor shaft temperature and provide automatic feedback regulation, meaning that the generator will shut off if the proximal shaft in contact with the patient's skin exceeds a temperature of 43°C.

NeuWave Medical

NeuWave Medical (Madison, WI) manufactures the Certus 140, a 2.45-GHz ablation system with tissue-specific probes, including the Certus^{LK} ablation probe and the recently released Certus^{PR} ablation probe (Figure 2-26). The Certus 140 system provides synchronized power delivery to the target tissue. It is the only CO_2-cooled ablation system on the market. The CO_2 cooling design allows for the added benefit of "sticking" the probe to the target tissue to prevent migration. The CO_2 cooling system also protects the device by limiting overheating of probe shaft and handle during ablation. It ensures that MW energy is effectively "choked" and stays at the tip of the probe for maximum ablation size and facilitates generation of up to 140 W of power on a single channel.

BSD Medical

BSD Medical (Salt Lake City, UT) microwave ablation system named the MicroThermX® consists of a generator and pump

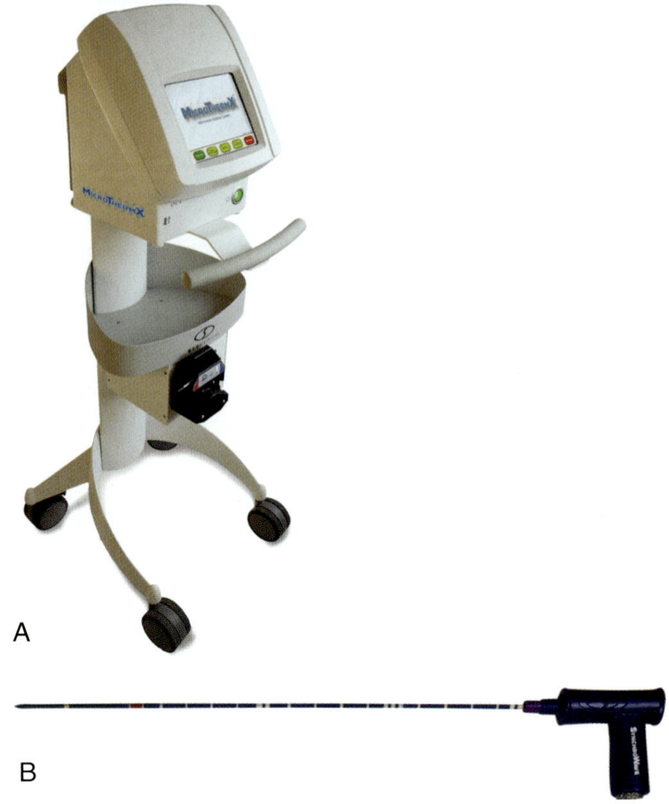

Figure 2-27 (A) BSD Medical microwave ablation system, MicroThermX®. (B) SynchroWave antenna. *(Courtesy BSD Medical.)*

(Figure 2-27). The MicroThermX® microwave ablation system includes a 915-MHz single generator and single amplifier system with coherent synchronous phased array capability that can accommodate up to three SynchroWave antennas (probes) in a nonparallel fashion. It is thought that this coherent synchronous phased array capability allows for large contiguous, more-consistent ablation zones when compared to asynchronous systems that use multiple amplifiers.

MedWaves

The MedWaves (San Diego, CA) system uses electromagnetic waves operating at a frequency of 915 MHz. The major difference between this device and others is its freedom from the need for irrigation and cooling (Figure 2-28).

Microsulis

Microsulis's Acculis (Hampshire, UK) Microwave Tissue Ablation (MTA) system consists of the Sulis VpMTA generator operating at 2.45 GHz and a power of 180 W. The Accu2i pMTA antenna creates a near spherical coagulation of up to 5.6 cm in 6 minutes at maximum power (Figure 2-29). At 2.45 GHz, the frequency of the Acculis MTA System, the energy will penetrate 2 cm into the tissue. This is the active microwave heating zone. The coagulation zone is largely spherical, with a slight elongation in the direction of the shaft.

HS Amica

The HS Amica (Rome, Italy) microwave system consists of a generator operating at 2.45 GHz and a power of 70 W. The Amica probe is designed with enhanced sonographic visibility and comes as 11, 14, and 16 gauge (Figure 2-30).

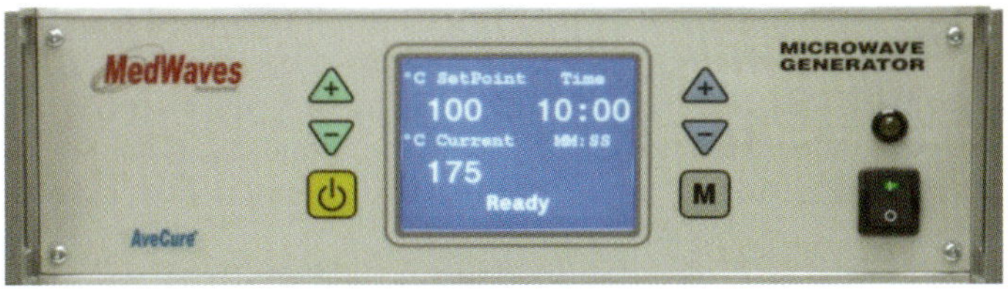

A

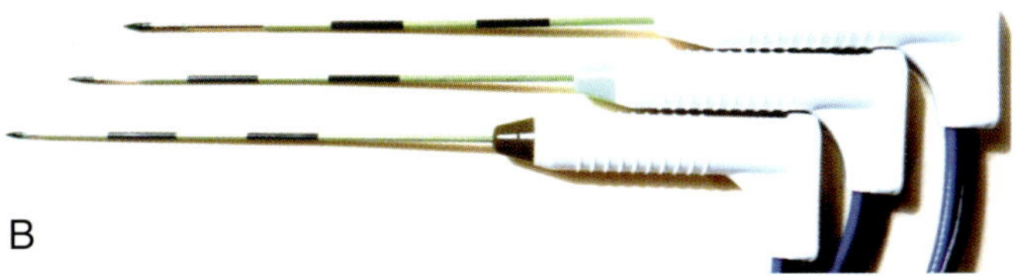

B

Figure 2-28 (A) MedWaves ablation system. (B) MedWaves antenna. *(Courtesy MedWaves.)*

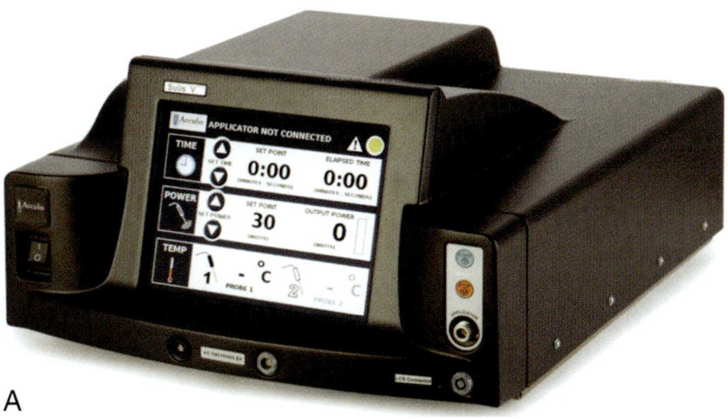

A

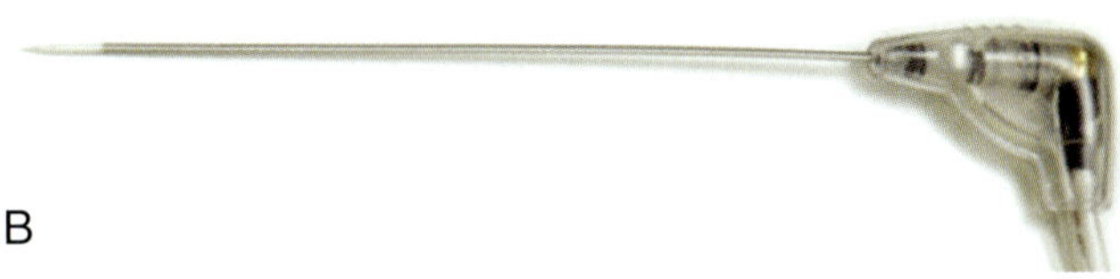

B

Figure 2-29 Microsulis's Acculis Microwave Tissue Ablation (MTA) system. (A) Sulis VpMTA generator. (B) Accu2i pMTA antenna. *(Courtesy Microsulis.)*

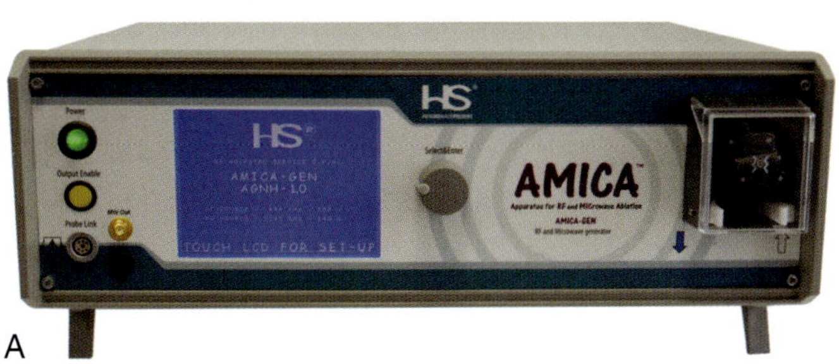

A

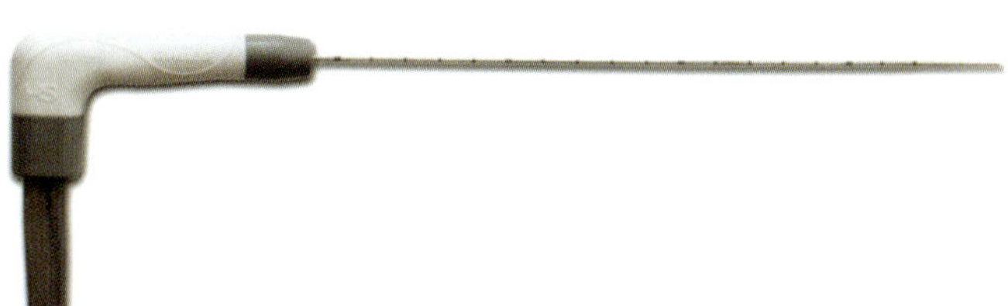

B

Figure 2-30 HS Amica microwave system. (A) Generator and built-in pump. (B) HS Amica antenna. *(Courtesy HS Amica.)*

Irreversible Electroporation Ablation

MECHANISM OF ACTION

Irreversible electroporation (IRE) is the newest commercially available percutaneous ablation technique. Its mechanism is entirely electric and nonthermal. IRE uses pulses of high electrical current to disrupt the lipid cellular membrane. Cellular membranes are changed by formation of multiple permanent, heterogeneous nanopores. Formation of permanent nanopores alters cellular components and causes cell death via both apoptosis and coagulation necrosis.[15-17] Nanopores occur when the membranous potential exceeds a threshold of 200–300 mV/cm.[18,19] Cellular energy is depleted by the presence of unregulated pores, with loss of homeostasis leading to eventual cell death.[21] Currently, it is unclear which mechanism, apoptosis versus coagulation necrosis, predominates in IRE ablation.[16,17]

One of the potential advantages of IRE is that it can ablate tissue without causing thermal damage.[20,21] IRE creates tissue ablation in a manner independent of heat generation or heat-sink effect.[16,17,22] IRE ablation uses ultra-short electric pulses with high current amplitudes to damage cell membranes, without affecting the extracellular scaffolding.[20,23] It has been found that tissue temperature changes are negligible even when using a larger number of ultra-short pulses or a smaller number of longer pulses with appropriate cooling delays between pulses.[24] This property gives IRE a theoretical advantage in that it should be less affected by the heat sink effect of vascular structures adjacent to target tissue.[25]

The high voltages associated with IRE can cause muscular activation. Therefore, a muscle relaxant, such as cisatracurium besylate, vecuronium bromide, or pancuronium bromide, is used as a neuromuscular blockade agent for both induction (150 μg/kg intravenously [IV]) and maintenance (30 μg/kg IV every 20 minutes as needed). Careful discussion with the anesthesiologist is prudent as respiratory weakness related to the neuromuscular blockage may complicate or delay extubation. Additionally, ventricular fibrillation can be caused by the high voltage of IRE ablation in lung and liver tumors in proximity to the heart. Therefore, an electrocardiogram gating synchronization mode is currently available in IRE generators in order to mitigate the risk of cardiac arrhythmia.

IRE is a safe and effective method of ablating tumors near large blood vessels without great risk of vascular damage, as IRE affects only cell membranes and its mechanism of action is not affected by nearby blood flow.[26] Use of ultra-short electric pulses makes the effective IRE ablation time very short, in the range of microseconds to milliseconds, when compared with other ablation techniques, which are in the range of minutes to even hours.[16]

EQUIPMENT

Two main types of IRE probes, monopolar and bipolar, connected to a NanoKnife Generator (AngioDynamics) (Figure 2-31, *A*), exist in the market.

Monopolar

Two monopolar probes are inserted into the lesion, where the electric current is conducted between the tips of the probes, resulting in IRE ablation. The monopolar probe consists of a

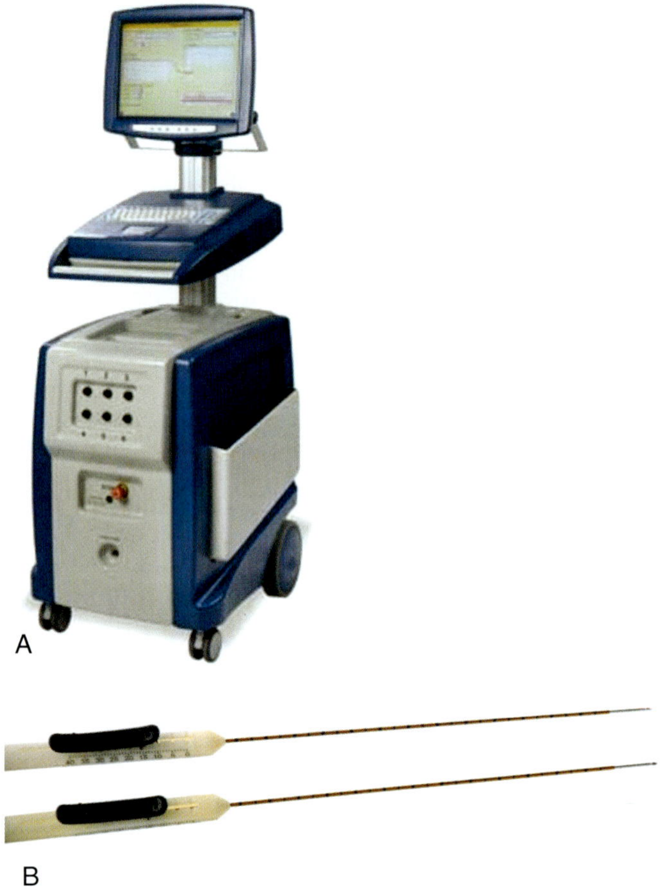

Figure 2-31 NanoKnife generator (A) and two monopolar probes (B) which are used together, the electric current is conducted between their tips, resulting in IRE ablation. *(Courtesy AngioDynamics.)*

19-gauge needle with a length of 15 cm (Figure 2-31, *B*). Applying 2500 V between the two probes spaced 15 mm apart causes an ablation zone measuring approximately 2 × 3 × 3 cm. The operator can insert up to six monopolar-type probes simultaneously to create a larger ablation area. This would ablate a tissue volume measuring approximately 3 × 3 × 5 cm in an average of 10 minutes of electroporation.

Bipolar

One bipolar-type probe, containing two distal poles, can be used to perform IRE ablation. The monopolar probe is composed of a 16-gauge needle with a length of 18 cm. Applying 2500 V between the two poles will result in an ablation zone measuring approximately 2 × 2 × 3 cm.

Chemical Ablation

MECHANISM OF ACTION

Chemical ablation is commonly performed using either acetic acid or ethanol, with similar or greater efficacy with intratumoral instillation of acetic acid when compared to ethanol.[27] Percutaneous chemical ablation is principally used for treating hepatocellular carcinoma in patients with cirrhosis.[28]

The treatment of primary hepatocellular carcinoma with chemical injection has been considerably more successful than its use in the treatment of liver metastases.[29] Chemical ablation is a viable option in many developing countries because of its simplicity and relatively lower cost. Thermal ablation has replaced chemical ablation because of the difficulty in achieving uniform diffusion of injected acetic acid or ethanol over larger tumors.

The injection of ethanol or acetic acid destroys tissue by diffusing into neoplastic cells, resulting in immediate cytoplasmic dehydration, protein denaturation, and consequent coagulation necrosis. In addition, ethanol enters the local circulation, leading to necrosis of the vascular endothelium and subsequent platelet aggregation, resulting in vascular thrombosis and ischemic tissue necrosis.[30] The mechanisms of action are similar for both acetic acid and ethanol, although some animal studies suggest that the diffusion abilities of acetic acid solutions may exceed those of ethanol, especially in fibrous tissues.[31]

EQUIPMENT

During chemical ablation, 100% ethanol or 15% acetic acid is injected directly into the tumor via needle under sonographic or CT guidance. The Quadra-Fuse multipronged injection system is an 18-gauge stainless steel injection needle that can be used for chemical injection and is manufactured by RexMedical (Austin, TX). The three tines of the needle are deployed in an umbrella fashion. Each of the three retractable tines (size: 27 gauge) has two through-holes, equivalent to four fluid exits, for a total of 12 points of simultaneous infusion (Figure 2-32). The RexMedical needle is available in 10, 15, and 20 cm needle lengths. There are two designs: the Quadra-Fuse needle that uses a five-tine array and the Quadra-Fuse ST with a two-array system.

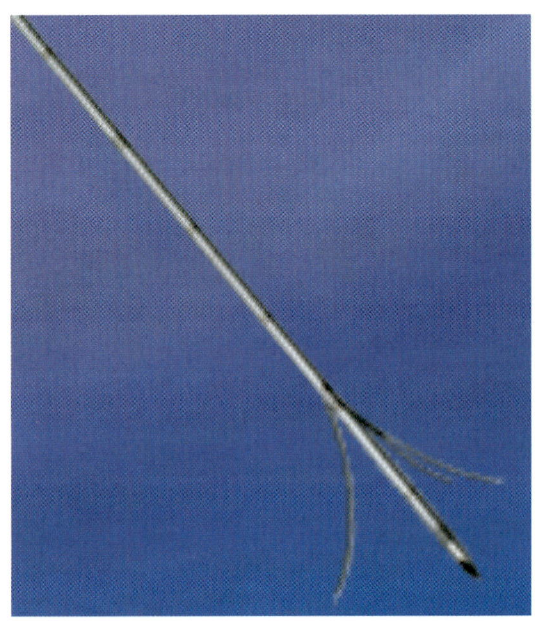

Figure 2-32 Quadra-Fuse multipronged injection 18-gauge stainless steel needle can be used for chemical injection. Each of the three retractable 27-gauge tines has two through-holes, four fluid exits, for a total of 12 points of simultaneous infusion. *(Courtesy RexMedical, Austin, TX.)*

Conclusion

Percutaneous image-guided tumor ablation with both thermal and nonthermal techniques constitutes an important tool in the treatment of many focal malignancies. This chapter provides an overview of the basic principles of percutaneous image-guided tumor ablation and describes the mechanisms of action and equipment that have been developed to ensure clinical success of this ablative therapy. The interventional radiologist should be familiar with these principles in order to apply them appropriately to optimize safety, efficiency, and efficacy.

REFERENCES

The complete reference list is available online at www.expertconsult.com.

3

Principles of Isolated Regional Perfusion of the Extremity or Liver

RICHARD E. ROYAL

KEY POINTS

- Regional perfusion is a method of delivering high-dose chemotherapy to a region burdened with cancer.
- Isolated limb perfusion and hepatic perfusion are traditional open surgical methods of regional therapy in treating melanoma confined to an extremity or the liver.
- Newer hybrid methods employ percutaneous techniques by interventional radiologists to gain access to the afferent and efferent blood flow of the limb or liver.

Introduction

Regional perfusion is a unique approach to treating cancer confined to a region or organ of the body. This includes procedures that attempt to deliver effective levels of chemotherapy to an area of the body that bears a malignancy.

The afferent and efferent blood supply of a region or organ is placed on a heart-lung bypass circuit in regional perfusion. The blood flow to this organ or region is then independent of the systemic circulation, so that the blood flow within the region or organ is "isolated." A high dose of chemotherapeutic agent is circulated through the isolated segment to treat the cancer while sparing the rest of the body from exposure to the agent. This increases the amount of chemotherapy delivered to the cancer cells, potentially to a range where the agent is more active while minimizing systemic toxicity from the treatment.

Two prototypic regional perfusion techniques are used to treat either cancers confined to the extremities or the liver. For each technique, the initially developed complex open operative procedure has evolved to a minimally invasive approach requiring the skills of multiple specialties. Classically, regional treatment of the extremities uses an open surgical procedure called an isolated limb perfusion (ILP). This procedure has evolved into a minimally invasive approach known as an isolated limb infusion. Similarly, regional treatment of hepatic cancers has evolved from an operation called an isolated hepatic perfusion to hepatic chemosaturation (formerly known as percutaneous hepatic perfusion or extracorporeal chemofiltration).

In each case, a complex open operative procedure has progressed into a hybrid procedure combining elements of image guidance done by interventional radiologists with intraoperative chemotherapy. This is best accomplished with a multidisciplinary approach combining the abilities of interventional radiologists, surgical oncologists, and anesthesiologists. For regional perfusion of the limb or liver, the hybrid procedure has not supplanted the open approach but rather provides an alternative to complex procedures with their own advantages and challenges.

RATIONALE FOR REGIONAL TREATMENT

There are theoretic advantages of regional perfusion strategies that include the following:

1. Minimizing systemic exposure and toxicity from the chemotherapeutic agent. By separating the blood flow to the organ or region of interest, chemotherapy can be intentionally delivered to the tumor-bearing area. Systemic exposure to the chemotherapeutic agent is limited to that amount that leaks into the systemic circulation. With no leak, the only toxicity is confined to the treated organ or region.
2. Chemotherapeutic agents are delivered to the tumor-bearing area at a more effective dose. The therapeutic index is the dose that causes toxicity in 50% of recipient patients divided by the dose that causes regression of tumor in 50% of those treated. For many chemotherapeutic agents, the latter dose is higher than the former so that the therapeutic index is <1. The dose can be escalated if exposure is limited to an organ or region that does not experience significant toxicity from the agent. This brings the therapeutic index to a level significantly greater than 1, resulting in increased efficacy.
3. The entire tumor-burdened organ or region is treated. This is in contrast to local resection, ablation, or selective embolization procedures. In some instances, a single lesion or oligometastatic disease may be effectively controlled with resection, ablation, or selective embolization. But regional perfusion can encompass a larger distribution and/or volume of tumor burden.

CANDIDATE CANCERS FOR REGIONAL PERFUSION

Regional perfusions, theoretically, are most applicable for cancers in which the disease is isolated to an upper extremity, a lower extremity, or the liver. Eradication of the cancer in these cases may result in prolonged disease-free survival. This usually includes a very narrow spectrum of clinical scenarios. By definition, only disease that is in the region of interest is treated by high-dose chemotherapy. But cancers are rarely confined to a region. Most cancers are confined locally to the primary site, metastatic to the regional lymph nodes, or systemically disseminated through hematogenous spread.

There are examples, however, where a regional approach makes sense. In the limb, advanced primary tumors or tumors with lymphatic spread may be susceptible to this approach. In the liver, advanced primaries or metastatic disease isolated to the liver, but not amenable to resection, may be candidates for regional perfusion.

In practice, only melanoma (cutaneous for limb regional perfusion, ocular for hepatic regional perfusion) has been adequately clinically investigated for this approach using single agent melphalan or melphalan-based combination therapies. Regional therapy to the limb or liver for other types of cancer should be considered investigational and completed on a research protocol.

When considering the range of cancers that can be treated with a regional perfusion, it is important to recognize that regional perfusion is a method of chemotherapy delivery and therefore the range of response is similar to systemic chemotherapy. It is not equivalent to ablative therapies like alcohol injection, radiofrequency ablation, or high-frequency focused ultrasound. If systemic chemotherapy kills one type of cancer, it cannot be expected to be equally efficacious if used for a completely different type of cancer, whereas ablative therapies may be used interchangeably against differing histologies.

Responses are dependent on the specific tumor's susceptibility to the chemotherapy used.

IN-TRANSIT METASTASES FROM CUTANEOUS MELANOMA

Melanoma often has its primary lesion in the upper or lower extremity and initially treated by wide excision and staging of the regional nodal basin.[1] In a small subset of patients, melanoma will recur as metastases within the lymphatic channels of the limb, either in a dermal or subcutaneous location. These can occur with or without nodal involvement, and without evidence of hematogenous distant spread. This disease pattern is referred to as satellite or in-transit metastases depending on the distance from the primary site (satellite lesions occur within 5 cm of the excised primary). Metastatic lesions can occur between the primary and draining lymph node bed, or on the limb, distal to the primary lesion as so-called retrograde in-transit lesions.

In-transit disease is an infrequent yet clinically significant pattern of spread from a primary melanoma. Between 1991 and 2001, a total of 1395 patients at the M.D. Anderson Cancer Center had their primary lesion treated with wide local excision and sentinel lymph node biopsy to assess the regional lymph node basin. Ninety-one patients, or 6.9%, subsequently developed in-transit melanoma.[2] Similar trials show an incidence of in-transit disease of 3.5%–8%.[3–5] The development of in-transit metastases portends a poor survival. In-transit metastases without lymph node metastases assigns the patient to American Joint Committee on Cancer (AJCC) stage 3A with a median survival approximating 5.5 years, and with nodal disease places the patient in stage 3C with median survival approximating 2.0 years.[6]

Although in-transit metastases can be excised, they often represent disseminated disease throughout the limb lymphatics. In rare instances, the limb can be surgically sterilized of disease through one or multiple operations leading to long-term cure. The most aggressive form of local control is amputation and can result in a 5- and 10-year survival rate of 40% and 20%, respectively.[7] Because systemic therapy provides only a modest objective response rate, more effective strategies of delivering chemotherapy such as regional treatment of the upper or lower extremity are adopted in an attempt to render these patients free of disease without the need for amputation.

OCULAR MELANOMA AND CANCERS FOR PERCUTANEOUS HEPATIC PERFUSION

Ocular melanoma represents an example of a cancer with a natural history favorable for regional treatment. Uveal melanomas develop in the vascular layer of the orbit, including the iris, ciliary body, and choroid. Although the primary lesion is in the eye, metastatic spread tends to be to the liver. In the collaborative ocular melanoma study, 361 of 1003 subjects with large uveal melanomas developed metastatic disease and of these 93% had hepatic metastasis.[8] Many patients die of hepatic failure from hepatic replacement with metastasis, in the absence of other disease. Regional treatment, therefore, has the potential to halt the life-threatening component of the metastatic disease.

Cancers metastatic to the liver or advanced primary hepatic cancers are likely to be susceptible to isolated hepatic perfusion or chemosaturation; however, current studies for these cancers are inadequate for perfusion to be a standard approach.

Gastrointestinal cancers that spread through the portal system to the liver have a natural history that is unique compared to other metastases from hematogenous spread. Patients with limited colon cancer metastases in the liver exemplify this point. When the disease is isolated to the liver, with minimal and anatomically favorable location, resection is often used to eliminate the metastasis. In selected patients treated with resection, 41% remain alive at 5 years following resection.[9] This suggests that colon cancer may spread hematogenously to the liver, but that hematogenous spread does not continue systemically in all cases.

Other cancers with portal spread may also be limited to hepatic metastases. Therefore liver-directed therapies are often used when metastatic disease exceeds the limits for resection. The role of regional perfusion therapy—either isolated hepatic perfusion or chemosaturation with percutaneous hepatic perfusion—for these histologies is yet to be defined and treatment of these cancers remains experimental.

Isolated Limb Perfusion

THE PROCEDURE

ILP, an operative technique for regional therapy delivered to a specific limb (Figure 3-1), is used to treat in-transit melanoma limited to either a lower extremity or an upper extremity. High-dose melphalan can be infused into the diseased limb with minimal systemic exposure to the chemotherapy, similar to other regional perfusions.

The regional artery and veins can be approached at several sites along the vessel depending on the distribution of disease in the limb. Vascular surgical principles for anticoagulation and vessel repair are applicable and must be followed as in any other vascular procedure.

In the lower extremity, cannulation can occur at the external iliac vessels, the superficial femoral vessels, or the popliteal artery and vein. The iliac approach is useful for disease that extends up to the groin crease, or when iliac nodes are involved. The external iliac vessels are approached through a retroperitoneal incision,

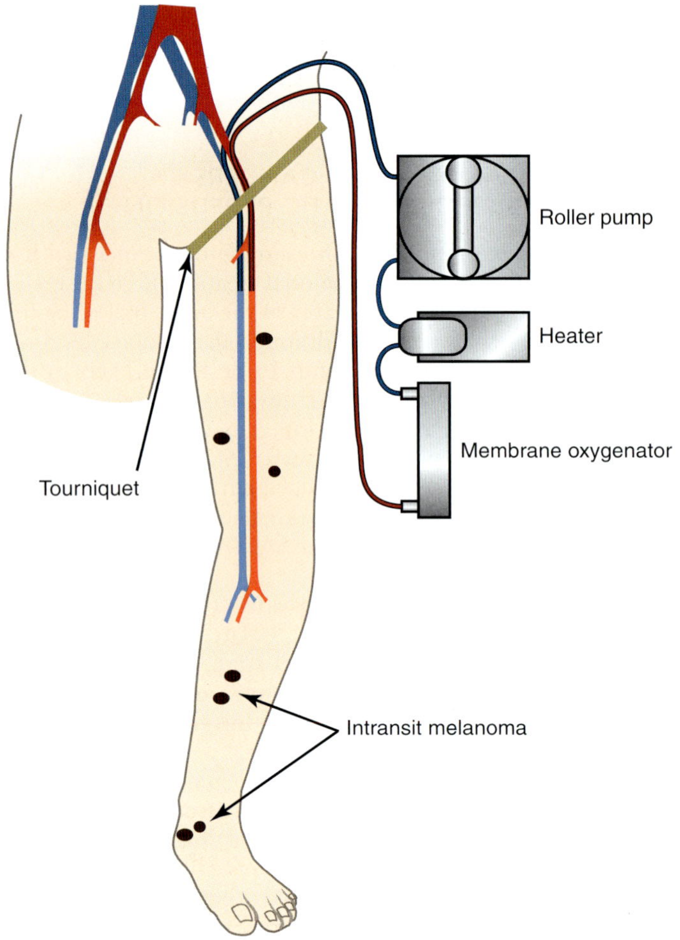

Figure 3-1 Diagram of circuit used for isolated limb perfusion. Cannula advanced into the exposed external iliac artery and vein are advanced below a tourniquet in the groin crease. The catheters are attached to a heart–lung bypass circuit that circulates blood through the limb. With the tourniquet inflated, the circulation is isolated to the limb, allowing administration of chemotherapy to the lower extremity without systemic exposure.

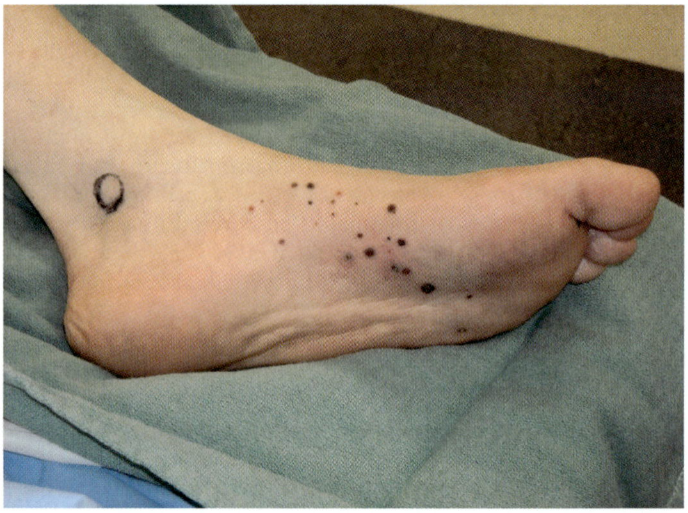

Figure 3-2 In-transit metastases from melanoma that is limited to the foot. Disease can be treated using a popliteal approach for isolated limb perfusion.

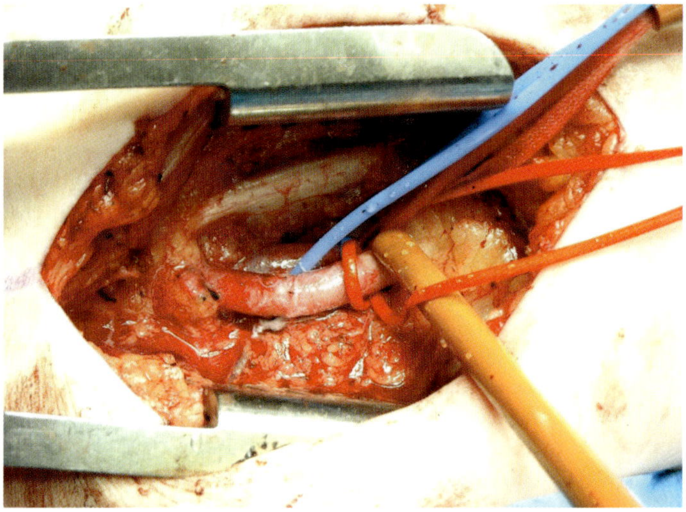

Figure 3-3 The popliteal artery and vein are dissected free for cannulation for isolated limb perfusion.

and a deep dissection is completed at the time of cannulation. This allows for the dissection of any deep lymph nodes with metastatic involvement at the time of perfusion. For disease in the distal one-third of the thigh and below, or when inguinofemoral lymph nodes are involved, the superficial femoral vessels can be cannulated. A superficial lymph node dissection is completed first and then the vessels are cannulated entering at the level of the common femoral vessels. For the iliac and superficial femoral approaches, the cannula must be advanced below the tourniquet. The popliteal vessels can be used for disease that is limited to a level below the knee (Figures 3-2 and 3-3). These are approached superiorly through the Hunter canal. The pneumatic cuff is inflated at a level above the incision (Figure 3-4).

In the upper extremity, vascular access can occur at the subclavian vessels through an infraclavicular approach or at the axillary vessels through an axillary incision. The cannula must be advanced to a level below the tourniquet for each approach.

All collateral vessels are surgically ligated for procedures where cannulation is above the tourniquet. This is especially important for an iliac approach. This is to prevent any leak of perfusate out of the limb into the systemic circulation, and conversely to prevent leak of systemic circulation into the limb.

After cannulation and application of a tourniquet, the limb circulation is placed completely on a heart–lung bypass circuit. In this circuit, the blood is circulated using a roller pump, heated using an external bath, and blood gas is maintained using a membrane oxygenator. Hyperthermia is established both by heating the perfusate and external warming of the limb. Chemotherapeutics are added to the circuit and circulated through the limb for a period of 60 minutes.

Leak is minimal with a pneumatic cuff used on the thigh. But in many patients, the disease extends high on the thigh, mandating iliac cannulation and a manual tourniquet at the groin crease; leak may occur across this tourniquet, exposing the patient to potentially toxic levels of chemotherapy. In addition, the systemic circulation can leak into the limb, increasing the blood loss when the limb blood is discarded at the conclusion of the case. Leak can be managed by tightening the tourniquet, and adjusting the flow into the limb. The arterial pressure in the limb is constant, not pulsatile because of the use of roller pumps.

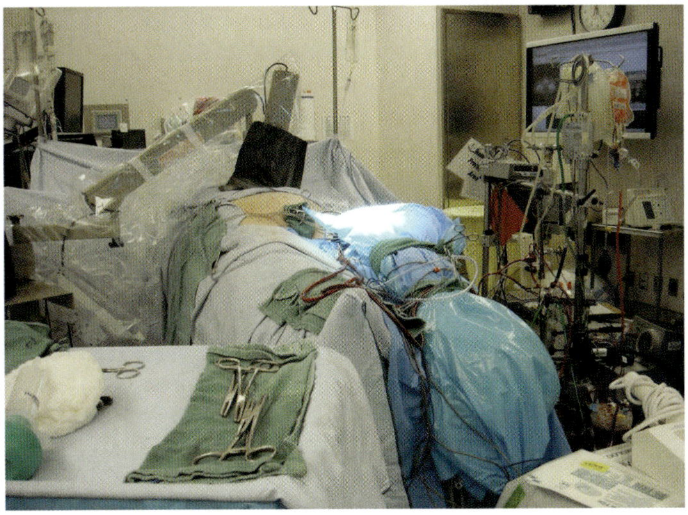

Figure 3-4 Isolated limb perfusion of the left lower extremity in the operating room. The patient's feet are facing the camera. The leg is wrapped in warming blankets to the patient's left. The heart–lung bypass machine is on the right side of the picture. A gamma probe is seen crossing the patient's chest sitting on the precordium. This is to measure for any leak of perfusate into the systemic circulation. A lead shield protects from any signal from the circulating tubing.

Increasing the blood pressure to above the systemic mean can minimize leak into the limb. Further, decreasing the flow, and thereby the limb blood pressure to below the mean arterial blood pressure, leak from the limb into the systemic circulation can be decreased.

Monitoring leak is important when a manual tourniquet is used. Several methods have been used to monitor leak, but the use of radioactive labeled autologous blood is most widely accepted. Separate aliquots of blood are labeled with ^{99}technetium; one with a defined dose, usually approximating 3.0 mCi, and one with 1/10th the dose, usually 0.3 mCi. A gamma-counter is placed over the heart to measure the level of radioactivity in the systemic circulation. After the limb circuit is established and the tourniquet inflated, the 0.3 mCi aliquot of blood is given systemically. The resulting increase in gamma counts/min over baseline establishes the change associated with a 10% leak. Then the 3.0 mCi aliquot is given in the limb circuit. Any leak can be measured by the gamma counter using the 10% leak as a standard. For melphalan, the dose used in limb perfusion tends to be 10 times the dose that could be given systemically, so greater than 10% leak can be extremely toxic to the bone marrow.

CLINICAL RESULTS

The Sydney Melanoma Unit studied 101 patients with melanoma of the extremity who were treated with ILP using melphalan and dactinomycin. Of the 87 patients available for evaluation, there was a 90.8% overall response rate, with 58 patients exhibiting a complete response. The median local recurrence-free interval after complete response was 21 months, with 32 patients eventually developing distant disease.[10] Long-term follow-up of 120 patients from Sydney who underwent ILP between 1984 and 1997 revealed that after an initial complete remission (CR) rate of 69.2%, there was a sustained CR rate of 33.7% (median follow-up of 199 months; 8–226 months).[11] The response rate increased to 56.6% when patients who underwent minor resection of recurrent or residual disease were included. Several groups have confirmed a high response rate to melphalan-based ILP for regional melanoma (Table 3-1).

In an effort to improve response rates and disease-free duration, several groups combined tumor necrosis factor (TNF) with melphalan in ILP (Table 3-2). In a single-arm trial, Leinard and associates in the Netherlands tested the combination of melphalan/TNF-α and interferon-γ delivered by ILP to patients with limb-restricted malignances including melanoma. Patients with melanoma showed a high response rate (overall response 100%, CR 90%) for in-transit disease.[12] Similarly, the NCI conducted a dose escalation trial of melphalan, TNF-α, and interferon-γ in 38 patients with biopsy-proven in-transit or satellite melanoma. Response rates were high, with a CR rate of 76% for the low TNF-α group (4 mg) and 36% for the high TNF-α group (6 mg).[13] In a subsequent multicenter phase II study run by the Dutch group, 64 patients with locally recurrent melanoma were randomized to receive melphalan/TNF-α with or without interferon.[14] The objective response rate was 91%–100% for the two groups.

A small multiinstitutional trial enrolled 103 patients with measurable in-transit lesions randomized to ILP with melphalan or melphalan/TNF-α/ interferon-γ. There were more CRs in the group receiving TNF-α (72% vs. 58%) with no statistical differences in overall response (81% vs. 96% respectively) or survival (disease-free survival 12 vs. 14 months, respectively, and 3-year survival 58% for both groups).[15]

The cumulative results of these studies led to cooperative group randomized multicenter trial comparing ILP with melphalan only or melphalan + TNF-α (ACSOG Z0020).[16] One hundred twenty-four patients with locally advanced extremity melanoma were enrolled and underwent treatment. Accrual was halted early when investigators found no difference in

TABLE 3-1 Response of Stage 3 Melanoma to Isolated Limb Perfusion With Melphalan

Group	N	Agents	Objective response	Survival	Toxicity
University of Erlangen 2006[10]	101	Melphalan Dactinomycin	90.8% (CR = 66%)	Median PFS: 21 mos.	Grades IV and V: 5%
Netherlands Cancer Institute, 2002[39]	202	Melphalan	CR = 56.1% (>75 years old) CR = 58.2% (<75 years old)	5-year survival: 37.0–40.6%	Grades III and IV 20.8%–23.7%
Tulane University, 1996[40]	468	Melphalan +/− Thiotepa +/− Dactinomycin		5-year survival: 21%	

CR, complete remission; PFS, progression-free survival.

TABLE 3-2 Evaluation of Melphalan/TNF-α Combination Therapy in Isolated Limb Perfusion for In-Transit Melanoma

Group	Agent(s)	N	Overall Response (%)	CR (%)
Lienard, 1992[41]	Melphalan/interferon-γ/TNF-α	29	29 (100)	26 (90)
Vaglini, 1994[42]	Melphalan/interferon-γ/TNF-α	11	7 (64)	7 (64)
National Cancer Institute, 1996[13]	Melphalan/interferon-γ/4 mg TNF-α	26	24 (92)	20 (76)
	Melphalan/interferon-γ/6 mg TNF-α	11	11 (100)	4 (36)
University of Pennsylvania 1999[15]	Melphalan	51	49 (96)	30 (58)
	Melphalan/interferon-γ/TNF-α	52	47 (91)	37 (72)
Lienard, 1999[14]	Melphalan/interferon-γ	33	30 (91)	23 (69)
	Melphalan/interferon-γ/TNF-α	31	31 (100)	24 (78)
ACOSOG, 2006[15]	Melphalan	58	36 (62)	14 (25)
	Melphalan/interferon-γ/TNF-α	58	40 (69)	15 (26)

CR, complete remission; TNF, necrosis factor.

response rates between the treatment groups. Analysis did show a slight improvement in the durability of the CR in the TNF-α group, though this was not a study end point. Many criticize this study for nonstandardization of the assessment of tumor response and the short duration of follow-up in the CR assessment. The response rates for this trial are dramatically lower than previous trials (see Table 3-4). In addition, the early cessation of this trial meant that a subgroup analysis on patients with bulky disease could not be completed. Many suggest that bulky disease appears to respond more rapidly and more frequently with the TNF-α combination.

Generally, overall objective response rates of 80%–90% with complete response rates of 50%–60% should be expected from melphalan-based ILP. These response rates, unfortunately, are rarely durable, with a median time to progression reported of 9–24 months. Long-term follow-up from the National Cancer Institute shows 5-year recurrence-free survival (in the field and out of the field) to be 18.0%.[17] Similarly, investigators from Australia report that at a median follow-up of 177 months, 18.5% of 108 patients are alive without disease.[10] Survival data are difficult to interpret though, because perfusion is applied to patients with various stages of disease and survival after perfusion stratifies by stage.[10,11] Series with a large proportion of early-stage disease will therefore show a prolonged survival for the study group that may not be reflective of survival in the whole population of patients typically treated with ILP.

Toxicity from melphalan-based ILP includes specific toxicity to the limb, as well as delayed effects from system exposure to melphalan.[18] Limb toxicity is defined by the Wieberdink classification (Table 3-3). Toxicity is dependent to some degree on the conditions of ILP. When hyperthermia is used, increased regional toxicity is measured at higher temperatures. Temperatures exceeding 42°C degrees results in high toxicity.[19] Additionally, systemic complications are dependent on systemic exposure to the drug.

TABLE 3-3 Wieberdink Classification of Acute Regional Toxicity

Grade	Description
I	No subjective or objective evidence of reaction
II	Slight erythema and/or edema
III	Considerable erythema and/or blistering; slightly disturbed motility permissible
IV	Extensive epidermolysis and/or obvious damage to the deep tissues, causing definite functional disturbances; threatening or manifest compartment syndromes
V	Reaction that necessitates amputation

Long-term complications of ILP have been analyzed in a group of patients at an average of 20 years following ILP. Of 312 patients treated with ILP during 1973–1983, 82 were alive at the time of their 2008 study and 39 agreed to be seen for extensive questionnaires and examination where the perfused limb was compared to the contralateral limb. All patients were without disease, and 13 patients continued to wear elastic stockings for lymphedema. At examination, 5 of 10 patients undergoing upper limb perfusion had limited motion at the shoulder, with 2 also exhibiting limited range of motion at the elbow. In the 29 subjects treated with lower extremity perfusion, there was some limitation in the range of motion in at least one joint (hip, knee, or ankle) for every patient. The findings tended to not be clinically significant, with 67% reporting no impairment of daily life due to the procedure.[20] Similarly, in a trial of patients undergoing adjuvant ILP with melphalan, 3.6% (15 of 420) had severe long-term limb complications from perfusion, including lymphedema, neuropathy, and vascular injury. This compares with 6.4% (10 of 156) severe long-term limb complications when treated with excision of primary with lymph node dissection in the same trial.[21]

ISOLATED LIMB INFUSION: AN ALTERNATIVE REGIONAL THERAPY FOR LIMB DISEASE

To simplify the technique of ILP, isolated limb *infusion* was developed (Figure 3-5). In this hybrid procedure, catheters are placed in the femoral vessels via the contralateral artery and vein preoperatively in the interventional radiology setting. Then, in the operation theater under general anesthesia, a pneumatic tourniquet is placed at the proximal limb and the blood within the circuit is circulated by hand using a syringe. This is a low-flow, low-pressure, normothermic, hypoxic circuit within the limb. Melphalan only or melphalan + actinomycin D is added to the circuit and circulated for 30 minutes, after which the leg is flushed and the effluent discarded. Severe physiological derangements occur during the period of filtration and both surgical decision making

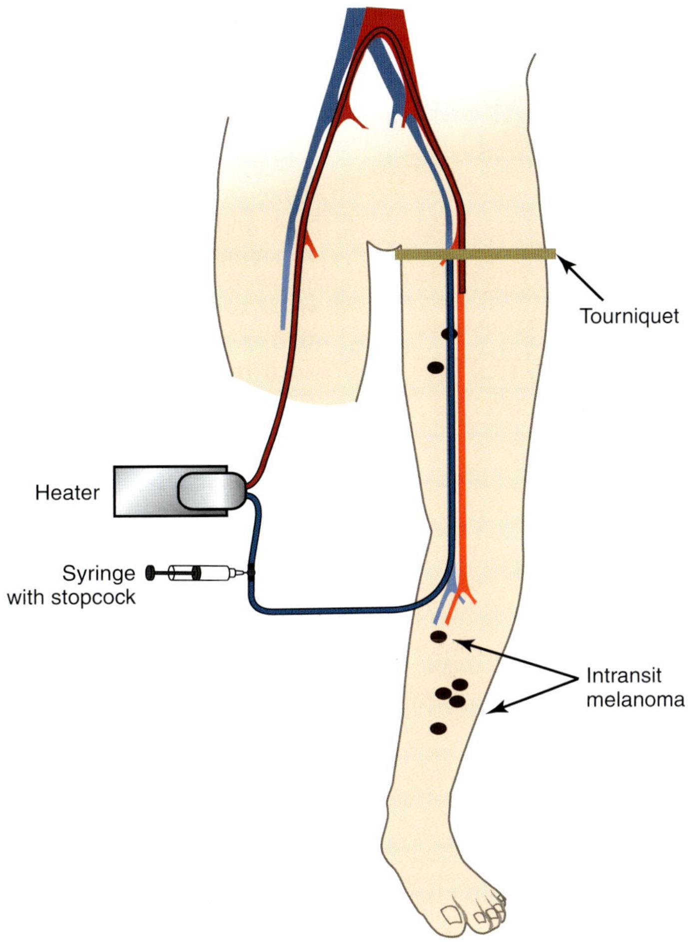

Figure 3-5 Diagram of circuit used for isolated limb infusion. Catheters placed by interventional radiology techniques are advanced into the midthigh. With the tourniquet inflated, the blood is circulated in the limb with a syringe stopcock setup. This is an ischemic low-flow perfusion.

about the intraoperative treatment and anesthetic management are crucial for a patient to survive the procedure.

Procedure in Detail

Isolated limb infusion first requires interventional cannulation of the superficial femoral artery of the affected limb. The artery is approached through the contralateral common femoral artery. An introducer is placed percutaneously and catheter advanced under fluoroscopic guidance across the aortic bifurcation down the arterial system of the affected lower extremity. If the upper extremity is involved, the catheter is advanced up the descending aorta, across appropriate arterial branches to end in the brachial artery of the diseased limb.

Classically, the venous catheter is advanced through the femoral vein that accompanies the arterial introducer. The femoral catheter is advanced parallel to the arterial catheter. But at the M.D. Anderson Cancer Center, we introduce the venous catheter in the popliteal vein of the affected lower extremity or in the basilic vein of the diseased upper extremity. The catheter is advanced along the direction of venous flow to end at the same level as the arterial catheter. In this manner, a shorter, lower-resistance catheter is used and the venous catheter does not traverse the vessel under the tourniquet (Figure 3-6).

In the lower extremity, a pneumatic cuff is then inflated at the level of the femoral triangle apex. In the upper extremity, it is inflated at the deltoid insertion. The blood is then circulated using a stopcock and syringe attached to a stopcock in the line exiting the venous catheter. Using the stopcock, blood is circulated through a heater and into the arterial line. Once a stable circuit is established, high-dose chemotherapy is infused into the limb. After infusion, circulation is resumed with the syringe-and-stopcock assembly. The chemotherapeutic agent is circulated for 30 minutes, and then all blood is flushed from the limb. The tourniquet is deflated and systemic circulation resumed. After reversing anticoagulation, the catheters are removed.

Clinical Results

This technique was initially championed by the Sydney Melanoma unit showing an overall response rate of 84% in 185 patients with a 38% CR rate. Median duration of response was 13 months, with a longer survival seen in patients experiencing a CR (53 months vs. 38 months).[27] The significance of this survival advantage is unclear though, because patients with a CR tend to have lower-stage disease than those who did not have a CR. Grade III and IV limb toxicity was noted in 53% and 5% of patients, respectively.

Studies in the United States have demonstrated a lower response rate with this treatment. The group at the Memorial Sloan Kettering Cancer Center conducted a single-arm

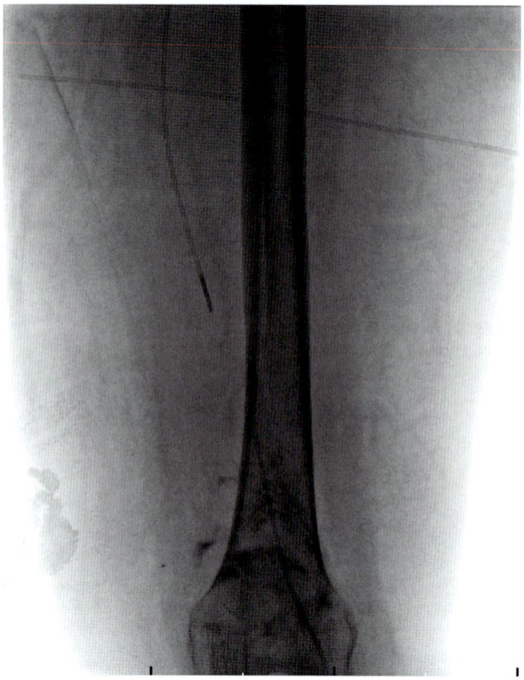

Figure 3-6 Radiograph of the left thigh following insertion of inflow and outflow catheters by interventional radiology. Horizontal radiopaque marker shows the planned level for the tourniquet. Arterial access is via the contralateral common femoral vein crossing over the aortic bifurcation to end below the tourniquet. The venous catheter for isolated limb infusion enters the popliteal vein via the popliteal space. Both end at the same level within the superficial femoral vessels.

phase 2 trial of melphalan and actinomycin D delivered using isolated limb infusion and reported response rates for 22 patients (21 with melanoma). The overall response rate was 50%, with a 23% CR rate. The median time to progression for CR was 12 months and PR 11 months.[23] The group at Duke University initially reported an experience with 61 patients with melanoma treated with isolated limb infusion. They measured an overall response rate of 44%, with a CR rate of 30%. The median duration of a CR was 12 months and 18% of patients experienced at least grade III toxicity.[24]

A randomized trial comparing isolated limb infusion and ILP has not been completed, but the trials to date suggest ILP mediates more responses in the limb with a higher rate of toxicity in the limb (Table 3-4). Both treatments have low durability with comparable times to progression.

With the exception of the recent American College of Surgeons Oncology Group (ACOSOG) trial, response rates have been uniformly high in all modern trials evaluating ILP for melanoma. Response evaluation was not standardized for the ACOSOG trial, and it has been criticized for inaccurate analysis of response. Following ILP, lesions that regress may leave behind areas of skin pigmentation that on biopsy show pigment laden macrophages without evidence of tumor (Figure 3-7). These lesions have completely regressed pathologically, but in the ACOSOG trial may have been counted as residual disease due to inexperience of the surgeons involved, and lack of clear guidelines for assessment of response.

Regional Perfusion of the Liver

ISOLATED HEPATIC PERFUSION: PROCEDURE IN DETAIL

Isolated hepatic perfusion is an open operative procedure. Overall, the liver is isolated from systemic circulation. Blood is circulated through the liver using a heart lung bypass set up, and high doses of chemotherapeutic agent is added to the hepatic circuit so that the agent is circulated only in the liver, not through the systemic circulation (Figure 3-8).

First, the liver is fully mobilized. The membranous portion of the falciform is divided. The peritoneal reflection surrounding the liver is divided including division of the full length of coronary ligament, triangular ligaments, and the inferior reflection at the hepatorenal space. The liver itself is then dissected out of the bare area bilaterally.

For some hepatic resections, the liver is dissected off the inferior vena cava (IVC). But for this procedure, the IVC remains with the liver and dissection needs to proceed at a more posterior plane. A retrocaval dissection is completed from the renal veins to the diaphragmatic hiatus. This requires ligation and division of the short lumbar and intercostal veins draining into the posterior aspect of the IVC. Also the phrenic veins must be ligated and divided from the superior portion of the IVC. This

TABLE 3-4 Response of Melanoma to Regional Treatment: Isolated Limb Infusion vs. Isolated Limb Perfusion

Group	N	Objective Response Rate (%)	PR (%)	CR (%)	Median TTP (Months)
Isolated limb Infusion					
Sydney Mel Unit, 2011[31]	91	85			
MSKCC, 2006[23]	22	50	27	23	
Duke University, 2011[32]	126	43	13	30	
Multiinstitutional, 2009[33]	128	64	33	31	24
Isolated limb perfusion					
ACOSOG, 2006[34]	124	61	38	23	
Padova, Italy, 2003[35]	37	99	31	66	
Lausanne, 1999[36]	64	95	22	73	
Glasgow, UK, 1996[37]	103	94	23	76	
National Cancer Institute, 1996[38]	38	97	50	47	
Duke University, 2011[32]	62	81	26	55	32

ACOSOG, American College of Surgeons Oncology Group; CR, complete remission; MSKCC, Memorial Sloan-Kettering Cancer Center; PR, partial remission; TTP, time to progression

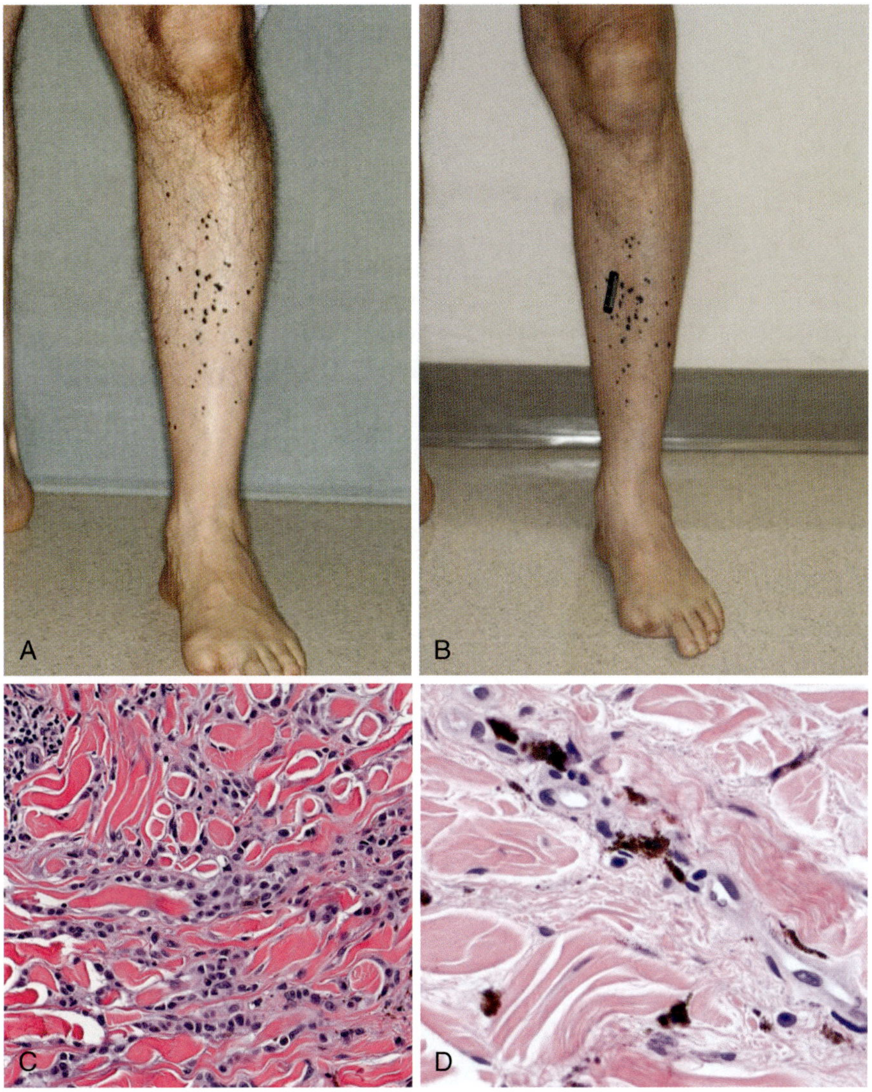

Figure 3-7 Complete response in the left lower extremity following isolated limb infusion with melphalan and actinomycin D. (A) Pretreatment photograph shows multiple in-transit lesions. A palpable mass is present at each site of pigmentation, and new lesions are visible each week. Toe amputation previously used to treat the subungual primary. (B) Appearance after complete response. Lesions are flat, but area of tattooing remains at previous sites of disease. (C) Biopsy of the pretreatment lesions shows melanoma at the level of the dermis and superficial subcutaneous tissue. (D) Posttreatment biopsy shows pigment-laden macrophages or melanophages remain in the area of tattooing, with no viable malignant cells. The continued presence of melanocytic pigment can complicate the assignment of response in individual lesions following regional treatment of the limb.

completely frees all other veins draining into the IVC except for major hepatic veins and small caudate tributaries that directly drain into the IVC. With this, only the hepatic blood flow drains into the retrohepatic IVC when the IVC is occluded above the renal veins.

The porta hepatis is also skeletonized. The course of the hepatic arteries and branches, the portal vein and branches, and the common bile duct are skeletonized, dividing all minor vascular tributaries and lymphatics. A less complete dissection can be used if provisions are made for clamping all possible draining structures.

Following this dissection, the liver remains tethered only by the IVC, portal vein and hepatic artery. Clamping these structures ceases all blood flow in and out of the liver. No vessels that could potentially communicate between the liver and the systemic circulation can remain intact.

An inflow cannula is placed into the gastroduodenal artery (GDA). A second outflow cannula is advanced into the retrohepatic IVC. The liver can then be isolated from system circulation by clamping the common hepatic artery, portal vein above the confluence of the splenic vein, and the cava both above the renal veins and below the diaphragm. Blood flow continues along the two small arteries that run along the common bile duct, and the flow in these can be controlled by clamping the bile duct itself.

Following that, the blood flow is supplied using a heart–lung bypass machine. Inflow is established through the GDA cannula and outflow from the retrohepatic IVC cannula. The blood is circulated, heated, and oxygenated by the heart–lung bypass setup. Blood pH drops significantly as it is circulated through the liver, and this must be monitored either by continuous arterial blood gas (ABG) monitoring of blood in the perfusion

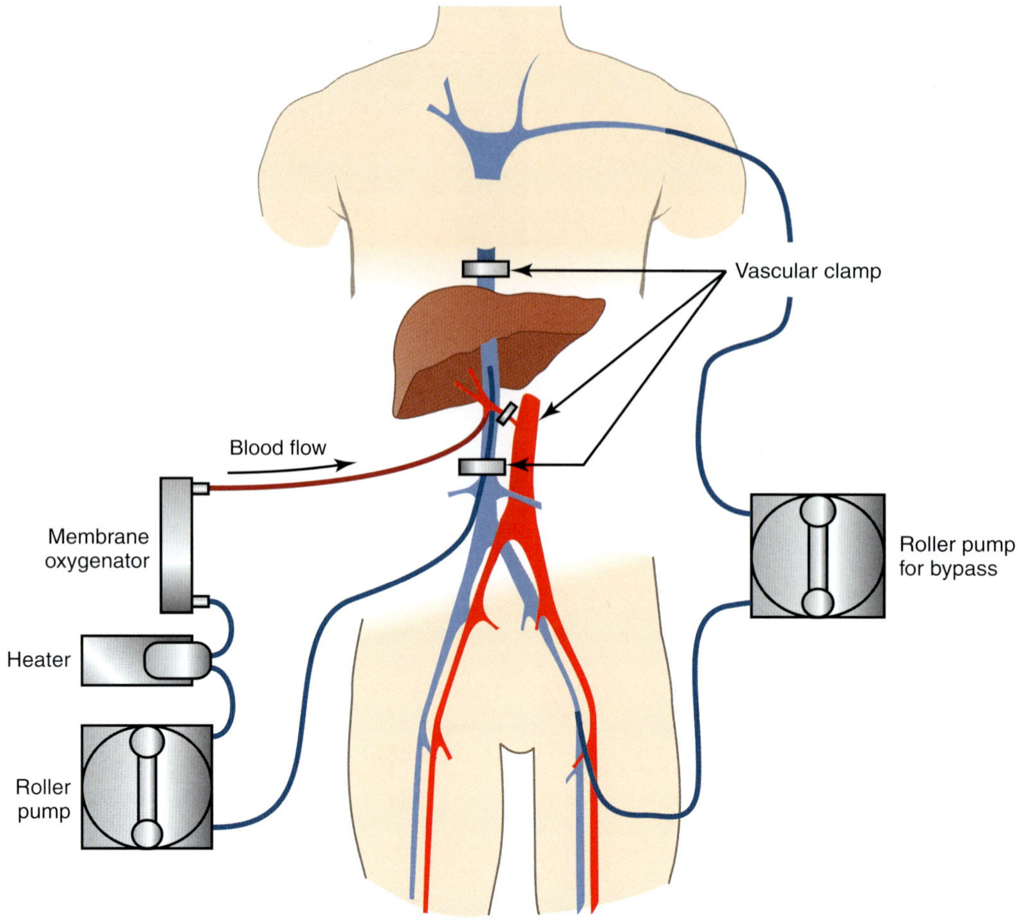

Figure 3-8 Diagram of the circuit for isolated hepatic perfusion. Two circuits are used for the procedure. On the right, a roller pump returns blood to the superior vena cava when the inferior vena cava is clamped. Blood from the fully dissected retrohepatic IVC flows through a bypass circuit with roller pump, heater, and oxygenator. Inline blood gas monitoring is used to titrate pH using a sodium bicarbonate drip.

circuit, or frequent rapid ABG testing. A sodium bicarbonate drip draining into the perfusion circuit can be titrated to maintain pH.

With the IVC clamped above the renal veins, a bypass circuit is also used to return infra hepatic blood to the superior vena cava. The circuit can drain from the saphenous or femoral veins and a roller pump used to advance this through an axillary or internal jugular vein.

With the liver on its own separate circulation, the liver can be heated to hyperthermic levels with minimal effects on a patient's core temperature. High-dose chemotherapy can then be added to the circuit. With no leak of blood flow to the systemic circulation, the dose of chemotherapy is limited by hepatic toxicity rather than systemic toxicity. The amount of increase over systemic dose varies by chemotherapeutic agent used.

Clinical Results

A technique for isolated hepatic perfusion was originally described by the group at Roswell Park Cancer Center. The procedure evolved through adaptation in 49 dogs, and then was used in 5 patients. Four were treated for metastatic gastrointestinal cancers and one for metastatic carcinoid. The circuit was similar to that described in the last section, except that the inflow cannula was advanced retrograde through the splenic artery and the upstream celiac artery clamped. Nitrogen mustard was used for perfusion and no toxicity was seen at the doses used. Response is not reported in this study completed before the advent of cross-sectional imaging. The one patient with a carcinoid tumor exhibited a decrease in serum serotonin.[25]

A small but select group of investigators have reported on the use of this technique in patients with metastatic ocular melanoma. Systemic toxicity is minimal while hepatic toxicity is frequent (Table 3-5).

CHEMOSATURATION WITH PERCUTANEOUS HEPATIC PERFUSION: PROCEDURE IN DETAIL

Rather than absolute vascular isolation, the minimally invasive equivalent of isolated hepatic perfusion maintains normal hepatic arterial and portal vein inflow into the liver. The hepatic vein drainage is relatively isolated and chemotherapeutic agent extracted from the hepatic venous effluent before returning the blood to the systemic circulation (Figure 3-9).

First, inflow catheters are advanced from a common femoral arterial introducer into the hepatic arterial supply to the liver. Chemotherapeutic agents must flow exclusively into the liver, so branches like the right gastric and gastroduodenal artery are embolized, or other provisions made to spare chemotherapeutic agent flow to any other upper abdominal organs. Melphalan inadvertently administered through the gastric arterial distribution

TABLE 3-5 **Isolated Hepatic Perfusion for Ocular Melanoma**

Group Reporting	*N*	Melphalan Dose	Hepatic Toxicity% (Grades III and IV)	Heme Toxicity% (Grades III and IV)	Objective Response Rate %	Median TTP (Months)	Median OS (Months)
Salgrenska University (Sweden) 1994	10	0.5 mg/kg + CDDP	NA	0	50	NA	4.5
National Cancer Institute (USA) 2000	22	1.5–2 mg/kg + TNF-α	68–82	18	62	9	11
National Cancer Institute (USA) 2003	29	1.5 mg/kg	65	NA	62	8	12
Leiden University (Netherlands) 2004	12	200 mg (≈3 mg/kg)	37	13	50	6.7	10
Salgrenska University (Sweden) 2008	27	0.5–2.0 mg/kg	26	NA	70	NA	12.5
Erasmus University (Netherlands) 2009	8	1 mg/kg	13	38	37.5	6	11

NA, not available; OS, overall survival; TTP, time to progression.

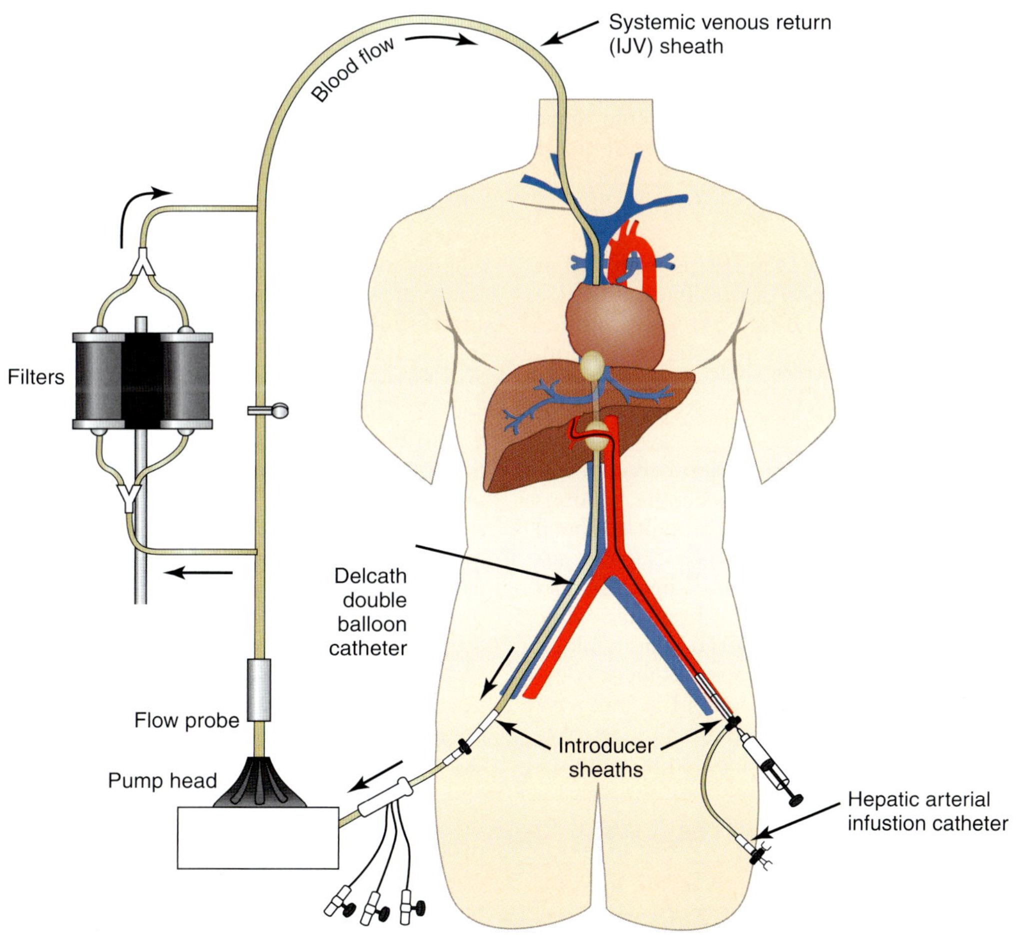

Figure 3-9 Diagram of the circuit used for chemosaturation using percutaneous hepatic perfusion. Chemotherapeutic agent flows into the hepatic arterial branches whereas native blood flow remains intact. Hepatic vein drainage is captured by a catheter in the IVC that uses two balloons to isolate the segment of vein. The blood is then filtered to remove the chemotherapeutic agent and returned via the internal jugular venous sheath. Chemotherapy exposure is concentrated in the liver using this regional perfusion system.

results in severe stomach toxicity and gastric ulceration. Anomalous hepatic arterial anatomy may be compensated for by using multiple catheters, or repositioning during arterial administration of chemotherapy.

After the branches are embolized and arterial catheters positioned, the venous catheter is advanced into the retrocaval IVC. The catheter for this is part of the Delcath system for hepatic chemosaturation. This catheter has an outer diameter of 16 French and is introduced through a femoral venous introducer. The catheter has two balloons, one distal near the tip of the catheter, the other located more proximally with a 7-cm fenestrated segment between the balloons. The catheter has four lumina, two for inflation of each of the balloons and two for blood flow. One of the blood flow lumens is used to bypass the occluded segment of vein and one to aspirate the blood out of the retrocaval IVC.

The catheter is advanced over a wire by a monorail design advancing the tip to the level of the right atrium. This is done over a guidewire through the bypass portion of the catheter. The distal catheter is inflated and the catheter is drawn back so that the balloon is wedged in the diaphragmatic hiatus. The IVC itself is quite distensible and the seal at this balloon is ensured by the diaphragm.

The inferior balloon is then inflated, isolating the hepatic venous drainage into the retrohepatic IVC. One or both renal veins may also drain into the isolated segment of the IVC, or the orifice of the renal veins may be occluded by the proximal balloon, neither of which is of deleterious consequence in normal anatomy. Other native branches drain into this segment of the IVC, including intercostal branches and the phrenic veins. But with the blood drawn out of the IVC, the volume of blood drawn by the Delcath system maintains antegrade flow in these veins, minimizing systemic exposure from retrograde flow in these tributaries.

With the inferior balloon inflated, the IVC is occluded at or above the renal veins. To facilitate IVC drainage, a bypass channel is present in the catheter. Blood enters a channel through a port located just proximal to the inferior balloon. It then travels through the bypass lumen exiting at the tip of the catheter. With this design, lower IVC blood can return to the atrium.

Blood from the retrohepatic cava is then aspirated continuously through the fenestrated segment between the balloons using a centrifugal pump and then pumped through activated charcoal filters returning to the circulation via a catheter advanced into the superior vena cava. High-dose chemotherapy can then be infused into the hepatic arterial branches, while maintaining normal hepatic arterial and portal venous blood flow. Some of the high dose of chemotherapeutic agent is extracted by the tumor and hepatic parenchyma in this first pass. After passing through the liver, the effluent entering the retrohepatic IVC is aspirated out of the cava and pumped through the filters, where a major portion of the chemotherapeutic agent is removed from the blood, and chemotherapeutic agent–poor blood is returned to the circulation.

After infusion of the chemotherapeutic agent is completed, the venous effluent is filtered to remove any agent still leaving the liver. It is important to provide continuous downward traction on the catheter during the entire filtration process. Without downward traction, the catheter can easily migrate superiorly out of its wedged position in the diaphragmatic hiatus. This releases the seal at this portion of the IVC, allowing for flow of the blood from the retrohepatic IVC into the atrium. The chemotherapeutic agent is not filtered out of this blood that leaks around the balloon and the systemic exposure to the chemotherapeutic agent, and subsequent toxicity is increased.

The period of filtration can be physiologically eventful for the treated patient. Other moieties in the blood, including clotting factors, antithrombin III, catecholamines, and platelets, can also be filtered out. Thus, the patient can experience profound anticoagulation, heparin resistance, and cardiovascular collapse. Close attention to blood pressure support and replacement of needed blood factors is paramount to safely complete this therapy. The level of intervention needed for blood pressure support is often profound, unlike any other procedure that is commonly encountered. The need to prepare for circulatory support cannot be overemphasized.[26] Improvement in the specificity of drug extraction by the filters is expected to decrease the physiologic volatility during this treatment.

Clinical Results

The approach for chemosaturation using percutaneous hepatic perfusion was developed in animals initially at Yale University. The M.D. Anderson Cancer Center completed a phase I dose escalation study of doxorubicin in subjects with nonresectable hepatocellular cancer using the chemofiltration approach. The maximum tolerated dose (MTD) for doxorubicin was defined as 120 mg/m^2. Pharmacokinetic studies demonstrated that the peak systemic concentration of the chemotherapeutic agent was 85.6% lower than levels in the hepatic venous effluent. These measurements confirmed that the carbon filters extracted chemotherapeutic agents not absorbed in the liver, minimizing systemic exposure. The second patient in this study experienced severe fatal hypotension when blood flow was directed through the carbon filters. Subsequently, the remaining nine patients on the trial were successfully managed with phenylephrine administered during the filtration period.[27] The group at Yale subsequently reported a single-institution phase II trial of 18 patients treated with 57 chemofiltration procedures using 90 or 120 mg/m^2 of doxorubicin. Four of 12 evaluable patients experienced a partial response to therapy, with a median survival of 23 months in the four patients. Pharmacokinetic studies demonstrated a hepatic extraction ratio of 60.3% of doxorubicin that remained constant despite the dose of chemotherapeutic agent used. The investigators conclude that the therapeutic index of doxorubicin is improved on the basis of this high extraction of the high-dose chemotherapy.[28]

Despite these early reports, hepatocellular carcinoma has not remained a focus for chemofiltration in Western literature. Owing to the success of operative isolated hepatic perfusion, the chemofiltration approach was then adapted by Alexander and the investigators at the National Cancer Institute (including this chapter's author) for the treatment of metastatic disease to the liver. In a phase I study, melphalan was infused into the arterial supply to the liver and venous effluent was captured and sent through activated charcoal filters using a centrifugal pump and circuit identical to that proposed for this study (Figure 3-10). Melphalan levels were measured in the venous effluent before the blood entered the filters, after the filters, and in the systemic circulation, in an effort to measure the efficiency of the filters in removing the melphalan. Filter extraction percentages ranged

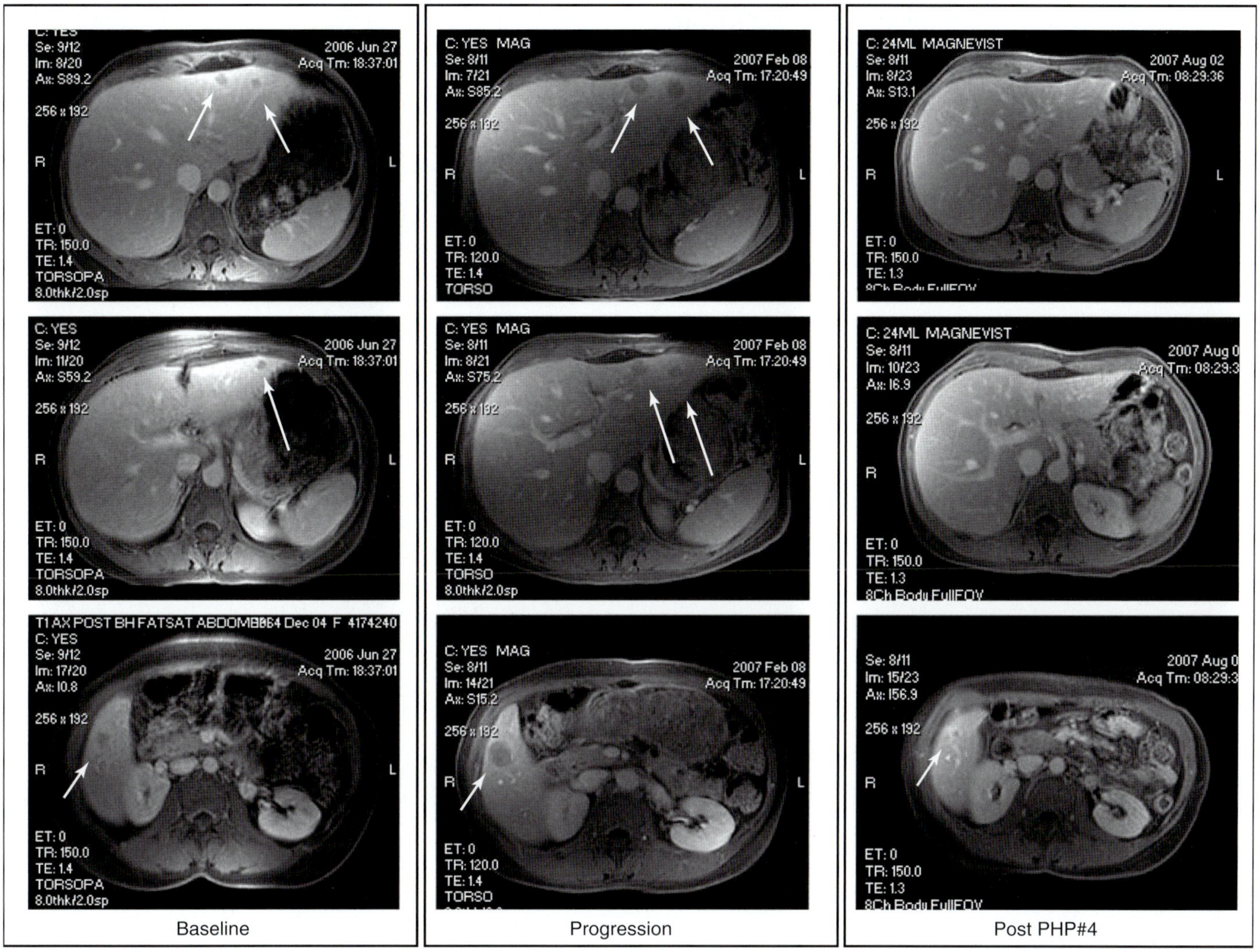

Figure 3-10 Response to chemosaturation using percutaneous hepatic perfusion. Selected axial images from a patient with metastatic ocular melanoma shows bilobar hepatic metastasis at baseline. These progress on a regimen of systemic chemotherapy as shown in the center panel. Partial response is evident following a total of four percutaneous hepatic perfusion procedures.

from 58.2% to 94.7%, with a mean of 77%. At the MTD for liver perfusion, filter efficiency was 78.5% with melphalan area under the curve (AUC) of 5.42 ± 2.04 μg/mL/h. This series of pharmacokinetic measurements demonstrates that the filters effectively extract melphalan from the venous effluent, albeit not completely.[29]

A multiinstitutional phase III trial using melphalan chemosaturation was completed for hepatic metastases from ocular melanoma. Patients were randomized to treatment with sequential hepatic chemosaturation with percutaneous hepatic perfusion, or best available care. Ninety three subjects with primarily ocular melanoma metastatic to the liver were enrolled, 44 in the percutaneous hepatic perfusion arm. Objective response was superior in patients treated with percutaneous hepatic perfusion (34.1% vs. 2%). Hepatic progression-free survival was superior in those treated with the percutaneous hepatic perfusion compared to best available care (245 days vs. 49 days). Those who progressed on best available care were allowed to cross over and receive chemosaturation procedures. This ethically necessary step negatively interfered with interpretation of overall survival because both groups could gain survival advantage from the treatment.[30]

Initial experience using melphalan hepatic chemosaturation for other histologies has shown promise. In 120 patients with metastatic colon cancer, 61% experienced an objective response from chemosaturation and the group experienced a 17.4-month median survival. In a separate report, median overall survival from treatment of metastatic neuroendocrine tumors is 40 months. Chemosaturation using percutaneous hepatic perfusion remains experimental for these types of cancer, and other agents may be more efficacious for these diseases than melphalan.

Summary

Regional perfusion is a method of delivering high-dose chemotherapy to a region of the body burdened with regional cancer. ILP and isolated hepatic perfusion are traditional surgical methods of regional therapy that are effective in treating melanoma confined to an extremity or the liver. Newer hybrid methods employ interventional radiology techniques to gain access to the inflow and outflow of the limb or liver. Isolated limb infusion simplifies the approach for ILP. Percutaneously placed catheters are used in an isolated limb to deliver high doses of melphalan-based chemotherapy. Similarly, chemosaturation or percutaneous hepatic perfusion employs the use of percutaneously placed catheters to perfuse the liver in a semi-isolated fashion.

Both of the hybrid techniques are under evaluation to define their place in the treatment of cancer, but all these procedures are effective in causing regional regression of tumors.

REFERENCES

The complete reference list is available online at www.expertconsult.com.

4 Principles of Radiotherapy

DAVID YOO | CHRISTOPHER WILLETT

KEY POINTS

- The clinical application of radiation oncology balances the dual goals of improved tumor control with reduced treatment-related morbidity.
- Over time, technological and biological advances have offered many opportunities to further reduce normal tissue complications and improve tumor control with radiotherapy.
- More recent and emerging technologies promise further improvements in the therapeutic ratio.
- Rational application and critical appraisal of these new technologies will remain essential responsibilities for the field of radiation oncology.

Introduction

The discipline of radiation oncology involves the therapeutic application of ionizing radiation in the management of benign and malignant diseases. In fact, x-rays were used to treat a patient with ulcerated breast cancer less than 2 months after their discovery in November 1895.[1] Therapeutic radiology, like its diagnostic counterpart, has undergone considerable evolution since then. Still, the practice of radiation oncology has at its core several fundamental concepts that have guided, and will continue to guide, management decisions.

Tumors and their neighboring organs will remain in proximity to one another. These tumors and their normal tissue counterparts will have varying responsiveness to ionizing radiation. Therefore, an ideal radiation treatment will balance optimal tumor control with acceptable acute side effects and late toxicities. Over time, new technological or biological advances will promise improved differentiation of these two populations, with better clinical outcomes. Some of these advances will actually work, shifting paradigms and reinforcing the ongoing need for rigorous testing before widespread adoption and changes to accepted standards of care.

With each new patient encounter, the radiation oncologist considers these concepts and determines the most appropriate treatment approach. A simplified algorithm is shown in Figure 4-1, showing the general thought processes and decision points involved. The global decisions regarding treatment and goals of therapy are usually reached within a multidisciplinary context with other medical providers and informed consent of the patients and their support networks. Once the decision has been made to incorporate radiation therapy into the treatment plan, the more specific questions regarding timing, dose, treatment volume, and technology are considered. The solid and dashed arrows between the various boxes represent the interrelated nature of these questions and how they may each in turn influence the decision-making process.

This chapter will briefly describe these concepts, along with specific clinical examples with various malignancies to illustrate the interplay between the decision points. We will focus on the therapeutic ratio, selection and definition of radiation target volumes, side effects and toxicity considerations, dose fractionation, and the impact of technological advances on these topics.

Therapeutic Ratio

The overriding goal in patient care is to optimize treatment efficacy while minimizing toxicity. This concept is represented by the therapeutic ratio (Figure 4-2). Depending on the tumor type and the surrounding normal tissues, a given amount of radiation dose will yield an expected range of both tumor control probability (TCP) and normal tissue complication probability (NTCP). The vertical white lines illustrate how an increase in dose (dashed line to solid line) leads to both higher tumor control and normal tissue complications. An example would be the dose escalation experience in prostate cancer. Multiple randomized trials have shown an improvement in prostate-specific antigen disease-free survival with higher doses of radiation at the cost of increased rectal and urinary complications.[2]

Ideally, the two curves can be further separated, with the same radiation dose providing extremely high TCP and low NTCP. Strategies that preferentially radiosensitize tumor cells and shift the curve left (dashed blue curve) may allow for improved TCP with the same physical dose. Alternatively, techniques that preferentially protect normal tissues (dashed red curve) may reduce treatment morbidity without compromising efficacy.

In clinical practice, agents that sensitize tumors often affect normal tissues as well, leading to improved outcomes at the cost of increased toxicity. Examples of this include the use of concurrent chemotherapy with radiation compared to radiation alone in the management of lung, head and neck, cervical, esophageal, and gastrointestinal cancers.[3-6] At the same time, radioprotection agents have had less clinical impact than expected. For example, the compound amifostine is U.S. Food and Drug Administration (FDA)-approved for mitigation of xerostomia in head and neck cancer patients treated with radiation alone.[7] In practice, very few centers now utilize this agent because of its cumbersome administration, its own toxicity profile, the superiority demonstrated of concurrent chemoradiation in head and neck cancer, and the subsequent development of new radiation technologies that better spare the parotid glands.

One example where technological advances may have improved the therapeutic ratio is the use of four-dimensional computed tomography simulation (4DCT) and intensity-modulated radiotherapy (IMRT) planning in locally advanced lung cancers.[8]

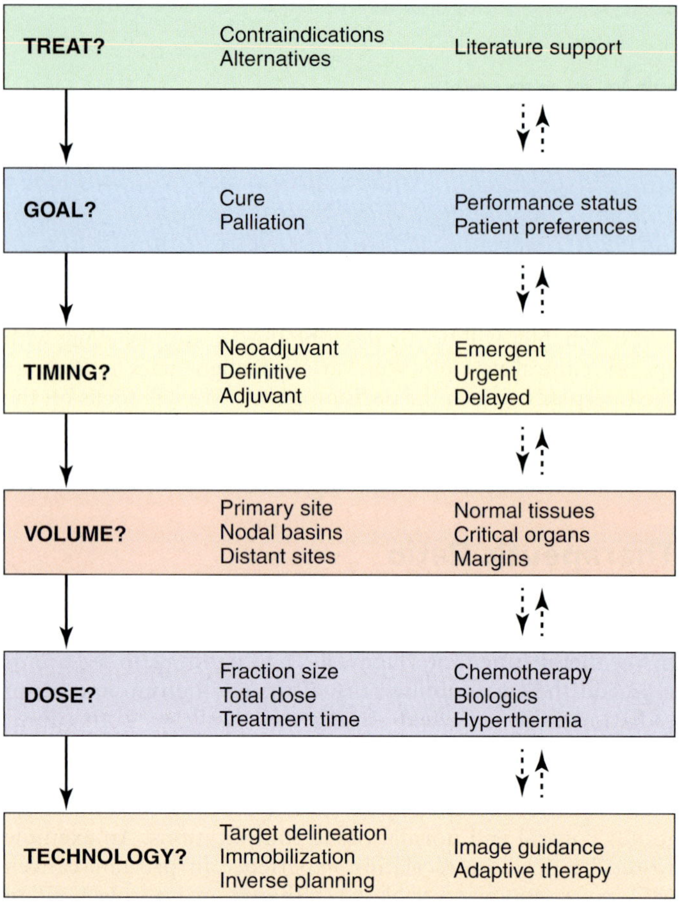

Figure 4-1 Treatment algorithm. This simplified algorithm shows the general questions when encountering a patient under consideration for radiation therapy. The questions are interrelated, as shown by the dashed arrows to the right. Technological advances can often redefine what is possible when it comes to treatment delivery. This, in turn, reemphasizes the importance of clinical investigations to demonstrate the safety and superiority of these new techniques.

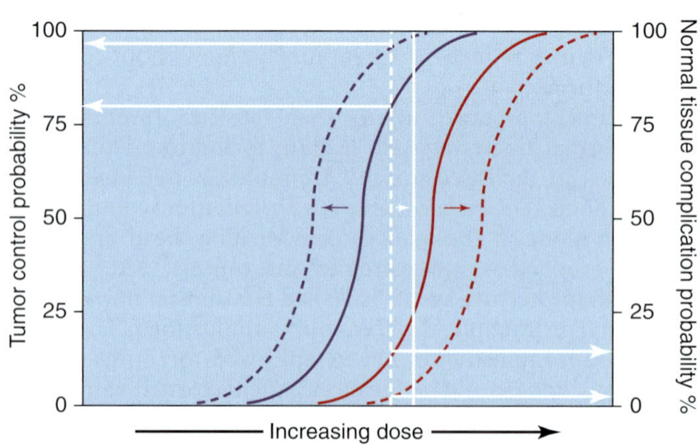

Figure 4-2 Therapeutic ratio. The blue solid curve represents tumor control probability (TCP), whereas the red solid curve shows normal tissue complication probability (NTCP). As radiation dose increases (dashed vertical line to solid vertical line), both tumor control and toxicity are likely to increase. The final dose chosen strikes the optimal balance between the two outcomes. Various strategies can be employed to separate the two curves. Factors that sensitize tumors to radiation may shift the TCP curve to the left (dashed blue curve), whereas agents that protect normal tissues may mitigate treatment-related toxicity, shifting the NTCP curve to the right (dashed red curve).

Simulation with 4DCT allows for capture of respiratory motion to avoid missing the tumor, whereas IMRT planning has the capacity to deliver more conformal dose distributions with reduction in high-dose normal tissue irradiation. In a retrospective series, the use of 4DCT/IMRT compared with conventional computed tomography (CT) and planning resulted in improvements in overall survival with decreased rates of radiation-induced pneumonitis.

Target Volumes

When radiation oncologists discuss treatment targets and volumes (Figure 4-3), they utilize definitions and acronyms developed by the International Commission of Radiation Units and Measurements (ICRU). The ICRU 50 report published in 1993 introduced the concepts of gross tumor volume (GTV), clinical target volume (CTV), and planning target volume (PTV).[9] The GTV represents grossly visible disease, either clinically or radiographically. The CTV represents areas of potential microscopic extension of disease from the GTV. These microscopic deposits may be in proximity to the primary tumor and/or dispersed throughout the relevant draining regional lymph node basins. The PTV includes sufficient margin around the CTV to ensure adequate coverage and accounts for various uncertainties such as patient/organ motion and daily setup errors.

Technologic advances such as 4DCT, which captures organ motion, and immobilization devices/onboard imaging modalities that can reduce setup errors, have helped characterize and eliminate some of these uncertainties. A modern linear accelerator treatment machine with onboard imaging and respiratory motion tracking capabilities is shown in Figure 4-4. The subsequent ICRU 62 report considered these advances with the addition of internal target volume (ITV) and setup margin (SM).[11] Now, PTV = CTV + ITV + SM. Further advances in diagnostic radiology with functional imaging modalities are providing potential biologic target volumes (BTVs) to further improve the therapeutic ratio.[12]

These target volume definitions help to determine how much technology and complexity is required to safely and effectively deliver the radiation treatments to optimize the therapeutic ratio. Depending on the clinical scenario, treatment plans may

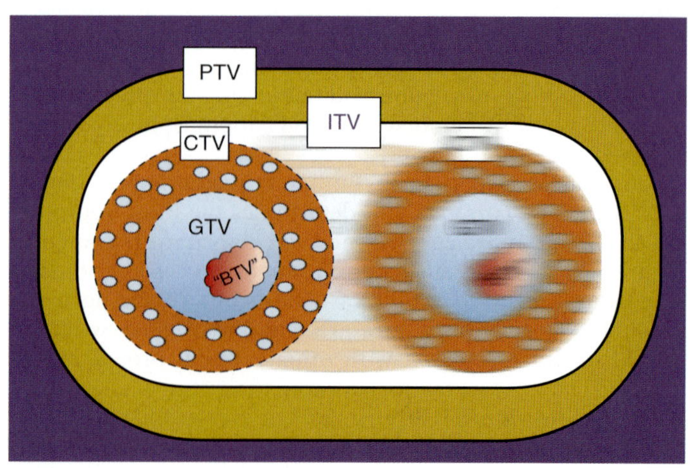

Figure 4-3 Target volume definitions in radiotherapy. BTV, biological target volume; GTV, gross tumor volume; CTV, clinical target volume; ITV, internal target volume; PTV, planning target volume.

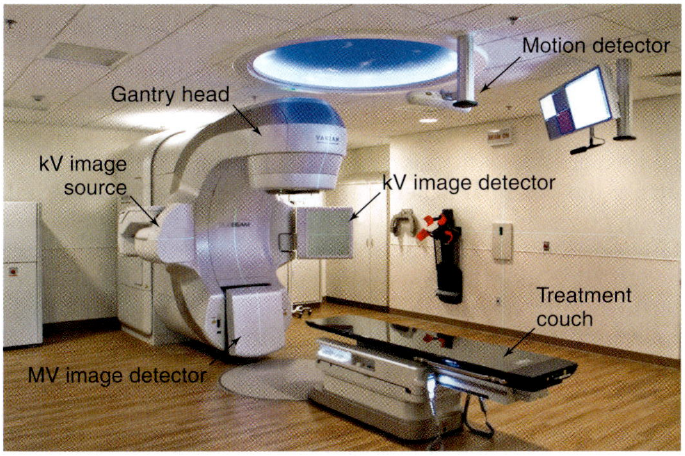

Figure 4-4 Linear accelerator treatment machine with onboard imaging and respiratory motion tracking devices. The radiation is delivered via the gantry head that can rotate 360 degrees. The treatment couch also rotates, allowing for various beam angle approaches. The kilovoltage imaging source and detector allow for acquisition of static portal images as well as cone-beam CT images to confirm patient setup. Megavoltage portal films may also be captured to ensure proper targeting. An infrared tracking device is seen in the ceiling, allowing for detection of respiratory motion.

vary from relatively straightforward beam arrangements to highly complex delivery methods with rigid immobilization and onboard imaging modalities. For example, Figure 4-5 shows representative treatment fields used to treat a patient with locally advanced rectal cancer. Typically, the plan involves a posterior–anterior (PA) beam and two opposed lateral beams for coverage. Tumor volumes and normal tissues are shown contoured on a slice-by-slice basis and projected onto the digital reconstructed radiographs. The primary tumor and nodal GTVs are shown in red. The iliac blood vessels have been contoured in turquoise as surrogates for sites of potential microscopic disease in the pelvic lymph nodes. Small bowel (magenta) and femoral heads (tan and blue) are also outlined. Panel A (PA) and panel B (left lateral beam) demonstrate the additional margins on the GTV superiorly, inferiorly, and laterally to account for microscopic disease in the mesorectum and pelvic nodes (CTV) and additional margin for setup uncertainties (PTV). Organ motion considerations are often moot given the size of the treatment fields. Still, patients undergo fluoroscopic evaluation with rectal contrast before treatment to ensure the fields adequately cover the intended volumes.

How do these target volumes fit into an algorithmic approach for rectal cancer as described in Figure 4-1? When the decision is made to treat a patient with locally advanced nonmetastatic rectal cancer, the goal is cure and generally involves therapy with surgery, radiation, and/or chemotherapy. Radiation therapy is often used in a neoadjuvant fashion, delivered preoperatively to the target volumes as outlined in Figure 4-5, prior to surgical resection. The extensive literature on this subject has described multiple fractionation regimens, including 5 Gray (Gy) × 5 daily treatments to a total dose of 25 Gy with radiation alone.[13] A more typical strategy employed at Duke involves 1.8 Gy daily fractions to a total dose of 50.4 Gy with concurrent chemotherapy.[14] These volumes are large, with up to 2-cm margins in all directions to account for any organ motion and setup uncertainties.

The radiation doses are dictated by the tolerance of the small intestines and by the fact that radiation therapy plays an adjuvant role to reduce locoregional recurrences following the primary treatment modality, which is surgical resection. Microleaf collimators help to shield the small bowel and femoral heads. Of note, the patient was also treated in the prone position with a belly board designed to further minimize the amount of small bowel irradiated by the lateral fields. Oftentimes, simple maneuvers or changes in patient position during simulation and immobilization can facilitate treatments without the need for advanced planning and delivery techniques.

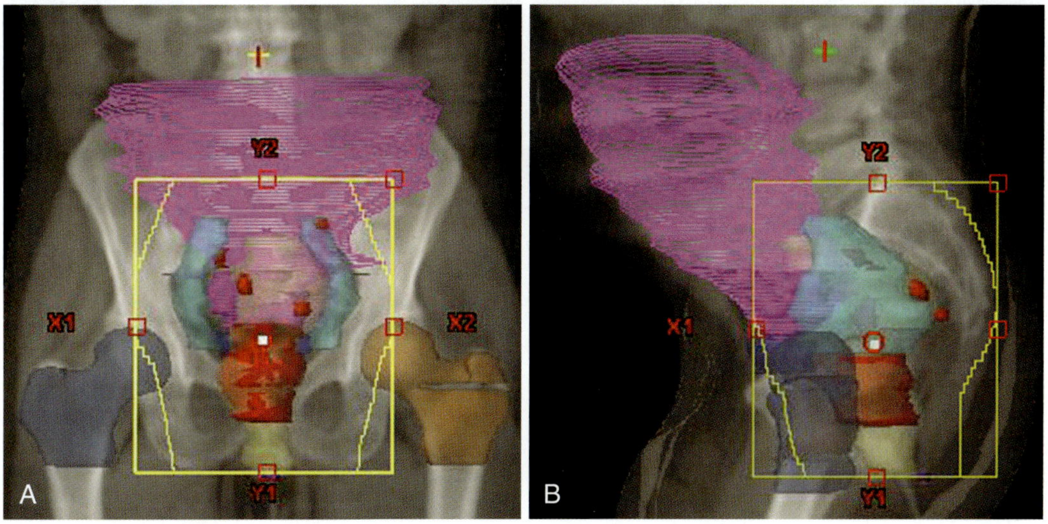

Figure 4-5 Three-dimensional treatment fields for rectal cancer. The beam apertures are custom-designed with multileaf collimators located in the head of the treatment machine to encompass the target volumes with adequate margin while sparing surrounding normal tissue structures. Normal tissues and tumor volumes are contoured and projected onto digital radiographic reconstruction—left femoral head (*blue*), right femoral head (tan), small bowel (*magenta*), bladder (*purple*), rectum (*yellow*), iliac blood vessels (*turquoise*), and gross tumor volume (*red*). (A) Posterior–anterior field. (B) Left lateral field.

Side Effects and Toxicity

Although some clinical scenarios may not benefit from the utilization of advanced technological breakthroughs, the field of radiation oncology remains dedicated to the rational application of these emerging technologies for any potential gains in the therapeutic ratio. One such example may be found in the evolution of adjuvant radiation therapy in the management of breast cancer patients. Breast conservation with lumpectomy followed by whole breast radiotherapy remains the current standard, with radiation reducing the risk of recurrence by two-thirds compared to surgery alone.[15]

Given the excellent survival and rates of cure, especially in early-stage breast cancer patients, there is growing awareness and emphasis on the potential late side effects of radiotherapy that may reduce the therapeutic ratio.[16] In particular, patients with left-sided breast cancers often had anterior portions of the heart within the tangential radiation treatment portals. This excess heart irradiation likely contributed to the increased risk of late cardiac morbidity and mortality seen in breast cancer survivors.[17] Subsequent techniques that tried to better shield the heart may have compromised target coverage and resulted in more recurrences under the heart blocks.[18]

With the advent of respiratory motion tracking, many left-sided breast patients are now simulated using breath-hold techniques (Figure 4-6). Panel A shows the merged CT images from a patient during both free-breathing and breath-hold at end-inspiration. Panel B shows the medial border of a typical tangential field for treatment of the whole breast. Portions of the heart can be seen within the treatment volume. In panel C, the heart has physically moved away from the chest wall, allowing the same tangent field to cover the breast while minimizing heart irradiation.

Because the late effects of radiation-induced changes to the heart may require 10–20 years to manifest, longer follow-up and experience with this breath-hold technique are required before the potential benefits of this change may be seen. Still, the hope would be that the benefits of radiation already seen in terms of locoregional control and survival would be further enhanced if more patients were no longer dying from subsequent cardiac complications. Other strategies being employed to minimize heart dose include treating patients in the prone position or the use of IMRT to minimize heart dose in treatment planning. A much more radical change currently under debate within the field is a redefinition of the appropriate CTV itself—from treating the whole breast to just the lumpectomy cavity alone.[19]

Despite the continuing refinement and focus on target volumes, the tolerance of the surrounding normal tissues often drives decisions regarding treatment. Acute side effects happen during therapy and are often transient, requiring supportive care, whereas late effects, as discussed, can develop months to years following radiation therapy and tend to be irreversible. The issue is further complicated by the fact that organs often have different expressions of toxicity with different time courses. For example, the skin may respond acutely to radiation with mild erythema and dry desquamation. With increasing doses, patients may develop moist desquamation and even ulceration. Late effects may include tanning changes, skin fibrosis and contracture, atrophy, telangiectasias, or permanent hair loss.

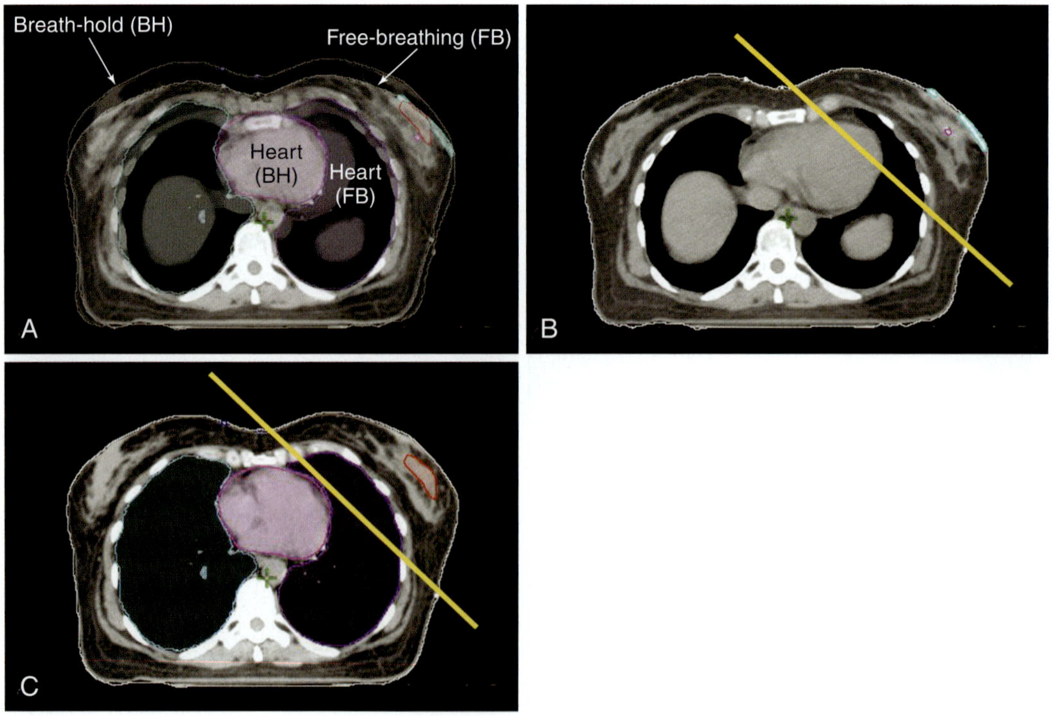

Figure 4-6 Utilization of breath-hold for treatment of left-sided breast cancer. (A) A merge of axial slices is seen from both free-breathing and deep inspiration breath-hold CT simulation scans. The outer body contour shows increased chest wall expansion with deep inspiration. (B) Free-breathing CT scan, with the thick yellow line representing the medial border of the tangential radiation fields used to treat the whole breast. In this scenario, a small portion of the left ventricle is within the radiation treatment fields. (C) The use of deep inspiration breath-hold allows the same radiation tangential fields to cover the left breast without irradiating the left ventricle.

Not all normal tissues are created equal. Some are organized in a parallel fashion, with multiple independent functional subunits.[20] For example, the kidney is composed of approximately 1 million separate nephrons, capable of performing their duties independently from their neighboring subunits. Therefore, organs arranged in parallel, such as the kidney, lung, and liver, may have significant portions surgically removed or irradiated beyond tolerance, with the remaining undamaged subunits able to maintain normal global organ function. Other tissues, such as the small bowel and spinal cord, are arranged in series, where excessive damage along any point may compromise the entire organ's function.

These differences have significant implications in treatment planning. When the target lies in proximity to a parallel structure, the dose parameters to avoid excessive toxicity are typically expressed in mean dose or volume percentages. For example, when evaluating lung cancer plans, a primary concern is the potential development of radiation pneumonitis. One well-studied dosimetric parameter is the volume of normal lung receiving at least 20 Gy (V20), with higher percentages associated with increased risk of pneumonitis.[21] For serial organs, the goal is to avoid any dose beyond the expected tolerance of that structure. With either the small bowel or spinal cord, the maximum dose is generally in the 45–50-Gy range for conventionally fractionated regimens.

Not all toxicities are created equal as well. Radiation-induced cataracts may develop after doses beyond 10 Gy to the lens. These can be easily removed surgically. Spinal cord myelopathy resulting in paralysis or blindness due to optic chiasm damage are irreversible catastrophic complications. Figure 4-7 shows a patient with nasopharyngeal carcinoma with intracranial extension treated with concurrent radiation and chemotherapy.[22] Panels A and B demonstrate the utility of magnetic resonance imaging (MRI)[23] in the delineation of both tumor and normal tissues compared to CT. The light-blue contour represents the 4400-cGy isodose line. This dose level with chemotherapy is felt to be sufficient for microscopic disease control in the cervical neck nodes. The yellow contour shows the 7000-cGy isodose line used for gross disease control.

This is an example of an IMRT plan, where the intensity of the beams is modulated during therapy to allow for more conformal dose distributions. The isodose lines show the radiation dose being shaped away from the bilateral parotid glands and the larynx in order to minimize long-term xerostomia and edema/dysphagia. More critically, panel C shows the proximity of the optic chiasm to the target volumes. Visual loss from radiation-induced optic neuropathy has been carefully studied and reviewed. The risk is very low when the maximum dose to the chiasm/optic nerves is less than 55 Gy at 1.8–2.0 Gy fraction sizes. The incidence rises to 3%–7% with maximum doses of 55–60 Gy and rises quickly beyond 60 Gy.[24] In this example, the chiasm has been contoured and expanded by 1 mm to allow for daily setup uncertainties (chiasm + 1 mm). During IMRT planning, priority was placed on covering the target volumes while keeping the dose to the chiasm + 1 mm structure less than 54 Gy.

Plan evaluation is performed by careful examination of the isodose distributions in the various axial, sagittal, and coronal planes and by review of a dose volume histogram (DVH) that shows the various structures and their associated dosimetric characteristics (panel D). Based on the plan, the expanded chiasm + 1 mm structure is receiving a maximum dose of 5334 cGy. In essence, this 5334-cGy dose represents the worst-case scenario if the patient's setup position is off by 1 mm every day toward the high-dose areas. The chiasm itself is receiving 4731 cGy. Other organs, such as the parotids, are arranged in a more parallel fashion. For these, the maximum dose has not been found to be as critical as the mean dose received. Generally, mean doses less than 26 Gy are associated with improved salivary function.[25] Given the need to balance cure with toxicity, and that patients are unlikely to die from xerostomia, target volume coverage is usually given priority over parotid gland sparing.

Over time, the typical tolerances of normal tissues to conventionally fractionated radiation have been meticulously gathered and reexamined.[26,27] The rapidly growing use of stereotactic techniques, which deliver much higher doses per fraction, has spawned significant discussion and research in the establishment of guidelines and tolerances of normal tissues to these larger doses. For example, the recommended optic chiasm tolerance for single fraction radiosurgery procedures is in the 10–12-Gy range.[24]

Dose Fractionation

In the earliest days of radiation therapy, treatments often involved a single large fraction of radiation. Any clinical responses were unfortunately accompanied by significant early and late toxicities.[1] Subsequent strategies employed more protracted courses of therapy, splitting the radiation treatment into multiple fractions with smaller doses. Classical experiments from the 1920s with rams' testes showed the ability of small daily radiation fractions to sterilize the animals without the resulting skin necrosis associated with single large doses. The radiobiology behind fractionation was best described by Withers and what he labeled the four Rs—repair of sublethal injury, cell repopulation, redistribution into more radiosensitive phases of the cell cycle, and reoxygenation.[28]

Nonmalignant cells are more adept at the repair of radiation-induced DNA damage than their malignant counterparts. Therefore, the use of multiple radiation fractions allows for killing of tumor cells, while giving the normal surrounding tissues time to repair sublethal damage. One potential drawback of protracted treatment courses is the opportunity for repopulation of both normal and cancerous cells. For this reason, more fractionated regimens typically require higher total doses to achieve similar degrees of tumor control. Still, with each subsequent fraction, the potential exists for more cancer cells to redistribute into the more radiosensitive G2/mitosis phase of the cycle, allowing for more effective radiation-induced cell kill. One final advantage of fractionation is the potential for reoxygenation of tumors during treatment progression, as hypoxic cells are much more radioresistant compared to normoxic cells.

Different fractionation regimens have been used in a number of clinical scenarios. For example, common prescriptions for the palliation of bone metastases include a single fraction of 8 Gy, 5 fractions of 4 Gy to a total dose of 20 Gy, 10 fractions of 3 Gy to 30 Gy, and 14 fractions of 2.5 Gy to 35 Gy.[29] To make comparisons between various schedules, radiation oncologists often speak in terms of the biologically effective dose (BED) of a particular treatment regimen. This equation takes into account a number of parameters, including total dose, fraction size, overall treatment time, and the relative sensitivity of the tissue to changes in fraction size.[30] This final factor is known as the alpha/beta ratio. Most tumors and normal tissues with

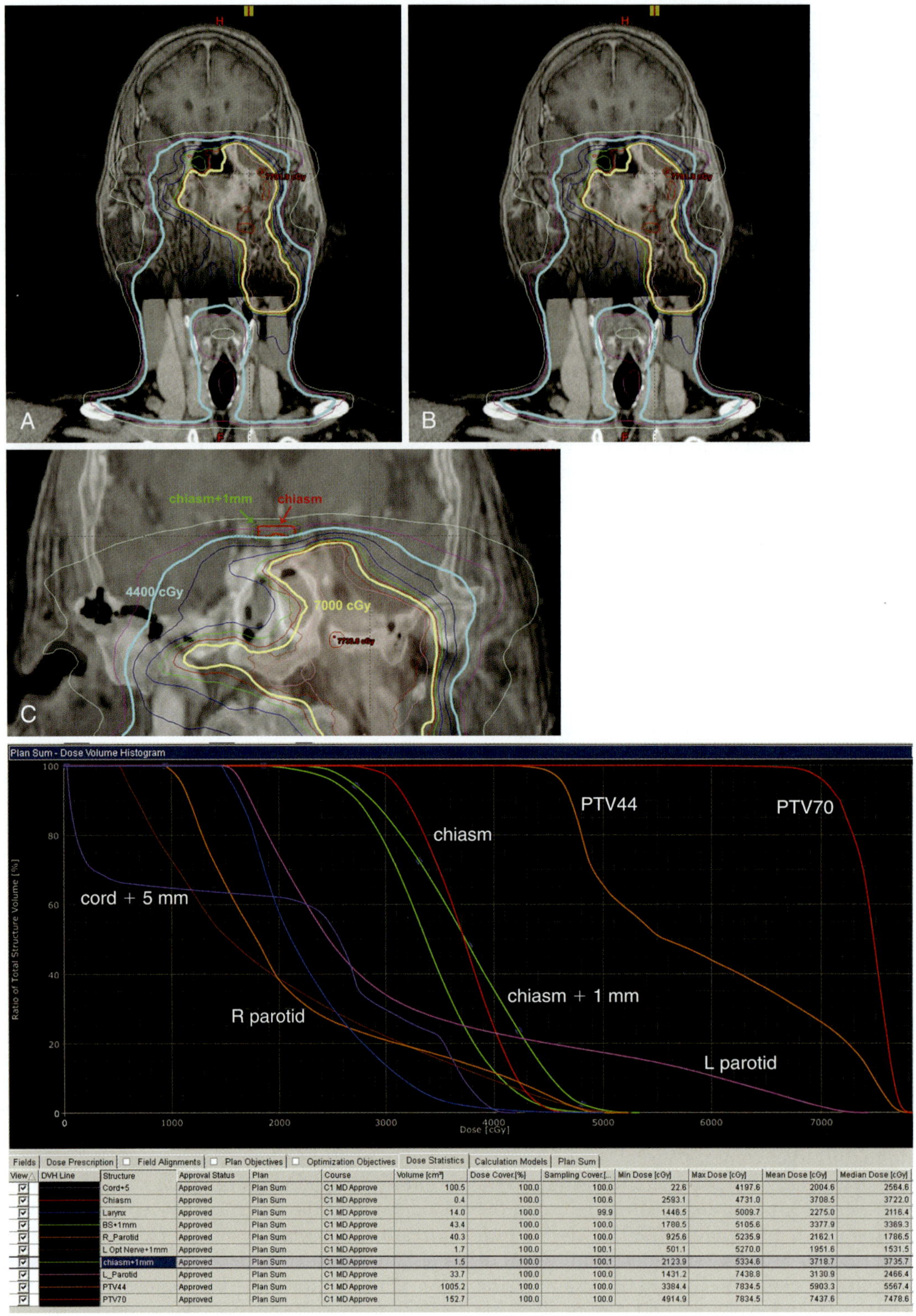

View	DVH Line	Structure	Approval Status	Plan	Course	Volume [cm³]	Dose Cover.[%]	Sampling Cover.[...	Min Dose [cGy]	Max Dose [cGy]	Mean Dose [cGy]	Median Dose [cGy]
☑		Cord+5	Approved	Plan Sum	C1 MD Approve	100.5	100.0	100.0	22.6	4197.6	2004.6	2564.6
☑		Chiasm	Approved	Plan Sum	C1 MD Approve	0.4	100.0	100.6	2593.1	4731.0	3708.5	3722.0
☑		Larynx	Approved	Plan Sum	C1 MD Approve	14.0	100.0	99.9	1446.5	5009.7	2275.0	2116.4
☑		BS+1mm	Approved	Plan Sum	C1 MD Approve	43.4	100.0	100.0	1788.5	5105.6	3377.9	3369.3
☑		R_Parotid	Approved	Plan Sum	C1 MD Approve	40.3	100.0	100.0	925.6	5235.9	2162.1	1786.5
☑		L Opt Nerve+1mm	Approved	Plan Sum	C1 MD Approve	1.7	100.0	100.1	501.1	5270.0	1951.6	1531.5
☑		chiasm+1mm	Approved	Plan Sum	C1 MD Approve	1.5	100.0	100.1	2123.9	5334.6	3718.7	3735.7
☑		L_Parotid	Approved	Plan Sum	C1 MD Approve	33.7	100.0	100.0	1431.2	7438.8	3130.9	2466.4
☑		PTV44	Approved	Plan Sum	C1 MD Approve	1005.2	100.0	100.0	3384.4	7834.5	5903.3	5567.4
☑		PTV70	Approved	Plan Sum	C1 MD Approve	152.7	100.0	100.0	4914.9	7834.5	7437.6	7478.6

D

Figure 4-7 Intensity-modulated radiation therapy (IMRT) for nasopharyngeal carcinoma. Isodose distributions from the IMRT plan are superimposed on coronal images from the CT (A) and MRI (B) simulation planning. The isodose lines show target volume coverage with sparing of the bilateral parotid glands and larynx. The light-blue 4400-cGy isodose line covers all areas of potential microscopic tumor spread, whereas the yellow 7000-cGy isodose line encompasses areas of gross disease. (C) The use of IMRT allows more precise coverage of target volumes while simultaneously sparing the optic chiasm. To account for potential setup errors that could result in exceeding organ tolerance, the chiasm is expanded by an additional millimeter (chiasm + 1 mm) for treatment planning purposes. (D) The dose volume histogram (DVH) displays the dose delivered to various normal tissues and target volumes.

rapid turnover (high alpha/beta ratios) are less impacted with changes in fraction size. Some tumors and more slowly proliferating tissues (low alpha/beta ratios) are much more sensitive to changes in fraction size, as seen with the optic chiasm.

To further illustrate this concept, consider a rapidly dividing lung cancer (alpha/beta ratio 10) adjacent to the spinal cord (alpha/beta ratio 2.5). Conventional 2-Gy fractions are used to treat over 20 sessions to a total dose of 40 Gy. If the fraction size is doubled to 4 Gy but the total dose is kept at 40 Gy, the tumor will receive the equivalent of 47 Gy in 2-Gy fractions (17% increase). However, the spinal cord will receive the equivalent of 58 Gy in 2-Gy fractions (44% increase). If the fraction size is doubled again to 8 Gy, the tumor will receive the equivalent of 60 Gy in 2-Gy fractions (50% increase), whereas the spinal cord will receive what feels like 93 Gy (133% increase). Because the risk of myelopathy rises to unacceptably high levels beyond 50 Gy, regimens using higher doses per fraction will need to go to a lower total dose that respects cord limits or employ techniques during patient simulation or treatment planning/delivery to shield the spinal cord from irradiation beyond tolerance.

The Impact of Technological Advances

The ability to return to larger fraction sizes has been considerably aided by the various advances in target delineation, immobilization, organ motion capture, treatment planning, image guidance, and verification. These advances can influence every step along the decision-making process as initially shown in Figure 4-1. As a case illustration, a 50-year-old woman presents with a 1-cm brain metastasis in the left temporal lobe. Should she be treated with radiation? Are there any contraindications to radiotherapy? Is neurosurgical intervention an option? What if she has newly diagnosed lung cancer with widespread systemic disease but without any neurologic sequelae? With no neurologic symptoms requiring palliation, initiation of systemic chemotherapy to address all her sites of disease may be the best option, with radiation therapy to the brain reserved for symptomatic progression.

If she is treated with radiation, is the goal curative or palliative? Historically, the development of brain metastases has represented incurable disease, with median survivals in the 2–7-month range with radiotherapy.[31] With improved systemic therapy and identification of more favorable prognostic factors, further stratification has been performed, with median survivals approaching 21 months in young healthy breast cancer patients whose tumors are positive for the hormone receptors and Her2-neu.[32] Some argue further for a paradigm shift, with more aggressive management of limited metastatic sites and the potential for cure in select patients with oligometastatic disease.[33] There is a growing body of literature regarding aggressive treatment of metastatic disease, initially with surgical resection and now with ablative radiation therapy techniques.[34,35]

Over time, treatment strategies for patients with brain metastases have changed in step with each technological advance. Before the development of stereotactic radiosurgery, patients with brain metastases not felt to be surgical candidates received palliative whole brain radiation. A typical fractionation regimen would be 10 daily fractions of 3 Gy to a total dose of 30 Gy over 2 weeks. With the advent of radiosurgery, institutions began to investigate the potential benefits of boosting residual metastases with large single fractions of 15–24 Gy after whole brain radiotherapy. More recently, the long-term neurocognitive side effects associated with whole brain treatment have led investigators to study the use of radiosurgery alone to target individual brain metastases. Despite multiple randomized studies and meta-analyses, the optimal treatment of brain metastases remains controversial and continues to evolve.[36]

The decision to treat patients with whole brain radiotherapy or radiosurgery (or both) has major implications for subsequent management choices. There are differences in treatment volumes, total doses, fractionation schedules, and techniques that necessitate varying degrees of patient immobilization, simulation scans, the number of treatment portals, the resources required for treatment planning, quality assurance, and delivery verification.

With whole brain radiation, a patient may be planned "clinically" on the treatment machine itself without a separate CT or MRI scan, immobilized with a piece of tape across the forehead, with two opposing 17 × 23-cm portals and a custom block placed in the field path to shield the eyes. The treatment plan may be calculated by hand. Portal images may be taken just prior to treatment to ensure adequate coverage of the intracranial contents. With a stereotactic radiosurgery case, the patient requires rigid immobilization in a custom thermoplastic frame system, with fine-cut CT and MRI scans performed and subsequently registered together. The lesion(s) and all normal tissues are contoured on a slice-by-slice basis and expanded by a 1–2 mm margin to account for setup uncertainties. Various plans with multiple beam arrangements and arcs are generated and evaluated for adequate target coverage and respect for normal tissue tolerances. The plan then undergoes stringent quality assurance. Just prior to treatment, the tumor location can be more precisely matched with orthogonal films and cone-beam CT images. An example of a stereotactic radiosurgery plan is shown in Figure 4-8. Panel A shows the four arc paths chosen to treat the lesion while minimizing dose to the brainstem and optic structures. Panel B shows the arc paths with the field apertures. The microleaf collimators move dynamically and conform to the shape of the lesion as it changes along the arc path. The resulting isodose distribution is shown, with a prescribed dose of 20 Gy.

As the field evolves and technology improves, institutions are already studying the feasibility of delivering synchronous simultaneous whole brain radiation with integrated boosts to multiple metastases while minimizing dose to the hippocampus to potentially reduce neurocognitive effects.[37] Whether this advance, or others to come, will lead to significant improvements in clinical outcome that justify their increased costs and labor utilization is not known. As health care expenditures come under further scrutiny, the field may find outside forces ultimately determining what constitutes standard of care.

One final example of a technological advance changing the practice of radiation oncology is that of stereotactic body radiation therapy (SBRT). For early-stage lung cancer, the standard of care is surgical resection. Definitive radiation therapy has been reserved for those patients unfit or unwilling to proceed with surgery. Historically, the use of conventional radiotherapy with daily 2-Gy fractions to a total dose of approximately 60 Gy has been associated with poor local control and overall survival.[38] Higher doses of radiation have been shown to consistently improve local control in lung cancer. With advances in patient immobilization, respiratory motion capture, and on-board imaging capabilities, SBRT has the ability to deliver very high focal doses of radiation while minimizing irradiation

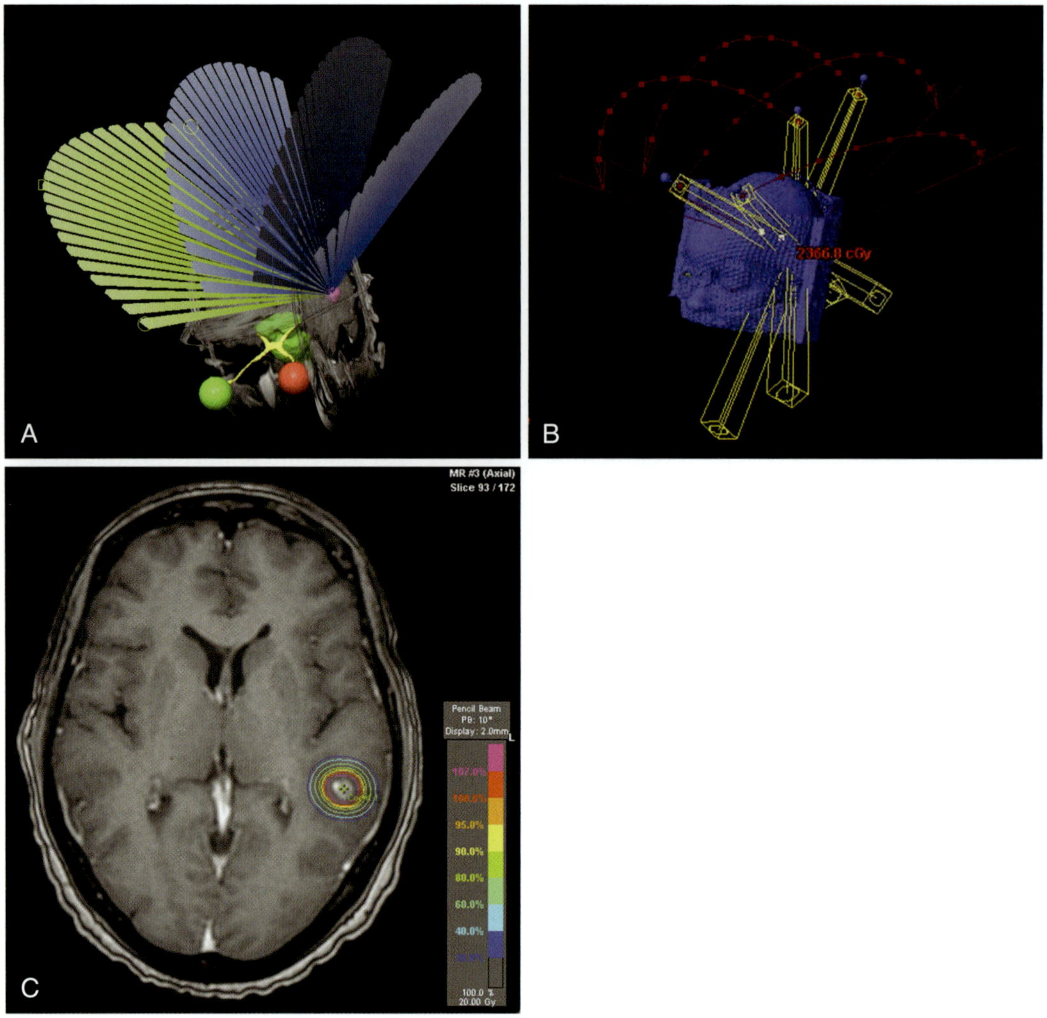

Figure 4-8 Stereotactic radiosurgery for brain metastasis. (A) The target volume is shown in purple. The optic structures and brainstem are also contoured. The fanlike structures show the paths of the four dynamic arcs used to deliver the radiation dose. (B) This reconstruction shows the beams and field apertures. As the gantry arm moves along the arc path, the micro multileaf collimators continuously change the field aperture shape to conform to the target volume. (C) The resulting isodose lines show the tight conformality of dose around the metastasis.

of surrounding normal tissues. Various fractionation regimens have been reported, from single doses of 34 Gy to five fractions of 10–12 Gy. This strategy has shown considerable improvements compared to historical series, with local control rates higher than 90%.[39] Overall survival numbers remain lower than those reported for surgical series, but that is not unexpected, given the competing risks in these inoperable patients. As the field continues to evolve, studies are underway examining the role of SBRT in operable lung cancer patients.

During simulation for an SBRT treatment plan, the patient undergoes a 4DCT scan to assess the degree of organ and tumor motion. Depending on the size and location of tumors, these lesions may or may not have significant excursion with respiration (Figure 4-9). Panel A shows sagittal views from each of the 10 phases of respiration captured by the 4DCT. After evaluation of tumor motion, the decision is made whether the patient is to be treated while breathing normally or with breath-hold. Patients unable to hold their breath (or unable to hear instructions) but with significant tumor motion can still be treated using respiratory gating techniques, where the radiation beam is turned on only during specific phases of the respiratory cycle when the tumor is within the treatment portal. Panel B shows a patient plan treated with free-breathing technique. The tumor was contoured on both the free-breathing images as well as the maximum intensity projection (MIP) CT images. The MIP data reconstructs the imaging information from all 10 respiratory phase CT scans and represents the degree of tumor motion due to respiration. This volume is then expanded by only 5 mm to generate a PTV. Excess toxicity has been reported with the use of 18 Gy × 3 fractions for centrally located tumors near the proximal bronchial tree.[40] As a result, this patient was treated per the protocol from the Radiation Therapy Oncology Group (RTOG) with 10-Gy fractions × 5 to a total dose of 50 Gy. Panel C shows the nine-field beam arrangement used to deliver the treatment. Just prior to each treatment, a cone-beam CT scan is obtained on the treatment machine to ensure the target volume is in right location (panel D). Finally, megavoltage cine images are obtained

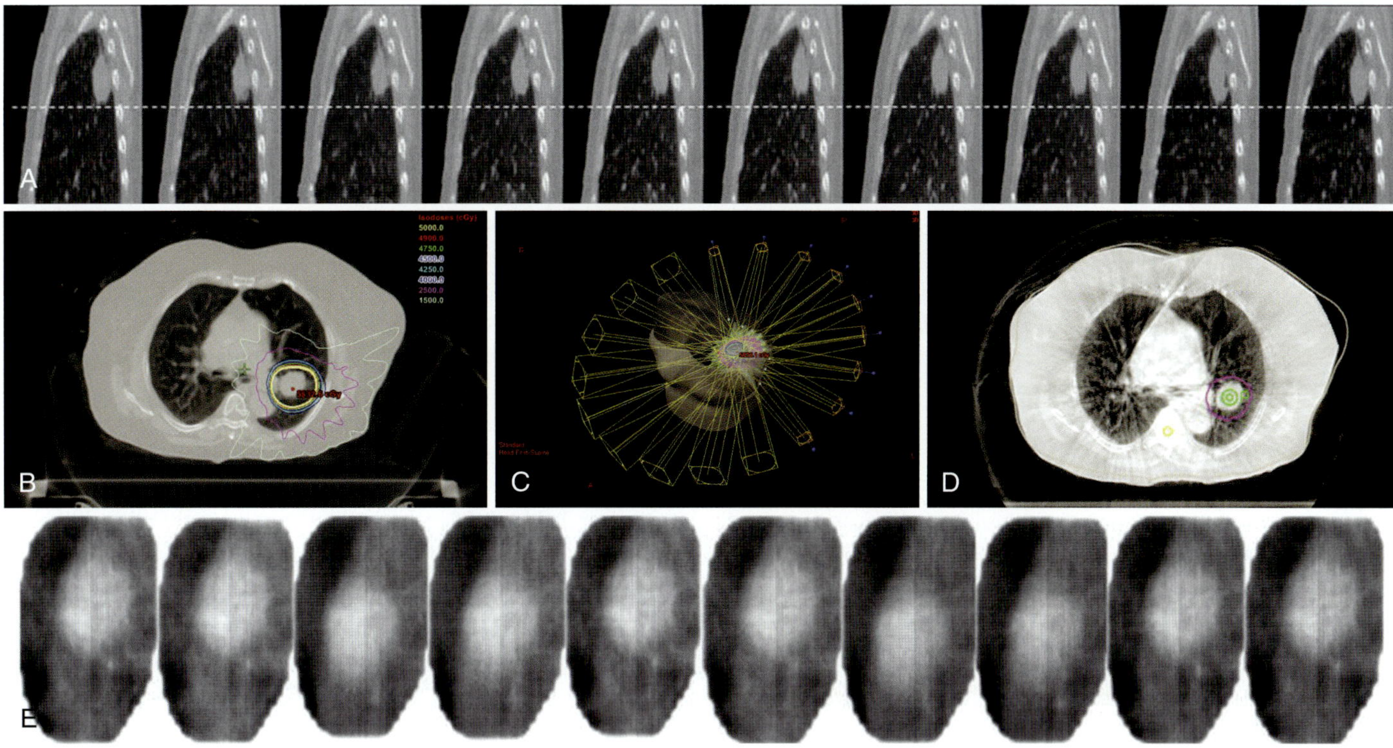

Figure 4-9 Stereotactic body radiation therapy (SBRT) for early-stage lung cancer. (A) Sagittal images from 10-phase four-dimensional CT scan (4DCT) demonstrate tumor motion during normal respiration. (B) Images from the4CT are used to generate a maximum-intensity projection (MIP) of the tumor mass from all phases of the respiratory cycle. The isodose lines from the SBRT plan are superimposed, showing target volume coverage. (C) The nine-field beam arrangement used for the treatment plan. (D) Cone-beam CT obtained on treatment table just prior to treatment to confirm accurate target localization. (E) Cine-megavoltage images acquired during treatment delivery from one of the nine fields to confirm tumor coverage throughout therapy.

during therapy to again confirm that the target volume remains within the treatment portals (panel E).

Summary

Technological innovations continue to change the field of radiation oncology. The dual goals of improved treatment efficacy and reduced toxicity remain at the core of the discipline. Investigators will continue to explore the potential benefits that come with each new generation of advances and ultimately how they can improve patient care.

REFERENCES

The complete reference list is available online at www.expertconsult.com.

5

Tumor Response for Image-Guided Interventions

SOPHIE CHHEANG | BRADLEY PUA | DAVID C. MADOFF

ASSESSMENT AND VALIDATION

KEY POINTS

- The pathologic endpoint for percutaneous thermal or ethanol treatment of unresectable tumors is coagulation necrosis. Similarly, the goals of transarterial therapy are cell necrosis and apoptosis.
- Although specific follow-up imaging protocols differ among practitioners and institutions, contrast-enhanced computed tomography (CT), positron emission tomography (PET), and magnetic resonance imaging (MRI) are the primary imaging modalities used.
- Because tumors can recur months or years after treatment, long-term imaging follow-up should be instituted.
- Suspicious findings for residual or recurrent tumor include nodular, scattered, eccentric enhancement about the ablation zone, ablation zone that does not completely encompass the tumor, heterogeneous or focally increased 18-F fluorodeoxyglucose (FDG) uptake, and increasing or new marked FDG uptake.

Introduction

Histopathology is the gold standard for assessing the impact of locoregional treatment of tumors. However, this is impractical except in cases such as treatment preceding organ transplantation or excision. Generally, one must assess treatment response using imaging, in spite of its limitations. Each imaging modality has its own particular advantages and disadvantages. In this section, we will review the mechanisms of tissue injury, the classic pathologic findings, and the imaging correlates that are seen with percutaneous thermal ablation and transcatheter arterial ablation of tumors in various solid organs.

Mechanisms of Tissue Injury and Histopatholic Assessment

RADIOFREQUENCY ABLATION

Much of the literature on locoregional tumor treatment focuses on the effects of radiofrequency ablation (RFA) on liver tumors. The concepts are largely applicable to other thermal ablative treatments and to other organ systems. In essence, successful targeted treatment of tumor entails the induction of cell necrosis or programmed cell death (apoptosis) using extreme heat.

Gross pathologic evaluation of the thermally ablated tissue typically reveals a localized hardening of the parenchyma, with a central "white zone" of coagulation and a surrounding "red zone" of hyperemia (Figure 5-1). The zone of coagulation mostly consists of coagulative necrosis, wherein intact nuclei are absent within cells, a finding that is consistent with cell death.[1] Capsular retraction can be seen if the tumor is subcapsular. In the chronic stage, the necrotic tissue hardens, undergoes volume loss, and is often surrounded by a thick fibrous capsule.[2]

RFA functions by imparting frictional energy to a tissue causing destruction (coagulative necrosis) through heat energy. In the most common system, a monopolar system, this energy is created by a rapidly alternating voltage current between the electrode placed within the target lesion (active electrode) and dispersive pads (reference electrode) placed on the patient's skin. This alternating electrical current, with frequencies in the range of 375–500 kHz, results in agitation of the surrounding tissue ions, resulting in tissue heating.[3,4] The density of this electrical current is greatest immediately surrounding the electrode, and diminishes with distance. Coagulation necrosis will occur if the tissue temperature is elevated and maintained at 60°C for several seconds. Therapeutic RFA strives to heat tissues in the range of 60–100°C.[3]

Immediately following RFA, conventional hematoxylin and eosin stain will not demonstrate significant change to the tissue other than subtle distortion of sinusoidal architecture.[5] This apparent false negative can be mediated by the use of specialized staining agents, such as the nicotinamide adenine dinucleotide stain, which will highlight devitalized tissue.[6,7] In the chronic phase, cytolysis and obscuration of the nucleus will result in an amorphous eosinophilic hepatocyte. Infiltration by fibroblasts and mononuclear cells are also seen. Eventually, a capsule of granulation and fibrous tissue forms around the ablation zone.[8,9]

Heat Sink Phenomenon

The "heat sink" phenomenon has been most often described in the setting of RFA. It refers to the reduction in tissue temperature due to the conductive effects of adjacent vessels, typically described as 3 mm or greater in diameter. It is one explanation for suboptimal treatment results and distortion of the ablation zone.

Techniques to overcome the heat sink effect include pharmacologically decreasing blood flow, temporary vascular balloon occlusion, intraarterial embolization, and the Pringle maneuver. The latter entails temporarily occluding the hepatic artery and the portal vein by compression during RFA at laparotomy.[1]

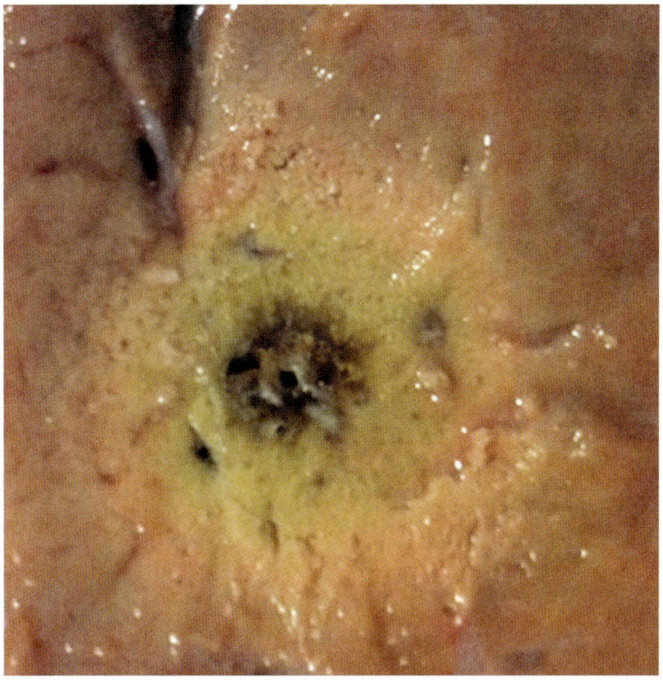

Figure 5-1 Gross pathologic specimen following unipolar microwave ablation (5 minutes at 65 Watts) of a resected bovine liver demonstrates the central white zone of coagulation (W) surrounded by a red zone of hyperemia (R). Central charring is also apparent.

CRYOABLATION

The mechanism of tissue injury in percutaneous cryoablation is variable and depends on several factors, including the rate and extent of freezing. Fast freezing rates result in direct tissue injury, whereby ice crystals form within cells. Slower rates result in ice crystals forming in the extracellular spaces resulting in cellular dehydration, leading to membrane damage.[10,11] Another mechanism of cryoablation-induced tissue injury is expansion of the microvasculature, leading to endothelial damage and subsequent thrombosis.[11,12] Additionally, sublethal freezing temperatures can lead to apoptosis (programmed cell death), a finding often seen in the periphery of the ablation zone.[11,13]

Like other thermal ablative technologies, coagulation necrosis is the desired histopathologic endpoint. Lethal temperature is considered to be within −40° to −50°C, although tumor cell survival has been reported after freezing to less than 50°C.[10] Most cryoablation protocols entail two freeze–thaw cycles, which compared to a single cycle, have been shown to result in a larger area of coagulation necrosis on pathologic specimens[14] and in a larger ice ball on imaging.[15]

Conceptually similar to the heat sink phenomenon described in RFA, cryoablation is limited by the delivery of warm blood by vessels adjacent to tumors, resulting in higher than desired temperatures. This is sometimes referred to as the "cold sink," and it can likewise result in variable size of the ablation zone and extent of the coagulation necrosis.[16,17]

MICROWAVE ABLATION

A relatively new treatment option for locoregional control of unresectable tumor is microwave ablation, which employs electromagnetic wavelengths in the frequency range of 900–2450 MHz. Rapid directional current changes in the microwave electrode causes surrounding water dipoles to oscillate, resulting in heat generation leading to cellular coagulative necrosis.[18] Unlike RFA, microwave ablation is not limited by the conductive properties of tissues, and therefore temperatures higher than 100°C can be more easily achieved, theoretically resulting not only in a larger area of coagulation necrosis but also in a more uniform ablation zone as the heat sink effect by regional vessels is less a factor.[18,19]

PERCUTANEOUS ETHANOL INJECTION

Owing to its ease of use and cost-effectiveness, percutaneous ethanol injection (PEI) remains a viable option in many parts of the world, particularly for the treatment of hepatocellular carcinoma (HCC) in cirrhotic livers. Coagulation necrosis is achieved by both direct and indirect mechanisms. Alcohol instillation will result in immediate cytoplasmic dehydration and protein denaturation. Indirectly, tumor death results following alcohol-induced vascular endothelial necrosis and subsequent thrombosis. Although it is not affected by heat sink, its success is largely limited by the difficulty in obtaining a uniform distillation of ethanol over a large tumor volume. As such, PEI is often not used in tumors with large size, heterogenous or dense composition, and in those without a capsule or pseudocapsule (the latter theoretically would aid in increasing intratumor concentration of alcohol).[20,21] Given the effectiveness and safety profile of RFA and other thermal ablative technologies, PEI has largely been replaced by these modalities in the treatment of HCC.[20,22]

TRANSCATHETER EMBOLIZATION

Exploiting the dual blood supply of the liver, transarterial therapy offers a unique adjunct to surgery and systemic chemotherapy. Most often described for nonresectable primary and secondary malignancies in the liver, transcatheter embolization can be further divided into three categories: arterial embolization, chemoembolization, and radioembolization. Extensive discussion of these techniques and their respective indications, risk profiles, and success rates is beyond the scope of this section. Detailed peer-reviewed literature abounds for the interested interventionalist. For our purposes, a short review of their mechanisms and imaging findings will be discussed.

Arterial Embolization

Akin to percutaneous thermoablative treatments, the goal of arterial embolization is cell necrosis. In this modality, occlusion of the terminal vasculature feeding the tumor results in ischemia and subsequent coagulation necrosis. Various agents have been used, including gelatin sponge, polyvinyl alcohol, or spherical embolic particles.[23] Extensive (>95%) coagulation necrosis can be seen within 3 days after complete embolization of the feeding artery (Figure 5-2).[24]

Chemoembolization

Technically similar to arterial embolization, chemoembolization also includes the injection of anticancer drugs with or without lipiodol (ethiodized oil) directly into the hepatic artery. In theory, the targeted delivery of chemotherapeutic agents would result in high local concentrations, thereby limiting the systemic toxicity associated with these drugs. However, there

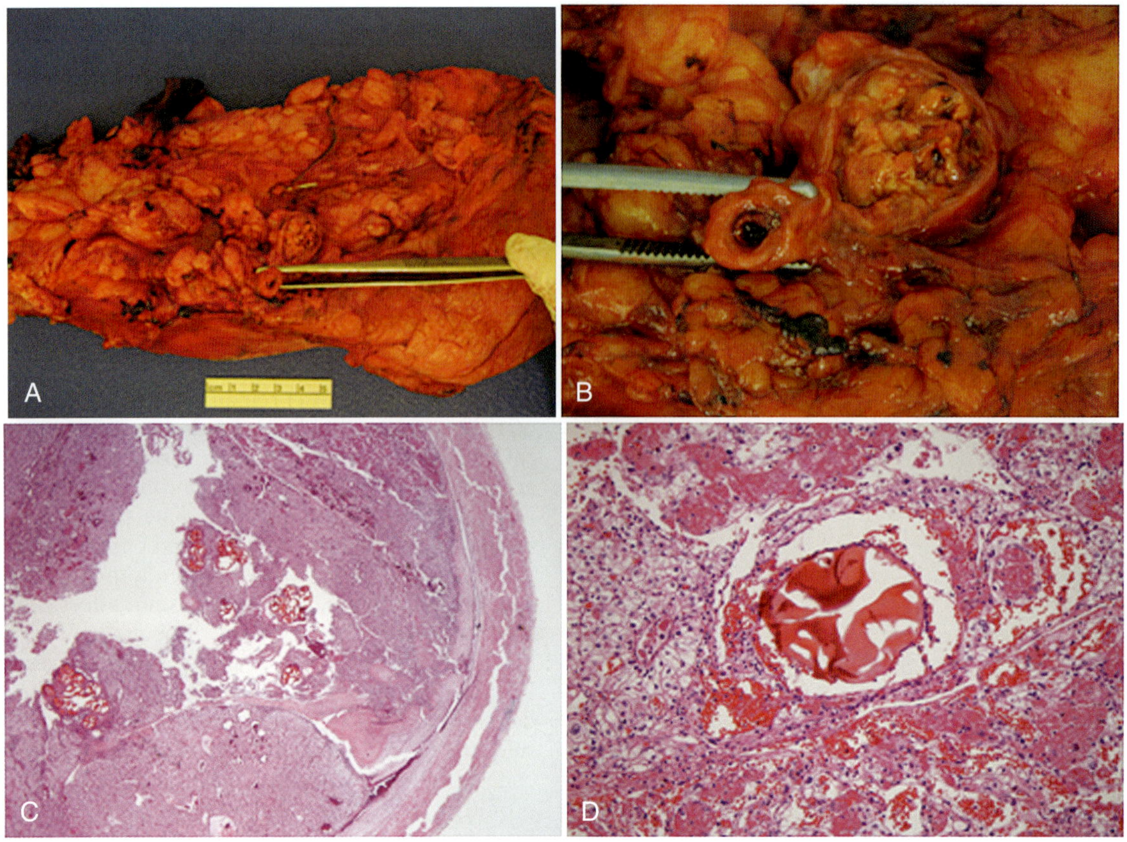

Figure 5-2 Gross and histologic evaluation of resected specimen following preoperative arterial embolization of renal cell carcinoma. (A) and (B) demonstrate a coil (*arrow*) within an occluded renal artery (*a*) adjacent to the vein (*v*). On low (C) and high (D) power hematoxylin–eosin stain, embolic (E) material is seen within the tumor microvasculature.

remains much debate as to the optimal chemotherapeutic to use, confounded by some authorities debating that bland embolization is equally as effective.[25,26] Special care is taken with patients with poor hepatic reserve as the toxicity of such high concentrations within the liver could result in irreversible hepatic failure if not properly controlled.

Radioembolization

Radioembolization represents a potential option in patients with limited hepatic reserve. To counter the potentially destructive effects of high concentrations of intrahepatic chemotherapy in the treatment of unresectable liver malignancies, radioembolization with yttrium-90 has been considered. Yttrium-90, a radioisotope with a half-life of approximately 64 hours, is a beta emitter with a maximum tissue penetration of about 1 cm. This limited tissue penetration allows extremely high levels of radiation (goal range of 125–150 Gy) to be selectively delivered to the tumors while regional hepatic and systemic toxicities are kept at acceptable levels.[23] Particles are delivered transarterially to the intended target in a fashion similar to other transarterial therapies. Appropriate dosing calculations need to be performed and pretherapy embolization of certain collateral vessels must be performed, which adds to the complexity of this therapy.

Imaging Assessment of Treatment Response

The primary modalities utilized to assess tumor and tissue response to locoregional treatment are computed tomography (CT), positron emission tomography (PET), magnetic resonance imaging (MRI), and ultrasonography. Each has its own advantages and limitations. With the increased utilization of ablative techniques, there is growing interest in identifying the optimal protocol for imaging follow-up.

At some centers, contrast-enhanced imaging is obtained immediately following completion of the procedure, especially for tumors with preprocedure enhancement. Otherwise, a common follow-up protocol is to obtain contrast-enhanced CT or MRI 1–6 weeks after the initial ablation and every 3–4 months thereafter. Some practitioners advocate more frequent follow-up in the first year following treatment, the time during which most local recurrence would manifest.[27]

Regardless of the imaging modality used, the margins, shape, and if applicable, enhancement pattern of the ablative zone should be described and the absence or presence of complications should be assessed. Because percutaneous treatments will inevitably include the ablated perilesional tissue, comparison of ablation zone size should be made to the cross-sectional measurements obtained postablation, rather than preablation.[27]

As with any technologically based treatment, newer-generation equipment as well as tuning and experience of current equipment will continue to improve. Thus, it is important to understand certain elements that are fundamental to ensuring an adequate ablation: (1) The imaging appearance and the amount of perilesional normal parenchyma to ablate to obtain an "A0" ablation; (2) The various thermal maps supplied with each electrode/cryoprobe in addition to changes of these zones when more than a single probe is utilized in unison; (3) Properly identify on postablation imaging both expected findings as well as what constitutes local tumor recurrence allowing prompt retreatment when necessary.

Much of this session will focus on CT, which is the most commonly used modality, although CT descriptors are often translatable to both MRI and ultrasonography.

COMPUTED TOMOGRAPHY

At most centers, CT is the primary modality used for immediate postprocedure imaging and follow-up after percutaneous ablation or transarterial embolization.[28] This is largely due to its wide availability, relatively low cost, and greater user experience. Depending on the target organ treated and pretreatment tumor imaging characteristics, the phase and protocol used when performing posttreatment follow-up will vary. For instance, when CT is performed following treatment of hepatic tumors, a common imaging protocol includes a triphasic CT that includes arterial, portal venous, and delayed phases allowing optimal comparison to pretreatment images.

Ablation Zone

In the immediate postablation setting, most practitioners obtain a scan to establish a new imaging baseline and to assess for treatment adequacy.

Following microwave ablation or RFA in the lung, ground-glass opacity surrounding the treated lesion is correlated with treatment success (Figure 5-3).[29-31] A circumferential margin of at least 5 mm is ideal to ensure complete tumor kill.[32] Conversely, areas lacking this opacity are associated with recurrence.[33,34] In solid organs, thermally ablated lesions generally appear as increased density in the center with poorly marginated peripheral hypoattenuation on immediate postprocedural noncontrast CT. Secondary to this poor margination, intravenous contrast administration is often used to more readily identify residual viable tumor, which can manifest as regions of enhancement, and therefore guide further therapy.[35]

When cryoablation is utilized in solid organs such as liver or kidney, the ice ball formed is often well depicted on intraprocedural CT as an area of low attenuation. It is important to understand that the entire circumference of this ice ball does

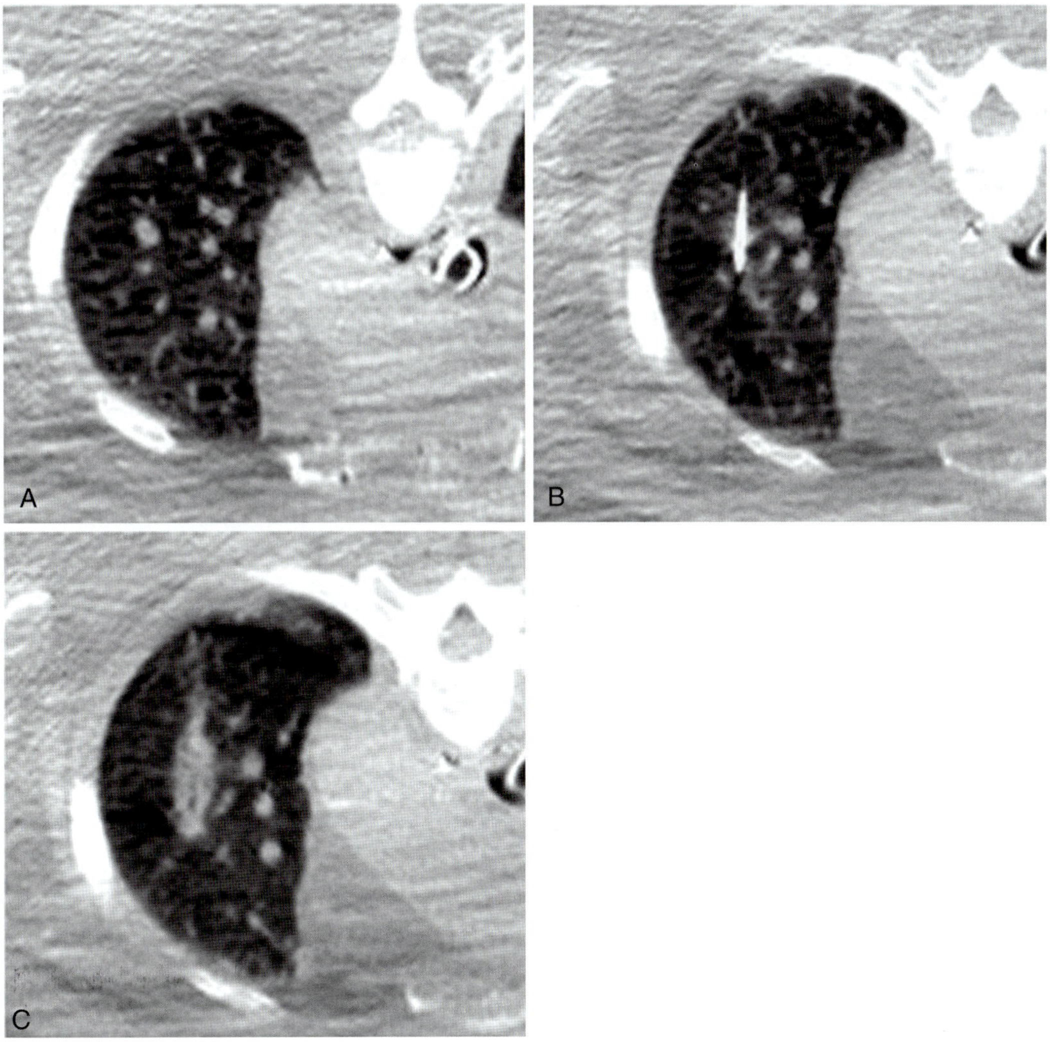

Figure 5-3 Preprocedure CT shows a round nodule in the left lung apex (A). The electrode is positioned within the center of the needle (B). Postablation CT shows the ground-glass ablation zone completely encompassing the prior nodule (C).

not often constitute "lethal" ice, or temperatures required to kill all viable tumor. This has been confirmed in a porcine model in liver, kidney, and lung.[17] The ice ball is often not well visualized in lung tissue secondary to the already low attenuation of the surrounding normal air-filled alveoli, making confirmation of complete treatment difficult. Therefore, it is of extreme importance to study and understand the isotherm maps for each cryoprobe used to both optimally treat the tumor and obtain adequate peritumoral margins.

Although most often spherical in shape, the RFA zone can also appear slender or irregular. This can be attributed to several etiologies, including the aforementioned heat sink effect, deformation by large hepatic vessels, insufficient radiofrequency power output, or movement of the electrode with patient breathing. Additionally, parenchymal infarction abutting the RFA zone can have the same attenuation as the ablated tissue, thus giving the impression of abnormal shape.[3]

If factors preclude obtaining an adequate treatment margin, such as juxtaposition to large portal or hepatic vessels in the liver, the patient should be closely observed with contrast-enhanced imaging for evidence of residual tumor.[36]

Contrast Enhancement

Contrast enhancement following treatment does not always correspond to residual tumor. In fact, enhancement of the periablation parenchyma seen on contrast-enhanced imaging is a pathologically proven benign physiologic response to thermal injury. Postulated etiologies for this phenomenon include psuedoenhancement, such as seen with renal cysts, or contrast escaping into surrounding tissues secondary to leaky capillaries secondary to treatment.[1] Initially, the response is reactive hyperthermia. This is followed by fibrosis and giant cell reaction.[37] This benign periablational enhancement, seen immediately following ablation, most commonly resolves within 1 month of treatment; however, it can be seen months afterwards owing to variability in imaging protocols, such as the injection rate and the scanning delay as well as perilesional inflammation.[3] This widespread variability complicates recommendations for appropriate timing of imaging follow-up.

In the kidney, minimal contrast enhancement (<20 HU) that is seen soon after ablation represents devitalized tissue on pathology,[38] compatible with treatment success.

Findings on contrast-enhanced CT has also been used to evaluate treatment outcome following RFA of unresectable pulmonary malignancies. Abtin et al. showed that imaging findings concerning for treatment recurrence include enhancement greater than pretreatment levels, nodular or central enhancement greater than 10 mm or 15 HU, or progressive enhancement (beyond 180 seconds) on multiphasic imaging.[39] As a corollary to this finding, Suh et al. showed that mean contrast enhancement dramatically decreases as soon as 1 month following treatment, which the authors attributed to injury to the local vasculature. Although this reduction in enhancement "recovered" somewhat on subsequent scans, the level of enhancement remained less than that seen on pretreatment scans, suggesting positive treatment outcome. This led the authors to conclude that CT densitometry can potentially play an important role in the noninvasive evaluation of thermally ablated pulmonary tumors.[40]

In the liver, an area of benign enhancement can be seen adjacent to the ablation zone. This is thought to be secondary to arterioportal shunting, which is often wedge-shaped or nodular in appearance. The pathogenesis is likely related to mechanical injury to the hepatic microvasculature from the treatment probe, which is seen both following biopsy and percutaneous ethanol ablation.[41,42] These shunts are typically small and resolve spontaneously, conferring little clinical significance.[43]

Benign periablational enhancement should be differentiated from the irregular peripheral enhancement that signals the presence of residual or recurrent tumor at the treatment margin. This pattern of enhancement is often described as scattered, nodular, or eccentric.[36,37] On CT, residual tumor is usually of high attenuation during the arterial phase and low attenuation during the portal venous and equilibrium phases, indicating washout. Because many hypovascular tumors exhibit delayed enhancement, portal venous or delayed imaging may be indicated.

Other Findings and Complications

Other imaging findings following thermal ablative therapy includes inflammatory stranding in the acute setting and fibrosis, scarring, and architectural distortion in the chronic setting. Scarring and fibrosis typically results in volume loss of the ablation zone, inclusive of the index tumor and of the treated parenchymal margin, over time. One study evaluating the CT findings following RFA of hepatocellular carcinoma reported mean volume changes of 79%, 50%, 27%, and 11%, at 1, 4, 16, and 19 months, respectively.[36] It is important to note that the absence of involution is not synonymous with treatment failure.

Air within the immediate postablation cavity or tract is a normal finding (Figure 5-4). This typically resolves within 1 month. Their presence is likely related either to the production of gas during tissue necrosis or to the introduction of air when the probe is advanced into the organ.[28,36] This finding often complicates diagnosis of superimposed infection. In one study, 4 of 14 patients with air pockets after microwave ablation was found to have hepatic abscesses, but all four patients presented with fever and pain that persisted for more than 2 weeks.[28] Of note, biliary obstruction has been reported as a predisposing factor for postprocedure hepatic abscess formation when transarterial chemoembolization of the liver is performed.[44]

Other reported complications from ablative therapy of liver malignancies include peritoneal hemorrhage, perforation of bowel loops, hepatic infarction, biloma formation, and tumor seeding along the needle track, the latter with an incidence rate approaching 0.6%, similar to that seen following percutaneous ethanol injection.[45–47] Of the potential complications, hepatic abscess, needle track seeding, and biloma do not occur in the immediate postprocedure period, and should be considered when suspicious findings are noted on follow-up imaging, either on ultrasonography, CT, or MRI. These findings include biliary tree anomalies, such as duct dilation, interval enlargement of the RFA zone (from the initial posttreatment baseline), or a "mural nodule in a cyst" pattern, representing the biloma and peripherally positioned portal vein.[3,48,49]

CT Imaging Considerations Pertinent to TACE

Iodized oil (Ethiodol or Lipiodol) is occasionally used in transcatheter arterial chemoembolization of liver tumors, and its unique imaging findings are discussed herein.

The association between iodized oil deposition and tumor necrosis has not been clearly described. Some studies suggest that dense retention of iodized oil has prognostic value, and

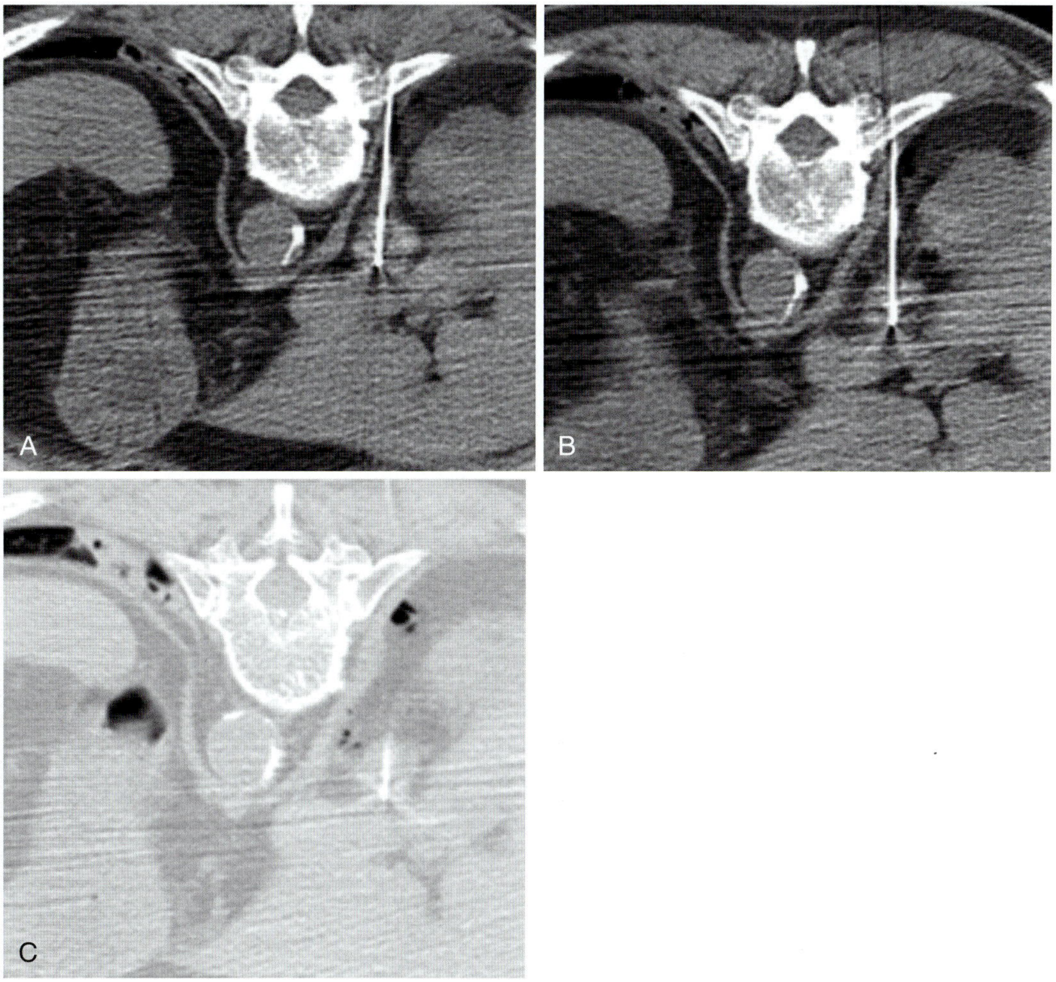

Figure 5-4 Periprocedural CT images demonstrate the ablation probe in the center of the right adrenal nodule (A, B). Air along the needle tract is noted, best seen in lung window (C).

indicates complete or near-complete tumor necrosis.[50,51] However, it has also been shown that iodized oil deposition does not always equate to cellular necrosis.[52] This may be due to the inherent difficulty in evaluating the post-TACE treatment zone on CT.

Beam hardening artifact from iodized oil can make detection of small foci of tumor difficult on CT, making it a less than ideal imaging modality to follow patients after TACE. The inherent high attenuation of iodized oil also limits evaluation of enhancement that could indicate the presence of viable cells.[53]

POSITRON EMISSION TOMOGRAPHY

The utility of PET in the evaluation of tumor burden or disease recurrence for a variety of neoplasms is well established. This is becoming true as well in the assessment of tumor recurrence following locoregional therapy of solid organ malignancies, particularly for the liver and the lung.[54,55]

Although not specific for cancer, 18-F fluorodeoxyglucose (FDG)-PET or PET/CT provides added diagnostic information as compared to CT or MRI imaging alone, as multiple reports have indicated.[54,56,57]

The optimal time to perform PET imaging is under question. One study suggests that the ideal time to do so is 24–48 hours following thermal ablation in both the liver and the lung, prior to the development of inflammatory changes that may manifest as false positives.[55] However, another study suggests that the optimum imaging time instead is at 3 months, thus limiting false positives secondary to uptake inflammation, which is generally maximal at 1 month.[58] Clearly, larger studies are indicated to establish the optimum imaging window and interval.

Ablation Zone

In the lung, it has been shown that after 2 months following thermal ablation, increased overall metabolic activity, central residual activity, or development of nodular activity about the ablation zone are signs suggestive of tumor recurrence.[39] In both the lung and the liver, periablation hyperemia can also demonstrate increased metabolic activity, but generally to a lesser extent than tumor.[55]

Likely more important than the standardized uptake value (SUV) value itself is the morphology of the uptake. Uptake that is diffuse, circumferential, and homogeneous more likely represents inflammation, whereas uptake that is heterogeneous and focal is likely related to tumor.[58]

FDG is excreted by the kidney and is generally not preferentially taken up by most renal cancers. As such, the utility of FDG-PET imaging in the postablation setting is equivocal in this case.[59] In the future, the development of tracers with avidity for renal cancers and the routine use of a diuretic to speed the excretion of the radiotracer could certainly shift the post-treatment imaging paradigm.[60]

Standardized Uptake Value

Although inflammation generally has lower SUVmax values than a tumor would, it can certainly manifest at levels of 5 and greater. Given that a maximum SUV value greater than 3 can reasonably be considered suspicious, the rate of false positivity could be unacceptably high. Therefore, maximum SUVs cannot by themselves serve as reliable differentiators of inflammation versus tumor. However, their temporal evolution may be more telling—that is, inflammation tends to show decreasing uptake whereas tumor tends to show the reverse.[58]

MAGNETIC RESONANCE IMAGING

MRI has been shown to have an 86% correspondence rate to CT in the evaluation of patients following thermal ablation of hepatic malignancies.[61] The choice of modality for imaging follow-up is often center specific. MRI is currently of limited utility following follow-up of thermally ablated lung lesions, secondary to motion and air artifacts. When MRI is utilized in other solid organs, the following sequences are usually obtained: unenhanced T1- and T2-weighted, and contrast-enhanced T1-weighted dynamic imaging.

Ablation Zone

In the liver, unenhanced T1- and T2-weighted sequences usually demonstrate heterogeneous signal intensity within the ablated zone, a variability that is both due to the uneven evolution of coagulation necrosis and to the host response to thermal injury over time.[35] The T1 signal is known to increase with time.[3] However, in the chronic stage, the radiofrequency zone typically manifests as homogeneous high T1 and low T2 signal intensity.[62]

Contrast Enhancement

Regardless of the technique used, viable tumor in the solid organ typically manifests as early intense enhancement.[63] Residual enhancement following arterial embolization is postulated to be related to collateralization or portal vein blood supply.[24] Granulation tissue is another potential confounding factor for peripheral enhancement, and is related to increased capillary permeability.[64]

MRI Imaging Considerations Pertinent to TACE

Compared to CT, MR imaging is likely of greater utility after TACE. In addition to the lack of ionizing radiation, it is unaffected by artifacts produced by iodized oil.

With histopathology as the gold standard, one study showed that the sensitivity and specificity of MRI (43% and 75%) is greater than that of CT (36% and 57%) in evaluating for residual or recurrent tumor following hepatic transarterial chemoembolization (TACE).[63] Another study reported a sensitivity of 72% and specificity of 91% for CT.[65] This apparently wide range in sensitivity and specificity is postulated secondary to varying tumor size and presence of arterioportal shunting as a cause of pseudolesions, resulting in false positive diagnosis.

Diffusion-Weighted Imaging

Diffusion-weighted MR imaging holds promise in evaluating the presence of viable cells following treatment. Cellular necrosis leads to increased membrane permeability, which allows water molecules to move freely, resulting in increased apparent diffusion coefficient (ADC) values.[66] Still largely within the realm of research, DWI imaging has not gained widespread acceptance in clinical practice, but its potential is clear.

ULTRASONOGRAPHY

Although ultrasonography has the advantage of not exposing the patient to ionizing radiation, in the United States it plays a limited role in the peri- and postprocedural evaluation of tumor response. Therefore, it will only be briefly discussed here.

The utility of grayscale ultrasonography in the thermal ablative therapies lie primarily in its ability to guide the placement of the treatment probe in real time. This would be pertinent only to solid organ tumors or peripheral lung lesions.

The "transient hyperechoic zone" seen during and immediately after RFA refers to the zone of increased echogenicity within and surrounding a tumor. Sometimes referred to as a "cloud" of echogenicity, it generally persists for approximately 30–90 minutes, and the physiology is thought related to the production of microbubbles of water vapor and other cellular products that result from tissue vaporization.[67,68]

As a modality to assess treatment response, ultrasonography is limited by its inability to adequately differentiate viable tissue from necrotic tissue. Postablation ultrasonography findings have not been shown to correlate sufficiently with the extent of tissue necrosis.[37]

There are, however, promising results for ultrasonographic contrast agents in detecting the presence of intratumoral microvasculature—viable tumor.[69] In general, residual viable tissue manifests as hypervascular foci within the treatment zone. In the absence of ultrasonographic contrast agents, these foci are generally better recognized with other imaging modalities, such as CT or MRI, as previously discussed.[61,70-73]

Conclusion

Although the technologies underlying percutaneous ablation and transcatheter arterial therapies have existed for many years, their use in the management of unresectable malignancies is only recently incorporated in patient management on a routine basis. Standard treatment protocols and follow-up imaging regimens remain to be delineated. Technological advances, treatment considerations, and controversies pertinent to the malignancies involving each organ system will be discussed further and in greater detail throughout this book.

REFERENCES

The complete reference list is available online at www.expertconsult.com.

6

Trends in Basic Science Research in Interventional Radiology

NANOTECHNOLOGY, STEM CELL, RNAi, AND RADIOGENOMICS

EDWARD W. LEE | MINZHI XING | STEPHEN T. KEE

Introduction

Research in interventional radiology has historically been driven by innovation and technological development leading to the conceptualization, investigation, validation, and application of a myriad of novel procedures into clinical practice.[1] The development of new techniques and therapies is critical to ensuring the continued success and relevance of interventional radiology as a subspecialty.[3] This has been reflected in the vision statement of the Society of Interventional Radiology Interventional Oncology Task Force, which states that there should be enhanced integration of image-guided oncologic technologies by 2015, along with new developments in genomics, proteomics, molecular imaging, and nanotechnology.[4] The rapid evolution of such transformative technologies has necessitated an expansion in the scope of scientific knowledge and technical skills required of interventional physician-scientists.[5] This chapter summarizes the background and current developments in these areas and outlines potential future research of particular relevance to interventional oncology (Figure 6-1).

Nanotechnology

Nanotechnology refers to the design, creation, and manipulation of structures on the submicroscopic scale, usually below 100 nm in size.[6] The use of nanotechnology in medicine, "nanomedicine" has demonstrated exciting potential for clinical use. The majority of current research is focused toward (1) novel methods of imaging and diagnostic techniques, (2) antimicrobial therapy, (3) micro-robotics, (4) cell repair, and (5) delivery of therapy through minimally invasive means.[7] More specifically, potential applications of nanotechnology in interventional radiology (IR) have been described in the areas of drug delivery, thermotherapy, vascular interventions, and implantable devices.

NANOTECHNOLOGY FOR SYSTEMIC AND LOCAL DRUG DELIVERY

Nanoparticles for drug delivery are engineered systems in the nanometer size range, and drugs can be attached to the surface of such particles or entrapped or encapsulated within them.[8] The advantages associated with nanoparticle use lie in its ability to increase drug efficiency and improve the therapeutic index of currently available drugs, reducing drug toxicity to improve side-effect profiles,[9,10] and controlled release to achieve therapeutic levels for an extended period of time.[11–13] They can also improve drug stability and solubility[9] and allow targeted drug delivery.[14] The potential to accommodate multiple types of drug molecules may allow for the development of systems for combined therapeutic and imaging applications.[12,14] The need for targeted drug delivery is particularly evident in interventional oncology, where it would be preferable for tumor to be exposed to high drug concentrations, while reducing systemic toxicity. As nanoparticles are able to pass through the fenestrations of the highly permeable tumor vasculature and are limited by tumor lymphatic systems, preferential collection of nanoparticles within the tumor interstitium may be achieved, and has been termed the enhanced permeability and retention (EPR) effect.[8,15,16]

The development of controlled or triggered intratumoral drug release in systemic chemotherapy is desirable as it can result in optimum drug delivery for longer periods, thus increasing efficacy of treatment.[11] Such targeting has extended beyond the use of the passive EPR effect, and active targeting based on molecular recognition of tumor has been described.[8] In terms of local drug delivery, direct intratumoral injection of chemotherapy-loaded nanoparticles in tumor-bearing mouse models has been observed to increase efficiency in impeding tumor development.[17] Local intratumoral injection of radiosensitizers to enhance radiotherapy such as gadolinium has similarly shown promise in inhibiting tumor growth and increasing life expectancy.[18] In the area of local thrombolysis of particular relevance to IR, nanoparticles modified with streptokinase and targeted to fibrin have been described.[19,20] Marsh et al. developed fibrin-targeted nanoparticles surface conjugated to streptokinase in vitro and found that they were able to lyse 90% of clots within 60 minutes of exposure, with substantially more potent fibrinolytic activity and the same degree of thrombolysis as a 1000-fold greater dose of free streptokinase.[19]

ULTRASOUND-MEDIATED DRUG DELIVERY

When used in combination with systemically administered encapsulated therapies such as drug-loaded microbubbles or nanoparticles, locally applied ultrasound has been shown to enhance drug transport through tissues and across cell membranes.[21,22] As a drug delivery method, it is noninvasive and may be controlled and focused locally, thereby limiting the drug interactions to the target tissue and sparing surrounding

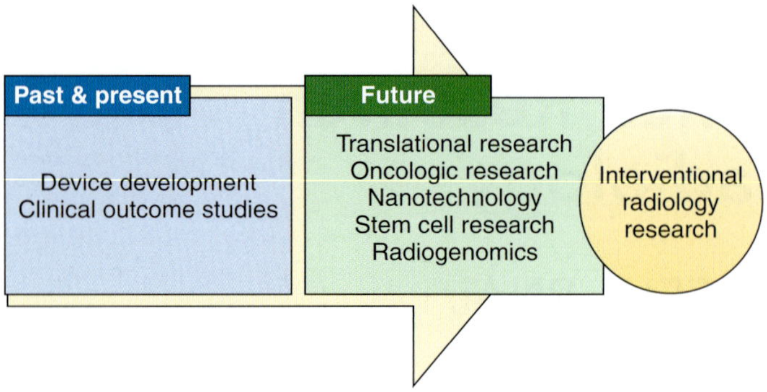

Figure 6-1 Schematic of changes in interventional radiology (IR) research. The IR research trends in the past and present mainly include the device development and clinical outcome in both retrospective and prospective studies. A new direction of IR research is IR incorporating and understanding more biology and pathophysiology behind the procedures and techniques, which includes translational research in vitro and in vivo with emphasis on oncologic research. Animal research will take a huge role in future IR research. IR will expand a spectrum of research involving nanotechnology, stem cell research, and theranostics, such as radiogenomics.

normal tissues from unwanted side effects.[21] An added major advantage is the targeting of deep tissues and the ability to be used through intraluminal, endoscopic, or percutaneous means to reach almost any site.[23] Dayton et al.[24] found in an in vitro study that ultrasonography, in combination with nanodroplets carrying the cytotoxic drug paclitaxel, resulted in significant cell death. In vivo studies using low-frequency ultrasonographic and polymeric micelles and liposomes encapsulating doxorubicin or fluorouracil have found statistically significant decreases in tumor size[25] and increased effects of drug on tumor growth.[26] Rapoport et al.[23] described the potential for multifunctional nanoparticles to function both as drug carriers and ultrasound contrast agents for enhanced visualization. Long-lasting contrast provided enhanced tumor visualization in conjunction with ultrasonography-mediated enhanced release of encapsulated doxorubicin and intracellular uptake of drug from nanoparticles.

NANOTECHNOLOGY AND THERMAL THERAPY

The use of thermal therapeutics such as radiofrequency ablation has become established clinical practice for certain tumors including solitary renal masses.[28] The minimally invasive nature of thermotherapy allows for treatment of tumors in sites where surgical resection is clinically impractical. However, this requires sufficient depth and penetration of tissues by the heating element. Current heating techniques do not discriminate between tumor and normal tissue, giving rise to potential damage to surrounding structures.[29] In addition, heating tissue to different degrees has different effects—hyperthermia (40°C–42°C) may render cells more susceptible to the cytotoxic effects of chemotherapy or radiation and can induce some degree of apoptosis,[30,31] whereas thermal ablation (>46°C) has a direct cytotoxic effect on cells, and can be used as a monotherapy for destruction of tumor cells.[31] A combination of hyperthermic effect of thermal ablation and use of nano-carrier of cytotoxic drugs may have enhanced therapeutic effects on the locoregional treatment of solid tumors, including hepatocellular carcinoma (HCC).

MAGNETIC THERMOTHERAPY

The capacity of magnetic nanoparticles to absorb energy from an alternating magnetic field and convert it to heat, forms the basis of magnetic thermotherapy.[31] The feasibility of this technique has been demonstrated in patients with locally recurrent prostate cancer.[32,33] Iron oxide nanoparticles in suspension were injected transperineally into the prostate gland of patients under transrectal ultrasound, and an alternating magnetic field was applied. Because of retention of particles within the gland, serial heat treatments could be performed after a single injection, with the achievement of hyperthermic temperatures achieved at relatively low field strengths. The technique could potentially be used as a combination therapy along with irradiation and implantation of iodine-125 (^{125}I) seeds, as the thermal dose achieved during the study would prove effective in such a setting.[33] The intraarterial route has also been examined as a means for selective magnetic hyperthermia of tumors. In a rabbit model for renal carcinoma, Takamatsu et al.[35] investigated the possibility of intraarterial selective hyperthermia using a transcatheter arterial embolization technique with a mixture of commercially available nano-sized magnetic particles (Ferucarbotran) and the embolic material lipiodol. Injection of this mixture into the renal artery under fluoroscopic guidance and exposure to an alternating-current magnetic field increased intratumoral temperatures to 45°C, which were sufficient for hyperthermia but not ablation. However, given the relative hypovascularity of the tumor, the authors hypothesized that much stronger selective hyperthermia might be achievable in a hypervascular tumor such as HCC.[35]

RADIOFREQUENCY ABLATION

Studies in the use of RFA in combination with chemotherapy for malignant tumors have shown improved efficacy as compared to either treatment alone.[4,36–39] Intravenous administration of a single dose of adjuvant liposomal doxorubicin in the rat breast cancer model increased the extent of coagulation necrosis induced with RFA compared with RFA alone.[38] Similar increases in tumor destruction have been seen in the use of liposomal doxorubicin in combination with RFA in a variety of focal hepatic tumors.[39] Ahmed et al.[37] studied the independent effects of three different chemotherapeutic agents, nanoparticle size, and liposomal circulation time on the same combinational RFA therapy in a rat breast tumor model. It was found that all combinations of RFA with liposomal chemotherapy resulted in significantly greater tumor necrosis than RFA alone. The extent of tumor destruction was greatly influenced by nanoparticle size, with liposomes 100 nm in diameter achieving optimal results. In addition, the use of a pegylated liposomal preparation with prolonged circulation time was demonstrated to significantly influence intratumoral drug accumulation and coagulation necrosis.[37] Thus, increasing drug circulation time and modifying nanoparticle properties may further enhance the efficacy of existing RFA and chemotherapeutic combinations.

NANOTECHNOLOGY IN VASCULAR INTERVENTIONS

Conventional drug-eluting stents function via disruption and delay of the natural healing response and limiting the growth of neointima, making late in-stent thrombosis a major concern[40] particularly in more complex lesions such as those in peripheral arterial disease. Thus, the development of endovascular stents with improved clinical characteristics remains imperative.[41] Nanoparticle-eluting stents have been described and could provide a novel platform for delivery of therapeutic agents to the vessel wall.[42] By utilizing electrodeposition coating to create a thin, uniform layer of biodegradable polymeric nanoparticles on stent surfaces, multiple agents within various nanoparticles may be delivered using a single stent.[42] Intracellular uptake of nanoparticles and retention within the cytoplasm or extracellular space may allow for sustained drug delivery within cells. Such a stent has been tested in a porcine coronary artery model, where it demonstrated good biocompatibility and efficient drug delivery, and could potentially be used in the delivery of proteins or genes that inhibit inflammation, smooth muscle cell proliferation, and thrombosis.[42] Polymer-based drug-eluting stents remain in contact with the arterial wall indefinitely, and the polymer is thought to induce local inflammation and potentially lead to late stent thrombosis and restenosis.[27,43] This could potentially be solved by the development of a biocompatible, noninflammatory medium for drug delivery to replace the standard polymer, and one study has demonstrated the efficacy and biocompatibility of a paclitaxel-eluting porous carbon-carbon nanoparticle-coated nonpolymeric cobalt chromium stent in a porcine model.[43]

The use of local and systemic intraarterial drug-laden nanoparticles has been reported to have good outcomes in tumor treatment.[44,45] Concurrent use of balloon angioplasty has been demonstrated to cause a marked increase in vascular permeability, thereby allowing nanoparticles to selectively enter the arterial wall at specific sites.[44] Doxorubicin-encapsulated nanoparticles administered intravenously have been shown to accumulate at sites of balloon stretch injury, with resultant inhibition of vascular smooth muscle proliferation and dose-dependent suppression of neointimal growth. Such an effect was not observed with administration of doxorubicin alone,[44] and the approach shows potential for increased penetration and localization of therapy. Combining ionic or antibody targeting with local delivery of drug-laden nanoparticles to the vessel wall may deliver sufficient drug concentrations to prevent restenosis while avoiding systemic toxicity.[46,47] A study involving the modification of nanoparticles for a resultant positive surface charge has demonstrated enhanced local uptake of such nanoparticles into the arterial wall, possibly because of increased ionic interactions with the negatively charged glycosaminoglycan-rich arterial wall.[46] In addition, in vitro studies by Lanza et al.[47] showed that tissue factor-targeted perfluorocarbon nanoparticles containing doxorubicin or paclitaxel significantly inhibited the proliferation of vascular smooth muscle cells in culture, with the functionalized nanoparticles showing enhanced potency compared with nontargeted nanoparticles or free drug. In addition, these nanoparticles could be formulated with gadolinium and were readily detectable on T1–weighted spin echo imaging, whereas quantification of the nanoparticles was possible using 19F spectroscopy. It follows that targeted therapeutic nanoparticles could potentially provide visualizable and quantifiable therapy to prevent restenosis (Figure 6-2).[47]

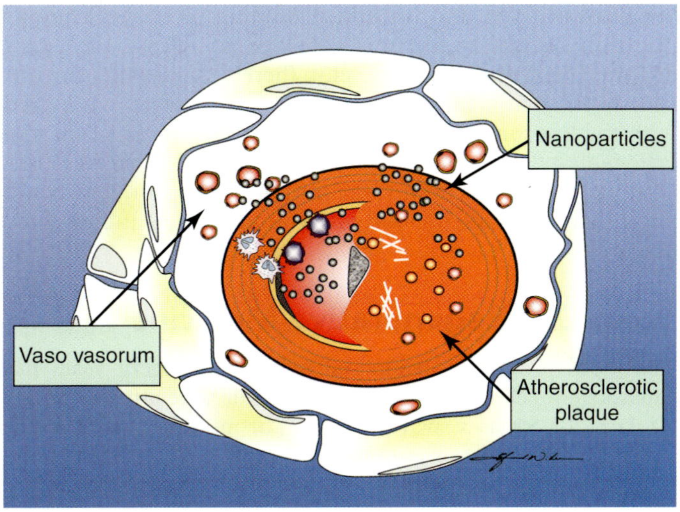

Figure 6-2 Nanotechnology in vascular intervention. Nanoparticles conjugated or encasing antiinflammatory drug can be delivered either percutaneously or endovascularly to the area of severe atherosclerosis. These nanoparticles travel through both the main vessel involved in atherosclerotic process and the vaso vasorum surrounding that vessel to effectively decrease the atherosclerotic process. Because of their size and potency, nanoparticles can affect all types of cells and matrix involved in atherosclerosis.

NANOTECHNOLOGY IN IMPLANTABLE DEVICES AND HEMOSTASIS

The use of nanoparticles loaded with dexamethasone as a drug-delivery coating for implantable devices has been shown to reduce local postimplantation inflammatory response and may potentially improve biocompatibility.[48] Several studies have examined the surface modification of nanoparticles with heparin without loss of the anticoagulant properties of heparin, and delivery of such nanoparticles has demonstrated prolonged clotting time of more than 200 seconds, as compared to 16.5 seconds with unmodified nanoparticles. Such an approach could potentially be used in the coating of interventional vascular devices, and hydrophilic surface modification of silicon catheters using a polymeric phospholipid monolayer has been shown to cause decreased platelet adhesion.[49] The potential for nanotechnology to improve hemostasis has been shown through the development of a novel self-assembling peptide that establishes a nanofiber barrier when applied and achieves local hemostasis within 15 seconds,[50] allowing the sealing of wounds in any wet ionic environment in the body. Its efficacy in achieving rapid hemostasis in brain, spinal cord, liver, skin, and even transection of the femoral artery has been demonstrated in a rat model such that bleeding could be stopped without the use of any conventional hemostatic methods such as pressure or cauterization. Additionally, the nontoxic, nonimmunogenic solution is also broken down into amino acids to serve as building blocks for tissue repair.[50]

ULTRASOUND-MEDIATED VASCULAR THERAPY

The application of focused ultrasound has been demonstrated to enhance clot lysis when used in conjunction with thrombolytic agents.[51–54] In addition, the use of microbubble-based contrast agents has also been shown to be effective for ultrasound-enhanced clot lysis,[55] even in the absence of a thrombolytic agent.[56,57] Tiukinhoy-Laing et al. showed that the use of echogenic liposomes in conjunction with ultrasound produced effective thrombolysis with the thrombolytic agent tissue plasminogen activator (tPA),[58] with retention of fibrin-specific properties of tPA and liposomal binding to fibrin. The application of ultrasound was observed to release the agent and mechanically disrupt the clot, thereby facilitating thrombolysis,[58,59] with improved thrombolytic effect compared with the liposomal drug alone or free tPA.[59] In addition, the echogenicity of the liposomes allowed them to serve as a contrast agent for improved visualization of the clot, and could potentially facilitate focused ultrasound therapy and directed drug release.[58,59]

Stem Cell Regenerative Medicine

The rapid progress in stem cell research in recent years has caused stem cell therapy to garner considerable attention, particularly for diseases such as diabetes or multiple sclerosis that are difficult to treat or considered incurable.[60] The role of the interventionalist in stem cell therapy lies mostly in targeted stem cell delivery via percutaneous, selective intravenous or intraarterial techniques, although this could potentially expand to include procedures prior to stem cell implantation such as the creation of engraftment territories or improvement of engraftment conditions via thermal ablation.[60]

Stem cells are capable of dividing and self-renewing indefinitely as well as differentiating into one or more cell types.[61] Embryonic stem cells (obtained from the inner cell mass of the blastocyst) are pluripotent, while adult stem cells (found in adult somatic tissue) are multipotent cells with more limited differentiation ability and the capacity to develop into cells of a specific organ, tissue, or organ system to potentially fulfill corresponding functions. Adult stem cells may be harvested from bone marrow, adipose tissue, and umbilical cord blood as autologous cells and are generally free of ethical controversy. Numerous studies have demonstrated the ability of stem cells to repair damaged tissue and restore function that would otherwise be irreversibly lost,[62,63] fueling further research for the use of such cells in lieu of organ transplantation or in the absence of alternative treatments. However, it has been noted that the type and extent of experimental data varies considerably between differing fields of clinical and experimental stem cell applications and across specific entities.[42] Since discrepancies in results within the field have mostly been attributed to methodologic differences such as variations in stem cell delivery route and timing, further in-depth knowledge in the areas of stem cell properties, harvesting, cell trafficking, engraftment bed receptiveness, engraftment efficiency and subsequent engraftment monitoring has been posited to be critical for future success in stem cell therapy.[42]

A noteworthy but poorly examined area of stem cell research is the utilization of stem cells as a medium for gene and drug delivery, based on the fact that viable stem cells have the ability to adjust, multiply, migrate, and communicate with adjacent cells. For example, Shah et al.[64] found that injected mouse neural precursor cells were able to migrate to the contralateral brain hemisphere and deliver cytotoxic tumor therapy to glioma foci and hence slow tumor growth.[64,65]

THE ROLE OF INTERVENTIONAL RADIOLOGY IN STEM CELL THERAPY

Successful stem cell transplantation generally involves adequate stem cell harvesting, trafficking to the target area (including cell homing and interstitial migration), full differentiation, and significant, ideally sustainable, contribution to organ function. Targeted stem cell delivery via interventional techniques may help overcome challenges currently associated with stem cell homing, which involves directed blood dispersion of stem cells. In the setting of liver cirrhosis and fibrosis, selective and direct stem cell release to the target organ by transcatheter intraarterial delivery may overcome potential mechanical barriers that have been postulated to exist for nonselective stem cell delivery techniques.[66] In particular, the recommendation by a renowned stem cell expert of recipient organ perfusion with donor cells "via a radiologically placed catheter" has been noted.[66] Further clinical studies have shown that hepatic regeneration may be enhanced with portal venous infusion of bone marrow-derived stem cells into portal vein branches prior to portal vein embolization and partial hepatectomy.[67] Furthermore, because nonselective systemic routes of administration have been implicated in some of the previously mentioned inconsistencies in experimental results due to differentiation of stem cells, the relevance of interventional radiology in performing selective delivery techniques (such as transportal administration) has been highlighted.[68–70]

CELL-BASED THERAPY FOR DIABETES MELLITUS

Although pancreatic transplant been used as a therapeutic option for the treatment of medically refractory diabetes mellitus, its limited donor supply, significant morbidity, and associated lifelong immunosuppression confer severe risks and disadvantages for the patient. In contrast, cell-based therapy is minimally invasive and more cost-effective, although the initial use of islet cells from brain-dead donors still possessed the problem of limited donor supply.[60] In evaluating the possible delivery routes of stem cell injection (including percutaneous intrasplenic, subcapsular renal, intraomental, subcutaneous, and into the celiac artery), intraportal venous delivery for cell engraftment has been described as technically most feasible, efficient, safe, and least complicated because of easy access.[74] This has particular implications in IR since percutaneous access to the portal vein for islet cell transplantation has replaced previous invasive surgical laparotomy-based cannulation,[75,76] with the preferred method being ultrasonographic guidance for puncture with the adjunct of fluoroscopic guidance.[77] It has been shown that intraportal venous infusion of islet cells may achieve effective control of blood glucose in type 1 diabetics for 1 year before disease recurrence.[78] Possible complications such as the occurrence of tract hemorrhage and portal venous thrombosis have been ascribed to the intraprocedural increase in portal venous pressure.[78,79]

The use of stem cell-based therapy has been examined in animal models, but has encountered problems because of the lack of a clearly identifiable type of pancreatic stem cell. Although embryonic stem cells have been transformed into cells with β cell properties, it is difficult to ascertain if these cells are capable of producing insulin or simply absorb it.[80,81] However, studies using rodent models have successfully shown success in curing or improving diabetes[82,83] and allowing the differentiation of hematopoietic and bone marrow-derived stem cells into functional islet cells.[84,85] As with other organs, pre-cell-transplantation in vitro differentiation of toti- or pluripotent cells into endocrine pancreatic cells appears most efficient.[60] The use of percutaneous intraportal venous delivery, as was observed in islet cell transplantation, appears to best integrate technical feasibility and low complication rates with engraftment efficiency.[60]

PERIPHERAL ARTERIAL DISEASE

Peripheral arterial disease has an estimated prevalence of 4.2%–35%[86] and progresses to critical limb ischemia in 4.3%–9.6% of cases, conveying quality of life indexes similar to terminal cancer patients and the eventual undesirable outcome of amputation.[86] For the investigation of treatment of critical limb ischemia, endothelial progenitor cells harvested from peripheral blood or bone marrow have been tested in numerous clinical trials. The initial study in 2002[87] in patients with chronic limb ischemia demonstrated the safety and efficacy of intramuscular injection of bone marrow cells and the achievement of significantly improved ankle-brachial pressure indexes, transcutaneous oxygen pressures, and pain-free walking times, with reduced rest pain at follow-up. Numerous further studies confirmed these results, with several showing improvement of endothelial function and increased blood perfusion as assessed with 99mTc tetrofosmin perfusion scintigraphy.[88–90] However, current data for stem cell utilization in peripheral vascular disease is limited by the lack of randomized controlled studies and longer-term clinical follow-up, and although the majority of studies chose the intramuscular route for delivery, the most efficient mode of stem cell delivery, optimal dose, and cell type and subtype for treatment of critical limb ischemia remain uncharacterized and should be the focus of future studies.

FUTURE PROSPECTS FOR STEM CELL RESEARCH

The distinct trends in stem cell research may define the future role of the interventional radiology in the area of stem cell therapy, with the most relevant areas of research being stem cell engraftment kinetics, optimal administration timing, and optimal delivery routes[60] via minimally invasive techniques. In addition, the use of thermal ablation and devascularization of malignant or dysfunctional tissue by RFA may potentially increase stem cell engraftment bed fertility, with periablational hyperemia providing the vascular environment for optimal stem cell trafficking to target areas and subsequent stem cell engraftment. An additional area for future investigation is the role of transarterial catheter-directed embolization for devascularization of dysfunctional tissue, with subsequent targeted transarterial cell delivery to improve stem cell trafficking efficiency compared to current peripheral intravenous cell administration techniques.[60]

RNA Interference and Small Interfering RNA

RNA interference (RNAi) is a sequence-specific, posttranscriptional gene silencing mechanism mediated by double-stranded RNA (dsRNA) that reduces the expression of endogenously expressed proteins. Such a mechanism may be harnessed for highly specific silencing of mutant, exogenous, or aberrant genes, and to develop novel drugs for the treatment of a wide range of diseases.[91] The development of RNAi for therapy is based on knowledge of small RNA biogenesis pathways, and the two main types of small RNAs involved in gene silencing are microRNAs (miRNAs) and small interfering RNAs (siRNAs). siRNA-based drugs have distinct advantages over conventional small-molecule or protein-based drugs, including high specificity, higher potency, and reduced toxicity.[92] However, barriers to the translational application of such drugs and the overall attainment of efficient RNAi such as specificity for the target gene, delivery to cell or tissues, durability of RNAi activity, and stability of the target mRNA and encoded protein have become increasingly evident.[92] Further important considerations for therapeutic RNAi are that gene silencing approaches rarely remove 100% of the transcript, off-target silencing may occur, and that each organ, cell type, and target transcript presents unique challenges.[91]

RNAi APPLICATIONS IN ONCOLOGY

In the treatment of cancer, siRNAs could possibly be used to inhibit expression of not only receptor tyrosine kinases but also antiapoptotic genes or other survival factors, tumor-promoting growth factors and the key participants in their signaling pathways, or genes essential for cell proliferation, including cyclins.[92] RNAi technology may be used to suppress oncogenic transcription factors that regulate key cell growth-promoting pathways and are not considered viable conventional drug targets, with the potential for these new drug targets to be designed to eliminate cancer stem cells within a tumor or within chemotherapy- or radiotherapy-resistant tumors. Although siRNA drugs are highly potent and not susceptible to drug-efflux, duration of gene silencing is limited by the dilution of siRNAs that occurs with each cell division, and in proliferating tumor cells, gene silencing lasts for less than a week. However, this may be long enough to suppress key oncogenes, antiapoptotic genes, or drug resistance genes to cause irreversible tumor cell death.[92]

RNAi APPLICATIONS IN TARGETING HEPATIC CANCERS

The liver was one of the first organs targeted in the development of RNAi-based therapies for cancer. Stable nucleic acid-lipid particles (SNALPs), a form of liposome, have been used to deliver siRNAs to suppress ApoB expression in the liver of both mouse and nonhuman primates, leading to impressive decreases in blood cholesterol levels.[93] The use of SNALPs to target PLK1 (a cell cycle protein crucial for the activating phosphorylation of many cell cycle proteins) led to cell cycle arrest and tumor cell apoptosis.[94] SNALP-formulated PLK1 siRNA treatment administered in mice with hepatic tumors showed significant improvements in survival.[95] An additional hepatic cancer application has been described using SNALPs to simultaneously deliver siRNAs to kinesin spindle protein (KSP) and vascular endothelial growth factor (VEGF). KSP is required for cell division, and VEGF is required for tumor cell growth. A Phase I trial using this approach has reported evidence of RNAi activity in biopsied tissue, and these initial studies, along with the first report of RNAi activity from exogenously applied siRNA complexes,[96] serve as important milestones in the development of RNAi delivery systems as cancer therapeutics.

OBSTACLES TO RNAi-BASED THERAPEUTICS IN ONCOLOGY

Although RNAi appears promising for use in cancer therapy, several barriers to its clinical use have been described.[97] Extracellular fluids contain RNA-degrading ribonucleases that cause siRNA breakdown, and this has been noted to be the key obstacle in many delivery approaches.[92] Although endocytosis via cell-surface receptors serves as a first step for entry into cells, a viable strategy for the release of RNA from the endosome needs to be developed.[92] By changing the nucleotide linkages at the ends to phosphorothioates that are resistant to exonuclease cleavage and using chemical modifications similar to those that reduce off-target effects, the half-life of siRNA in extracellular fluids and serum may be extended to several days without significantly affecting gene silencing activity.[92,98]

An additional major barrier to RNAi-based therapeutics is intracellular delivery, since siRNA does not cross cell plasma membranes and is not taken up by cells, thereby presenting a problem in terms of systemic intracellular delivery, particularly for disseminated disease.[92] Multiple delivery strategies have been investigated with varying success, including chemical conjugation of RNA to small molecules capable of binding cell surface receptors heavily expressed in cancer, incorporating siRNA into nanoparticles or liposomes that may be modified for cell-specific targeting, and binding siRNA to peptides that facilitate cell membrane penetration, and fusing the small RNAs to aptamers (structured pieces of RNA that recognize cell surface receptors).[92,93,99] Although RNAi may not be able to achieve efficient gene silencing in all tumor cells in a given population, RNAi-based therapeutics may be able to cause differentiation or death of the highly malignant subpopulation of tumor-initiating cells that may be responsible for tumor resistance, relapse, and possibly metastasis that are often resistant to conventional cytotoxic therapies.[92] Given the complementary nature of these therapies, it follows that combining RNAi-based therapeutics and conventional cytotoxic drugs has the potential to achieve more effective outcomes.

Gene Therapy

Gene therapy, defined as the insertion of a gene into recipient cells, was initially considered only as a treatment for patients with congenital metabolic defects or late-stage malignancy.[100] However, with the identification of DNA sequences in the human genome, increased interest has been directed toward gene therapy for the development of new therapeutic options.[101] Gene therapy allows for the expression of a chosen transgene, which could either be a deficient protein (such as in genetic abnormality) or a protein with therapeutic effects (such as in cancer treatment). Successful gene therapy is dependent on effective delivery of the desired gene to the appropriate target and achieving the appropriate expression to achieve the desired clinical response. The technique is applicable in a myriad of diseases for which clinical trials have been performed, such as retinoblastoma,[102] coronary artery disease,[103] peripheral vascular disease,[104] HIV/AIDS,[105] and cancer.[106] However, complications related to the use of viral vectors such as insertional mutagenesis and immune responses to the vector have been described.[101] Such risks could be avoided with non-viral gene transfection using plasmid DNA-based injections alone or in combination with physical and chemical techniques, although these have been found to be less efficient than viral vectors.[107,108] The need for nonviral gene transfection techniques with similar efficacy profiles to that of viral vectors without the inherent side effects has shifted the focus to physical and chemical approaches.

GENE ELECTROTRANSFER

The technique of gene electrotransfer refers to electroporation-assisted gene transfer via the application of short electric pulses to cells or tissues, thereby conferring membrane permeability for previously non-permeant molecules. This has been demonstrated to be a safe and efficient method of nonviral gene transfection,[109] and administration of the appropriate electric pulses allows the cell membrane to reseal within minutes for restoration of equilibrium. Besides gene transfection in muscle,[110] where it is most frequently used, gene electrotransfer has been demonstrated a number of other organs including the liver,[111] kidney,[112] bladder,[113] testis,[114] tumor,[115] and skin.[116,117] Because gene transfection only occurs where the plasmid is injected and the electric pulses are delivered, the specific location of gene transfection is known and may be manipulated to affect the duration of response. Gene transfection in rapidly dividing cells such as keratinocytes allows for short-term transfection due to faster cell turnover, whereas transfection in muscle cells, which rarely divide, gives rise to long-term transfection and hence expression of the transgene.[110]

GENE ELECTROTRANSFER IN CANCER TREATMENT

Studies investigating gene electrotransfer for the production of anticancer proteins have focused on plasmids coding for tumor antigens such as prostate-specific antigen (PSA),[118] carcinoembryonic antigen (CEA),[119] vascular endothelial growth factor (VEGF) (via the antiangiogenic effect of VEGF antibodies),[120] or cytokines such as interleukin-12,[121] although research for further proteins with anticancer effects is ongoing. Preclinical studies with anticancer vaccines and antigens have shown promising results, with the ability to elicit an immunologic response and induce production of cytotoxic T cells and various other cytokines. Furthermore, the combination of plasmid injection and administration of electric pulses is more efficient than injection of naked DNA alone.[101]

Few studies have examined the effect of gene electrotransfer to skin on tumor growth. Gene electrotransfer to the skin of the gene AMEP, which codes for an antiangiogenic and antimetastatic molecule (metargidin), has been shown to be effective in reducing the number of metastases of B16 melanomas in mice.[122] Lladser et al.[123] transfected mice with a plasmid coding for a survivin vaccine (a tumor antigen involved in inhibition of apoptosis and upregulated in a vast number of malignant cell lines[124]) prior to inoculation with tumor, and found this decreased tumor growth, while gene electrotransfer to skin with the survivin vaccine after the inoculation of tumor cells did not reduce tumor growth compared to controls. In addition, in vivo gene transfection by intradermal plasmid injection in the peritumoral area of soft tissue sarcoma has been shown to be capable of producing an antitumor response.[125]

GENE ELECTROTRANSFER IN WOUND HEALING

A potential application of gene electrotransfer is to deliver therapeutic molecules that would accelerate the healing of large wounds. Although the local administration of growth factors has been shown to facilitate wound healing, the short half-life of growth factors and need for repeat injections makes it less attractive as a therapeutic option.[126] Gene electrotransfer allows for the attainment of higher local concentrations of growth factors and would allow for long-term production, thus optimizing the conditions for wound healing. This technique has been investigated using a variety of growth factors in ischemia,[127] septic wounds,[126] and in diabetic animal models.[128–130] Results of these studies have shown that delivery of a molecule such as VEGF may induce cell proliferation, promote cell migration and differentiation, as well as induce angiogenesis and inhibit apoptosis, thereby promoting wound healing.[127]

Radiogenomics

Radiogenomics involve the correlation of diagnostic imaging to cellular and molecular genomic data via the association of radiologic phenotypic traits with underlying gene expression.[131] Its primary goal is the utilization of noninvasive tissue imaging as a substitute for invasive biopsy-based gene expression profiling (Figure 6-3).[132]

DIAGNOSTIC TECHNIQUES IN THE POSTGENOMIC ERA

The conventional reference standard for diagnostic imaging has intrinsically been its correlation to gross and histopathologic features of disease,[131] with the aim of achieving the equivalent of in vivo microscopy. Recent remarkable advances in acquisition time and temporal and spatial resolution of new-generation cross-sectional tools such as high-field magnetic resonance imaging (MRI), multidetector-row CT (MDCT), and position emission tomography/computed tomography (PET/CT) have vastly improved image correlation to histopathology and enabled diagnostic imaging to move closer to this reference standard.[133–136] However, there has been a fundamental shift away from the classical radiologic-pathologic relationship because of the development of new in vitro molecular diagnostic techniques, in parallel with increasing evidence that conventional imaging may be used to elucidate genomic properties of disease.[131]

Such a shift has been most apparent in the field of oncology. The development of high-throughput molecular methods such as gene-expression microarrays and next-generation sequencing has permitted an enhanced understanding of underlying tumorigenic mechanisms with unprecedented detail and precision.[131] Gene expression signatures, each comprising up to hundreds of genes, have been shown to be useful in improving diagnostic classification, clinical course prediction, and assessment of therapeutic responses in cancer,[34,137–141] with the potential identification of key pathways involved in any given molecular phenotype.[142] A broad spectrum of cancer types including lymphoma, lung, breast, brain, renal, melanoma, colon, and prostate have undergone genomewide expression analysis, with the identification of distinct molecular subclasses previously undetectable by histopathology alone.[143]

UTILITY OF IMAGING AS A SURROGATE FOR GENE EXPRESSION PROFILING

Although gene expression profiling has proven useful for determining underlying molecular mechanisms, it requires invasive tissue biopsy techniques and specialized equipment, making the process unfeasible for widespread clinical adoption.[128,144] In contrast, diagnostic imaging provides a safe and reliable method of characterizing tissue morphology in situ, and already plays an established role in oncologic management as the primary basis for clinical staging, prognostication, and developing guidelines on modality and intensity of therapy.[135,145,146] Although distinct radiologic phenotypes have been observed in histologically similar tumors,[34] diagnostic imaging has a perceived lack of ability to depict detail at the molecular level. To overcome this, several studies have introduced novel methods for correlating the specific features of tumor morphology and physiology from noninvasive imaging with specific patterns of gene expression on a genomewide scale.[147–149] These unique radiological tumor phenotypes or "radiophenotypes" have been proposed to have the ability to serve as surrogates for gene expression signatures, informing a more precise diagnosis of tumor subtype and molecular biology.[132] Furthermore, the fusion of conventional imaging techniques with molecular techniques such as functional genomic assays offers the potential for rapid

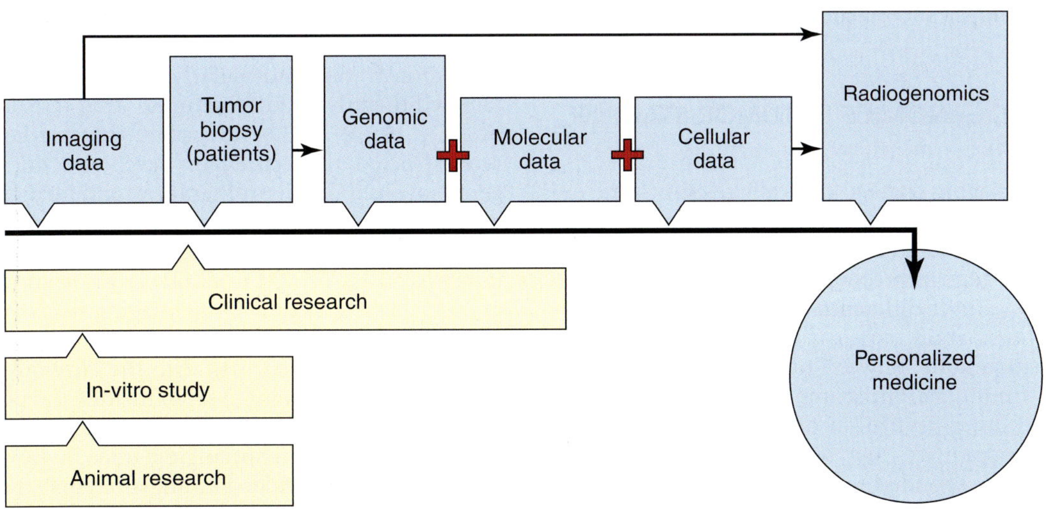

Figure 6-3 Radiogenomics. Radiogenomics is defined as the correlation of diagnostic imaging to cellular and molecular genomic data via the association of radiologic phenotypic traits with underlying gene expression. Radiogenomics can be utilized in a wide spectrum of research from in vitro study to clinical research. Its primary goal is the utilization of noninvasive tissue imaging as a substitute for invasive biopsy-based gene expression profiling. Ultimately, radiogenomics in conjunction with theranostics will provide "personalized medicine."

clinical translation of high-throughput technology, providing global gene expression information to illustrate the molecular state of the cell more accurately than current histopathology-based approaches.[132]

The creation and use of association maps in particular allows the defining of molecular targets of diagnostic interest and the optimization of imaging trait prediction.[131] Segal et al.[148] studied global gene expression programs in HCC using systematic correlational analysis with a large number of specific imaging phenotypes, creating such association maps between imaging features and gene expression patterns that allowed the linking of genomewide gene expression variability in HCC with its imaging appearance. It was determined that a large fraction of the gene expression program could be captured from a small number of imaging traits, with an average of three (and a maximum of four) traits required to predict a given expression program's variation. By creating a global association map, the relative expression level of a particular gene in any given liver tumor could be roughly determined by mapping the gene back to a specific gene expression module and defining its associated network of imaging phenotypes that describe similar liver tumors.[148] This established that a classifiable, systematic relationship between the imaging appearance of HCC and their underlying large-scale gene expression patterns exists. The utilization of this approach to different tumor types could determine levels of biological activation or repression and potentially lead to clinical use as a "noninvasive biopsy" to elucidate the molecular phenotype of tumors.[132]

The potential for translating such an approach into clinical practice was examined by Diehn et al.[149] by linking imaging phenotypes obtained from MRI of glioblastoma multiforme (GBM) to important known gene-expression modules related to established physiologic processes in GBM. In addition to confirming Segal's observation that a large proportion of a tumor's molecular heterogeneity could be reconstructed via a small number of imaging traits, it was noted that the specific gene expression modules could be represented by single imaging traits, suggesting specificity in the radiophenotype-gene expression module relationship.[149] The utilization of this approach to different tumor types could determine levels of biological activation or repression and potentially lead to clinical use as noninvasive biopsies to elucidate the molecular phenotype of tumors.[132]

UTILITY OF RADIOGENOMICS IN TUMOR STAGING AND PROGNOSIS

The correlation of imaging traits to clinically relevant gene expression profiles has the potential to redefine existing diagnostic and tumor staging paradigms. A study by Kuo et al.[147] found that a liver-specific gene expression program known to be closely associated with liver differentiation[140] was highly correlated with the tumor margin score radiophenotype, which delineated the transition zone between tumor and surrounding liver tissue. High tumor margin scores corresponded to poor differentiation and down-regulation of the liver-specific program, whereas tumors with low scores were more highly differentiated and corresponded to up-regulation of the liver-specific program. Tumor margin scores were also found to correlate with a gene expression program associated with venous invasion in HCC. Further integration of these data with histopathology found that tumors with high tumor margin scores also fared worse according to the HCC diagnostic criteria in terms of tumor, node, metastasis (TNM) staging, and increased likelihood of venous invasion. Segal et al.[148] also reported correlations of the increased HCC tumor margin score to the upregulation of genes associated with extracellular matrix remodeling and increased tumor invasiveness.[148] It has thus been proposed that the tumor margin score radiophenotype could potentially be used in HCC diagnostics as a surrogate for both gene expression programs and histopathology.[132] In this way, radiogenomics allows for the conversion of information from images into global gene expression patterns to define patient groups and recognize the underlying molecular mechanisms associated with particular radiophenotypes.[131]

Furthermore, because microscopic venous invasion in HCC is well established as a poor prognostic indicator,[150] similar radiophenotype correlates of venous invasion gene expression programs and histologic venous invasion may be able to serve as independent surrogates for prognostication. Diehn et al.[149] demonstrated the potential use of radiophenotypes as molecular surrogates for inherent tumor gene expression programs that are independent predictors of survival. Significant radiogenomic overlap was reported between a predefined survival-associated gene expression program and a unique "infiltrative" phenotype pattern of T2 edema. Survival analysis demonstrated that the patients with the infiltrative radiophenotype had significantly worse survival than those who did not. Further confirmation by testing on an independent data set of patients with GBM demonstrated the ability to stratify patients based on the presence or absence of this infiltrative radiophenotype alone into multiple prognostic groups possessing significant differences in overall survival. Tumors with the infiltrative phenotype were also more likely to have multiple tumor foci, suggesting that the upregulation of the infiltration-associated genes may increase invasion of tumor cells into surrounding parenchyma.[149] These results illustrated the potential for the use of radiogenomics for identifying molecular surrogates of prognostic biomarkers and allow for patient stratification and prognostication.[131,132]

UTILITY OF RADIOGENOMICS IN ASSESSING OPTIMAL THERAPY

Drug response gene expression programs could potentially be associated with noninvasive imaging phenotypes for use in demonstrating molecularly distinct subsets of tumors for targeted therapy and determining drug resistance. In the study of HCC, Segal et al.[148] described three radiophenotypes that reconstructed the expression level of a module comprising genes involved in cell proliferation, and further showed that the expression level of VEGF—a driver of tumoral angiogenesis—covaries with these cell cycle genes and is predicted by the same imaging traits. Using the available association map, clinicians are thereby able to define the imaging traits on CT and predict approximate VEGF expression levels in a tumor[131] for specific anti-VEGF therapy such as with the antibody bevacizumab.[151] Further applications in research include the possibility of using CT alone for patient selection of high expression levels of angiogenesis genes in antiangiogenesis therapy trials.[131]

The increased understanding of signal transduction pathways in cancer allows for the development of novel targeted therapies; thus there is a need for simultaneous development of biomarkers for identification of patients in whom such targeted therapy is effective.[131] The study by Diehn et al.[149] showed that a radiogenomic approach could be used to identify an image biomarker of epidermal growth factor receptor (EGFR) expression that is commonly dysregulated in GBM, thus identifying patients most amenable to targeted anti-EGFR therapy. Using the GBM radiogenomic association map to identify the "contrast necrosis" phenotype that was highly associated with an EGFR gene-expression program, they were consequently able to select patients with GBM who overexpressed the EGFR protein from this MRI phenotype.[149] Kuo et al.[147] studied six imaging traits on conventional contrast-enhanced CT that could be associated with a previously defined doxorubicin response gene expression signature.[152] The HCC "tumor margin score" radiophenotype was found to show significant association with the doxorubicin response gene program, and tumors associated with greater doxorubicin resistance on the basis of gene expression tended to have higher tumor margin score, with relative specificity confirmed on comparison of this radiophenotype against a more broad multidrug resistance gene expression program. As doxorubicin is a routine component of transarterial chemoembolization (TACE), such associations have the potential to inform existing interventional management of HCC. Along with the previously described findings of this study, it was determined that HCC with a high tumor margin score on CT tended to activate multiple gene-expression programs corresponding to an aggressive phenotype that was also reflected by histopathology and clinical staging.

Although future validation studies are still required, the results of these preliminary studies highlight the concept that the radiogenomic approach appears robust and scalable, with the capability to integrate macroscopic information from routine clinical imaging to the molecular and microscopic levels, and would potentially inform the assessment of optimal oncologic therapy and associated interventional techniques.[131,132]

REFERENCES

The complete reference list is available online at www.expertconsult.com.

PART

2

Gastrointestinal Oncology

DAVID C. MADOFF | RAVI MURTHY

7

Surgical Management of Hepatocellular Carcinoma

SER YEE LEE | MICHAEL D. KLUGER | DANIEL CHERQUI

KEY POINTS

- Patients with cirrhosis are at highest risk of developing hepatocellular carcinoma (HCC) and screening with sonography every 6 months is recommended.
- Early-stage HCC should be treated by resection, liver transplantation, or ablation. The best modality depends on tumor size and location, number of tumors, liver function status, future liver remnant, organ availability, as well as patient's fitness for surgery.
- Curative anatomic liver resection is the optimal treatment for HCC in noncirrhotic patients and in selected patients with Child-Pugh Class A cirrhosis, with small solitary tumors. Laparoscopic liver resection has benefits in selected cases.
- Patients who are not suitable for resection and meeting the Milan criteria should be considered for liver transplantation (living or cadaveric). Bridge therapy with locoregional treatments should be utilized during transplant evaluation and waiting time.
- Patients who are not surgical candidates should be treated with loco-regional approaches such as ablation and transarterial therapies. Transarterial therapies include bland embolization, chemoembolization, and radioembolization.
- Inoperable patients may be offered systemic treatment with antiangiogenic drugs, such as sorafenib. The role of systemic treatment in an adjuvant setting remains to be determined. Inclusion in trials of new drugs should be encouraged.
- Because of multiple treatment options, multidisciplinary team/conference is the indispensable platform for best comprehensive care.

Introduction

Hepatocellular carcinoma (HCC) is the most common primary malignancy of the liver. Surgical management of this deadly cancer remains a challenge for all involved in the care of patients diagnosed with it. It is the second most common cause of cancer-related death in the world in men and sixth in women.[1,2] The mortality per year in HCC is close to its incidence worldwide, emphasizing the high fatality rate of this aggressive disease.[1] Liver cirrhosis, irrespective of the etiology, is an established major risk factor for HCC. Chronic hepatitis B and C are recognized as the main risk factors for HCC, with risk being escalated in the presence of coinfection with hepatitis B virus (HBV) and hepatitis C virus (HCV).[3]

The Barcelona Clinic Liver Cancer (BCLC) classification is one of the widely used and accepted classification; it stratifies patients according to outcome, avoids the use of a single scoring system for all patients, and simultaneously links it with treatment strategy (Figure 7-1).[4] The BCLC classification is constructed in the setting of cohort and randomized controlled studies; it has also been validated in different settings and establishes treatment recommendations for all stages of HCC.[4,5] Patients with early-stage HCC are treated by resection, liver transplantation, or ablation, and prognosis can be refined for all these procedures according to different variables. It considers variables related to tumor size, liver function status, physical status, as well as cancer-related symptoms.

Treatment Strategy

Surgery, including surgical resection and liver transplantation, is currently the mainstay and treatment of choice for HCC. In general, the principles of surgery for HCC after the patient is evaluated to be medically fit for general anesthesia and major surgery are as follows. Liver resection is indicated as a potentially curative procedure if the patient has an adequate liver function (generally Child-Pugh Class A without portal hypertension) and the tumor is resectable with an adequate future liver remnant of at least 20% in a noncirrhotic liver or at least 30%–40% in patients with Child-Pugh Class A cirrhosis. For patients with chronic liver cirrhosis being considered for major resection, preoperative portal vein embolization (PVE) should be considered as an option to induce hypertrophy in the future liver remnant, to minimize risk of postoperative liver failure (Figure 7-2). Patients with HCC meeting the United Network for Organ Sharing (UNOS) criteria should be considered for liver transplantation (living or cadaveric). Situations that are beyond these criteria are controversial (e.g., resectable multifocal disease, patients with resectable tumors who are Child-Pugh Class A within the UNOS criteria) such that a multidisciplinary tumor board should be the platform for decision making.

Patients who are not candidates for potential cure or not medically suitable for major surgery, should be treated with loco-regional approaches. These are broadly classified into ablation techniques and transarterial embolization. Systemic chemotherapy should only be recommended to patients with unresectable HCC in a context of a clinical trial. There are modest but promising results in phases III trials using sorafenib (Nexavar) in both the Western and Asia Pacific regions when compared to best supportive care.[6,7] The details of loco-regional treatment and systemic treatment for advanced HCC are beyond the context of this chapter, and only surgical management will be discussed.

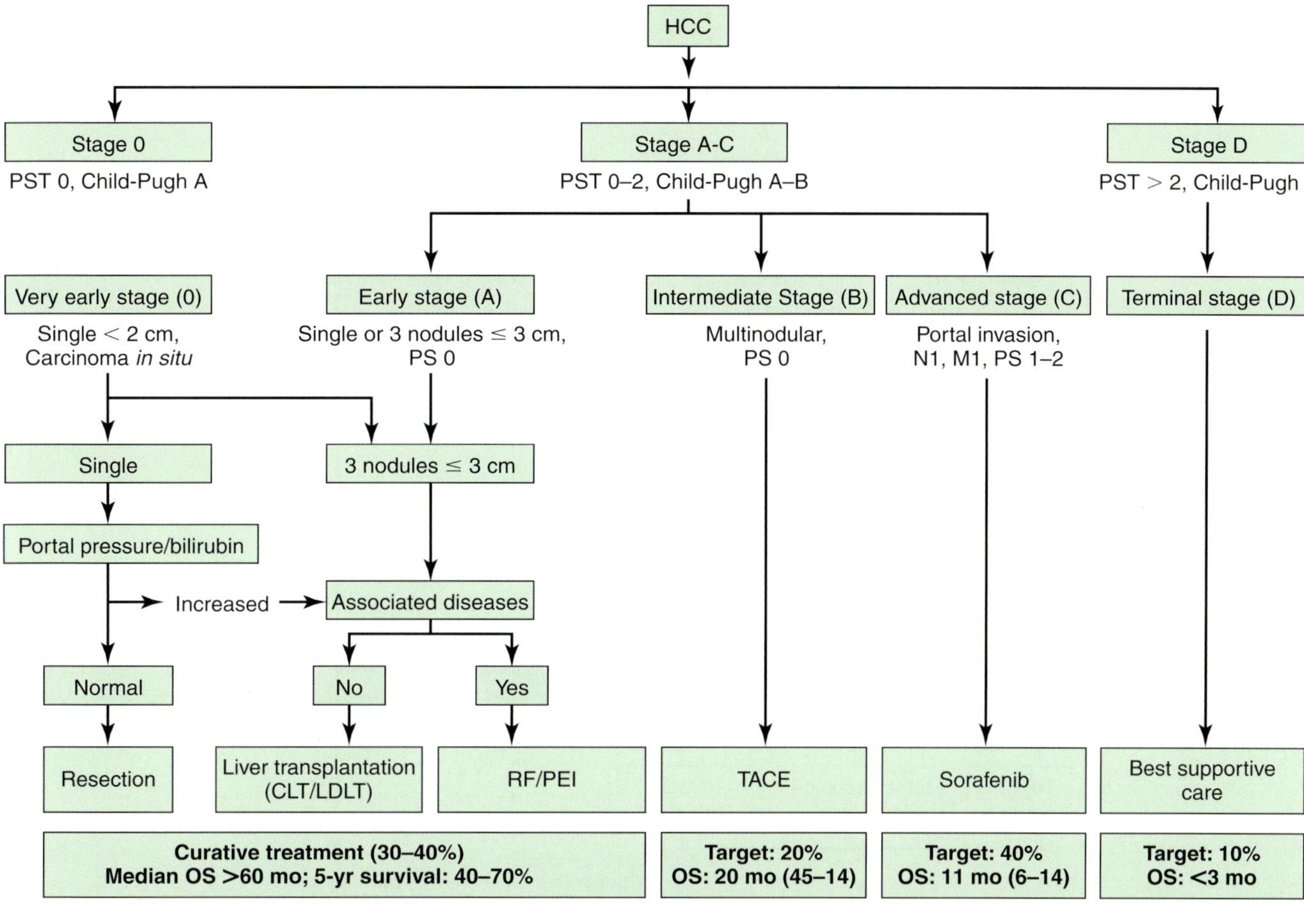

Figure 7-1 Barcelona Clinic Liver Cancer Staging classification 2011. *(From European Association for Study of Liver, European Organisation for Research and Treatment of Cancer. EASL-EORTC clinical practice guidelines: management of hepatocellular carcinoma.* Eur J Cancer. *2012;48(5):599-641.)*

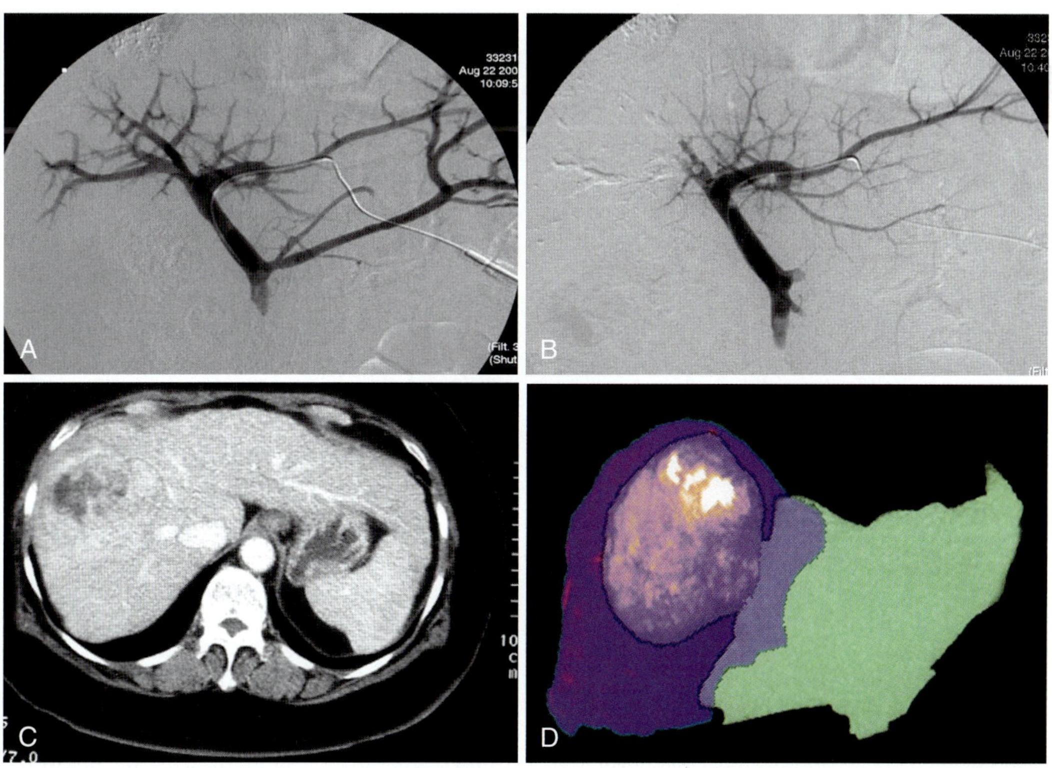

Figure 7-2 Portal vein embolization and hypertrophy of future liver remnant. (A) Portal vein embolization. (B) Post–portal vein embolization. (C) Left lobe hypertrophy on computed tomography. (D) Volumetric assessment of hypertrophy of the left lobe.

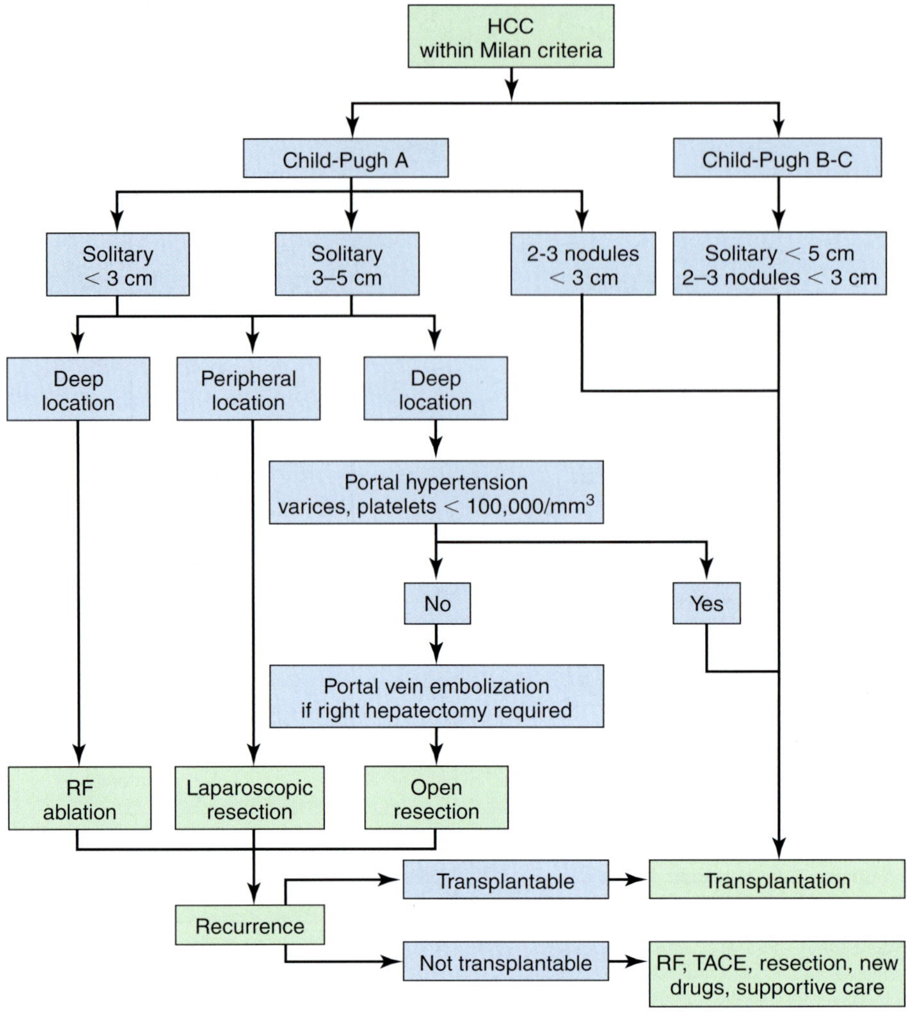

Figure 7-3 Algorithm for management of hepatocellular carcinoma within Milan criteria used at Henri-Mondor Hospital, Paris. *(From Cherqui D, Laurent A, Mocellin N, et al. Liver resection for transplantable hepatocellular carcinoma: long-term survival and role of secondary liver transplantation.* Ann Surg. *2009;250:738-746.)*

A general approach to treatment of HCC within Milan criteria is shown in Figure 7-3.[8] Our suggested approach is one example and is useful for conceptualizing the various treatment options that are available for individual patients but not negating the importance of a multidisciplinary HCC tumor board decision. Attempts to generate algorithmic approaches to the treatment of HCC are difficult because new treatments and indications for various treatments are evolving rapidly. A discussion of these issues and an overview of surgical therapies for HCC are summarized.

Comprehensive Multidisciplinary Care

Considering the complexity of the disease and the armamentarium of treatment options available, a multidisciplinary team should be the platform for all decision making in patients with HCC. The multidisciplinary HCC team should be inclusive of hepatobiliary/liver transplant surgeons, hepatologists/gastroenterologists, medical oncologists, dedicated liver radiologists, interventional radiologists and pathologists, and all relevant allied health care professionals.[9] The team should meet regularly at a tumor board and liver transplant meeting with a review of the patients' clinical status, radiologic images for surgical planning, and histopathology if available, after which an individualized treatment plan is decided by consensus. The meeting also provides an opportunity for the multidisciplinary HCC team to periodically review the latest relevant literature for an evidence-based management. Recommendations may be adapted to local regulations, team's experience and ability as well as consideration of balancing cost and benefits.[10]

Preoperative Assessment

Patient assessment is key in the selection of candidates for liver resection or liver transplantation. As HCCs often present at a late stage, surgical resectability is a primary concern. Once it has been established that curative resection is indicated, resectability can be determined by various factors, including patient, disease, and technical factors. General patient factors include assessment of comorbidities for medical fitness for general anesthesia and major surgery. Specific patient and disease factors determined from two aspects: anatomic feasibility and volumetric tolerance. The main principle lies in the technical ability to leave a liver remnant with adequate function for sustaining life but consistent with low perioperative morbidity and mortality, acceptable long-term outcome in survival, and good quality of life. Relative contraindications to partial hepatectomy include significant medical comorbidities and/or extrahepatic disease. The golden rule for partial hepatectomy is to ensure enough liver parenchyma with a satisfactory blood supply (hepatic artery, portal vein, and hepatic vein), and biliary drainage remains after resection so that the patient does not develop postoperative liver failure. Contraindications of liver resection are situations in which the tumors have invaded the biliary confluence or invaded the three hepatic veins or the portal bifurcation. Any scenario in which bilioenteric anastomosis to the remaining bile ducts cannot be constructed is also considered as a relative contraindication to resection.[11] A multidisciplinary team approach is recommended to validate the decision.

The ability of the nonpathologic liver to regenerate after liver resection is good and a remnant functional normal liver tissue as little as 20% to 25% may be sufficient.[12,13] The ratio of remnant functional liver to the initial total liver tissue may be difficult to estimate because of the size of the tumor or number of tumors (e.g., satellite nodules); the volume of these tumors should be excluded when determining the volume of the total liver. There are studies that utilize volumetric ratio without considering the total liver volume, but uses the percentage of total body weight instead.[14] It has been shown that there is a risk of postoperative liver failure when the remaining functional liver ratio falls to less than 0.5% of total body weight. Computed tomography (CT) of the liver is usually applied to measure liver volumes. Most surgeons will not advocate resection if the estimated volume of functional remnant liver is either less than 20%–25% of the total liver volume or less than 0.5% of total body weight. In the West, many centers rely mainly on the Child-Pugh classification (Table 7-1), but as a single assessment, it has significant variations and may underestimate the degree of cirrhosis.[15] As a result, some centers include the clinical signs and radiologic evidence of portal hypertension to guide risk, and a study has shown that hepatic vein pressure of more than 10 mm Hg is a predictor of postoperative liver decompensation.[16] Model for End-stage Liver Disease (MELD) is a prospectively developed and validated chronic liver disease severity scoring system that uses a patient's laboratory values for serum bilirubin, serum creatinine, and the international normalized ratio for prothrombin time (INR) to predict survival (Figure 7-4). It has been universally adopted by UNOS in 2002 and many parts of the world as a prioritizing tool for liver transplantation. Other than Child-Pugh scoring, MELD and liver function test, some studies have validated the use of indocyanine green clearance (ICG) as an objective adjunct in assessing liver function; in Asia, some institutions use ICG selectively for patient with tumors that are borderline resectable. In patients with "borderline resectability," one safer option is to induce hypertrophy in the remaining functional liver via PVE to reduce the risk of postoperative liver failure. Compensatory hypertrophy of the contralateral lobe is generally observed in a period of 3–6 weeks (see Figure 7-2). Some studies report a high feasibility rate for this strategy and report a mean gain in liver volume of more than 40%, thus increasing the volumetric feasibility for liver resection.[17]

TABLE 7-1 Chronic Liver Disease Classified Into Child-Pugh Classes A, B, and C

	1 Point	2 Points	3 Points
Albumin (g/L)	>35	28–35	<28
Bilirubin (μmol/L)	<34	34–50	>50
INR	<1.7	1.71–2.20	>2.20
Ascites	None	Slight	Moderate
Encephalopathy	None	Grade 1–2	Grade 3–4
Points	**Class**	**1-y Survival**	**2-y Survival**
5–6	A	100%	85%
7–9	B	81%	57%
10–15	C	45%	35%

Model for End-Stage Liver Disease (MELD) Score

The MELD score for determining prognosis and prioritising for receipt of liver transplants is calculated using the following formula:
3.78 × Ln serum bilirubin (mg/dL) + 11.2 × Ln INR (mg/dL) + 9.57 × Ln serum creatinine (mg/dL) + 6.43
where Ln is the natural logarithm.

Notes for calculation of the MELD score:
1. *If the patient has undergone dialysis twice within the last 7 days, then the value for serum creatinine to use in the calculation should be 4.0mg/dL*
2. *Any value <1 is given a value of 1 (e.g. if bilirubin is 0.8, a value of 1.0 is used)*

Figure 7-4 Model for End-stage Liver Disease (MELD). *(Copyright © 2012 Singapore Health Services Pte Ltd.)*

Patients with significant comorbidities should be reviewed by the anesthetic team for evaluation of preoperative risk factors related to general health status (American Society of Anesthesiologists [ASA] score) or associated significant comorbidities to optimize preoperative status.

Surgery

Curative liver resection is the optimal treatment for HCC in noncirrhotic patients and patients with Child-Pugh Class A cirrhosis. This is the treatment of choice for HCC in noncirrhotic patients, who account for about 5% of the cases in Western countries and for about 40% in Asia.[9] A patient ideally suited for resection is one with a localized HCC confined to the liver without radiographic evidence of invasion of the hepatic vasculature, well-preserved hepatic function, and no evidence of portal hypertension (Figure 7-5).[18,19] Notwithstanding aggressive surgical policies, the majority of patients have HCC or liver disease too extensive to permit resection with curative intent. In high-incidence regions of the world, only a minority of the patients are candidates for standard resection, about 10%–15% of newly diagnosed patients and, in low-incidence areas, between 15% and 30% of patients are potentially resectable.[20]

INTRAOPERATIVE STAGING

Intraoperative ultrasonography (IOUS) may improve the selection of patients for potentially curative resection.[21] Intraoperative ultrasound can accurately determine the size of the HCC and detect portal or hepatic vein involvement, which precludes resection. In a study that included 91 patients with HCC who underwent IOUS prior to resection, and no surgery

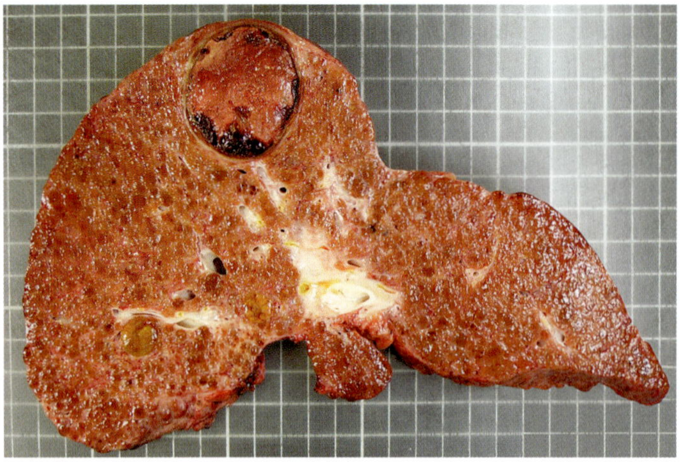

Figure 7-5 Solitary hepatocellular carcinoma in the background of liver cirrhosis without vascular invasion.

was performed in 16% because of unresectable disease.[21] Another advantage of IOUS to the surgeons is the identification of major intrahepatic vascular structures, which can be used to guide nonanatomic or segmental resections.[22] Intraoperative ultrasound can be done before resection in open surgery or via a laparoscopic technique.

SURGICAL TECHNIQUE

Hepatocellular carcinoma has a predilection for invading the portal vein, leading to intrahepatic metastasis, providing the basis for the preference for anatomic resection, along with the principles of surgical oncology. In the noncirrhotic liver, an anatomical resection should be performed, following Couinaud segments (Figure 7-6). Anatomic liver resection is achieved by selective ligation of the inflow portal triad and ligation of dominant outflow hepatic veins to the segments or segment resected.[23] If subsegmental resection is planned, IOUS enables precise identification of the intrahepatic vessels during segmentectomy.[24] For cirrhotic patients, the technical approach can be modified, with resection encompassing the least amount of nonmalignant

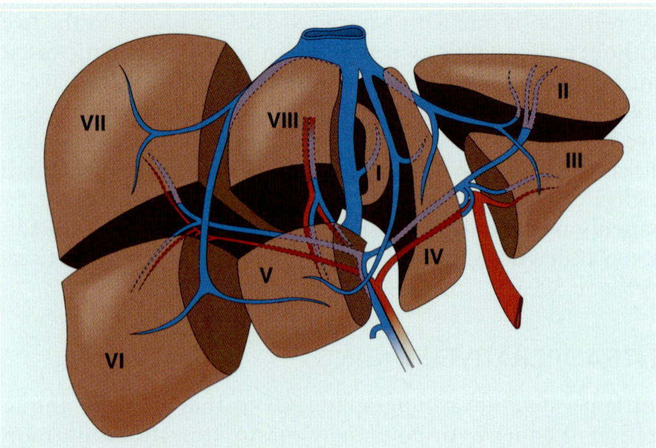

Figure 7-6 Couinaud segments of the liver. Segments 2, 3, 4a, 5, and 6 are most amenable to laparoscopic resection. *(From Iwatsuki S, Sheahan DG, Starzl TE. The changing face of hepatic resection.* Curr Probl Surg. *1989;26(5):287-379.)*

parenchyma feasible, so as to maintain satisfactory postoperative liver function. Importantly, both anatomic and wedge resection are acceptable as long as there are adequate clear margins of at least 1 cm. Anatomic resections aiming at 2-cm margins provide better survival outcome than narrow resection margins less than 1 cm.[25] The potential for liver regeneration is impaired in cirrhotic patients; thus, resection is generally more conservative. However, some patients maintain adequate functional liver reserve even after a formal hemihepatectomy, particularly if preoperative PVE is used to induce compensatory hypertrophy in the future liver remnant.[26]

Surgical techniques have improved over the past decade as a result of advances in surgical techniques and better experience. These include equipment for parenchymal transection, for example, ultrasonic dissector (CUSA, Tyco Healthcare, Mansfield, MA) and the Hydrojet (Hydro-Jet, Erbe, Tubingen, Germany) and various surgical staplers for pedicle or vascular transections.[27] Operative maneuvers include vascular occlusion techniques like the intermittent use of the Pringle maneuver for vascular inflow occlusion as an alternative to total vascular occlusion (clamping of the portal vein, hepatic artery, and the inferior vena cava [IVC]).[28] Intermittent Pringle occlusion (e.g., 15 to 20 minutes of clamping with 5 to 10 minutes of unclamping) is well tolerated by cirrhotic patients for up to a total of an hour and is better tolerated than continuous clamping.[29,30] Intraoperative anesthetic management (e.g., low central venous pressure maintenance) and immediate postoperative care have been optimized. These strategies have led to a decrease in blood transfusion from about 80% to less than 10% in two decades.[31,32] The conventional approach to resection of large right-sided HCC consisted of complete mobilization of the right liver followed by vascular control and then tumor resection.

Some surgeons have advocated a "no touch" technique or the anterior approach to resection of HCC. This approach utilizes initial anterior parenchymal transection of the liver parenchyma down to the IVC, and ligation of the inflow and outflow vessels before mobilization of the liver. The advocates hypothesize that the separation of the right liver and the tumor from the IVC before mobilization avoids prolonged rotation and displacement of the liver and manipulation of the tumor, thus reducing the risk of vascular rupture. In addition, division of the vessels before tumor manipulation theoretically minimizes the potential for tumor cell dissemination caused by tumor compression.[33,34] The liver hanging maneuver described by Belghiti describes the elevation of the posterior aspect of the liver by gently lifting the liver with a surgical tape passed between the anterior surface of the IVC and the liver parenchyma. This liver hanging maneuver during transection can be useful for improving exposure, especially when addressing large, right-sided tumors involving the diaphragm (Figure 7-7).[35]

Centrally located HCC (segments 4, 5, and 8) can be technically more challenging (Figure 7-8). Extended hemihepatectomy is the treatment of choice if potentially curative surgery can be undertaken safely. However, this conventional approach can be associated with high perioperative morbidity and mortality rates due to inadequate residual functional liver parenchyma.[36] An alternative segment-oriented approach, central hepatectomy, has been proposed in which the central liver segments 4 and/or 5, and 8 (with or without segment 1) are removed and the lateral sectors remain intact.[37] Current literature indicate that the available data suggest that central hepatectomy (mesohepatectomy) is an alternative to extended hemihepatectomy for centrally located

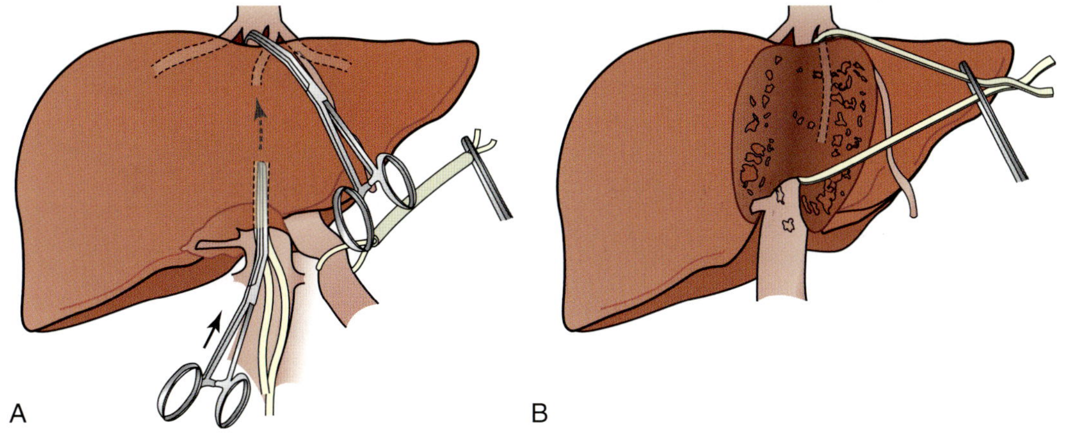

Figure 7-7 Liver hanging maneuver. (A and B) Steps in performing the liver hanging maneuver. *(From Belghiti J, Guevara OA, Noun R, Saldinger PF, Kianmanesh R. Liver hanging manoeuvre: a safe approach to right hepatectomy without liver mobilization.* J Am Coll Surg. *2001;193:109-111.)*

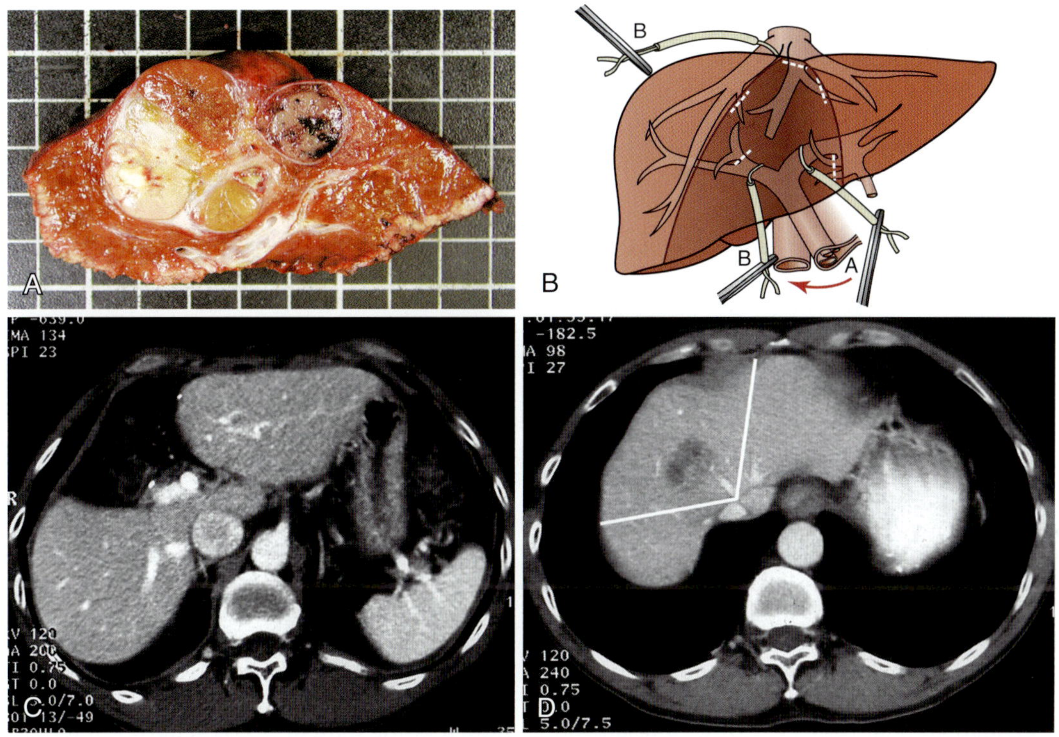

Figure 7-8 Central hepatectomy, segments 4, 5, and 8. *(B, From Chouillard E, Cherqui D, Tayar C, et al. Anatomical bi- and trisegmentectomies as alternatives to extensive liver resections.* Ann Surg. *2003;238(1):29-34.)*

tumors, providing acceptable oncologic outcomes with less liver parenchymal loss.[37] However, it is a complex and technically demanding procedure that requires two hepatic resection planes and bilateral biliary reconstruction.[38] Consequently, this translates to a higher risk of bile leak and bleeding as well as long-term biliary stricture and biliary dysfunction. Along the same principles, anatomic bi- or trisegmentectomy is also a safe alternative to extensive liver resection in selected patients with selective vascular occlusion (Figure 7-9).[37]

LAPAROSCOPIC LIVER RESECTION

The success of minimally invasive surgery and experience in resection of benign hepatic tumors along with advances in surgical technology has driven interest in laparoscopic approaches to surgery for HCC.[39,40] Development of advanced energy devices for parenchymal transection, for example, harmonic scalpel (Ultracision; Ethicon), which is a thermofusion device (Ligasure; Tyco Healthcare) also assisted in the advancement of laparoscopic liver resection. Indications and contraindications for laparoscopic liver resection are also well defined (Table 7-2, see Figure 7-6).[41] Liver resections, including major hepatectomies, are now performed by laparoscopy in specialized centers.[42,43] Preliminary results in the literature suggest that laparoscopic liver resections are associated with fewer postoperative general complications, less intraoperative bleeding, less postoperative analgesic demand, and reduced hospital stay when compared to open procedures.[44] Some series, with small

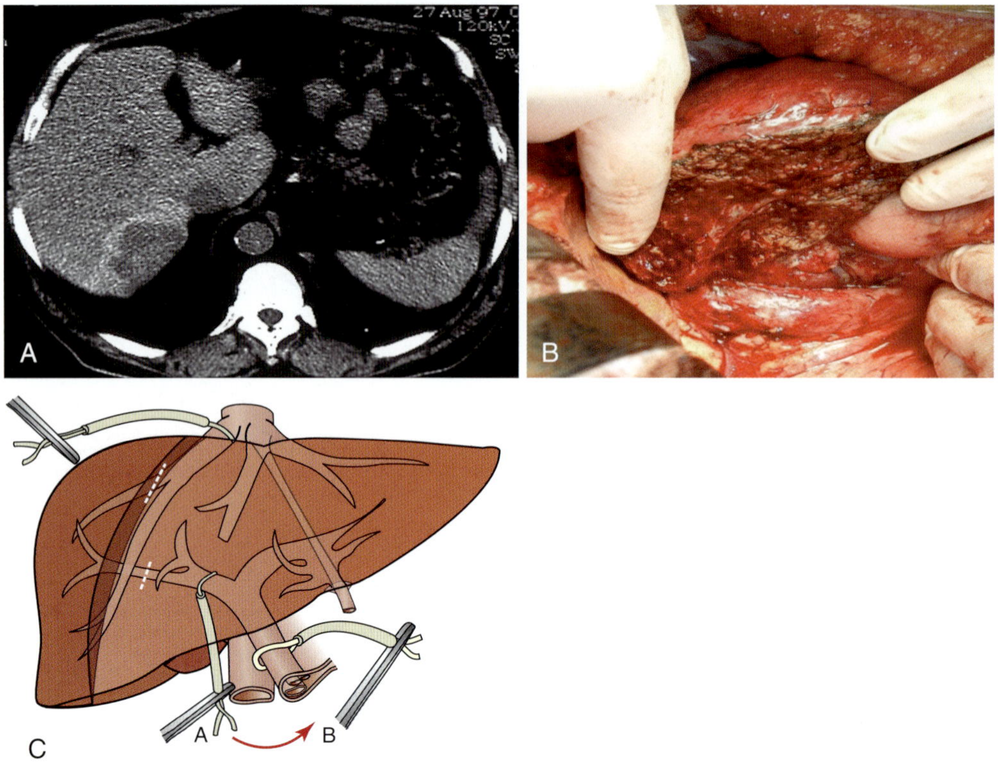

Figure 7-9 Right posterior sectionectomy of segments 6 and 7. *(C, From Chouillard E, Cherqui D, Tayar C, et al. Anatomical bi- and trisegmentectomies as alternatives to extensive liver resections.* Ann Surg. *2003;238(1):29-34.)*

numbers of patients undergoing liver resection for HCC, show that the benefit of laparoscopic over open procedures seems to be greater than in other indications of liver resection. Especially in cirrhotic patients, there is less liver mobilization and the amount of intraoperative intravenous fluid is reduced. Because of the minimal insensible fluid loss as compared to an open procedure, the third space fluid accumulation is reduced and this resulted in fewer postoperative ascites. Moreover, as a result of the significantly smaller wounds, abdominal wall complications were also decreased by the use of laparoscopy.[45,46] Most importantly, patient safety and oncologic outcomes must be of highest priority in the consideration of laparoscopic liver surgery. It is also highly technically demanding and should be undertaken only in high-volume centers with a program of graduated procedural complexity.[39]

POSTOPERATIVE MANAGEMENT AND PERIOPERATIVE MORBIDITY AND MORTALITY

There have been significant improvements in surgical and anesthetic techniques as well as perioperative management of patients with HCC, leading to significant reductions in the morbidity and mortality rates after partial hepatectomy. Even in institutions reporting a significant percentage of complex hepatectomies, perioperative mortality is approaching 1% to 3% in patients without underlying liver dysfunction.[47-49] After surgery, patients are monitored in the operating theater recovery room and subsequently transferred to the intensive care unit overnight or a high dependency unit for close monitoring. Subsequently they can be transferred to the general ward according to the patient's clinical condition. Postoperative care is primarily supportive in nature; it includes judicious fluid management, perioperative antibiotic prophylaxis, proton pump inhibitors, early mobilization, chest physiotherapy, and early enteral nutrition when possible. The extent of postoperative morbidity is related to the extent of surgical resection and patients' preexisting comorbidities.[50] Major postoperative complications include liver failure, bleeding, bile leak, intraabdominal sepsis, pneumonia, and pleural effusion; minor complications include wound infection, urinary tract infection, etc. Resection can now be achieved in experienced centers with a mortality rate of less than 5%.[49,51] Presence of cirrhosis is the most important predictor of postresection liver failure and early mortality. The 30-day postoperative mortality for cirrhotic patients is about 15%, compared to about 5% for noncirrhotic patients.[52] Generally, obesity is a risk factor for increased postoperative morbidity after major surgery, but in hepatic resection, as shown by one study, this is mainly related to minor abdominal wall complications and severe morbidity rates and mortality are not significantly different when compared to nonobese patients, even in cirrhosis or after major hepatectomy.[53] Intraoperative blood loss in excess 1500 mL and postoperative infection of any type are identified factors that might lead to postoperative liver failure in cirrhotic patients. Thus, as mentioned earlier, mortality can be minimized by appropriate selection of patients and meticulous surgical technique, including preoperative volumetry and PVE when appropriate, in the setting of a multidisciplinary team approach.[54] Patients with chronic hepatitis B or C and active viral replication are also treated by appropriate antiviral therapy before and after surgery by a hepatologist preferably. Postdischarge follow-up management includes liver function tests, α-fetoprotein, and CT or magnetic resonance imaging (MRI) at 3 months initially and then every 6 months.

TABLE 7-2 Indications and Contraindications for Laparoscopic Partial Hepatectomy

INDICATIONS
Location: Segments 2 through 6
Pathology
Benign and malignant neoplasms
Cystic lesions
Parasitic lesions

Size
Lesions <5 cm
Left lateral section lesions of any size not in proximity to major vascular
structures
Pedunculated neoplasms of any size not in proximity to major vascular structures

RELATIVE CONTRAINDICATIONS
Location
Lesions near the inferior vena cava, hilum, or distal hepatic veins
Multiple or bilateral lesions
Segments 1, 4a, 7, or 8

Pathology
Coagulopathy or thrombocytopenia
Moderate to severe portal hypertension
Previous operation, especially upper abdominal

Size
Laparoscopic approach requiring a larger parenchymal resection than would be necessary via an open approach
Nonpedunculated benign and malignant neoplasms >5 cm

ABSOLUTE CONTRAINDICATIONS
Gallbladder cancer and hilar cholangiocarcinoma
Inability to obtain a surgical margin that would otherwise be possible in an open resection
Patient unable to tolerate an open operation or pneumoperitoneum
Insufficient surgeon training

From MD Kluger, D Cherqui (2012). Minimally invasive techniques in hepatic resection. In Blumgart's Surgery of the Liver, Pancreas and Biliary Tract, 5th ed., pp. 1530. Elsevier Saunders.

TABLE 7-3 Survival Outcomes After Surgical Resection for HCC

			SURVIVAL RATE AT		
Author	**Year**	***n***	**1 y**	**3 y**	**5 y**
Arii et al.	2000				
HCC <2 cm, CP-A		1318	96%	NA	72%
HCC <2 cm, CP-B		502	92%	NA	56%
HCC, 2–5 cm, CP-A		2722	95%	NA	58%
HCC, 2–5 cm, CP-B		1548	95%	NA	45%
Zouh et al.	2001	2366	83%	61%	50%
Poon et al.	2001	241	82%	62%	36%
Nagasue et al.	2001	100	97%	61%	50%
Kanematsu et al.	2002	303	84%	67%	51%
Belghiti et al.	2002	300	81%	57%	37%
Chen et al.	2002	252	80%	54%	34%
Wayne et al.	2002	249	83%	NA	41%
Yeh et al.	2002	218	63%	42%	32%
Ercolani et al.	2003	224	83%	63%	43%
Chen et al.	2004	525	NA	34%	17%
Capussotti et al.	2005	216	NA	51%	34%
Hasegawa et al.	2005	210			
Anatomic resection		156	95%	84%	66%
Non-anatomic resection		54	93%	66%	35%
Sasaki et al.	2006	418			
Hepatitis B-positive		67	NA	80%	62%
Hepatitis C-positive		351	NA	78%	69%
John et al.	2006	100	75%	37%	22%
Nathan et al.	2009	788	NA	NA	39%
Yang et al.	2009	260	87%	56%	38%

CP, Child-Pugh classification; HCC, hepatocellular carcinoma; NA, not assessed.

Data from Takayama T. Surgical treatment for hepatocellular carcinoma. Jpn J Clin Oncol. 2011;41(4):447-454. Epub 2011 Mar 16.

LONG-TERM OUTCOMES OF SURGICAL RESECTION

The long-term outcome following curative resection of HCC has improved through the decades. A recent large review of surgical long-term outcomes looking at 17 studies of a total of more than 13,000 patients revealed a 1-year survival rate ranging from 67% to 97%, a 3-year survival rate ranging from 34% to 84%, and a 5-year survival rate ranging from 17% to 72% (Table 7-3).[55] Survival can be estimated based on the pathologic AJCC stage. In a series of 557 patients undergoing curative resection of HCC at four centers, 5-year survival rates, based on the TNM staging system, were as follows: Stage I (T1)—55%; Stage II (T2)—37%; Stage III (T3a, T3b, T4)—16%.[56] As demonstrated, there is a wide variability in outcomes, and the majority of this variability can be explained by patient selection.

PROGNOSTIC FACTORS

Prognostic factors for survival following resection have been extensively studied. They can be broadly classified to patient, tumor, and liver-related factors. For patient factors, age was shown in some studies but not consistently in other studies to be an independent risk factor. It appears that age-related coexisting comorbidities may confound advanced age as a negative prognostic factor.[15,57]

The most important tumor-related prognostic factors are degree of vascular invasion (macro- and microvascular), tumor number and size, and resection margin status. Other negative prognostic factors include absence of a tumor capsule, preoperative α-fetoprotein (AFP) levels >10,000 ng/mL, and poor histologic grade of differentiation.[48,58,59]

Both intrahepatic and extrahepatic spread of HCC is more common with tumors larger than 5 cm, particularly when associated with vascular invasion.[20] In a large study of liver resections over the same period, the authors compared more than 1000 patients on each arm with HCC less than 5 cm and more than 5 cm, and found the 5-year survival rates to be significantly better for patients with smaller tumors.[60] Nonetheless, there are also studies that indicate 5-year survival rates ranging from 25% to 35% in selected patients undergoing resection for large HCC in excess of 10 cm in diameter.[61] However, although increasing tumor size is associated with increased risk for vascular invasion, large, solitary tumors without vascular invasion have the same prognosis as small solitary tumors without vascular invasion. Gross or microscopic invasion of branches of the portal or hepatic veins is associated with a lower probability of survival following resection.[20] The width of surgical margins remains debatable; some studies show that a 2 cm negative margin confers better results whereas most accept clear margins of at least 1 cm to be adequate.[25] The clear consensus remains that the failure to obtain R0 status is an independent poor indicator.[15] About 10% of HCC presents with spontaneous tumor rupture, the presence of a tumor rupture suggests a high likelihood of peritoneal seeding and usually translates to a poor outcome. If the bleeding stops or can be controlled by interventional methods, for example, arterial embolization, and the patient is hemodynamically stable, a formal staging and evaluation with a view for a proper anatomic resection should aimed for.[62] Several retrospective series suggest a lower but beneficial long-term survival rate following resection in such cases.[62,63]

Liver-related factors include the severity of underlying liver dysfunction and whether there is active hepatitis. Preoperative liver dysfunction and cirrhosis are important negative prognostic factors; the long-term outcome is approximately halved in cirrhotic patients and this difference may be related in part to the higher frequency of multicentric HCC in cirrhotic patients.[64,65] In patients with cirrhosis related to HBV or HCV infection, active hepatitis is also shown to be a poor prognostic factor.[66] Generally, the severity of cirrhosis, rather than the presence of a small, early-stage HCC is the limiting factor for long-term survival in cirrhotic patients with HCC.

Combination Therapy

There is a role for combining surgery and loco-ablative treatment for selected patients with HCC, especially with the advent of laparoscopic techniques. Laparoscopic or open surgical ablation may be necessary in patients with deeply located HCC, locations not accessible to percutaneous puncture (segments 7 and 8), or superficial nodules adjacent to bowel or diaphragm. Surgical ablation may also be potentially safer in patients with a high risk of bleeding from coagulopathy, which is not uncommon in cirrhotic patients. Advantages of a surgeon's involvement include the ease and freedom of probe insertion at various angles for optimal ablative field facilitated by the mobilization of the liver if necessary, either via laparoscopic or open approaches. Moreover, with the surgical approach, the Pringle maneuver can be used to temporarily interrupt the portal vein and hepatic artery blood flow to facilitate heat ablation of large hypervascular HCC and tumors near major blood vessels to minimize the heat sink effect.[67] Last, laparoscopy and laparoscopic intraoperative ultrasonography can provide an opportunity for detection of peritoneal metastasis and extrahepatic invasion that may be missed even with extensive preoperative imaging.[21]

In patients with multiple HCCs, multiple resections is possible but is often limited by the amount of residual liver and as a result, extensive resection entails a higher risk of liver failure for patients with cirrhosis. Hence, in the management of multifocal HCC, combined use of resection (for the large tumor) and radiofrequency ablation (RFA; for the smaller tumors) is a reasonable option for the achievement of complete tumor clearance in a single general anesthesia sitting. Thus, loco-regional therapy in combination with surgery widens the applicability of surgical intervention for the HCC.[68] Liver-directed loco-regional therapy can serve as a bridge to transplant, to halt, or downstage HCC for liver transplant consideration.

Liver Transplantation

Hepatocellular carcinoma is the only solid organ cancer treated by transplantation, and liver transplantation is theoretically the optimal treatment for HCC if not for the lack of donor organs. In theory, it is better than surgical resection as it not only removes the HCC—the underlying cirrhosis, thus minimizing the risk of HCC recurrence—but also prevents any future morbidity from liver cirrhosis. In 1963, the first human liver transplantation was performed by Tom Starzl and his team but this did not gain wide acceptance until the mid-1980s with the advent of effective immunosuppressants.[69] Earlier selection criteria for liver transplantation were poor and ill defined, resulting in unsatisfactory outcomes, with recurrence rates of approximately 50% and 5-year survival rates of 40%.[70] Bismuth and his team first rationalized the role of liver transplantation for HCC according to tumor characteristics in 1993, and in 1996 Mazzaferro et al. published a study that identified and defined tumor characteristics that are associated with superior outcomes after liver transplantation, known as the Milan criteria.[71] This has been adopted by many countries and is the current UNOS criteria (one lesion less than 5 cm or a maximum of three lesions less than 3 cm in diameter each) for liver transplantation.[9] In 2001, Yao et al. proposed an expanded selection criteria, known as the University of California in San Francisco (UCSF) selection criteria (a single lesion of 6.5 cm or up to 3 lesions, none of which are larger than 4.0 cm, with a maximum combined tumor size of 8.0 cm), in these patients, they reported a 1-year survival of 90% and 5-year survival of 75%, comparable with the Milan criteria results.[72]

The introduction and subsequent verification of the MELD score, based on serum bilirubin and creatinine and the international normalized ratio of the prothrombin time, adopted as the tool for organ prioritizing, led to improvements in organ allocation, especially considering the large number of HCC patients considered for liver transplantation (see Figure 7-4).[73,74] The issue is in achieving the right balance between HCC and non-HCC recipients. Based on the radiologic assessment of the number and size of the HCC lesions, MELD exception points are awarded for HCC, with the expectation that liver transplantation is accomplished in a reasonable period of time. When MELD allocation was first introduced, it was agreed that mortality was not the appropriate end point for HCC candidates, but instead tumor expansion beyond the Milan criteria would necessitate dropout from the wait list. As a result, candidates with HCC within the Milan criteria and with T2 lesions were initially assigned 29 points at the time of the initial listing, with incremental points granted every 3 months.[75] This initial point allocation was decreased to 24 in 2003 and to 22 in 2005. The current exception points for HCC are based on the 3-month pretransplantation mortality rates. For patients with the Milan criteria who currently receive a MELD score of 22, unless their calculated MELD score is otherwise greater and for each 3-month interval that they remain on the waiting list, a greater number of exception points are awarded based on an expected increase of 10% for the 3-month pretransplantation mortality rate (e.g., first extension: 25 points for 25% mortality).[9] The challenges encountered in HCC and organ allocation relate closely to the appropriate degree of MELD exception points that should be assigned to HCC patients so that the number of transplantations done for HCC patients are reasonable compared to other indications. The system should have an acceptable and comparable mortality from all indications while awaiting transplantation and ensure that the survival outcomes are similar after transplantation; thus, there are ongoing studies validating the current MELD exception points for HCC.[76]

There is always a waiting period between listing and transplantation. This varies significantly among programs and countries but if the waiting time is long enough, the HCC will grow and develop major contraindications to be beyond the criteria for transplantation.[77] The rate of exclusion on the waiting list may be as high as 25% if the waiting list is longer than 12 months.[77] If extended listing criteria are used, the patients with more advanced HCC will be included and as a result, the dropout rate will be even higher and this will translate into poor survival figures on an intention-to-treat analysis. Studies have shown that if the dropout rate due to HCC advancing is 25% at 1 year, this will translate into a 60% survival rate for patients with HCC listed for transplant, based on an intention-to-treat analysis basis.[77,78]

Hepatocellular carcinoma growing beyond the criteria for transplantation has led to many efforts in bridge therapy, especially in centers where there is a shortage of donor organs and waiting period is typically more than 6 months.[79] Downstaging of HCC with loco-regional therapy that aims to reduce the size and/or number of HCC lesions is widely utilized.[69] Studies have shown that successful HCC downstaging can be achieved in up to 70% of the patients treated in a protocol with one or more therapeutic modalities, including transarterial chemoembolization (TACE), RFA, or percutaneous ethanol injection (PEI). Subsequently, successful liver transplantation was accomplished in nearly half of these patients.[80] In 2010, an international consensus conference reported guidelines for liver transplantation for HCC; it stated that bridging strategies might be appropriate for patients with UNOS T2 lesions (one nodule 2–5 cm or three or fewer nodules each ≤3 cm) who are likely to wait 6 months or longer. However, there is no evidence that bridging strategies are of any benefit in patients with UNOS T1 tumors (<2 cm).[69] The role of salvage liver transplantation after liver resection of HCC is less clear. Several centers have reported their experience in transplantation after liver resection for HCC and advocated this as a form of bridging therapy.[81]

One solution to reduce waiting time and dropout rate is to increase the number of donor organs; naturally, living donor liver transplantation (LDLT) has been shown to be an alternative to cadaveric liver transplantation. LDLT is a complex procedure that is associated with a morbidity of 20%–40% and a donor mortality of 0.3%–0.5%.[9,82] A decision analysis study considering the risk of dropout, the donor mortality, and expected survival of recipient has shown that if the waiting time on the list exceeds 7 months, LDLT is cost effective; this protocol was adopted by the European Association for the Study of the Liver (EASL).[10,83] A recent retrospective study noted that the disease-free survival following LDLT was lower than that of cadaveric liver transplantation, and LDLT recipients had a higher rate of HCC recurrence within 3 years than deceased donor orthotopic liver transplantation (OLT) recipients; however, there was no difference in mortality or the combined outcome of mortality or recurrence.[84]

The development of LDLT has driven the discussion about expansion of the tumor burden criteria for HCC patients further. Because transplantation can be done with much less delay, it has been proposed by some that living donation might be a valid option for those patients whose HCC stage does not allow listing for cadaveric liver transplantation.[9] However, there is no current data to support utilizing such expanded criteria.[85]

The main issue in LDLT is donor safety, because the risk of complications or mortality, even if small, cannot be downplayed.

TABLE 7-4 Results After Liver Transplantation for HCC

Author	Number	Mortality (%)	Recurrence (%)	5-y OS (%)	5-y DFS (%)
Molmenti, 2002	790	—	—	44	—
Leung, 2004	144	—	15	47	43
Todo, 2004	316	11.1	13	—	—
Hwang, 2005	312	18.7	18	—	—
Zavaglia, 2005	155	11	6	72	—
Duffy, 2007	467	—	21	52	—
Mazzaferro, 2009	1,556	—	20	73	59
Vibert, 2010	153	2	33	72	69
Sandhu, 2011	287	—	15	75	70

DFS, disease-free survival; HCC, hepatocellular carcinoma; OS, overall survival.

Data from Cauchy F, Fuks D, Belghiti J. HCC: current surgical treatment concepts. Langenbecks Arch Surg. *2012;397(5):681-695.*

The risks and benefits need to be openly discussed and understood by all parties involved in such cases.[86] In 2005, the Vancouver Forum, convened under the auspices of the Ethics Committee of The Transplantation Society, brought together leaders in organ transplantation to develop an international standard of care for the live organ donor that addressed the ethnics and concepts in LDLT, in addition to issues of informed consent, responsibilities of the transplant team, live donor selection, autonomy and satisfaction, and procedural safeguards.[87]

Survival after liver transplantation has progressively improved over the decades. Excellent 5-year posttransplant patient survival of at least 70% has been reported from many centers (Table 7-4).[48,88,89] This can be attributed to advances in the surgical technique, perioperative and posttransplant intensive care management, and the introduction of better immunosuppressive drugs.

Summary

Hepatocellular carcinoma is the second most frequent cause of cancer-related death in the world. Patients with cirrhosis of whatever etiology are at highest risk of developing HCC, and screening with ultrasonography every 6 months is recommended in certain high-risk groups. Patients with small solitary tumors and good/normal liver function are the best candidates for surgical resection. Liver transplantation is most beneficial for individuals who are not good candidates for resection, especially those within Milan criteria.[9] Donor shortage greatly limits the applicability of liver transplantation, and development of LDLT helps to some extent. Comprehensive multidisciplinary approach should be the platform for decision making and care of all HCC patients.

REFERENCES

The complete reference list is available online at www.expertconsult.com.

8

Interventional Management of Hepatocellular Carcinoma

AKHILESH K. SISTA | DAVID C. MADOFF

KEY POINTS

- Image guided techniques are the most common invasive therapy for unresectable hepatocellular carcinoma (HCC).
- Level 1 evidence supports survival benefit chemoembolization.
- New embolic devices may offer benefits not currenlty realized.

Background

Hepatocellular carcinoma (HCC) is the fifth most common cancer worldwide and the third most common cause of cancer-related death. Although the highest prevalence is still in sub-Saharan Africa and Asia, the incidence in the United States is rising along with the rise in hepatitis B and C and the longer survival of cirrhotic patients.[1] As novel therapeutic options have emerged and been refined, the manner in which HCC is treated has changed dramatically compared with just two decades ago. The approach to a patient with HCC has been reasonably standardized as a result of several international guidelines.[2-4] Now, there is a reproducible algorithm that determines whether a patient undergoes transplantation, surgical resection, ablation, transarterial treatment, or systemic chemotherapy (Figure 8-1). It should be noted that a minorty of HCC patients can be treated with resection or transplantation, and percutaneous ablation and transarterial techniques have emerged as essential therapies in the treatment algorithm for HCC.

This chapter focuses on these ablative and transarterial techniques. Percutaneous ethanol injection (PEI) was introduced in the 1980s as the first effective ablative technique.[81] Since then, the thermal systems radiofrequency (RF), microwave (MW), and cryoablation have gained wide acceptance, with the most data having been gathered for RF ablation (RFA). The newest method, though largely experimental in the treatment of HCC, is irreversible electroporation (IRE).

Transarterial therapy for HCC was first reported in the late 1970s.[5-7] In the 1980s, several reports discussed the feasibility of combining embolic and chemotherapeutic agents.[8-10] Two seminal randomized controlled trials in 2002 were the first to demonstrate a survival benefit in patients with unresectable HCC treated with transarterial chemoembolization.[11,12] Phase 1 and 2 clinical trials on doxorubicin eluting embolic beads in the treatment of unresectable HCC were conducted in the mid 2000s in an attempt to standardize the procedure and improve the pharmacokinetic profile of chemoembolization.[13-15] During the past 10 years, nonocclusive alternatives to transarterial embolization (TAE)/transarterial chemoembolization (TACE) have received growing interest. The following pages discuss the technical details of these approaches, their indications, complications, and their relative value in the treatment of unresectable HCC.

Percutaneous Ablation

The technical details of the various percutaneous ablative techniques named above can be found in Chapter 2. The discussion here will focus on workup and preoperative imaging, data-based patient selection, complications, and postprocedural care and imaging.

PATIENT PREPARATION AND PREOPERATIVE IMAGING

Either magnetic resonance imaging (MRI) or computed tomography (CT) with arterial and portal contrast phases should be obtained to identify the location, number, and size of tumors to be treated. The imaging is essential to determine whether the lesions are amenable to ablation. The case should be explicitly discussed with the referring physician or tumor board, and the patient's disease stage should be characterized by the combination of imaging findings, laboratory results, and functional status. Blood product replacement should be performed if the international normalized ratio (INR) is >1.5 and the platelets are <50,000/mm^3. Aspirin and/or clopidogrel should be held at least 5 days prior to the procedure if possible. Imaging will also guide whether ultrasonography, CT, or a combination will be used to ablate the lesion(s).

ABLATIVE TECHNIQUES

Radiofrequency Ablation

As stated above, most of the data on percutaneous techniques has been generated for radiofrequency ablation (RFA), so the current recommendations primarily apply to this ablative modality (Figure 8-2). RFA relies on thermal heat created by an electrical current passing through the electrode embedded in the tumor. Patients who should be considered for RFA are those with very-early-stage and early-stage HCC. Very early stage is defined as having a performance status of 0, being Child-Pugh Class A, and having a single tumor <2 cm in size. The treatment options for these patients are surgical resection and ablation, and the decision is made based largely on anatomic location. Lesions that should be resected include those in a subcapsular or perivascular distribution, as ablation is occasionally unsafe and

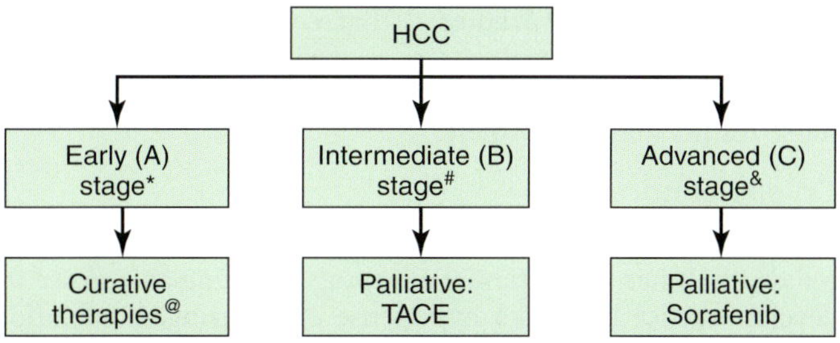

* Solitary HCC, 3 nodules < 3 cm
\# Multinodular, unresectable, Child-Pugh A or B, performance status (PST) 0
& Portal vein invasion, N1, M1, PST 1–2
@ Transplantation, resection, ablation

Figure 8-1 Hepatocellular carcinoma treatment allocation. *(Adapted from Bruix J, Sherman M, Practice Guidelines Committee, American Association for the Study of Liver Disease: Management of hepatocellular carcinoma,* Hepatology *42(5):1208–1236, 2005.)*

less effective in these respective locations. Presuming the patient is a good surgical candidate (normal liver function, absence of portal hypertension), the 5-year survival rate following anatomic resection is >75%.[82,83] Livraghi et al. conducted a retrospective analysis of 218 very-early-stage HCC patients treated with RFA and found an overall 55% 5-year survival rate, which climbed to 68% in patients whose initial tumor was deemed resectable, indicating a favorable comparison to surgery.[84] Cho et al.[85] simulated a randomized trial between resection and RFA based on previous data and concluded that RFA followed by resection (if necessary, in the event of local failure) had a nearly identical survival to primary resection. In conclusion, the current recommendations favor surgical resection in patients with very-early-stage disease; however, for nonresectable tumors, RFA offers excellent 5-year survival and spares significantly more hepatic parenchyma than anatomic resection.

Early-stage HCC patients, defined as having intact liver function (Child-Pugh Class A or B) and a solitary tumor 2–5 cm or 3 tumors <3 cm, can undergo resection, transplantation, or ablation. The decision as to which to pursue is highly patient and tumor specific. Head-to-head comparisons between RFA and resection have been conflicting, with one randomized trial[86] demonstrating essentially no difference, and the other favoring resection.[87] Other factors to consider are the size of the tumor; lesions greater than 3 cm are not as effectively treated at the margins by RFA.[88] As stated above, the heat-sink effect caused by vessels adjacent to the lesion limit the effectiveness of RFA. Other technologies, including MW ablation, may overcome some of these limitations of RFA, but further studies are required for confirmation.

Contraindications include diffuse or infiltrative tumors, those with vascular invasion, and distant disease. Relative contraindications include proximity to the gallbladder and gastrointestinal viscera, and a central location. Iatrogenic cholecystitis is usually temporary. The colon is most susceptible to thermal damage, possibly because of its fixed position and thin wall. A central tumor position has a higher risk for biliary tract violation.

The estimated mortality rate is 0.1%–0.5%, with major complication rates ranging from 2% to 3%.[94] Complications include thermal burns, intraperitoneal hemorrhage, bile duct

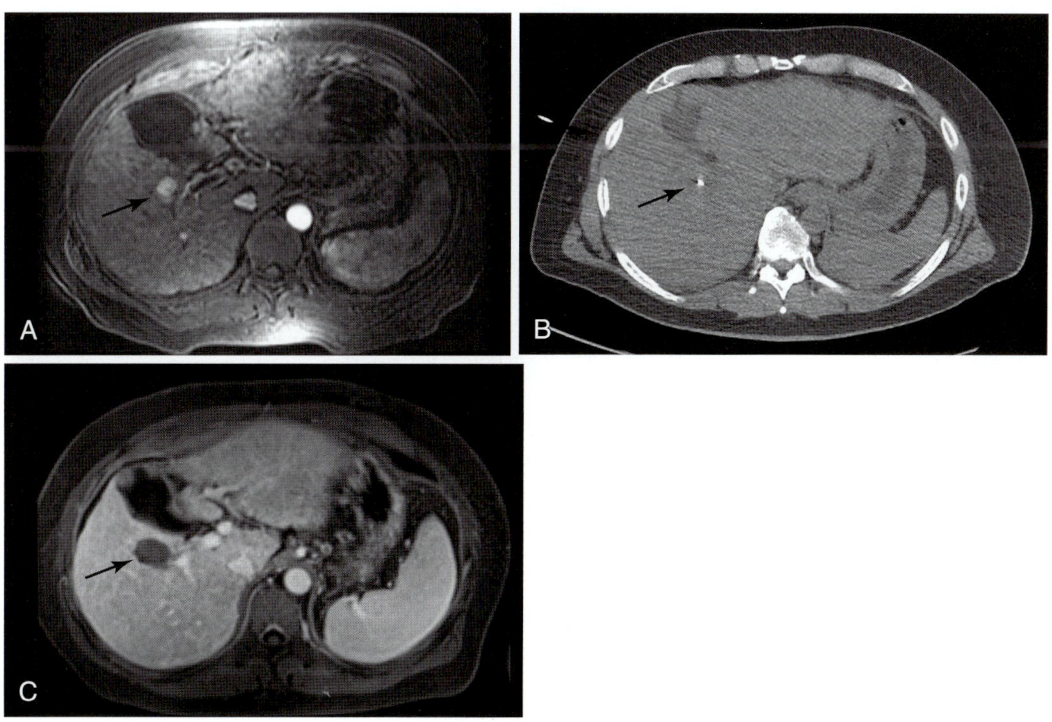

Figure 8-2 Radiofrequency ablation (RFA) of hepatocellular carcinoma (HCC) adjacent to the gallbladder. (A) Preablation contrast-enhanced magnetic resonance imaging (MRI) demonstrates a hypervascular HCC (*arrow*) adjacent to the gallbladder. (B) Intraoperative computed tomographic image demonstrates the tip of the RFA probe (*arrow*) in the lesion. (C) Postoperative MRI 3 months later demonstrates a hypointense well-circumscribed ablation zone with no residual or new disease.

injury, and visceral injury. Special note should be made of tumor tract seeding, estimated to have a 0.5% incidence,[95] for which many practitioners ablate the tract itself.

Percutaneous Chemical Injection

PEI is the oldest of the percutaneous ablative techniques. It relies on the dispersion of ethanol within the lesion, which results in coagulation necrosis. When compared to RFA for early-stage HCC, PEI shows a less favorable survival profile.[90] It also has been shown to have higher recurrence rates,[93] postulated to be secondary to inhomogeneous infiltration of a lesion and the inability to create an ablation margin that would encompass satellite lesions. However, in patients with very-early-stage HCC, PEI can be effective when tumor location makes the lesion unresectable or suboptimal for RFA.[89] It is also much less costly than the thermal ablative technologies.

Percutaneous acetic acid injection works on a similar principle to PEI, with the theoretical benefit compared to PEI of being able to dissolve intratumoral septations and achieve higher homogeneity. It compares favorably with PEI, but has not been widely adopted.

Microwave Ablation

MW technology causes local excitation of water molecules to generate tissue heat via friction, and is capable of creating much higher intratumoral temperatures than RFA (Figure 8-3). Moreover, MW ablation is capable of creating a larger ablation zone and is not affected by adjacent vasculature. That being said, the one randomized trial that compared MW ablation with RFA failed to demonstrate a survival benefit.[91] However, MW technology has improved markedly since this trial, and those results may be obsolete.

Cryoablation

Cryoablation relies on freezing temperatures to induce tumor cell death. It has the potential advantage of being able to see the developing "ice ball" as a hypodense oval during the ablation. However, it suffers from having very limited data to support its use in the setting of HCC. A 2011 study demonstrated a 60% 3-year survival in 40 patients with a 70% local control rate; however, the major complication rate was 12%.[92] It should be noted that Child-Pugh class and tumor size were not controlled for, so the relevance of this study to early-stage HCC is questionable.

Irreversible Electroporation

IRE is predicated on membrane disruption and subsequent cell death in the treated area. Its theoretical advantages are precision and nonthermal tumor kill, allowing for treatment of lesions adjacent to vasculature without injury to these vessels. No significant data are yet available to evaluate this upcoming technology in the setting of HCC.

POSTPROCEDURAL MANAGEMENT AND IMAGING

Patients should be kept in the hospital overnight for pain control and monitoring. Most patients can safely be discharged the

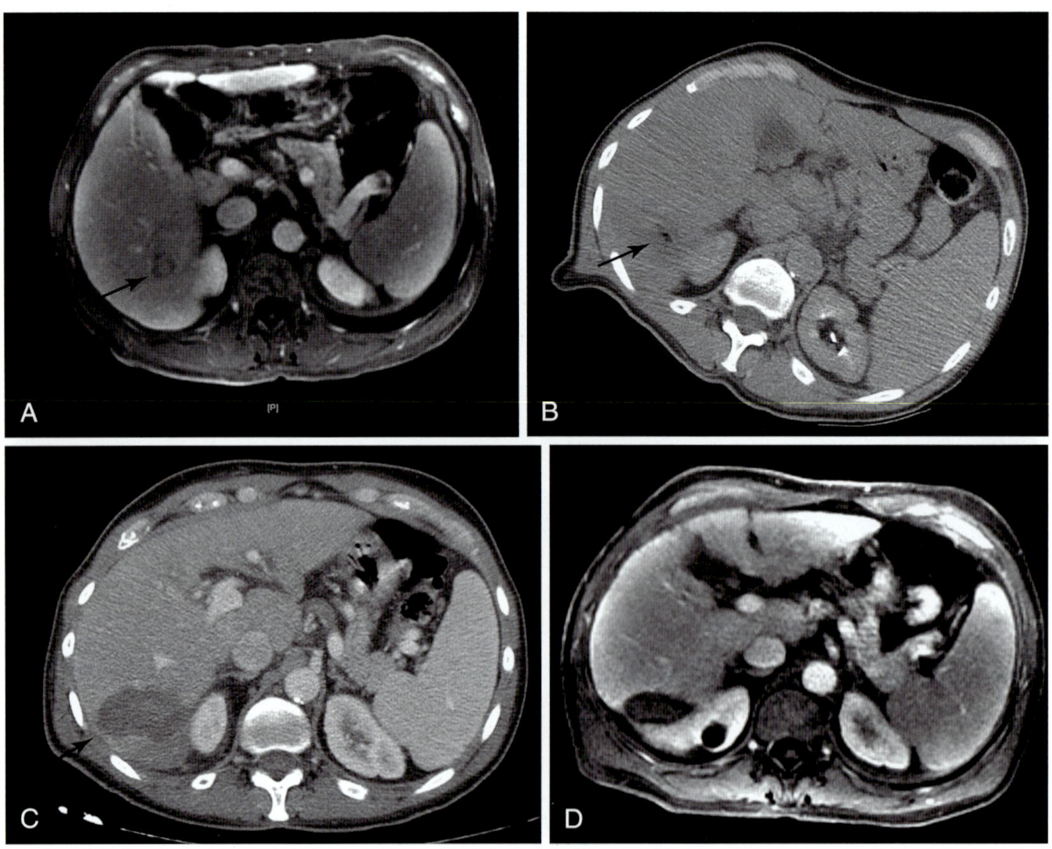

Figure 8-3 Microwave ablation of segment 6 hepatocellular carcinoma (HCC). (A) Preablation MRI demonstrates a nodular enhancing HCC (*arrow*) in segment 6. (B) Intraoperative computed tomographic (CT) image demonstrates the developing ablation zone (*arrow*). (C) CT obtained 3 days after the procedure shows a large ablation zone, including the ablation tract, with a smooth rim of hyperenhancement, consistent with reactive hyperemia. (D) Contrast-enhanced MRI 1 year after the ablation demonstrates a hypointense, nonenhancing ablation zone consistent with complete treatment.

day following the procedure. Some practices will obtain contrast-enhanced cross-sectional imaging several days after the procedure. It should be noted that a benign hyperenhancing smooth rim is often seen at this time, representing reactive hyperemia (Figure 8-3, *C*). This appearance should not be confused with residual tumor. A 1-month postablation scan is the standard, at which time nodular or irregular enhancement can be signs of residual tumor. Repeat ablation or alternative modalities can then be considered.

Transarterial Embolization and Chemoembolization

CLINICAL INDICATIONS

Table 8-1 lists the circumstances under which TACE is employed. The most common indication is for the treatment of unresectable HCC. Figure 8-1 demonstrates the Barcelona Clinic Liver Cancer (BCLC) schematic and highlights the patients who are most appropriate for transarterial therapies. As shown in the algorithm, those patients with Child-Pugh Class A or B, with unresectable intermediate-stage tumors, are the most appropriate candidates according to several society guidelines.[2-4]

The BCLC recommendation comes primarily from the two randomized clinical trials mentioned above that demonstrated a survival advantage for patients with unresectable HCC treated with conventional transarterial chemoembolization (cTACE) compared with best supportive care.[11,12] It should be noted that three other randomized controlled trials failed to show a survival benefit in patients treated with cTACE.[33-35] Several meta-analyses that were subsequently conducted supported the role of cTACE in treating unresectable HCC.[36,37] When understanding these data, it is important to note that patient selection likely accounted for the differences between the positive and negative trials. In the positive studies, patients were less than 75 years old, did not have portal vein thrombosis, had no hepatic decompensation (ascites, encephalopathy, variceal bleeding), and had preserved liver function.[38] Of note, the largest case series comes from Japan, in which data collected for more than 8000 patients demonstrated a mean survival of 34 months.[39]

Several trials have examined bland embolization in the setting of unresectable HCC. Bruix et al. demonstrated no survival advantage when 80 patients were randomized to receive bland embolization; however, these patients received embolic treatment that is not considered standard of care in most institutions, including proximal deployment of steel coils.[40] In contrast, other studies using bland embolization have shown a meaningful survival benefit. Covey et al. demonstrated 86%, 74%, and 47% survival at 1, 2, and 3 years, respectively, in patients with mostly Okuda stage I disease with recurrent HCC after resection.[41] The largest study was conducted by Maluccio et al., who reported a median survival of 21 months and 1-, 2-, and 3-year survival rates of, respectively, 66%, 46%, and 33% overall, and 84%, 66%, and 51% when patients with portal vein invasion or extrahepatic disease were excluded.[42]

Drug-eluting bead (DEB)-TACE has also shown efficacy in the treatment of unresectable HCC. Poon et al. conducted phase 1 and 2 clinical trials examining safety and efficacy in patients with unresectable HCC and showed that a dose of 150 mg of doxorubicin was tolerable with a response rate (partial plus complete) of 70%.[43] Varela et al. demonstrated a 1- and 2-year survival of 92.5% and 88.9% at 1 and 2 years in patients with unresectable HCC treated with DEB-TACE.[13] Malagari et al. reported on 71 patients with unresectable HCC and Child-Pugh Class A or B disease treated with DEB-TACE and showed an overall response rate of more than 80% and a 30-month survival of 88%.[44] The first phase 2 trial in the United States demonstrated 1- and 2-year survival rates of 65% and 55% in 20 patients.[15]

Transarterial therapies have also been used to improve the treatment efficacy of RFA. Limitations of RFA include higher recurrence in tumors greater than 3 cm and poor efficacy for tumors close to hepatic vessels secondary to a heat sink phenomenon. Transarterial techniques have been used in combination with RFA in both of these circumstances. Maluccio et al. compared surgical resection with combination RFA and transarterial embolization and found a trend toward improved survival in the combination group, although this finding was not statistically significant.[45] Morimoto et al. found slower tumor progression in patients with solitary HCCs between 3 and 5 cm treated with both RFA and TACE than in those treated with RFA alone.[46] Combination therapy may also be of value in patients with recurrent HCC after surgical resection, with lower intrahepatic recurrence compared with RFA or TACE alone.[47]

The transplant population represents a special category of unresectable HCC patients. For patients within the Milan criteria for transplantation, transarterial methods have been used to maintain their tumors within the size and number required for transplantation. Although the survival benefit has not been firmly established, some studies have noted that a better response to transarterial therapy is associated with higher posttransplant survival.[48] In select patients, transarterial therapy has successfully downstaged tumors so that these patients could be listed for transplant. Several studies have shown similar posttransplant survival in patients who were successfully downstaged and transplanted to those who were always within the Milan criteria before transplant, with one study demonstrating a 70% success rate in downstaging tumors and a 4-year posttransplant intention to treat survival of 69%.[49]

Combining transarterial techniques with surgical resection has also been explored. In a prospective study randomizing patients with tumors larger than 5 cm to upfront cTACE or surgical resection, no difference in survival was detected. However, those patients who responded to cTACE and ultimately underwent surgical resection had a longer survival than those

TABLE 8-1 Clinical Circumstances Under Which TAE, cTACE, or DEB-TACE Are Used

Current
Unresectable, intermediate stage HCC, Child-Pugh class A or B*
Combined with percutaneous ablation
Bridge to transplantation
Downstaging for transplantation
Combined with surgical resection
FUTURE/ONGOING
Combined with systemic therapy

*Current recommendation

cTACE, conventional transarterial chemoembolization; DEB, drug-eluting bead; HCC, hepatocellular carcinoma; TACE, transarterial chemoembolization; TAE, transarterial embolization who did not respond, suggesting that transarterial therapy response may be predictive of a good outcome after resection.[50]

COMPARISON OF TECHNIQUES

Currently, there is no consensus on which of the techniques are most efficacious in the treatment of HCC for the indications listed above. The strongest evidence supports cTACE in the treatment of intermediate unresectable HCC, as stated previously. However, this evidence is far from conclusive. The following paragraphs compare the three major techniques: cTACE versus TAE, cTACE versus DEB-TACE, and TAE versus DEB-TACE.

cTACE versus TAE

The two aforementioned randomized trials in 2002[11,12] demonstrating a significant survival benefit of cTACE over supportive care for unresectable HCC legitimized cTACE as the embolization method of choice for this disease. However, no direct large-scale comparison between bland embolization and cTACE has been performed. The Barcelona study,[12] which treated patients with both cTACE and bland embolization, was halted early and was not powered to detect a difference between the two embolic therapies. A meta-analysis looking at pooled data of bland and cTACE treated patients demonstrated similar 2-year survival between the groups.[36] A retrospective analysis published in 2006 demonstrated similar survival rates at 6 months, 1 year, and 2 years to those seen with cTACE.[42]

The underwhelming clinical evidence for cTACE over bland embolization has made some suggest that it is the embolic effect rather than the chemotherapeutic effect that predominates in transarterial tumor kill. Several lines of evidence favor this theory. First, lipiodol has embolic properties of its own.[20] Moreover, pharmacokinetic studies have shown that lipiodol poorly "retains" chemotherapeutic drugs, and that the systemic doses from cTACE are similar to those seen with systemic infusion.[13] Proponents of bland embolization also argue that it results in less pruning of the hepatic arterial circulation compared with cTACE because of the lack of chemotherapeutic toxicity on the endothelium.[51] This argument has yet to be validated prospectively, however. They also cite the lack of systemic toxicity that bland embolization offers.

Overall, there is no strong evidence to recommend one embolic strategy over the other when comparing bland embolization to cTACE.

cTACE versus DEB-TACE

Drug eluting beads operate on the principle that both tumor ischemia and cytotoxicity are necessary for maximal tumor kill. They also arose out of a desire to create uniformity during embolization that is not seen with cTACE. Moreover, DEB-TACE aims to reduce some of the systemic toxicity and side effects seen with cTACE.

Several comparisons between DEB-TACE and cTACE have been made. The PRECISION V trial[52] demonstrated a reduction in drug-related adverse events and liver toxicity in the DEB-TACE arm, as well as a trend toward higher rates of complete response, objective response, and disease control in the DEB-TACE arm, and a statistically significant improvement in tumor response in patients with more advanced disease. However, no survival advantage was seen between the 2 groups.

Larger multicenter randomized controlled trials are needed to convincingly support the use of one technique over the other.

DEB versus Bland Embolization

The crux of this comparison is whether the addition of drug elution from similar-sized beads results in better tumor response and overall survival. There are relatively few trials, however, that have looked at this question. Malagari et al. compared 84 patients with HCC who received either bland embolization or DEB-TACE, and found a longer time to progression in the DEB-TACE arm and higher recurrence rate in the bland embolization arm.[53] Limited head-to-head survival data have been collected.

The question as to which of these three techniques is superior has yet to be answered. Randomized trials comparing standard methodologies for each are underway and will potentially offer some clarity.

PATIENT PREPARATION AND PREOPERATIVE IMAGING

Relevant cross-sectional imaging, either magnetic resonance or computed tomography with arterial and portal contrast phases, should be reviewed to delineate the location of tumors and the extent of tumor burden. Moreover, the cross-sectional imaging will determine patency of the portal vein, the presence of extrahepatic disease, and arterial anatomy. The indication for embolization, whether it is to palliate or bridge to transplantation, should be explicitly discussed with the referring physician or tumor board. Important laboratory values to obtain or review include liver function tests (esp. serum bilirubin), serum creatinine, a complete blood count (including hemoglobin and platelet counts), and coagulation parameters (i.e., INR). Although practices vary, if the INR is >1.5 and the platelets are <50,000/mm^3, blood products should be administered before the procedure. If the patient has a history of biliary tree manipulation or ductal dilation, there is a higher risk of postembolization liver abscess formation, and prophylactic antibiotics should be administered preprocedurally. A history of contrast allergy should prompt appropriate premedication to prevent a contrast reaction during the procedure.

The patient's medication history should also be carefully reviewed. If possible, the patient should be off any antiplatelet agent (aspirin, clopidogrel) for 5 days before the procedure to avoid complications of arterial puncture.

Contraindications to transarterial therapy are listed in Table 8-2. A relative contraindication is portal vein thrombosis. However, Georgiades et al. demonstrated that cTACE could safely be performed in patients with portal vein thrombosis.[54] Other contraindications are related to poor hepatic function and decompensation, including Child-Pugh Class C disease, elevated bilirubin, and depressed serum albumin. No definite cutoff can be cited, although many practitioners become wary above a bilirubin of 2.0 mg/dL. Tumor biology also clearly affects the outcome of patients treated with transarterial therapies, with tumors >5 cm, tumor involving >50% of the liver, bilobar disease, more than three nodules, and elevated α-fetoprotein (AFP) conferring worse outcomes.[38,55]

PROCEDURAL TECHNIQUE

After access is gained most commonly via the common femoral artery, abdominal aortography is performed to determine the

TABLE 8-2 Contraindications to TAE/TACE

ADVANCED LIVER DISEASE
Child Pugh Class C
Moderate-severe ascites
Encephalopathy
Active gastrointestinal bleeding
Bilirubin >2*
Hypoalbuminemia (<2.5 mg/dL)*
Active transaminitis
Performance status >2
SYSTEMIC PARAMETERS
Neutropenia†
Cardiomyopathy†
Renal insufficiency

Partially adapted from Liapi E, Geschwind JF: Transcatheter arterial chemoembolization for liver cancer: is it time to distinguish conventional from drug-eluting chemoembolization? Cardiovasc Interv Radiol *34:37–49, 2011.*

*Relative contraindication; different practices have different thresholds

†Potentially exacerbated by doxorubicin administration, n/a for TAE

TACE, transarterial chemoembolization; TAE, transarterial embolization

arterial anatomy. This step can be omitted at the discretion of the interventionalist if the procedure is a repeat embolization; however, given that tumors parasitize the vasculature, if a significant time has elapsed between treatments, repeat aortography should be considered. Aortography will uncover the origins of the celiac artery and superior mesenteric artery (SMA), determine whether hepatic arterial anatomy is conventional or aberrant, and identify other potentially significant branches such as the left gastric artery, intercostal arteries, or the inferior phrenic arteries. Moreover, stenoses can be either visualized or inferred based on direction of flow (e.g., reversal of flow in the gastroduodenal artery implies a celiac stenosis). Third, the angle of the origin and the course of the celiac artery or the SMA can be identified to guide catheter choice.

The celiac artery can be engaged with a number of 4- or 5-French catheters. The cobra, Sos, or Simmons catheters are used most commonly. Assuming conventional anatomy, the catheter is advanced into the common hepatic artery, where digital subtraction angiography (DSA) in multiple planes can be performed to delineate relevant anatomy. Contrast injections of approximately 3–5 mL/s, for a total volume of 15–20 mL, can determine the course of the hepatic arterial branches and the supply to hypervascular hepatomas. Alternatively, if available, contrast-enhanced cone-beam computed tomography (CBCT) could be employed to derive similar information, with three-dimensional postprocessing of the acquired images adding powerful anatomical insights. A recent publication demonstrated that CBCT did not significantly add to the radiation exposure during a case and could adequately substitute for multiple DSA runs.[56] During these contrast injections, careful attention should be paid to arteriovenous shunting, given that particles may pass through these shunts and embolize to the lung. Additionally, extrahepatic branches to bowel should be recognized so that they may be either bypassed or prophylactically coil embolized.

Once the number and distribution of the tumors are identified, an embolization strategy can take shape. An important factor to consider is the patient's liver function. If the serum bilirubin is >2, a superselective approach is most prudent to minimize further damage to uninvolved hepatocytes. This superselective approach also has the advantage of concentrating the dose of the agent to maximize tumoricidal effects. However, if multiple tumors are present, several territories feed a single tumor, and/or if the patient's liver function is good, a less selective approach may be attempted.

The combination of a microcatheter and microwire is then used to select the branches to be embolized. If conventional TACE is chosen (Figure 8-4), then a mixture of the chemotherapeutic agent and lipiodol, typically in a 1:1 or 2:1 ratio, is given until one of several endpoints, including 2–5 beat stasis or portal venous staining, is observed. It should be noted that there is marked worldwide variation in the cytotoxic agents used, ranging from single-agent doxorubicin to combination infusion of doxorubicin, mitomycin C, and cisplatin. The practitioner can elect to give Gelfoam or embolization particles after the infusion of the lipiodol/chemotherapeutic drug, although the embolic effects of lipiodol may be sufficient to make this second step unnecessary. If DEB-TACE is selected (Figure 8-5), the doxorubicin-laden beads are mixed with a saline-to-contrast ratio of 1:1 and infused until the same endpoints are observed. Administration should be reasonably slow, as slow as 1 mL/min. There is no definitive data supporting the use of a particular bead size currently, although studies are ongoing. A trend toward smaller beads (100–300 μm) can be attributed to the ability to create a more distal embolization. Care should be taken to avoid reflux to prevent nontarget embolization. The amount of drug used is variable, but ranges from 50 to 150 mg of doxorubicin. If bland embolization (Figure 8-6) is selected, 40–500-μm particles can be used with static endpoints at the discretion of the practitioner.

If CBCT is available (Figures 8-4, *D* and 8-5, *D*), a posttreatment noncontrast acquisition can be useful to determine uptake of lipiodol within the tumor if cTACE was employed. Although not as conspicuous, contrast staining of the tumor after DEB-TACE or TAE can also be seen with a noncontrast acquisition.

After catheter removal, the arteriotomy site can be closed with either a closure device or via manual compression.

POSTEMBOLIZATION CARE AND FOLLOW-UP IMAGING

The overall complication rate for the above transarterial therapies is 4%–7%, with a 30-day mortality of ~1%.[20] Postembolization syndrome (PES), consisting of nausea, abdominal pain, and fever, occurs in a majority of patients, with data suggesting that cTACE is associated with more severe PES.[52] This syndrome is thought to be secondary to a combination of tissue ischemia and inflammation. Other complications include liver abscess formation, liver infarction, cholecystitis, and nontarget embolization to the gastrointestinal tract with ulcer formation. Liver abscess formation, as mentioned previously, is most commonly seen in patients with preexisting biliary disease or biliary manipulation, and is thought to be secondary to bile duct ischemia compromising bacterial clearance.

Most practices will elect to keep a patient overnight for pain and nausea management. Typical discharge medications include an antiemetic, medications for pain control (usually abdominal pain), and stool softeners. Postembolization pain can be expected for up to 1 week postprocedure.

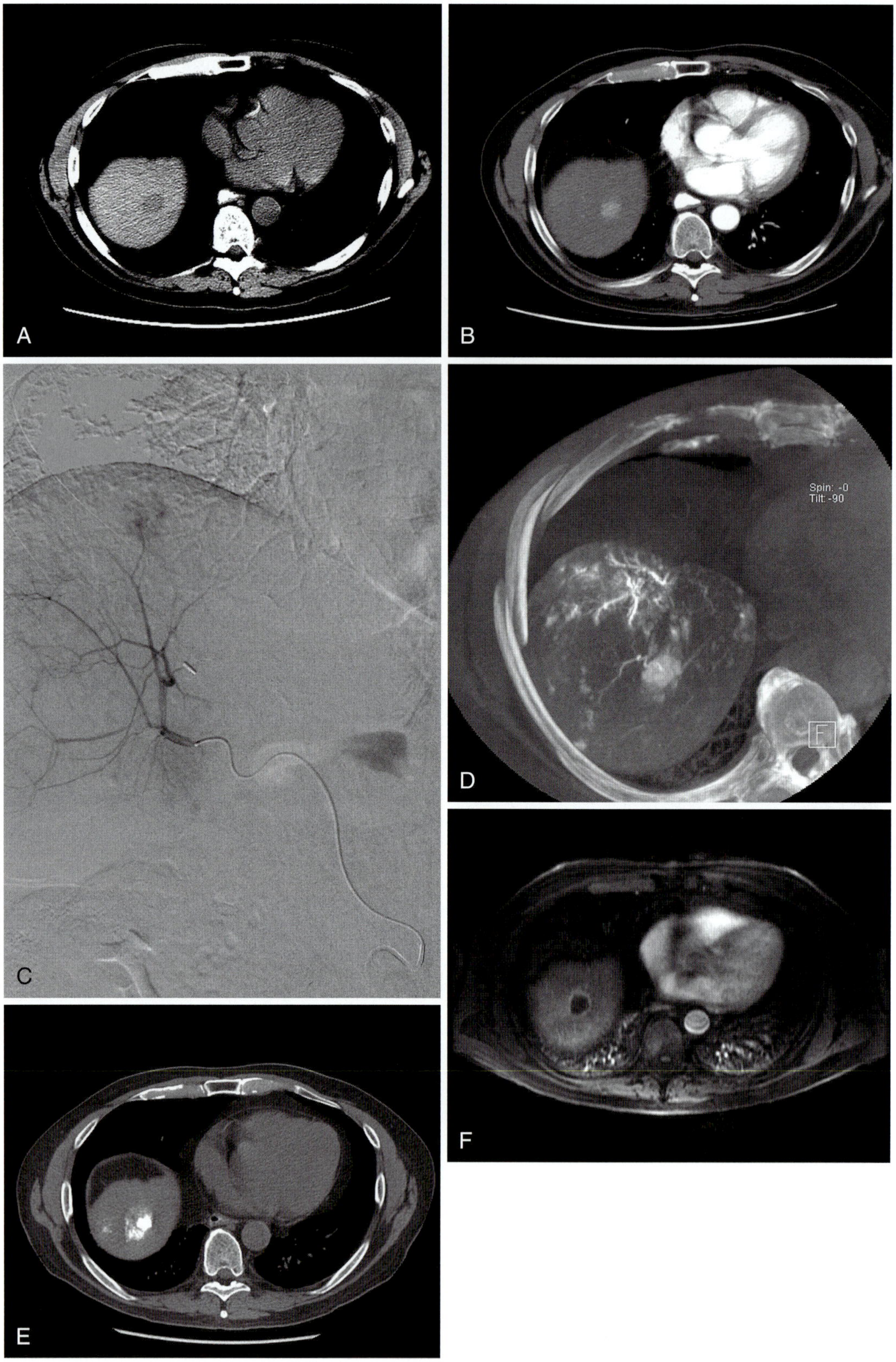

Figure 8-4 65-year-old man with known hepatocellular carcinoma (HCC). Initial therapy via left hepatectomy now with recurrence in the remnant. (A and B) Axial computed tomography (CT) without and with intravascular contrast. Focal hypoattenuating area in the right lobe enhancing with intravascular contrast consistent with and representing known solitary HCC. (C and D) Hepatic arteriography; digital subtraction angiography and axial reconstructed cone-beam CT. Demonstrate focal area of increased vascular density in the right lobe corresponding to the abnormality seen on preprocedure CT. (E and F) Lipiodol transarterial chemoembolization (TACE) follow-up. Axial CT demonstrates focal deposition and retention of lipiodol within known HCC. Liver acquisition and volume acquisition magnetic resonance imaging demonstrates lesion without gadolinium-based enhancement indicative of adequate therapy.

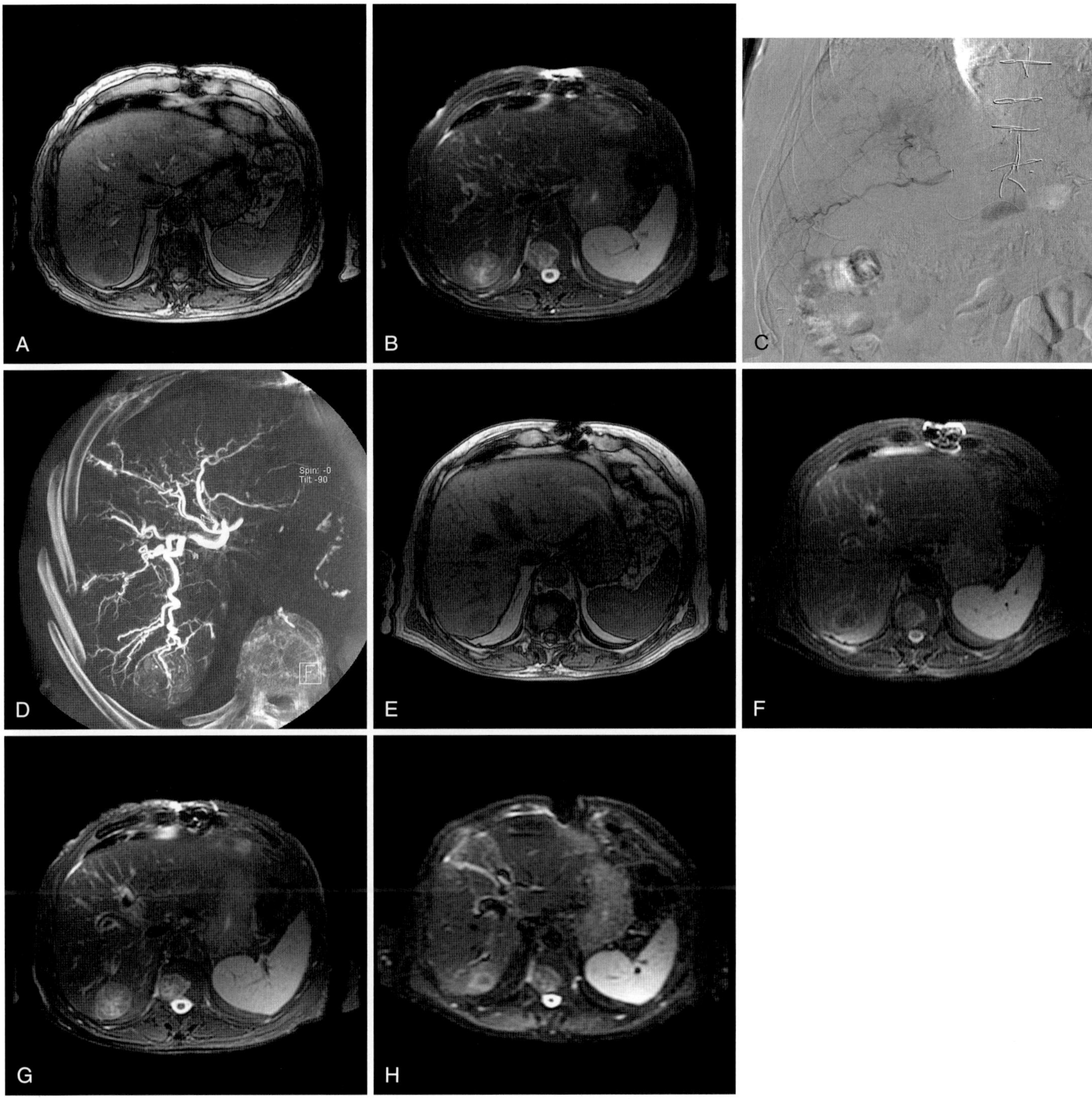

Figure 8-5 85-year-old man with history of large-cell lymphoma, prostatic cancer, and recently diagnosed with hepatocellular carcinoma in the right lobe of the liver. Treated with drug-eluting bead and transarterial chemoembolization (DEB-TACE). (A and B) T1- and T2-weighted magnetic resonance (MR) images demonstrate a well-circumscribed mass in the right lobe of the liver representing the patient's biopsy-proven hepatocellular carcinoma (HCC) pretherapy. (C) Right hepatic selective arteriography. A solitary hypervascular focus consistent with multiple arterial afferents is noted. (D) Axial reconstructed cone-beam computed tomographic (CT) images with hepatic arterial contrast enhancement. Solitary, well-circumscribed focus corresponding to the HCC lesion seen on MRI is noted. (E and F) T1- and T2-weighted MR images demonstrate decrease in the size of the mass in the right lobe of the liver post DEB-DOX. (G and H) Diffusion-weighted MRI demonstrated drastically decreased diffusion into the lesion, indicating posttherapy effect.

Follow-up imaging, either contrast-enhanced multiphase MR or CT, can be performed from 4 to 6 weeks to 3 months after the procedure to assess for residual, recurrent, or new disease. Previously, RECIST and WHO criteria were employed to determine treatment response. More recently, the EASL and mRECIST criteria have been gaining greater acceptance because they take into account tumor enhancement as a measure of response.[57]

If another embolization is indicated after the 3-month period, a reassessment of the patient's liver function, including the serum bilirubin, is necessary to gauge the likelihood of worsening hepatic function after a repeat embolization.

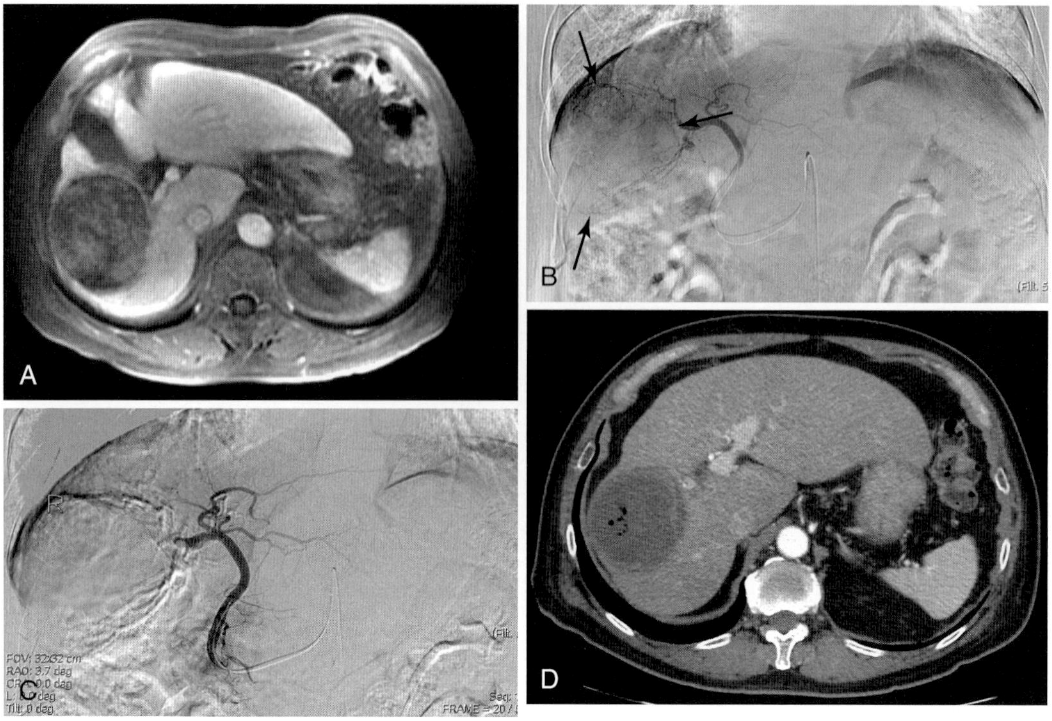

Figure 8-6 Bland embolization of large right lobe hepatocellular carcinoma in a 72-year-old man. (A) Contrast-enhanced magnetic resonance imaging demonstrating large right hepatic lobe mass. (B) Right hepatic arteriogram demonstrating the arterially enhancing mass, margins delineated by arrows. (C) Postembolization with 100-μm bland particles demonstrates no arterial enhancement. (D) Computed tomography performed 1 month after embolization demonstrates no residual enhancement, with foci of air indicative of tumor necrosis.

OTHER TRANSARTERIAL APPROACHES

Radioembolization

Radioembolization refers to the intraarterial administration of ^{90}Y-loaded beads that lodge in the arteriolar circulation supplying tumors and deliver tumoricidal radiation. It evolved out of the inability of external beam radiation to deliver high doses without causing radiation hepatitis.[58] In contrast to external beam radiation, which can only deliver 30–35 Gy of radiation before causing clinically significant hepatotoxicity, intraarterial ^{90}Y can deliver up to 150 Gy.[58,60] Moreover, ^{90}Y beads lodge preferentially in tumor vasculature and have a limited treatment zone, thus maximizing radiation to the tumor and minimizing it to the hepatic parenchyma. Histologic studies have demonstrated accumulation in tumoral arterioles at a concentration greater than 50 times that in adjacent normal liver.[59]

^{90}Y is a pure beta emitter, with a half-life of 64.2 hours, decaying to stable ^{90}Zr.[61] This fact, combined with the maximal penetration of electrons 10 mm from the delivered beads, makes patient isolation unnecessary. Two radioembolic beads are commercially available: resin-based SIR spheres (Sirtex Medical, Lake Forest, IL) and glass-based TheraSpheres (MDS Nordion, Ottawa, Ontario, Canada). These <50-μm beads both encapsulate ^{90}Y and prevent leakage of the radioisotope. TheraSpheres carry approximately 50 times more dose per bead than SIR spheres, so much fewer beads are required to deliver a similar dose. SIR spheres are U.S. Food and Drug Administration approved for the treatment of colorectal cancer metastases in combination with 5-FU. TheraSpheres received a humanitarian device exemption for the treatment of HCC in 1999.

Radioembolization has been used in multiple clinical settings. Similar to the transarterial therapies discussed earlier, several papers have demonstrated efficacy for unresectable HCC. The largest series in the United States, published by Salem et al., included 291 patients with unresectable HCC.[63] The authors found that the overall time to progression was 7.9 months. Patients with Child-Pugh Class A disease had a 17.2-month average survival, whereas those with class B disease had a 7.7-month survival. Other nonrandomized studies have demonstrated median survivals of approximately 20 months for early-stage patients and approximately 11 months for intermediate-stage patients (using Child-Pugh and Okuda staging).[63,64]

There are limited studies comparing radioembolization and chemoembolization. Several have demonstrated that the two approaches confer similar survival and tumor response.[65,66] Given that ^{90}Y microspheres are thought to be less embolic than the agents used in TACE and TAE, radioembolization may be safer in patients with extensive portal vein thrombosis. It should be noted, however, that main portal vein *tumor* thrombus, even in a safely treated patient, carries a poor prognosis, with an average survival between 3 and 6 months.[67] Radioembolization may also have an advantage over chemoembolization in downstaging tumors to within the Milan criteria, as demonstrated by Lewandowski et al.[68]

An interesting application of radioembolization is in the treatment of early-stage disease with a curative intent, given that 90% of ^{90}Y-treated tumors less than 3 cm and two-thirds of tumors between 3 and 5 cm show complete pathologic necrosis (so-called radiation segmentectomy).[69] Additionally, it has been observed that treatment of a lobe results in atrophy of that lobe and hypertrophy of the contralateral one, a characteristic that may aid in resection.[70]

When considering a patient for radioembolization, the tumor stage, liver function, renal function, performance status, α-fetoprotein level, coagulation parameters, and goals of treatment must be taken into consideration, most reliably achieved through a multidisciplinary board. Pretreatment imaging should include a contrast-enhanced CT or MR that defines the burden of disease and allows for dosimetry calculation. Those patients with poor hepatic reserve are less likely to tolerate a whole liver treatment. Other patients at high risk include those with disease affecting >50% of the liver, albumin less than 3 mg/dL, or bilirubin greater than 2 mg/dL.[71] Patients with impaired pulmonary status should also be examined carefully, because a significant lung shunt fraction is more likely to cause life-threatening radiation pneumonitis in this group. Prior external beam radiation therapy is also considered a contraindication.

Calculating the activity of radioactive particles to be administered is different for the two types of microspheres. Both techniques, however, require the calculation of liver volumes, obtained from cross-sectional imaging acquired prior to or during the procedure (i.e., cone-beam CT). The desired dose is anywhere between 80 and 150 Gy. For TheraSpheres, only the treated volume of liver is used, without accounting for tumor burden/volume. The activity required for a given dose is calculated using the following[72]:

$$A\ (\text{GBq}) = D\ (\text{Gy}) \times [\text{target liver mass (kg)}]/50.$$

The actual dose delivered to the liver takes into account how much is shunted to the lung (and therefore not retained in the liver) and the residual activity left in the vial, captured by the following formula[72]:

$$D\ (\text{Gy}) = 50[A\ (\text{GBq}) \times (1 - \text{LSF})(1 - R)]/M\ (\text{kg}),$$

where A is activity, D is dose, LSF is lung shunt fraction, and R is residual. For example, if the interventionalist wishes to treat a lobe with a volume of 1000 mL, assuming a density of 1.03 g/mL, with 100 Gy, the activity required from the manufacturer is

$$(100 \times 1.03)/50 = 2.06\ \text{GBq}.$$

The dose actually delivered to the liver, assuming a lung shunt fraction of 7% and a vial residual of 1%, is

$$D = 2.06 \times 50 \times (1 - 0.07) \times (1 - 0.01)/1.03 = 92.1\ \text{Gy}.$$

The SIR sphere calculation takes into account tumor volume and body surface area, in addition to liver volumes[73]:

$$A(\text{GBq}) = \text{body surface area } (m^2) - 0.2 + (\%\text{tumor involvement}/100).$$

Planning for the procedure is very different between the two types of microspheres. TheraSphere particles arrive in predetermined activity vials, so the dose calculation needs to take into account the daily decay; this gives the interventionalist some flexibility in scheduling the procedure. On the other hand, SIR sphere vials have a precalibrated activity of 3 GBq, and usually have to be used within 24 hours after arrival.

Dose determination for either of these microspheres must take into account hepatic function. For example, a patient with poor hepatic reserve and a single tumor confined to a segment can be treated in a segmental fashion. However, if the same patient has multiple tumors requiring a lobar or whole liver treatment, there is a higher likelihood of inducing liver failure. On the other hand, whole liver or lobar treatment can be safely administered to a patient with multifocal/multilobar HCC and preserved hepatic function.

The procedure itself (Figure 8-7) can be divided into two steps: a "mapping" step, during which essential arterial anatomy is identified and extrahepatic branches to critical viscera are prophylactically embolized, and an administration step, during which the radioembolic beads are infused. The puncture and catheterization techniques described above are identical, and will not be described further. Aortography is especially important during the mapping step, as anatomic variants (e.g., replaced right hepatic artery, accessory left hepatic artery), extrahepatic tumoral arterial supply (e.g., intercostals, inferior phrenic arteries), and visceral branches are preliminarily identified. Once the main hepatic arterial supply is catheterized, DSA and CBCT are vital tools. Critical branches to identify include the gastroduodenal artery, the right gastric artery, and pancreatic and duodenal branches arising from the common or proper hepatic arteries, and occasionally from branches of the proper hepatic artery (right and left hepatic arteries). Additionally, the falciform artery, if present, needs to be recognized. Depending on which lobe is to be treated, some or all of these arteries will need to be prophylactically embolized with coils to prevent nontarget embolization. During the mapping phase, extrahepatic arteries that supply the tumor are also coil embolized to allow for redistribution of blood flow from arteries that are to be treated. This is to avoid incomplete treatment of tumors that may derive some or most of their arterial supply from extrahepatic sources. At the conclusion of the mapping study, cone-beam CT is useful to ensure that the distribution to be treated contains the tumor. Moreover, it can be used to calculate liver volumes for dosimetry. Once the area to be treated has been defined, technetium^{99}-labeled macroaggregated albumin (~1–5 mCi) is injected into the artery to calculate a lung shunt fraction.

Typical lung shunt fractions, in the absence of underlying pulmonary disease, that are acceptable are approximately 10% for TheraSphere treatment and 20% for SIR sphere treatment, with a maximum dose to the lung of 30 Gy during an individual session and 50 Gy over a lifetime.[74] If fractions are higher, radioembolization should potentially be aborted. Several other techniques prior to or during the administration step (below) can be utilized in an attempt to prevent shunting of radioembolic particles, including balloon occlusion of the hepatic veins and bland embolization prior to administration of ^{90}Y-microspheres to reduce the shunt, although these techniques have not been validated.

The second step is the actual administration. Occasionally, if difficulty was encountered during the mapping study while catheterizing some of the more challenging branches (often the right gastric artery), catheterization of these branches can be reattempted prior to administration. Once the microcatheter (typically a 2.8-Fr microcatheter) is in position, the SIR spheres or TheraSpheres are administered under fluoroscopic observation, paying close attention to possible reflux. Differences in the microspheres are most obviously seen during administration; far more SIR sphere particles are injected for the same dose than TheraSphere particles. Given the much lower number of TheraSpheres administered, embolic effects and stasis are rarely

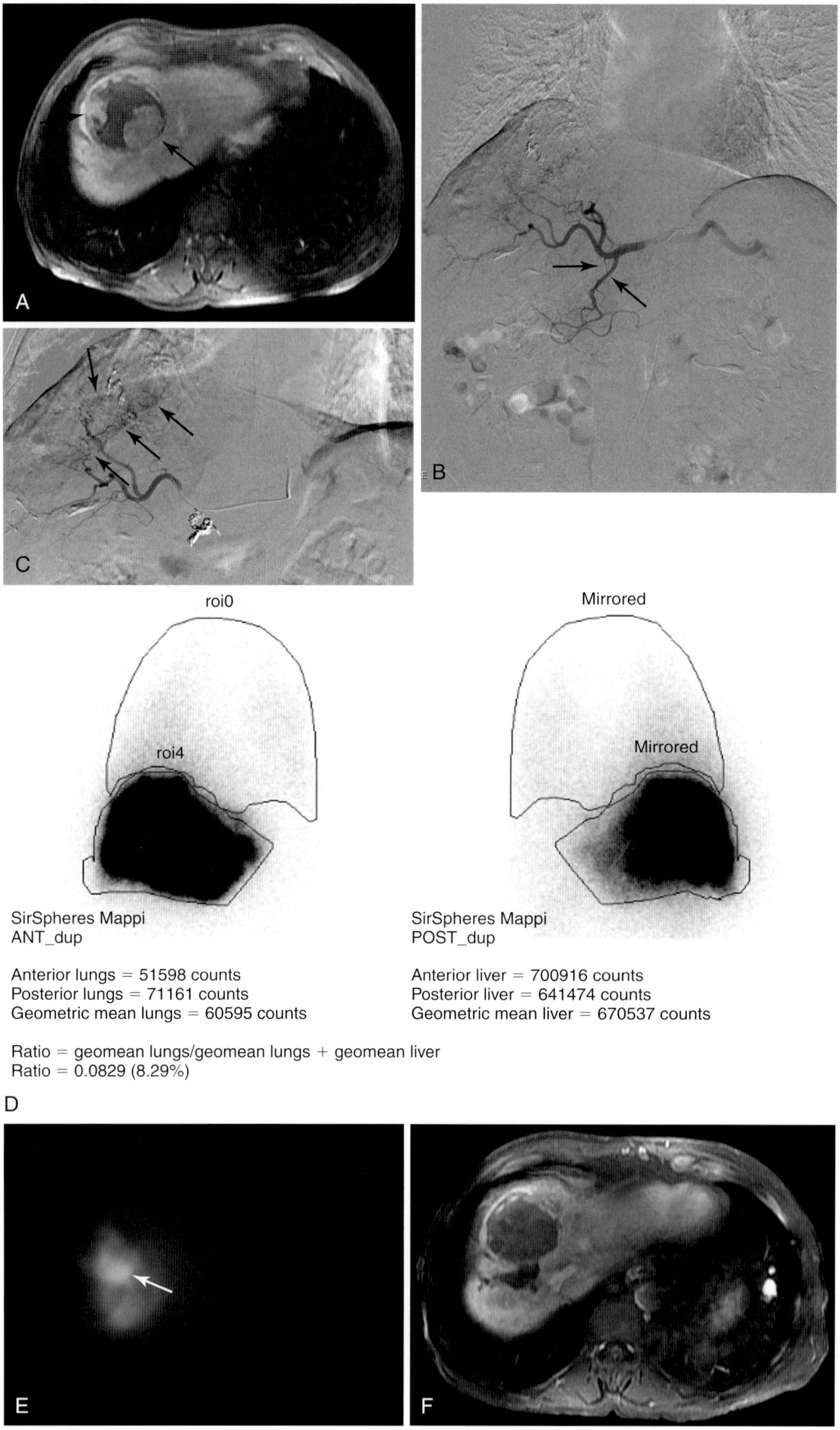

Figure 8-7 Yttrium-90 radioembolization treatment of multifocal/multilobar hepatocellular carcinoma in a 68-year-old man. (A) Large cystic and solid hepatocellular carcinoma (HCC) in right hepatic lobe with multiple nodular enhancing components (*arrows*). (B) Right hepatic arteriogram demonstrating the gastroduodenal and right gastric arteries (*long* and *short arrow*, respectively). (C) After coiling of the gastroduodenal artery and right gastric arteries, right hepatic arteriogram demonstrates multiple enhancing HCCs in the right hepatic lobe. (D) Scintigraphy after injection of 4.1 mCi of Tc-MAA demonstrates mostly hepatic uptake, with a lung shunt fraction of 8.29%. (E) Single-photon emission computed tomography after administration of Yttrium-90 microspheres demonstrates increased uptake within the nodular component of the tumor (*arrow*). (F) Contrast-enhanced MRI obtained 3 months after treatment demonstrates resolution of nodular enhancement seen on pretreatment MRI.

seen. In contrast, SIR spheres are more likely to cause stasis, and the full desired dose might not be delivered in this scenario.

The procedure itself is usually very well tolerated, with little to none of the postembolization syndrome seen with TAE or TACE. Gastrointestinal ulcer formation from nontarget embolization occurs in less than 2% of cases. Radiation pneumonitis is more common with higher lung shunt fractions and repeat sessions. Hepatotoxicity is the most common adverse event, complicating approximately 15% of radioembolic procedures.[38]

Patients on discharge should receive adequate medication for pain control, nausea, and constipation. Follow-up care should include repeat imaging at 4–6 weeks posttherapy to assess for treatment efficacy, residual, or new disease. A 1-month clinic visit is also warranted to assess the patient's functional status. Basic laboratory data and tumor markers can also be obtained at this time.

A special note should be made for whole liver treatment. It is generally discouraged to treat the whole liver from the common hepatic artery or proper hepatic artery, even if branches such as the right gastric artery and gastroduodenal artery have been coil embolized. The reason is that numerous small branches arising from these arteries supplying bowel and pancreatic tissue may not be visualized. Instead, whole liver treatment, whether administered on the same day or in multiple sessions, should be performed with separate microcatheters in each distribution (e.g., one from the right hepatic artery and a second from the left).[71]

Radiolabeled lipiodol is another form of transarterial delivery of radiation. Given that lipiodol is 37% iodine by weight and has a unique ability to concentrate within hepatomas, it is not surprising that several investigators have examined the effect of ^{131}I-labeled lipiodol delivery on tumor response and survival. Data are limited; however, one study showed a trend toward improved survival in patients treated with adjuvant postoperative intraarterial ^{131}I-labeled lipiodol compared with those who were not.[75] A randomized controlled multicenter trial demonstrated similar survival in patients treated with ^{131}I-labeled lipiodol versus TACE for unresectable HCC.[76] The main advantage of this approach is that it is well tolerated compared with cTACE. Its major drawback is the requirement for the patient to be in isolation after the procedure because of the long half-life and gamma emission of ^{131}I.

Chemoinfusion, or the exclusive administration of cytotoxic drugs into the liver without lipiodol or an embolic agent via a permanently placed catheter in the hepatic artery, has been primarily used in the setting of metastatic disease to the liver. One study that examined its use in the setting of unresectable HCC found no survival difference between chemoinfusion and chemoembolization.[77]

Future Directions

Clinical trials are underway to examine combined systemic therapy and transarterial therapy. Two agents, one used for monotherapy in advanced HCC (sorafenib) and an antiangiogenesis molecule (bevacizumab) are being added to chemoembolization and/or radioembolization to determine if the combination results in better tumor response, slower tumor progression, and longer survival than the individual approaches. The rationale behind combining bevacizumab and chemoembolization is to reduce the recruitment of blood vessels in the setting of induced tumor ischemia. Given sorafenib's efficacy in the treatment of advanced HCC, several trials are underway to evaluate TACE plus sorafenib versus placebo. One recent phase 2 trial reported acceptable safety in 35 patients treated with sorafenib with disease control rates of 95% and 100% (RECIST and EASL respectively).[78] Just as "radiosensitizing" chemotherapy is being used for external beam radiation, chemotherapeutic agents are being considered in conjunction with radioembolization for the treatment of HCC.[61]

Gene therapy targeting tumors offers an intriguing area of future research. Intraarterial delivery of both viral and nonviral vectors (nanocomposites, iodized oil) may improve, respectively, the safety profile and concentration of these two approaches.[79]

New cytotoxic drugs may have higher efficacy against HCC than those traditionally used, especially considering that the current cytotoxic agents were not chosen based on data. One interesting approach is the intraarterial delivery of 3-bromopyruvate to specifically target tumor glycolysis.[80]

Finally, advances in imaging, including magnetic resonance diffusion imaging, that look at both functionality and anatomy, will augment current imaging paradigms. Concomitantly, better definition of treatment response and outcomes taking into account both tumor size and necrosis will allow for improved assessment of current and novel techniques to treat HCC.

REFERENCES

The complete reference list is available online at www.expertconsult.com.

9

Systemic Therapy in Advanced Hepatocellular Carcinoma

CELINA ANG | DWIGHT OWEN | GHASSAN K. ABOU-ALFA

KEY POINTS

- Cytotoxic chemotherapy has not proven effective in hepatocellular carcinoma (HCC). Sorafenib is the only approved agent for advanced, unresectable disease.
- Current studies are evaluating a wide range of targeted agents covering the spectrum of molecular aberrations in HCC. Currently, there are no effective alternatives for sorafenib-refractory HCC.
- The combination of sorafenib and chemoembolization has not been shown to improve clinical outcomes. Combined systemic and liver-directed therapy in HCC remains investigational.

Introduction

Research and therapeutic development in advanced hepatocellular carcinoma (HCC) have evolved in recent years. New insights into the genetics and molecular biology of HCC have transformed the way it is studied and treated.

The management of HCC is generally determined by disease extent and performance status with the additional consideration of hepatic function. The prototypical Barcelona Clinic Liver Cancer (BCLC) algorithm considers these variables in separating patients into discrete groups for which specific lines of therapy are prescribed.[1] However, these categories are more fluid in daily clinical practice, especially for locally advanced disease considered unresectable. These patients may be treated with locoregional and/or systemic therapies at different times during the clinical course rather than pursuing a strictly linear therapeutic sequence. The growing reality of an interdisciplinary management approach is reflected by the proliferation of clinical trials studying combined modality therapy.

This chapter will discuss the management of locally advanced HCC that is no longer amenable to surgical and liver directed ablative therapies, as well as metastatic disease. An overview of systemic therapies currently being investigated in HCC will be presented in addition to a discussion of aspects that are important for the interventional radiology domain.

Staging

The challenge of managing HCC arises from the dual nature of the disease: the malignancy itself and the underlying cirrhosis. Before embarking on any course of treatment, an assessment of the hepatic functional reserve is imperative, in view if its prognostic implications, and its impact on the management plan. The most commonly used scoring system for cirrhosis in clinical practice is the Child-Pugh classification, which uses three laboratory (serum bilirubin, albumin, international normalized ratio [INR]) and two clinical (ascites, encephalopathy) variables. Each variable is graded according to its severity. The total grades of all five variables are added and make up a score that ranges from the least decompensated category (A), through moderate (B), to the most decompensated (C) liver.[2]

The key limitation of the Child-Pugh scoring system is its lack of any cancer-related parameters, which obviously are key contributors to HCC patients' prognosis.[3]

The objective of a staging system is to provide prognostic information that helps the clinician devise a management plan appropriate for the anticipated clinical outcome. Several different staging systems have been developed for HCC that include the purely anatomic American Joint Committee on Cancer/Union Internationale Contre le Cancer (AJCC/UICC) TNM (tumor, node, metastasis) system to a variety of hybrid anatomic and functional systems such as the BCLC algorithm. Given that each of these systems were developed in populations of varying ethnicities, risk factors for cirrhosis, and treatment approaches, their general applicability and predictive potential, especially for patients with locally advanced or unresectable HCC, is a continued subject of debate. Although the BCLC algorithm is considered to be the most comprehensive of the hybrid staging systems and has been validated prospectively,[4,5] its discriminatory power among patients with advanced HCC is limited. A single-institution review of the different systems found that the Cancer of the Liver Italian Program (CLIP) which was developed in patients with hepatitis C, the Chinese University Prognostic Index (CUPI) developed primarily in patients with hepatitis B, and the Groupe d'Etude et de Traitement du Carcinome Hepatocellulaire (GETCH) best predicted outcomes in patients with advanced HCC, whereas the BCLC and sixth edition TNM systems were not informative in this setting.[6] These findings were consistent with an earlier study showing that the CLIP system outperformed the BCLC and Okuda systems in the palliative setting.[7] Thus, although the BCLC algorithm serves as an important roadmap for prognostication and management, outcomes of patients with locally advanced or metastatic HCC may be better estimated by the CLIP, CUPI, or GETCH systems if the dominant underlying risk factor is hepatitis C, hepatitis B, or alcoholic cirrhosis, respectively.

Systemic Chemotherapy

Several classes of chemotherapy agents exist, each exerting its cytotoxic effects through one or several of these mechanisms: alkylating agents, platinums, and topoisomerase inhibitors cause DNA strand breakage; fluoropyrimidines and other antimetabolites inhibit DNA synthesis; taxanes and vinca alkaloids prevent microtubule formation and cell division. Unlike molecularly targeted agents that will be discussed later, chemotherapy represents a less discriminatory form of therapy; normal cells rely on the same mechanisms to maintain DNA integrity, proliferate, and survive as their cancerous counterparts and are therefore subject to the same cytotoxic effects. Many of the toxicities of chemotherapy drugs result from the collateral damage incurred to normal cells in addition to cancer cells.

Studies of single-agent chemotherapy in HCC began during the 1960s–1970s. One of the earliest agents to be tested was doxorubicin (also known as adriamycin), from the anthracycline family of alkylating agents. In 1975, a phase 2 trial reported a striking objective response rate of 79% and median survival of 8 months.[8] Subsequent studies of doxorubicin were unable to replicate these results; response rates ranged from 15% to 20% and median survival was only 4 months. Phase 3 studies also did not show doxorubicin to be superior to other chemotherapy regimens.[3]

Clinical trials of 5-fluorouracil, a fluoropyrimidine used in the treatment of many gastrointestinal malignancies, as well as newer agents such as the topoisomerase I inhibitor irinotecan and the antimetabolite gemcitabine failed to produce durable response and survival outcomes.[3] Although combination regimens such as gemcitabine + oxaliplatin (GEMOX) and oral 5-fluorouracil (capecitabine) + oxaliplatin (CAPOX) appeared to be more active on the basis of phase 2 data, their impact on survival has not been assessed in phase 3 studies.[3] The strategy of combined chemoimmunotherapy has also been studied in advanced HCC. Interferon α-2b (IFN) was combined with cisplatin, doxorubicin, and 5-fluorouracil (PIAF) in a phase 2 study.[9] Median survival was 8.9 months. Notably, 26% of patients had a partial response, 12% were converted to resectable disease, and 8% of patients had a pathologic complete response. PIAF was associated with significant hematologic toxicities; 34% of patients had grade 3/4 leukopenia, 22% had grade 3/4 thrombocytopenia and two patients died of neutropenic sepsis. Despite the considerable toxicities, the compelling clinical and pathologic responses reported in this study led to a phase 3 trial comparing PIAF with doxorubicin, which was still considered the most effective chemotherapy agent at the time.[10] The primary endpoint, overall survival, was not statistically significantly different between the study arms (8.7 vs. 6.8 months, $P = .83$). Response rates were higher but not statistically significant in favor of PIAF (20.9% vs. 10.5%, $P = .06$), and one patient on each arm had a pathologic complete response. There was a significantly higher incidence of neutropenia, thrombocytopenia, and hypokalemia of any grade on the PIAF arm; however, there were no treatment-related deaths.

The limited impact of chemotherapy on responses and survival in HCC has several potential explanations. HCC tumors have been shown to overexpress the multidrug resistance gene-1 (*MDR-1*) and P-glycoprotein drug extrusion molecule.[3] Furthermore, the therapeutic index of chemotherapy, especially chemoimmunotherapy, is narrowed in a patient population with limited end-organ reserve. For these reasons, chemotherapy has been supplanted by molecularly targeted agents in HCC, though it may still be useful as an adjunct to these agents. The combination of sorafenib and doxorubicin has shown promising activity[11] and will be discussed below.

Targeted Therapies

In most cases, the initiating step in hepatocarcinogenesis is liver injury due to hepatotoxins, viral hepatitis, or other insults, leading to chronic inflammation, cirrhosis, and the formation of dysplastic nodules and ultimately HCC (Figure 9-1). These steps are accompanied and driven by amplifications in oncogenes, losses in tumor suppressor function, and changes in signaling pathways that are normally responsible for maintaining hepatohomeostasis. Among the myriad factors that have been implicated in this process are the receptor tyrosine kinases (RTKs) including the epidermal growth factor receptor (EGFR) family, insulinlike growth factor receptor (IGFR), vascular endothelial growth factor receptor (VEGFR), and c-met. Interactions between these cell surface molecules and their specific ligands cause a conformational change in the RTK, leading to phosphorylation of their intracellular domains, and downstream activation of signaling cascades including the Ras/Raf/Mek/Erk (MAP kinase) and PI3K/Akt/mTOR cascades.[12] Signal transmission through these intracellular conduits results in the transcriptional activation of genes that govern cell growth, proliferation, the evasion of apoptosis, angiogenesis, and invasive and metastatic capabilities. Established HCC tumors also continue to evolve and acquire additional aberrations that enable their survival through compensatory changes in the same pathways, or through the co-optation of associated networks. Therapeutic disruption

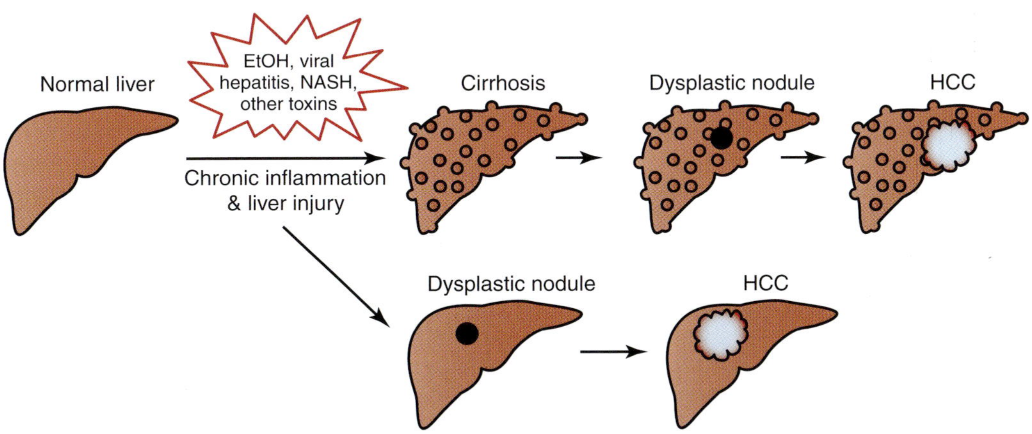

Figure 9-1 Pathogenesis of hepatocellular carcinoma

of tumor cell signaling circuitry at its different levels is actively being studied in HCC.

RECEPTOR TYROSINE KINASES

Epidermal Growth Factor Receptor

The EGFR superfamily consists of four RTKs: EGFR, c-erbB-2, c-erbB-3, and c-erbB-4, which regulate key cellular functions including proliferation, survival, angiogenesis, and motility. Recognition of the primacy of EGFR as an oncogene in multiple malignancies has made it a leading therapeutic target. Aberrant EGFR activity in HCC appears to be primarily the result of overexpression, which also appears to correlate with more aggressive disease characteristics.[3,12] Anti-EGFR agents undergoing active clinical trial assessment in HCC include small-molecule tyrosine kinase inhibitors (TKIs) and anti-EGFR monoclonal antibodies.

Small-molecule TKIs target the intracellular signaling domain of the EGFR, preventing the activation of downstream cascades and the transcription of genes that promote malignant behavior. Three anti-EGFR TKIs have been assessed in HCC: erlotinib, gefitinib, and lapatinib.

Erlotinib, a selective inhibitor of EGFR/ErbB-1/Her-1, was evaluated in two phase 2 studies that enrolled fit patients with locally advanced/metastatic HCC, 70%–80% of whom had Child-Pugh A liver function. The first study enrolled 38 patients, 50% of whom previously received systemic therapy.[13] Progression-free survival, defined as the proportion of patients without disease progression by Response Evaluation Criteria in Solid Tumors (RECIST) guidelines or death, at 6 months was 32%. Nine percent of patients had a partial response lasting 2–11 months, 50% had stable disease, and median survival was 13 months. Similar findings were noted in a phase 2 study that enrolled 40 patients who were naïve to systemic therapy.[14] Although no objective responses were observed, 43% of patients had stable disease; progression-free survival at 4 months was 42.5% and median survival was 10.8 months. The most common grade 3/4 toxicities with erlotinib were fatigue, diarrhea, skin rash, nausea, vomiting, anorexia, and transaminitis, which occurred in up to 13% of patients. In both studies, neither the presence nor the intensity of tumor EGFR immunoreactivity correlated with responses, and the relationship between cutaneous toxicity and clinical outcomes was not explored.[13,14]

Gefitinib did not exhibit clinically relevant activity in a phase 2 study conducted in 31 patients with advanced disease naïve to systemic therapy.[15] Although treatment was well tolerated, there was only one partial response, and 7 patients had stable disease for a disease control rate of 26%. Median progression-free and overall survival were 2.8 and 6.5 months, respectively

The dual EGFR/c-erbB-1 and c-erbB-2/Her-2 inhibitor, lapatinib, was evaluated in a phase 2 trial conducted in a mixed population of patients with advanced HCC and biliary tract carcinomas.[16] The practice of evaluating therapies in studies that include both HCC and biliary tract carcinomas is fading away as we learn more about the different biology of those two diseases. Regardless, the Ramanathan study did not show any activity in the HCC subgroup; 5% of patients had an objective response, and median progression-free and overall survival were 2.3 and 6.2 months, respectively. Results were somewhat better in another phase 2 trial that enrolled 26 patients with advanced HCC, 19% of whom were previously treated.[17] Although there were no objective responses and median progression-free survival was only 1.8 months, 40% of patients had stable disease (lasting >3 months in six patients and >1 year in two patients) and median overall survival was 12.6 months. Factors associated with improved survival included the development of a skin rash, infection with hepatitis C, and the presence of ≥20 EGFR intron 1 $(CA)_{n16\text{-}23}$ repeats within tumor cells instead of <20 repeats.[16]

Cetuximab is a chimeric monoclonal antibody that binds to the extracellular domain of the EGFR, preventing receptor-ligand interactions as well as intracellular domain phosphorylation. In a phase 2 study of cetuximab in HCC, there were no objective responses although 17% of patients had stable disease lasting a median of 4 months.[18] Median progression-free and overall survival on that study were 1.4 and 9.6 months, respectively. Tumor EGFR expression did not correlate with responses to cetuximab. In another phase 2 study, 44.4% of patients had stable disease with a median time to progression of 8 weeks.[19] Among patients who maintained stable disease for >8 weeks, the median time to progression was 22.5 weeks. Sixty percent of responders exhibited an upregulation of cell cycle inhibitory proteins compared to only 14% of nonresponders. The relationship between the development of skin rash, *KRAS* and *BRAF* mutation status, and responses to cetuximab has not been explored in HCC.

Taken together, anti-EGFR agents failed to show any meaningful activity in advanced HCC, although there appear to be subgroups of patients who might derive greater benefit from these agents compared to the unselected population. Characterization of these subgroups remains a work in progress.

Insulinlike Growth Factor

Obesity, dyslipidemia, type 2 diabetes, and nonalcoholic steatohepatitis (NASH) are features of the metabolic syndrome that is a recognized risk factor for the development HCC.[20] The link between the metabolic syndrome and HCC is thought to be mediated by insulin, insulinlike growth factor (IGF) ligands and their receptors, in concert with reactive oxygen species, proinflammatory cytokines, and activation of the c-Jun amino-terminal kinase 1 (JNK1). These complex interactions result in a final common pathway of hepatocellular inflammation, apoptosis, compensatory proliferation and, ultimately, hepatocarcinogenesis.[20] Targeting of the IGF axis using small-molecule TKIs and monoclonal antibodies is currently being evaluated in HCC.

A phase 2 study of the anti IGF-1 receptor (IGF-1R) antibody, cixutumumab (IMC-A12), in advanced HCC was terminated for inefficacy after 24 patients were enrolled.[21] The primary endpoint, progression-free survival at 4 months, was 30% and median overall survival was 8 months. There were no objective responses, 29% of patients had stable disease, and 41% progressed. Therapy was complicated by grade 3 and 4 hyperglycemia in 46% of patients. High serum IGF binding protein-1 levels correlated positively with progression-free survival. The combination of cixutumumab and sorafenib in patients with advanced HCC naïve to systemic therapy is undergoing evaluation in both a phase 1 and phase 2 study (www.clinicaltrials.gov, NCT00906373, NCT01008566).

BIIB022 and AVE 1642 are two other anti-IGF-1R antibodies undergoing evaluation in HCC. A phase 1B study of sorafenib and BIIB022 has been completed and results are pending (www.clinicaltrials.gov, NCT00956436). The combination of AVE1642 and sorafenib was found to be safe and tolerable in a phase 1 study that also reported stable disease lasting a median of 13 weeks in 85% of patients.[22]

OSI-906 is an oral dual inhibitor of IGF-1R and the insulin receptor.[23] A randomized phase 2 study in advanced HCC was terminated by the sponsor (www.clinicaltrials.gov, NCT01101906), but another phase 2 study assessing the combination of OSI-906 and sorafenib is ongoing (www.clinicaltrials.gov, NCT01334710).

c-Met and the Hepatocyte Growth Factor

The c-met receptor tyrosine kinase and its cognate ligand, hepatocyte growth factor (HGF), are potent mitogens that coordinate hepatogenesis in the developing embryo and promote regeneration and maintain the integrity of the mature liver.[24] In preclinical models, aberrant c-met expression demonstrates tumorigenic potential, and inactivation of c-met/HGF signaling has shown antitumor activity.[3,12] Although data on the clinicopathologic characteristics and outcomes associated with c-met overexpression in human HCC are conflicting,[3,12] c-met targeting is actively being evaluated in clinical trials. Tivantinib (ARQ197), an oral non-ATP-competitive c-met TKI, is currently being studied in a phase 1B study of patients with Child-Pugh A or B cirrhosis and HCC, with preliminary data demonstrating acceptable toxicity[25] (www.clinicaltrials.gov, NCT00802555). A phase 1 dose escalation study of ARQ197 and sorafenib in HCC has shown that the combination is well tolerated and may be active in treatment-naïve as well as pretreated disease[26] (www.clinicaltrials.gov, NCT00827177).

Several hybrid antiangiogenic and c-met inhibitors have also been developed and are being studied in HCC. Results from the HCC subset of a phase 2 discontinuation study of cabozantinib (XL184), a dual c-met/VEGFR-2 inhibitor were recently presented.[27] Seventy-eight percent of patients experienced tumor regression with cabozantinib and median progression-free and overall survival were 4.4 months and 15.1 months, respectively. Tumor regression was associated with a ≥50% decrease in AFP from baseline in 35% of patients, and outcomes were not affected by prior therapy with sorafenib. Of note that tumor c-met expression was not assessed. Foretinib, another c-met/VEGFR-2 inhibitor, is also being studied in a phase 1/2 trial (www.clinicaltrials.gov, NCT00920192).

INTRACELLULAR SIGNALING CASCADES

Receptor tyrosine kinases such as EGFR, IGF-1R, c-Met, and, as will be later discussed, VEGF exert their biological effects by activating a complex network of intracellular signaling pathways. Two of the most extensively studied pathways in oncology are the Ras/Raf/Mek/Erk or MAPK/ERK cascade and the PI3K/Akt/mTOR cascade, both of which have been implicated in the pathogenesis of many malignancies.

In HCC, both the MAPK/ERK and PI3K/Akt/mTOR pathways are constitutively active. Aberrant MAPK/ERK activity may be induced by the effects of hepatitis B or C viral proteins on Raf kinase among other mechanisms. In addition, ERK 1/2 activation has also been associated with more aggressive disease behavior and poorer survival.[12] Likewise, upregulation of various markers of mTOR activity has been associated with less favorable histopathologic features, more advanced disease, and both a shorter overall survival and time to recurrence after resection for HCC.[3,12] Activation of the PI3K/Akt/mTOR pathway has been documented in 40%–50% of HCC tumors. Mutations, downregulation, and deletions of the PTEN tumor suppressor gene are among the hypothesized mechanisms of PI3K/Akt/mTOR dysregulation in HCC.[12]

Targeting the MAPK/ERK Pathway

Functional Ras molecules are generated through posttranslational farnesylation of their C-termini.[28] In preclinical studies, farnesyltransferase inhibitors exhibit chemopreventive properties and have been shown to reduce the proliferative and metastatic potential of HCC cells through inhibition of Ras as well as PI3K/Akt activation.[28] A phase 1B trial of the farnesyltransferase inhibitor lonafarnib (SCH66336) with or without gemcitabine in advanced primary liver cancers was recently terminated for unspecified reasons (www.clinicaltrials.gov, NCT00020774).

Farnesyl can also be manufactured through the mevalonate biosynthesis pathway, of which HMG CoA reductase is a component. Statins, which inhibit HMG CoA reductase, have been associated with a decreased incidence of HCC, particularly in diabetic patients and those infected with hepatitis B.[20,29] Randomized phase 2 and 3 clinical trials of sorafenib with or without pravastatin in advanced HCC are currently recruiting (www.clinicaltrials.gov, NCT01075555, NCT01418729).

Selumetinib (AZD6244), a selective Mek1/2 inhibitor, was studied in a phase 2 trial that was terminated for inefficacy.[30] No objective responses were seen, though 35% of patients had stable disease. Both the median time to progression and PFS were 1.4 months, and median survival was 4.2 months. Toxicities were mild; grade 3 and 4 elevations in liver enzymes, hyperbilirubinemia, fatigue, hyperglycemia, hypokalemia, and hyponatremia each occurred in 5% of patients.

A phase 1/2 clinical trial of selumetinib and sorafenib is currently ongoing (www.clinicaltrials.gov, NCT01029418). Another MEK inhibitor, BAY 86-9766, is also being combined with sorafenib in a phase 2 trial (www.clinicaltrials.gov, NCT01204177).

Targeting the PI3K/Akt/mTOR Pathway

Clinical experience with mTOR inhibition in advanced HCC suggests disease-stabilizing activity in both the first-line setting and after progression on sorafenib.[31] Phase 1/2 and 3 trials examining RAD001 monotherapy in the first- and second-line settings have been opened (www.clinicaltrials.gov, NCT00390195, NCT00516165, NCT01035229), along with combination regimens of RAD001 with bevacizumab, sorafenib, or pasireotide (www.clinicaltrials.gov, NCT00467194, NCT01005199, NCT01488487). Temsirolimus is also being assessed in combination with sorafenib in phase 1 and 2 studies (www.clinicaltrials.gov, NCT01335074, NCT01013519) and with bevacizumab in a phase 2 trial (www.clinicaltrials.gov, NCT01010126).

ANTIANGIOGENESIS

Angiogenesis is a complex, multifaceted process orchestrated by a myriad of growth factors and stimuli; vascular endothelial growth factor (VEGF), platelet-derived growth factor (PDGF), basic fibroblast-derived growth factor (bFGF), angiopoietins, and their cognate receptors as well as the oxygenation status of the tumor milieu are recognized contributors. Several of these factors have been found to be overexpressed and/or dysregulated in preneoplastic liver and established HCC.[32] Systemic antiangiogenic therapies are a rapidly evolving area of research in HCC.

The Different Types of Antiangiogenics. VEGF signaling is the most extensively studied of the angiogenic pathways. Binding of VEGF to its cognate receptor, VEGF-R, induces intracellular signaling cascade activation and the transcription of genes controlling angiogenesis, mitogenesis, and survival. In HCC, baseline elevations in serum VEGF have been shown to correlate with unfavorable clinical and disease characteristics, and may also have independent prognostic value.[33] Anti-VEGF agents are believed to exert their effects through several mechanisms: the disruption of blood vessel formation leading to tumor cell hypoxia and necrosis, and/or normalization of the vasculature which allows for more effective drug delivery to the tumors they feed.[32]

Anti-VEGF(R) Agents

Bevacizumab is a humanized anti-VEGF A monoclonal antibody that is U.S. Food and Drug Administration (FDA) approved for the treatment of advanced colorectal cancer, renal cell carcinoma, nonsquamous non-small-cell lung cancer and glioblastoma. In a phase 2 trial conducted in patients with localized HCC, objective responses were observed in 13% of patients, including one complete response. Median progression-free survival was 6.9 months and survival at 1 and 3 years was 58% and 23%, respectively. Hemorrhagic toxicity was a concern; 11% of patients experienced higher than grade 3 events and there was one fatal episode of variceal bleeding, prompting an amendment requiring that patients with a history of varices or evidence of varices on imaging undergo pretreatment endoscopies.[34]

Ramucirumab is a recombinant human mAb that targets the VEGFR-2 receptor, preventing binding with VEGF. In a phase 2 first-line trial, ramucirumab produced a disease control rate of 50%, including partial responses in 3% of patients, and median progression-free survival was 4.3 months. Median progression-free survival was shorter in patients with Child-Pugh B liver function (2.8 months) than in those with Child-Pugh A liver function (4.2 months). Grade 3 adverse reactions included hypertension in 12%, gastrointestinal bleeding in 7%, infusion-related reactions in 5%, and headaches in 2% of patients.[35]

Cediranib (AZD2171) is an oral small molecule inhibitor of VEGFR. Two phase 2 trials of cediranib in advanced, unresectable HCC were opened, one of which was suspended for unspecified reasons (www.clinicaltrials.gov, NCT00427973). In the second trial, 84% of patients had grade 3 toxicities consisting primarily of hypertension, fatigue, and anorexia, resulting in a high attrition rate of 29%.[36] Efficacy data are pending.

Targeting Basic Fibroblast Growth Factor

Upregulation of basic fibroblast growth factor (bFGF) can initiate tumorigenesis and is a purported mechanism of acquired resistance to VEGF inhibition.[37] Brivanib is an orally administered dual inhibitor of VEGF and FGF signaling. In a phase 2 first-line study conducted in 55 patients with advanced HCC, the objective response rate was 7.2%, including one complete response, and 40% of patients had stable disease.[38] Median and 6-month progression-free survival were modest at 18.2% and 2.7 months, respectively, and median overall survival was 10 months. Patients who experienced disease control had a longer survival time (15.2 months) than those who progressed (5.1 months, hazard ratio [HR] 0.56). Toxicities were modest; grade 3/4 hepatic dysfunction or decompensation, hypertension, hyponatremia, pancreatitis, weakness, diarrhea, clinical deterioration, and asthenia occurred in 1.8%–3.6% of patients.

Brivanib continues to be investigated in phase 2 and 3 trials in the first-line setting (www.clinicaltrials.gov, NCT00355238, NCT00858871) as well as in patients with hepatic function (www.clinicaltrials.gov, NCT00437424). Second-line studies of brivanib have yielded negative results and will be discussed under "Therapy After Progression on Sorafenib."

Platelet Derived Growth Factor

The PDGF family of RTKs encompasses PDGF-α, PDGF-β, FLT3, KIT, and CSF-1R. Together, PDGF and VEGF play complementary roles in angiogenesis; the former initiates the development of immature blood vessels and the latter recruits pericytes to stabilize and fuse them. The modulatory effects of PDGF on the tumor microenvironment also promote tumor progression and survival.[39] Linifanib (ABT 869) is an oral TKI of both PDGF and VEGF signaling[39] that is undergoing investigation in a number of malignancies including HCC. A phase 2 study reported a 4-month progression-free survival of 32% and an objective response rate of 7%.[40] Time to radiographic progression and overall survival were 5.4 and 9.7 months, respectively. Child-Pugh A patients had better survival and response outcomes than Child-Pugh B patients. Therapy was generally well tolerated with the main side effects being diarrhea and fatigue; grade 3/4 toxicities included fatigue and hypertension that occurred in 14% and 18% of patients, respectively. One patient with Child-Pugh B liver disease died of an intracranial hemorrhage that was possibly related to linifanib. Patients who are able to tolerate extended therapy with linifanib (>48 weeks) appear to derive additional benefit in the form of disease control.[41]

A phase 3 trial of linifanib vs. sorafenib in advanced HCC naïve to systemic therapy is currently underway (www.clinicaltrials.gov, NCT00517920).

MULTITARGETED ANTIANGIOGENIC TKIs

Sorafenib

Sorafenib is an orally administered multitargeted inhibitor of the VEGFR, PDGFR, Flt-3, and Raf kinases that was initially evaluated in a phase 2 trial conducted in fit patients with advanced HCC and Child-Pugh A/B liver function.[42] Although the study was negative in regard to the primary endpoint as only 2.2% of patients had a partial response, 33.6% had stable disease for at least 4 months. This was commensurate with a median time to progression of 4.2 months and median overall survival 9.2 months, both of which compared favorably to the historical controls at the time.[9] Grade 3 and 4 toxicities attributable to sorafenib consisted of diarrhea, fatigue, and hand–foot syndrome occurred in 5.1%–9.5% of patients. The apparent disconnect between objective response and survival benefit was highlighted also by the fact that many patients' tumors actually increased in size. Further analysis revealed that the increase in size was accompanied by an increase in central tumor necrosis among patients benefitting from sorafenib.[42,43]

The results of this phase 2 trial led to two multicenter phase 3 studies of sorafenib versus placebo in advanced HCC: the SHARP trial conducted mainly in the Western hemisphere[44] and the Asia-Pacific trial.[45] The SHARP trial enrolled 602 patients, with advanced HCC and Child-Pugh A cirrhosis. With a median time on treatment of 5.3 months, a significant improvement in median overall survival (10.7 vs. 7.9 months,

HR 0.69, $P < .001$) was reported in favor of sorafenib. Response rates by RECIST remained almost inexistent, with 2% of patients achieving a partial response yet 71% of patients having stable disease. The most common toxicities leading to sorafenib dose reductions and/or discontinuation were fatigue, diarrhea, abdominal pain, hand–foot skin reaction, rash or desquamation, and liver dysfunction in 3%–8% of patients. Serious hepatobiliary adverse events, bleeding events, and cardiac ischemia/infarction occurred with similar frequency in both the sorafenib and placebo arms. The SHARP trial was important as the first statistically powered study to prove an overall survival benefit with sorafenib in HCC. Overall survival, calculated as the time from randomization to death, is a more definitive endpoint than progression-free survival because it is not subject to different interpretations and investigator bias.

The Asia-Pacific trial by Cheng et al.[45] enrolled 271 patients with advanced HCC and Child-Pugh A cirrhosis in a 2:1 randomization of sorafenib versus placebo. Median overall survival again improved in favor of sorafenib (6.5 vs. 4.2 months, HR 0.68, $P = .014$) though only 3.3% of patients had a partial response. Reported toxicities were similar in frequency to those reported in the phase 2 and SHARP trials.

In all three trials of sorafenib, survival outcomes were significantly improved with sorafenib despite negligible response rates. These observations have led investigators to question the validity of using conventional RECIST or World Health Organization (WHO) guidelines for characterizing responses to antiangiogenic agents. In addition to the potential relevance of tumor necrosis as reported by Abou-Alfa et al.,[42,43] the American Association for the Study of Liver Diseases (AASLD) and the European Association for the Study of the Liver (EASL) have proposed modified RECIST (mRECIST) guidelines which use changes in intratumoral arterial enhancement to define responses to antiangiogenic agents.[46] In phase 2 studies of brivanib, the proportion of patients classified as clinically benefitting from therapy (i.e., objective response or disease stabilization) was consistently higher using mRECIST as opposed to modified WHO criteria, corresponding to longer progression-free survival and time to progression.[37,38] Although these disparate results are intriguing, a caveat of the mRECIST guidelines is that changes in arterial enhancement may only reflect the effects of the drug on the tumor vasculature and not actual antineoplastic activity.[46] The ongoing debate over response definitions highlights the limitations of endpoints such as progression-free survival and time to progression that rely on radiographic criteria to define a progression "event." In addition, because death is also considered an "event," progression-free survival can also be influenced by factors unrelated to the study therapy or even the neoplasm itself. This is especially important in HCC where the underlying cirrhosis is as important in driving the clinical course. Validation of these novel response assessment tools against a "hard" endpoint like overall survival is needed in order to provide more definitive answers about their predictive and prognostic capabilities. In addition, an improvement in symptoms in parallel with radiographic responses would also be a valuable correlate.

Although the magnitude of benefit with sorafenib was similar between the two phase 3 trials, median overall survival was notably longer in the SHARP population compared to the Asia-Pacific population at 10.7 and 6.5 months, respectively. A head-to-head comparison of the demographic and clinical characteristics of the SHARP and Asia-Pacific populations revealed that nearly 30% more patients in the SHARP study had an ECOG PS of 0 than in the Asia-Pacific study. Moreover, more patients in the Asia-Pacific than in the SHARP group had extrahepatic metastases and BCLC stage C disease. More recently, a phase 3 trial comparing first-line sunitinib to sorafenib in advanced HCC also showed, in an exploratory analysis, that the magnitude of overall survival benefit with sorafenib compared to sunitinib was greater in non-Asians (15.1 vs. 9.3 months)) than in Asians (8.8 vs. 7.7 months). Sorafenib also significantly improved progression-free survival and time to progression in non-Asians compared to sunitinib, but there was no difference among Asians.[47] The ethnogeographic differences in response to sorafenib may be the result of regional and cultural variations in the treatment of HCC, with Asian patients being more likely to undergo surgery or embolization for a higher disease burden than Western patients before systemic therapy is considered.[48] The shorter survival in the Asia-Pacific study is therefore thought to be likely due to the fact that patients in Asia were generally less fit, had more advanced disease, and therefore derived less benefit from sorafenib than their Western counterparts.

A more plausible explanation for the differences in outcome that is based on the ethnicity of the patient and the etiology of the disease has surfaced as a critical one based on the results of the two studies as well as others. In the phase 2 and SHARP studies, 29%–48% and 17%–19% of patients were infected with hepatitis C and B, respectively.[42,44] In contrast, >70% of patients in the Asia-Pacific study had hepatitis B compared to only 4%–11% who had hepatitis C.[45] A retrospective subset analysis of the phase 2 study by viral etiology reported a trend toward longer survival among patients with hepatitis C (12.4 months) than with hepatitis B (7.3 months).[49] The beneficial effects of sorafenib were also confirmed in the subset of hepatitis C patients enrolled in the SHARP study; median overall survival was 14 months versus 7.9 months with placebo.[50] Furthermore, in the phase 3 trial of sunitinib versus sorafenib, patients with hepatitis C had superior survival when treated with sorafenib instead of sunitinib irrespective of ethnicity (17.6 vs. 9.2 months, HR 1.52, $P = .0165$). There was no difference in survival between sunitinib and sorafenib among patients infected with hepatitis B.[47] The outcomes of patients infected with hepatitis B in the SHARP trial have yet to be reported.

The differential outcomes with sorafenib in patients with hepatitis B and C are intriguing but puzzling. A potential explanation is that the hepatitis C viral core protein can activate Raf-1 kinase in HCC cells,[51] theoretically sensitizing them to sorafenib. However, hepatitis B X protein can also activate the Raf/Mek/Erk pathway,[12] yet the data indicate that outcomes with sorafenib are consistently better in patients who have hepatitis C. It is unlikely that changes in individual pathways can explain the differential viral–drug interactions observed; other variables including pharmacogenomics, activation of parallel pathways that enhance or counteract drug effects, among other considerations are likely at play.

Although sorafenib is well tolerated in the Child-Pugh A population, its safety in Child-Pugh B patients continues to be of concern. A subgroup analysis of the phase 2 sorafenib study reported higher rates of hepatic decompensation in Child-Pugh B compared to Child-Pugh A patients.[52] Grade 3 and 4 hepatobiliary toxicities in the Child-Pugh A and B groups were hyperbilirubinemia (14% and 53%), encephalopathy (3% and 13%), and ascites (3% and 5%). This translated to a shorter treatment duration as well as shorter survival in Child-Pugh B (3.2 months) than in Child-Pugh A patients (9.5 months).[52]

Similar findings have been reported from the phase 4 Global Investigation of Therapeutic Decisions in Unresectable HCC and of Its Treatment with Sorafenib (GIDEON) registry study.[53] Compared to their Child-Pugh A counterparts, Child-Pugh B and C patients were generally less tolerant of sorafenib. Although the frequencies of drug-related toxicities was similar, Child-Pugh B and C patients were treated for a shorter duration, were more likely to develop hepatic and serious drug-related adverse events, and also experienced a lesser survival benefit on sorafenib. The study investigators suggested that patients with a score of B7/8 had outcomes comparable to those of Child-Pugh A patients, with a more distinct decrease in benefit among those with a score of B9.[53] However, definitive conclusions cannot be drawn given that GIDEON is an uncontrolled postmarketing study that is still in progress.

Based on a phase 1 study of sorafenib pharmacokinetics in patients with hepatic dysfunction, patients with a serum bilirubin ≤1.5 × upper limit of normal (ULN) can safely initiate sorafenib at the full dose of 400 mg twice daily whereas those with a bilirubin 1.6–3 × ULN should be considered for a 200 mg twice daily dose. Sorafenib at 200 mg once daily was recommended for patients with an albumin <2.5 mg/dL and any bilirubin level. There was no safe dose identified for patients with a bilirubin >3 × ULN.[54]

Sunitinib

Sunitinib is a multitargeted TKI of VEGFR, PDGFR, c-Kit, and Flt-3 kinases. Several phase 2 studies of sunitinib in HCC have reported modest antitumor activity; partial response rates range from 2% to 3%, 35% to 50% of patients have stable disease, median time to progression is 1.5–5.3 months, and overall survival is 8.0–9.8 months.[55–57] Based on these results, a first-line phase 3 study comparing sunitinib with sorafenib in a predominantly Asian population was opened, but was terminated early because of excessive serious toxicities on the sunitinib arm.[47] There was a nearly sixfold increase in grade 3/4 hematologic toxicities and 17% more patients had grade 3–5 bleeding events on sunitinib than sorafenib. Furthermore, 18% of patients on sunitinib died of treatment-related causes compared to 2% of patients on sorafenib. Median overall survival was inferior with sunitinib compared to sorafenib (7.9 vs. 10.2 months, HR 1.3, $P = .001$). Subset analyses did not reveal any ethnic, etiologic, or other subgroups showing superior outcomes with sunitinib over sorafenib.

Combined Systemic Therapies

As monotherapies, most of the biologic agents evaluated in HCC result in a median survival of less than a year. Combination regimens are being actively evaluated in an effort to improve survival beyond the 1-year threshold. Two of the most promising regimens—sorafenib plus doxorubicin and bevacizumab plus erlotinib—are highlighted.

SORAFENIB AND DOXORUBICIN

At the same time the SHARP trial was launched, a randomized double-blinded phase 2 study of doxorubicin plus sorafenib and doxorubicin plus placebo in patients with advanced HCC and Child-Pugh A cirrhosis also opened to accrual.[11] In an exploratory comparison, the combination of doxorubicin plus sorafenib showed pronounced increases in median time to progression (6.4 from 2.8 months, $P = .02$), progression-free survival (6.0 from 2.7 months, $P = .006$) and overall survival (13.7 from 6.5 months, $P = .006$) compared to doxorubicin plus placebo. The apparent synergy between these drugs is thought to result from the downstream effects of sorafenib on Raf kinase and multidrug resistance genes that sensitize HCC cells to the effects of doxorubicin,[11] though these hypotheses have not been tested clinically. Obviously this theory needs to be tested clinically. A multicenter phase 3 trial of sorafenib plus doxorubicin versus single agent sorafenib is currently underway (CALGB 80802, www.clinicaltrials.gov, NCT01015833). This is a very important trial, as it is the first national phase 3 trial in HCC that is led by the National Institutes of Health. The commitment to that study is reflective of the increasing incidence of HCC in the United States.

BEVACIZUMAB AND ERLOTINIB

The rationale for combining bevacizumab and erlotinib is based on the known downstream interactions between VEGFR and EGFR signaling, which can undermine anti-EGFR therapy.[3] A phase 2 trial assessing the combination of bevacizumab and erlotinib in 40 patients with treatment naïve advanced HCC reported a median progression-free survival of 9.0 months and median overall survival of 15.7 months.[58] Twenty-five percent of patients had an objective response and 37.5% had stable disease. The most common grade 3/4 adverse event was fatigue at 20%, followed by diarrhea, hypertension, elevated transaminases, and gastrointestinal hemorrhage, which occurred in 10%–15% of patients. In an updated report of the trial that included an additional 19 patients with BCLC stage C disease as well as patients previously treated with sorafenib, median progression-free and overall survival were 7.2 months and 13.7 months, respectively.[59] Objective responses occurred in 24% of patients, and 56% had stable disease. Toxicities were similar to the original phase 2 study. High plasma levels of proangiogenic factors and the absence of a skin rash were associated with poorer outcomes.

A phase 3 trial comparing bevacizumab and erlotinib versus sorafenib the first-line setting for advanced HCC is currently underway (www.clinicaltrials.gov, NCT00881751).

OTHER COMBINATION REGIMENS

Bevacizumab has been combined with chemotherapy in several phase 2 studies. First-line bevacizumab with capecitabine and oxaliplatin resulted in median progression-free and overall survival times of 6.8 and 9.8 months, respectively. Three-quarters of patients experienced disease control, including 20% with partial responses. The regimen was well tolerated, with grade 3/4 toxicities limited to fatigue and neuropathy.[60] Similarly, bevacizumab plus gemcitabine and oxaliplatin produced a median progression-free survival of 5.3 months, median overall survival of 9.6 months, and partial responses in 20% of patients.[61]

Cetuximab has also been studied in combination with chemotherapy doublets. A phase 2 trial of cetuximab with gemcitabine and oxaliplatin (GEMOX) reported median progression-free and overall survival times of 4.7 and 9.5 months, respectively. Twenty percent of patients had a partial response lasting 2–14 months and 40% had stable disease. Trends towards improved disease control and progression-free survival were observed among patients who developed a grade 2–3 cetuximab-related skin rash.[62] The combination of cetuximab with capecitabine and oxaliplatin (XELOX) appeared to be less active; although 71% of patients had stable disease, 12.5% of patients had objective responses and median progression-free and overall survival were 3.3 and 4.4 months, respectively.[63]

Compared to prior studies of XELOX and GEMOX, the addition of bevacizumab or cetuximab to either of these chemotherapy doublets does not appear to improve response or survival outcomes. Although definitive conclusions cannot be drawn from cross-study comparisons, the data do not warrant further testing of these regimens in phase 3 clinical trials.

Therapy after Progression on Sorafenib

There are presently no standard therapies for HCC that has progressed on sorafenib. A number of second-line trials are ongoing, and several have been completed although none of them have yielded results that will impact clinical practice in the foreseeable future. Fit patients with preserved hepatic function and sorafenib-refractory HCC should be offered the option of participating in a clinical trial.

Second-line bevacizumab and erlotinib were evaluated in a phase 2 study based on the rationale that the combination might abrogate compensatory proangiogenic mechanisms that result in sorafenib resistance.[65] All patients progressed on therapy with a median time to progression of 1.8 months and median survival of 4.4 months, resulting in early termination of the study.[64]

A phase 2 trial of second-line brivanib was performed given that upregulation of FGF is thought to be the mechanism of acquired resistance to antiangiogenic therapies like sorafenib.[37] The study reported a median time to progression and overall survival of 2.7 and 9.8 months, respectively. Approximately 45% of patients had disease control, though 41.3% progressed. A decrease in serum AFP by >50% from baseline was associated with longer survival at 10.8 months compared to 7.3 months in patients without a decrease.[37]

Results from the phase 3 placebo-controlled BRISK-PS (Brivanib Study in HCC patients at Risk Post Sorafenib) trial of second-line brivanib were recently reported.[65] Although the primary endpoint of overall survival was not met, there were statistically significant improvements in time to progression (4.2 vs. 2.7 months, $P = .0001$) and response rates (12% vs. 2%, $P = .0032$) over placebo.

Second-line antiangiogenic therapy is also being evaluated in the phase 3 REACH study using ramucirumab (www.clinicaltrials.gov, NCT01140347).

Strategies to target alternative, nonangiogenic pathways are also undergoing therapeutic evaluation in sorafenib-refractory HCC. The phase 3, placebo-controlled EVOLVE-1 study is currently assessing mTOR inhibition with everolimus (www.clinicaltrials.gov, NCT01035229).

More recently, results from a randomized, placebo-controlled phase 2 study of two dose levels of tivantinib in the second-line setting were reported.[66] Tivantinib significantly improved median time to progression over placebo (1.7 vs. 1.5 months, HR 0.64, $P = .04$). Median overall survival was 6.2 months in the placebo arm and 6.6 months in the tivantinib arm and was not statistically significant. Outcomes were further analyzed according to tumor c-met expression levels as determined by immunohistochemistry. Patients with high tumor c-met expression had a significantly higher risk of death from HCC than those with low tumor c-met levels. However, patients with high c-met derived greater benefit from tivantinib with respect to disease control and overall survival than patients with low c-met (7.2 months and 3.8 months, respectively; HR 0.38, $P = .01$). Grade ≥3 anemia and neutropenia occurred in 16%–21% of patients at the 360-mg QD dose level, necessitating a reduction to 240 mg QD, which resulted in more manageable toxicities without compromising efficacy.

Arginine deprivation therapy with pegylated arginine deiminase (ADI-PEG 20) capitalizes on the auxotrophy of HCC cells since they lack the enzyme necessary for its synthesis. Preclinical as well as clinical studies have shown promising antineoplastic activity in HCC.[67,68] A phase 3, placebo-controlled, second-line trial of ADI-PEG in HCC is currently underway (www.clinicaltrials.gov, NCT01287585).

Combined Modality Therapy

Growing knowledge of the biological effects of systemic antiangiogenic and liver-directed ablative therapies has fueled interest in combined modality therapy. The rationale for combining systemic antiangiogenic therapy with transarterial chemoembolization (TACE) is based on several considerations. Transarterial embolization–induced cytotoxicity and hypoxia leads to the secretion of proangiogenic factors like VEGF, PDGF, and bFGF within hours of the procedure, peaking by 24 hours and gradually declining over subsequent days.[69] The release of these factors may enable malignant progression postembolization. In a prospective study, 75% of patients with elevated serum VEGF postembolization developed distant metastases within 3 months compared to 0% of patients who had decreased serum VEGF levels.[70] Given sorafenib's antiangiogenic properties, coadministration with hepatic arterial embolization could theoretically enhance cytotoxicity and also decrease the risk of distant spread.

The safety of combining sorafenib and doxorubicin-eluting bead TACE (DEB-TACE) was evaluated in a phase 2 study that enrolled 35 fit patients, 89% of whom had Child-Pugh A liver function and liver-confined disease.[71] One-third of patients also had partial portal vein thrombosis. Sorafenib was commenced 1 week before DEB-TACE and was administered continuously through up to four DEB-TACE treatments over a 6-month period. Eighty-three percent of toxicities during the first cycle were grade 1 or 2 events consisting of fatigue, anorexia, myelosuppression, transaminase elevation, hand–foot skin reaction or dryness, and pain. Grade 3 and 4 events occurred in 17% of patients and mainly consisted of fatigue and elevated transaminases. The grade, incidence, and profile of toxicities were similar during subsequent cycles. Patients received a median of two (range 1–5) DEB-TACE treatments and a median of 71 days (range 4–620) of sorafenib. The most common reason for sorafenib interruptions or dose reductions was hand–foot skin reaction. The objective response and disease control rates using conventional RECIST guidelines were 4% and 95%, respectively, and were 58% and 100%, respectively using mRECIST guidelines.

A Japanese and Korean phase 3 study randomized patients with advanced HCC who had achieved an objective response after TACE with epirubicin, cisplatin, doxorubicin, and mitomycin C to either sorafenib or placebo.[72] The study did not meet its primary endpoint of improving time to progression (5.4 vs. 3.7 months, HR 0.87, P = .252). Overall, 1- and 2-year survival were similar between the arms.[72]

The multicenter randomized phase 2 SPACE (sorafenib or placebo in combination with transarterial chemoembolization (TACE) for intermediate-stage hepatocellular carcinoma) trial enrolled 307 patients with BCLC stage B disease and Child-Pugh A liver function.[73] Sorafenib was initiated on a continuous schedule, with DEB-TACE administered within the first week of sorafenib, then at months 2, 6, 12, and 18. The option of additional DEB-TACE treatments between months 6–12 and 12–18 was also permitted. The addition of sorafenib to DEB-TACE did not improve median time to progression (5.6 months) relative to placebo (5.5 months, HR 0.797, P = .072). Median survival was not different between study arms (HR 0.898, P = .295). Responses were assessed using modified RECIST guidelines. In addition, the study introduced the novel endpoint of time to untreatable progression, which was defined as a failure to have an objective response after two DEB-TACE treatments, clinical deterioration, disease progression, and/or hepatic functional decline. This resulted in a very conservative treatment schedule reflected by the shorter duration of treatment received by patients on the sorafenib arm compared to placebo (median 21 weeks and 27 weeks, respectively), and lower proportion of patients on sorafenib who received >1 DEB-TACE treatment than on placebo (62% and 79%, respectively). In particular, non-Asian patients were more likely to discontinue sorafenib or DEB-TACE than Asian patients. The negative results of these studies are somewhat surprising given the compelling preclinical rationale. Reasons for these are several-fold. In the phase 3 trial by Kudo et al., most patients did not begin taking sorafenib until >9 weeks after TACE, thus missing the opportunity to suppress the rise in VEGF during the immediate posttreatment window.[72,74]

Interpretation of the SPACE trial is more complex and must consider the choice of endpoint, treatment schedule, as well as the potential contribution of regional differences in treatment culture and philosophy. Although the treatment schedule and stopping rules were developed with safety in mind, they might have been too restrictive, resulting in the unintended consequence of undertreating some patients, particularly those who had stable disease or a transient clinical/hepatic decline who might have benefitted from further treatment on recovery. Furthermore, modified RECIST guidelines have not been validated for the evaluation of responses to antiangiogenic and targeted therapies. These issues underscore the importance of endpoint selection and response assessment tools given their influence on the study conduct and subsequent interpretation of results.

The combination of TACE and sorafenib continues to be evaluated in the placebo-controlled phase 3 ECOG 1208 trial (www.clinicaltrials.gov, NCT01004978). The efficacy of this trial will be determined using the more global, and arguably more clinically relevant, primary endpoint of progression-free survival.[74].

Taken together, the existing data indicate that combining sorafenib and TACE is feasible and acceptably safe, but does not improve disease control or survival in patients with HCC. This approach should only be used in the investigational setting. The standard of care for advanced HCC remains systemic therapy.

Biologic Correlates

Biomarker identification for the purpose of predicting responses to therapy, prognostication, and therapeutic targeting is a key theme in oncologic research. Aside from serum AFP, no biomarkers have been validated or are routinely used in the management of HCC.

In the phase 2 sorafenib study by Abou-Alfa et al., pretreatment tumor specimens were immunostained for pERK, a downstream effector of Raf. There was a significant difference in time to progression between patients whose tumors demonstrated high-intensity pERK staining and those with low intensity staining (P = .00034). In addition, an 18-gene blood cell RNA panel distinguished "progressors" and "nonprogressors" with 100% accuracy.[42]

The results of plasma biomarker analyses from the SHARP study were recently published.[33] Although none were predictive of sorafenib sensitivity, time to progression and overall survival tended to be longer in patients who received sorafenib and had high s-c-Kit and low hepatocyte growth factor levels at baseline. High baseline levels of the proangiogenic factors VEGF and Ang-2 were strongly and independently associated with a poor prognosis.

Imaging correlates may also serve as surrogate biomarkers as suggested by the data indicating a potential role for tumor necrosis in predicting clinical benefit from sorafenib.[42,43] In the phase 2 sunitinib study by Zhu et al., decreases in vessel permeability on DCE-MRI and circulating cytokine and c-Kit levels were significantly associated with improved survival. In contrast, high levels of cytokines, angiogenic proteins, and progenitor cells were associated with a poor prognosis.[55] Bevacizumab was found to induce decreases in tumor vascularity on DCE-MRI, plasma VEGF-A, and chemokine levels as well as in vitro angiogenic activity in the phase 2 study by Siegel et al., although these changes were not correlated with clinical outcomes.[34] Similarly, responses to doxorubicin and sorafenib showed a trend toward a significant association between AUC180, a marker of tumor vascular density and permeability, on DCE-MRI.[75]

The biomarker analysis from the second-line tivantinib study[66] was especially noteworthy. As previously discussed, although patients with high tumor c-met had a poorer prognosis, their outcomes on tivantinib were superior with respect to disease control and progression-free and overall survival compared to patients with low tumor c-met. Although these observations were derived from a small number of patients, they suggest that tivantinib may be able to reverse the natural history of c-met high HCC, and has the potential to become the first biomarker-driven therapy in this disease.

Conclusion

Clinical nihilism toward the study and management of advanced HCC has been replaced with enthusiasm in recent years as our knowledge of the mechanisms underlying the pathogenesis and maintenance of this disease continues to expand. These advancements have allowed us to take advantage of the growing array of molecularly targeted agents that have become available, providing our patients with an unprecedented variety of experimental options. Although sorafenib remains the only FDA-approved drug for HCC, there is lot of work currently underway evaluating single agents, combination therapies, and second-line therapies with already several suggestions of improved median overall survival as high as 18 months. Nuances with respect to the tolerance and efficacy of sorafenib and other targeted therapies in different patient populations are now becoming apparent, as is the need for more accurate and sensitive response assessment tools. In the absence of data demonstrating clinical benefit, combined modality therapy with TACE and sorafenib should remain an investigational approach, and patients with advanced HCC not amenable to regional therapies, like patients with metastatic disease, should be treated systemically. Biomarker development, molecular enrichment, and subgroup identification are crucial research objectives that will hopefully enhance and optimize the management of patients with advanced HCC.

REFERENCES

The complete reference list is available online at www.expertconsult.com.

10

Cholangiocarcinoma: Diagnosis, Management, and Prognosis

JENNIFER ZHANG | MICHAEL N. MAVROS | TIMOTHY M. PAWLIK

KEY POINTS

- Although relatively rare, cholangiocarcinoma is the second most common primary hepatobiliary malignancy in the United States, and its incidence is increasing.
- Surgical treatment remains the cornerstone of curative therapy. Resection frequently requires a major procedure but can be done with relatively low morbidity and near zero mortality.
- Locoregional therapies have an important role in the management of cholangiocarcinoma, with radiation therapy more commonly used for hilar cholangiocarcinoma and intraarterial therapy possibly having a role for intrahepatic cholangiocarcinoma.
- The prognosis of cholangiocarcinoma remains poor. Five-year survival following resection ranges from 25% to 40%. More effective systemic and locoregional therapies are needed.

Introduction

Cholangiocarcinoma is an epithelial carcinoma of the bile ducts, which can be divided anatomically into intra- and extrahepatic. Intrahepatic and extrahepatic cholangiocarcinoma are distinct entities that have different considerations with regard to diagnosis, staging, and treatment. Intrahepatic cholangiocarcinoma (ICC) arises directly from the hepatic ducts within the liver, whereas extrahepatic cholangiocarcinoma (ECC) can include both hilar and distal bile duct cancers.[1] We herein review the management of ICC and extrahepatic hilar cholangiocarcinomas, also known as Klatskin tumors.

Epidemiology and Risk Factors

Cholangiocarcinomas are relatively rare in the United States. Cholangiocarcinoma is, however, the second most common primary hepatobiliary malignancy after hepatocellular carcinoma.[1,2] Around 25% of cases involve the common/hepatic bile duct, and the remaining are intrahepatic, nonperihilar tumors.[3,4] Cholangiocarcinoma is the ninth most common gastrointestinal cancer and it accounts for approximately 13% of cancer-related deaths worldwide (3% in the United States).[1]

The incidence of cholangiocarcinoma varies widely with geography. The reported incidence is highest in Southeast Asia (96 per 100,000) and lowest in Australia (0.1 per 100,000).[1] In the United States, the incidence is approximately 1 per 100,000 for both ICC and ECC.[1,2] The incidence of ICC has been increasing over the past 30 years worldwide,[1,2,5] and this increase does not seem to be solely attributable to improvements in diagnostic modalities or better pathologic characterization of the disease.[6,7] In the United States, age-adjusted incidence of ICC increased from 0.32 in 1975 to 0.85 per 100,000 in 2000, and has not yet reached a plateau. At the same time, incidence of ECC has declined.[6]

The prevalence of cholangiocarcinoma is approximately equal between the two genders, with a slightly higher prevalence in males.[1,4] Almost all patients are older than 50 years at the time of diagnosis, with most patients in the United States diagnosed in their sixth decade of life.[1] Asian Americans and Hispanics have a 2.5 times and 1.8 times, respectively, increased incidence of cholangiocarcinoma compared with non-Latino whites in the United States.[5]

Cholangiocarcinoma is associated with conditions that result in chronic biliary inflammation and cholestasis. For example, the risk of cholangiocarcinoma has been associated with primary sclerosing cholangitis and inflammatory bowel disease, biliary fluke infestations, hepatitis (due to hepatitis B and C virus or alcoholic steatohepatitis), and cirrhosis. In addition, biliary malformations, hepatolithiasis, carcinogens (i.e., thorotrast), as well as chronic conditions like diabetes mellitus or HIV infection have also been reported to be associated with a higher risk of cholangiocarcinoma.[1,5-6,8,9]

In the United States, one of the most common risk factors for cholangiocarcinoma is primary sclerosing cholangitis (PSC). PSC can cause fibrosis and stricture formation. Patients with PSC often present with cholangiocarcinoma at a younger age—often up to two decades earlier than non-PSC patients.[4] On average, the diagnosis of cholangiocarcinoma usually occurs 2.5 years after the diagnosis of PSC.[1,5] In contrast, the increased incidence of cholangiocarcinoma in Southeast Asia is associated with increased infection rates with *Clonorchis sinensis* or *Opisthorchis viverrini*.[9] The World Health Organization has labeled both of these organisms as grade 1 carcinogens. Humans can become infected by both types of flukes through ingestion of raw or undercooked seafood.[1,5]

Patients with malformations such as choledochal cysts or Caroli disease are also at increased risk of cholangiocarcinoma. Choledochal cysts are cystic dilations of the biliary tract, and Caroli disease is associated with multiple intrahepatic cysts. Both are associated with an approximately 10%–15% lifetime risk of cholangiocarcinoma.[1,5] Hepatolithiasis is another well-recognized risk factor for cholangiocarcinoma. In these cases, the stones are usually found in proximity to the tumor site. Some authors have reported a 10% lifetime risk of cholangiocarcinoma with hepatolithiasis.[1,5] Thorotrast, a past radiocontrast agent, and dioxins also increase the risk of cholangiocarcinoma. Both hepatitis B and hepatitis C are considered potential risk factors for ICC but not ECC.

Tumor Markers and Molecular Pathogenesis

The biomarkers carbohydrate antigen 19-9 (CA 19-9), carcinoembryonic antigen (CEA), and carbohydrate antigen 125 (CA 125) are often used during the diagnostic workup for cholangiocarcinoma. These markers are, however, not specific for cholangiocarcinoma and may be elevated in other conditions, including cholangitis, hepatolithiasis, or other malignancies such as colorectal cancer. The sensitivities of CA 19-9, CEA, and CA 125 have been reported to be less than 70%.[10] The sensitivity and specificity of CA 19-9 is higher among patients with PSC at 78.6% and 98.5%, respectively.[11] However, even in PSC, CA 19-9 does not prove to be an effective screening tool.[11] In areas with high incidences of liver fluke infestations, serum or stool tests, as well as urinary 8-*oxo*-7,8-dihydro-2′-deoxyguanosine levels may be potential screening tests.[12]

Biliary fluke infestation and hepatolithiasis have aided in the study of the molecular pathogenesis of cholangiocarcinoma. Specifically, biliary flukes can cause mechanical and toxic damage to bile ducts, causing chronic inflammation of the biliary epithelia leading to carcinogenesis. Similarly, hepatolithiasis can also cause biliary inflammation and bile stasis, leading to increased exposure of carcinogenic bile acids. Biliary injury and inflammation leads to the release of cytokines, which increases the production of nitric oxide (NO) and reactive nitrogen oxide species (RNOS) through the expression of inducible nitric oxide synthase in epithelial cells. NO and RNOS can cause DNA mutations and inactivate DNA repair proteins.[13] Through a multistep process, normal biliary epithelium can be transformed into hyperplastic, dysplastic, and eventually malignant epithelium. Notably, two distinct precursors have been identified for cholangiocarcinoma: biliary intraepithelial neoplasia and intraductal papillary mucinous neoplasia of the liver.[14,15] Several growth factors or cytokines have been found to increase biliary proliferation. These factors include hepatocyte growth factor, transforming growth factor α (TGF-α), endothelial growth factor, leukocyte inhibitory factor, and interleukin 6 (IL-6).[16]

Pathologic and Morphologic Classification

There have been many classification systems proposed to describe the pathologic and gross appearance of ICC and ECC. For ICC, the Liver Cancer Study Group of Japan's (LCSGJ's) classification scheme proposed dividing cholangiocarcinoma into three morphologies: mass forming, periductal infiltrating, and intraductal growth types (Figure 10-1).[17,18] In the mass-forming type, a nodular, gray-white lesion or mass is typically found in the hepatic parenchyma (Figure 10-2, *A*).[19] The mass is generally solid and well defined, with significant variations in size. The center of the mass can often be necrotic or fibrotic, with rare calcifications. The periductal infiltrating type grows along the bile duct wall and appears as a concentric thickening that is ill defined and frequently not recognized (Figure 10-2, *B*).[19] The bile ducts may appear to be strictured, narrowed, or obstructed, resulting in stasis of bile. The liver often appears green and enlarged.[18] Both the intra- and extrahepatic bile ducts are often involved in the periductal-infiltrating type. Intraductal-growing cholangiocarcinoma is characterized by intraluminal papillary tumors of the bile ducts that partially obstruct and dilate the ducts.[19] The projections form sessile or polypoid masses covered with columnar epithelial cells. The papillary tumors produce mucin that is often retained within the tumor or may leak out into the bile duct, leading to obstructive jaundice in excessive cases.[18] Traditionally, ECC has been described as nodular, sclerosing, and papillary, corresponding to mass-forming, periductal infiltrating, and intraductal-growing types of intrahepatic cholangiocarcinoma, respectively.[20]

In contrast, hilar cholangiocarcinomas are typically classified anatomically based on the location within the biliary tree using the Bismuth-Corlette classification, types I-IV (see Figure 11-2).[1,21] Type I cholangiocarcinoma begin distal

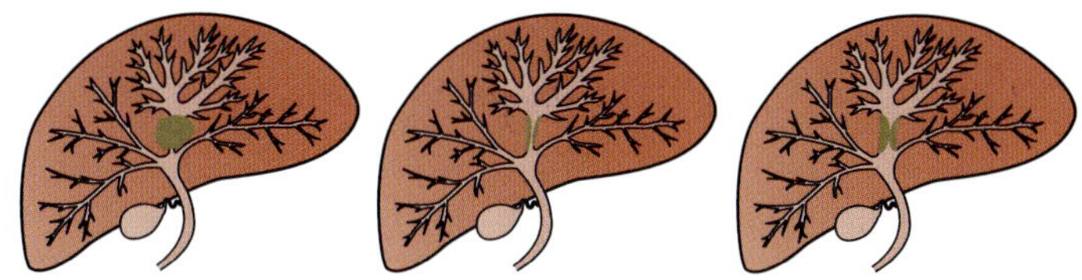

A B C

Figure 10-1 Schematic representation of the gross morphologic classification system for intrahepatic cholangiocarcinoma. (A) Mass forming. (B) Periductal infiltrating. (C) Intraductal growing. *Used with permission from Blechacz B, Komuta M, Roskams T, Gores GJ: Clinical diagnosis and staging of cholangiocarcinoma,* Nat Rev Gastroenterol Hepatol *8:512–522, 2011.*

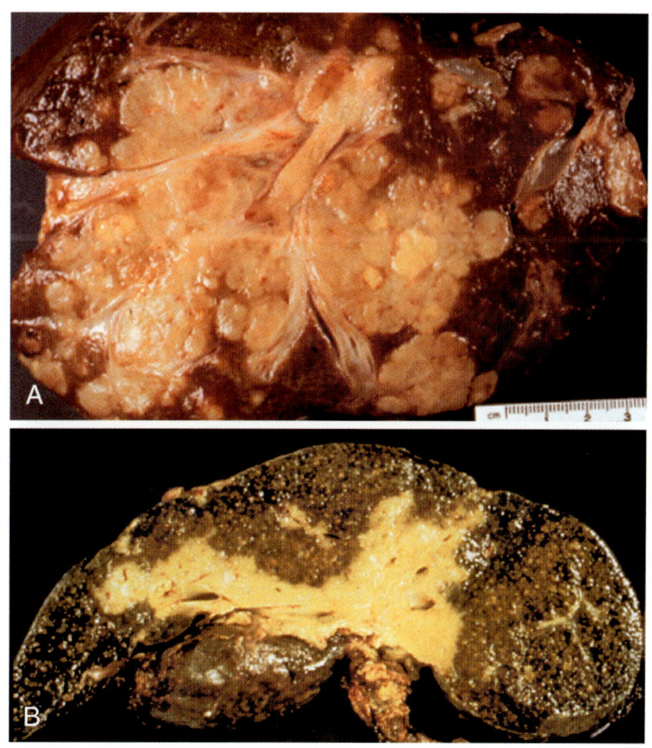

Figure 10-2 (A) Intrahepatic cholangiocarcinoma usually arises as a solitary mass forming liver. (B) In contrast, hilar cholangiocarcinoma usually presents as a mass/stricture that leads to biliary obstruction and intrahepatic biliary dilation; in some instances, the scarring of the bile duct may be indistinguishable from hilar scarring due to primary sclerosing cholangitis. *From Iaccobuzio CA, Montgomery E:* Gastrointestinal and liver pathology, *ed 2, Philadelphia, 2012, Saunders, Fig. 20–24.*

to the confluence of the right and left hepatic ducts, involving the common hepatic duct. Type II cholangiocarcinoma affect the confluence of the right and left hepatic ducts. Type IIIa cholangiocarcinoma involve the junction of the right and left hepatic ducts along with part of the right hepatic duct, and type IIIb also involves the junction and part of the left hepatic duct. Type IV cholangiocarcinoma include tumors that are multifocal or affect the union of the right and left hepatic ducts along with both the right and left hepatic ducts.

Overview: Intrahepatic Cholangiocarcinoma

PRESENTATION AND DIAGNOSIS

The presentation of ICC is often nonspecific and delayed. Symptoms may include abdominal pain, fever, night sweats, cachexia, and general malaise. Symptoms of biliary obstruction, such as jaundice and pruritus, are uncommon in ICC and usually signify very advanced disease. Often asymptomatic patients are diagnosed during routine evaluation of liver function tests.[3,22-25]

The diagnosis of cholangiocarcinoma relies on a combination of laboratory, cytology, and imaging studies. Laboratory studies include liver function tests, which can indicate biliary tract obstruction with elevated bilirubin, as well as possible elevation in alkaline phosphatase or γ-glutamyltransferase; however, it is not uncommon for patients to have a normal battery of laboratory exams.[24] CA 19-9 may be useful, especially among patients with PSC. As noted, one study of 218 PSC patients reported sensitivity and specificity of 78.6% and 98.5%, respectively, using a CA 19-9 cut-off value ≥129 U/mL.[11] However, a different study using the same cut-off reported a 37% false-positive rate.[26] Other cut-off points have yielded similar results in two smaller studies. A CA 19-9 >180 U/mL had a sensitivity of 66.7% and specificity of 97.7% in a study of 55 PSC patients, whereas the respective values in a study of 37 PSC patients were 89% and 86% for a CA 19-9 >100 U/mL.[27,28] For patients without PSC, the sensitivity and specificity were 53% and 76% for CA 19-9 >100 U/mL.[29] CEA can also be elevated in patients with intrahepatic cholangiocarcinoma.

Both computed tomography (CT) and magnetic resonance imaging (MRI) are used routinely in the evaluation of cholangiocarcinoma. However, their specificity is low. Dynamic CT or MRI may be useful in distinguishing between ICC and hepatocellular carcinoma (HCC).[30] Approximately 80% of ICC will take up contrast progressively throughout both the arterial and the venous phase, whereas HCC enhances rapidly during the arterial phase and washes out quickly in the delayed venous phase.[31] The utility of positron emission tomography (PET) in the workup of ICC remains unclear. One study showed that in 4 of 11 (36%) patients with ICC, PET was able to identify distant metastases that were not found on CT or MRI, even though it was not superior in detecting regional lymph node metastases.[32] Similar results were seen in a study from the Memorial Sloan-Kettering Cancer Center (MSKCC), which reported that PET scan identified metastatic disease in 24% of patients that eventually altered management. PET-CT does not appear to be superior in assessing the primary liver lesion.[33] Evaluation of extrahepatic disease is extremely important in the workup process and may drastically affect the management plan, and therefore PET should be strongly considered (Figure 10-3).[30]

STAGING

There is no consensus on the best staging system for ICC. Although factors such as tumor number, tumor differentiation, lymph node metastases, vascular invasion, and preoperative CA 19-9 have all been shown to be associated with survival, the effect of other factors such as tumor size and serosal invasion

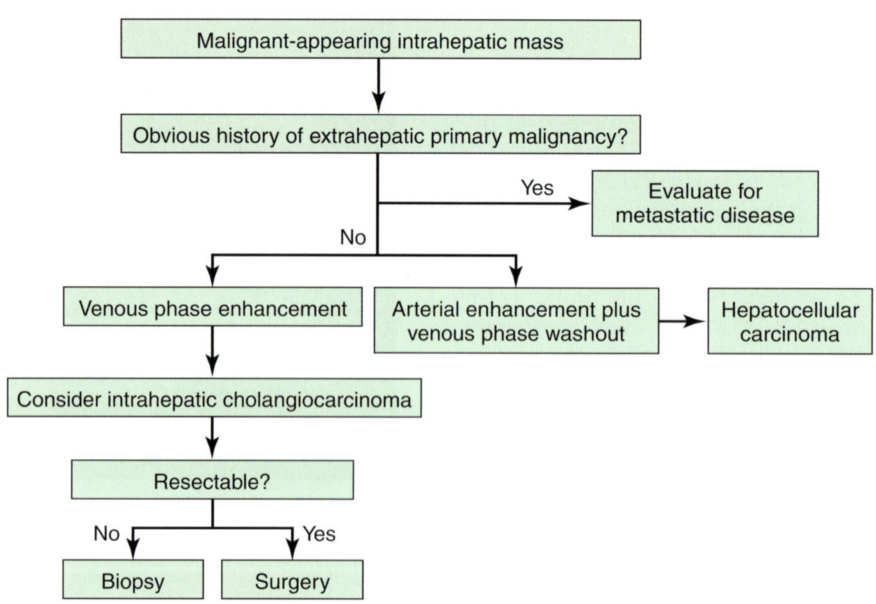

Figure 10-3 Algorithm for the diagnosis of intrahepatic cholangiocarcinoma. *Used with permission from Blechacz B, Komuta M, Roskams T, Gores GJ: Clinical diagnosis and staging of cholangiocarcinoma,* Nat Rev Gastroenterol Hepatol *8:512–522, 2011.*

TABLE 10-1 AJCC/UICC TNM Staging System 7th Version for Intrahepatic Cholangiocarcinoma

TNM classification	
Tx	Primary tumor cannot be assessed
T1	Solitary tumor without vascular invasion[a]
T2a	Solitary tumor with vascular invasion[a]
T2b	Multiple tumors, with or without vascular invasion[a]
T3	Tumor perforating the visceral peritoneum or involving local extrahepatic structures by direct invasion
T4	Tumors with periductal invasion[b]
Nx	Regional lymph nodes cannot be assessed
N0	No regional lymph node metastasis
N1	Regional lymph node metastasis[c]
M0	No distant metastasis
M1	Distant metastasis
Stage groupings	
Stage I	T1 N0 M0
Stage II	T2 N0 M0
Stage III	T3 N0 M0
Stage IVA	T4 N0 M0, any T N1 M0
Stage IVB	Any T Any N M1

[a]Includes major vascular and microvascular invasion.
[b]Includes tumors with periductal-infiltrating or mixed mass-forming and periductal-infiltrating growth pattern.
[c]Nodal involvement of the celiac, periaortic, or caval lymph nodes is considered to be distant metastasis (M1).
Used with permission from Blechacz B, Komuta M, Roskams T, Gores GJ: Clinical diagnosis and staging of cholangiocarcinoma, *Nat Rev Gastroenterol Hepatol* 8:512–522, 2011.

on survival is controversial. Currently, there are three main staging systems utilized for ICC: the American Joint Cancer Committee/Union Internationale Contre le Cancer (AJCC/UICC) TNM (tumor, node, metastasis) staging system seventh version (Table 10-1), the LCSGJ, and the National Cancer Center of Japan (NCCJ) staging system. The biggest difference between the three staging systems resides in the disparate criteria for the T stages (Table 10-2).[33]

Nathan et al. showed that the T stages of the AJCC/UICC sixth edition staging system failed to correlate well with survival and therefore proposed a new staging system, which was subsequently adopted in the seventh edition of the AJCC/UICC.[34] A recent independent study validated the seventh version of the AJCC/UICC system showing a strong correlation between the new proposed T stages and survival in nonmetastatic ICC.[35] Other groups such as the LCSGJ have proposed alternative staging systems using tumor size >2 cm, multiple tumor nodules, and vascular/serosal membrane invasion as negative prognostic factors. However, the LCSGJ staging system has been shown to have poor prognostic discriminatory power.[34] Similarly, another staging system proposed for mass-forming ICC that was based on regional lymph node metastases, multiple tumors, symptom manifestations, and vascular invasion[36] was shown to be somewhat poor.[34] As such, the seventh edition AJCC/UICC staging system is currently the preferred staging system for ICC prognosis.

SURGICAL TREATMENT

The use of staging laparoscopy at the time of surgery in order to detect metastatic disease remains controversial. Several groups have shown evidence of potential benefit for patients who undergo staging laparoscopy and have advocated its routine use. In a French study, the authors showed that 36% (4/11) of ICC patients were found to have metastatic disease upon laparoscopy.[37] They noted 67% accuracy for detection of hepatic and peritoneal metastasis in patients with ICC, since 4 of the remaining 7 were found to have unresectable disease owing to peritoneal metastasis, vascular involvement, or distal lymph node spread at the time of laparotomy. Both the yield and the accuracy for ICC exceeded that for hilar cholangiocarcinoma; however, laparoscopy was unable to detect lymph node metastasis or vascular invasion, which contributed to a significant false-negative rate. In a separate study from the MSKCC, the authors reported a 27% yield for

TABLE 10-2 Comparison of T Subclassifications Among the Staging Systems for Intrahepatic Cholangiocarcinoma

	NCCJ Okabayashi et al.	LCSGJ Nathan et al.	AJCC/UICC 6th Edition	AJCC/UICC 7th Edition
Primary Tumor (T)				
T1	Solitary tumor without VI	Solitary tumor without VI, any size	Solitary tumor without VI, any size	Solitary tumor without VI
T2	Solitary tumor with VI	Multiple tumors and/or VI, any size	Solitary tumor with VI, or multiple tumors <5 cm	T2a: Solitary tumor with VI T2b: Multiple tumors with or without VI
T3	Multiple tumors with or without VI	Extrahepatic extension	Multiple tumors >5 cm or major VI	Direct invasion of adjacent organs (except gallbladder) or with perforation of visceral peritoneum
T4			Direct invasion of adjacent organs (except gallbladder) or with perforation of visceral peritoneum	Periductal invasion

Abbreviations: AJCC/UICC, American Joint Cancer Committee/Union Internationale Contre le Cancer; LCSGJ, Liver Cancer Study Group of Japan; VI, vascular invasion.
Used with permission from Poultsides GA, Zhu AX, Choti MA, Pawlik TM: Intrahepatic cholangiocarcinoma, *Surg Clin North Am* 90:817–837, 2010.

laparoscopy.[38] Metastatic disease was found in 6 of 22 (27%) patients, whereas 5 of 11 (45%) with unresectable disease remained unidentified with laparoscopy. Despite these studies, the evidence to support routine use of laparoscopy to evaluate patients with ICC is still lacking.

Complete surgical resection is the only option that offers a potential cure for ICC. The contraindications to surgical resection for ICC are similar to most other cancers involving the liver: diffuse bilobar involvement, peritoneal and/or distant metastases, presence of major vascular invasion, advanced fibrosis/cirrhosis, or a small liver remnant.[39,40] In addition, presence of retropancreatic or paraceliac nodal metastases and direct invasion of adjacent organs are contraindications for surgery.

At the time of surgery, resection often requires a major procedure. Specifically, anywhere from 50% to 80% of resectable patients will require an extended hepatectomy in order to achieve an R0 resection.[41-44] In addition, approximately 20%–40% will also need bile duct resection and reconstruction.[43,44] The role of routine lymphadenectomy was traditionally controversial, but now many groups advocate for it.[35,45] De Jong et al. reported that up to one-third of patients may have lymph node metastasis and that therefore lymphadenectomy may not only help with local control but also provide important prognostic information.[45] Similar to other solid gastrointestinal-hepatopancreatobiliary malignancies, lymphadenectomy probably does not provide a substantive survival benefit. Shimada et al. noted no difference in survival or overall recurrence between patients who underwent routine lymphadenectomy and those who did not.[46] Another study comparing patients who underwent routine formal lymphadenectomy versus patients who had lymph node sampling found no difference in overall survival.[47] However, because of the staging and prognostic value of lymph node metastasis, as well as possible decrease in locoregional recurrence, routine lymphadenectomy at the time of resection should be strongly considered.[45]

Survival following resection of ICC has been reported to range from 25% to 40%.[34,45,48-50] Poor prognostic indicators include lymph node metastasis, positive margins, vascular invasion, multiple tumor sites, periductal-infiltrating types, bilobar disease, and elevated markedly elevated CA 19-9.[40,51-55] Survival based on AJCC seventh edition T stage is shown in Figure 10-4.

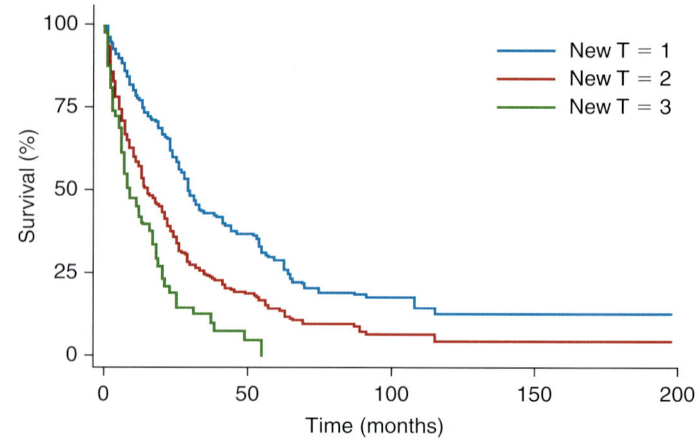

Figure 10-4 Stratification of survival according to AJCC 7th edition T stage. T1: solitary tumor without vascular invasion; T2: solitary tumor with vascular invasion or multiple tumors; T3: tumor perforating the visceral peritoneum or involving the local extrahepatic structures by direct invasion. *Used with permission from Edge SB, Compton CC: The American Joint Committee on Cancer: the 7th edition of the AJCC Cancer Staging Manual and the future of TNM,* Ann Surg Oncol *17:1471–1474, 2010.*

LOCOREGIONAL THERAPY

The role of adjuvant radiation therapy in the treatment of ICC is undetermined. Although a few retrospective studies have suggested a benefit for patients with completely resected cholangiocarcinoma,[56-58] others have not found a benefit.[3] Interpretation of these studies is difficult given their retrospective nature and because patients with ICC and ECC are often included. As such, routine adjuvant radiation therapy is not commonly utilized, but should be strongly considered in patients with positive surgical margins. Other types of locoregional therapy have not been well studied.

Several small studies have examined the role of intraarterial therapy for unresectable ICC and have shown some modest improvement in survival.[59-64] Because most patients with ICC present with large tumors that may be central in location, thermal ablation is often not a therapeutic option. External beam radiotherapy may be beneficial for some patients with unresectable disease. One study found that the use of radiation therapy for inoperable disease was associated with some survival benefit,[65] whereas a different study reported that radiotherapy also can lead to improved quality of life and relief of jaundice in some patients with ICC.[66]

SYSTEMIC THERAPY

Because of the high number of patients who present with locally advanced or metastatic disease, there is a significant need for effective systemic therapy for cholangiocarcinoma. The traditional single agents used include 5-fluorouracil (5-FU), gemcitabine, oxaliplatin, and docetaxel. Recently, a phase III randomized controlled trial evaluating chemotherapeutic agents in biliary tract cancers known as the ABC-02 trial was reported.[67] This study noted that the combination of gemcitabine plus cisplatin significantly increased progression-free survival compared with gemcitabine-only group (11.7 months vs. 8.1 months, respectively). Adverse effects were similar between the two groups except for an increase in neutropenia in the combination therapy group, which did not lead to increased neutropenia-associated infection.[67] The combination of gemcitabine plus a platin-based therapy is now considered the standard of care for treatment of metastatic and locally advanced cholangiocarcinoma for most patients. Oxaliplatin may be used in the place of cisplatin in patients with poor performance status; other gemcitabine combinations under investigation include gemcitabine–capecitabine[68,69] and gemcitabine–irinotecan.[70]

The role of such treatment in the adjuvant therapy for patients with resected disease is less clear. Adjuvant therapy should be considered in patients with lymph node metastasis, given the higher incidence of recurrence and worse overall prognosis for this subset of patients.

Overview: Hilar Cholangiocarcinoma

PRESENTATION AND DIAGNOSIS

In contrast to the often asymptomatic presentation of ICC, patients with hilar cholangiocarcinoma frequently present with jaundice, pruritus, dark urine, pale stools, and sometimes cholangitis.[3,39] Symptoms of fatigue, malaise, and weight loss may also be part of the presenting symptomatology. Whereas laboratory exams can be normal in many patients with ICC, most patients with hilar cholangiocarcinoma will present with elevations in direct and total serum bilirubin, alkaline phosphatase, and sometimes γ-glutamyltransferase. Transaminase levels and prothrombin time may initially be normal, although later in the course of the disease these studies can increase due to chronic hepatocellular damage. As discussed in the diagnosis of ICC, tumor markers can be indicative, but not diagnostic of cholangiocarcinoma. CA 19-9 has a sensitivity and specificity of 76% and 92%, respectively, in determining the difference between nonmalignant and malignant strictures.[29] The addition of CEA can also improve detection.

Diagnosis of hilar cholangiocarcinoma relies on multiple methods of assessment (Figure 10-5).[30] Ultrasonography is often the first mode of imaging used to evaluate a patient with jaundice, but is of little help except in identifying biliary dilatation. Cross-sectional studies are essential. Imaging with contrast is necessary for determination of vascular involvement, location of the bile duct obstruction, and tumor extent.[39] It is usually preferable to obtain cross-sectional imaging prior to stenting, as bile duct stents can obscure definition of the extent of disease. It is also important to determine the existence and extent of hepatic atrophy due to biliary obstruction and portal vein encasement, which can be suggestive of a malignancy.[39] CT has traditionally been the initial cross-sectional imaging obtained and was traditionally deemed inferior to MRI. With the introduction of multidetector CT (MDCT), the resolution and detection accuracy of CT has drastically improved. On CT imaging, hilar cholangiocarcinomas can appear as either a focal or ill-defined mass with vascularity changes ranging from hypovascular to hypervascular on delayed imaging.[71] Most clinicians believe that MRI and magnetic resonance cholangiopancreatography (MRCP) are still superior to CT in the diagnosis and determination of resectability of hilar cholangiocarcinoma.[72] In addition to evaluating the location of the stricture and the extent of vascular involvement, MRI can also determine the presence of choledocholithiasis and hepatolithiasis. MRCP can provide information similar to invasive procedures such as endoscopic retrograde cholangiopancreatography (ERCP) or percutaneous transhepatic cholangiography (PTC). The accuracy of MRI combined with MRCP is generally high, from 78% to 96%.[73,74] As with ICC, the use of PET scan in the management of hilar cholangiocarcinoma still remains to be elucidated. Although PET is not as accurate as CT in the detection of hilar cholangiocarcinoma,[75] PET may be most useful in detecting

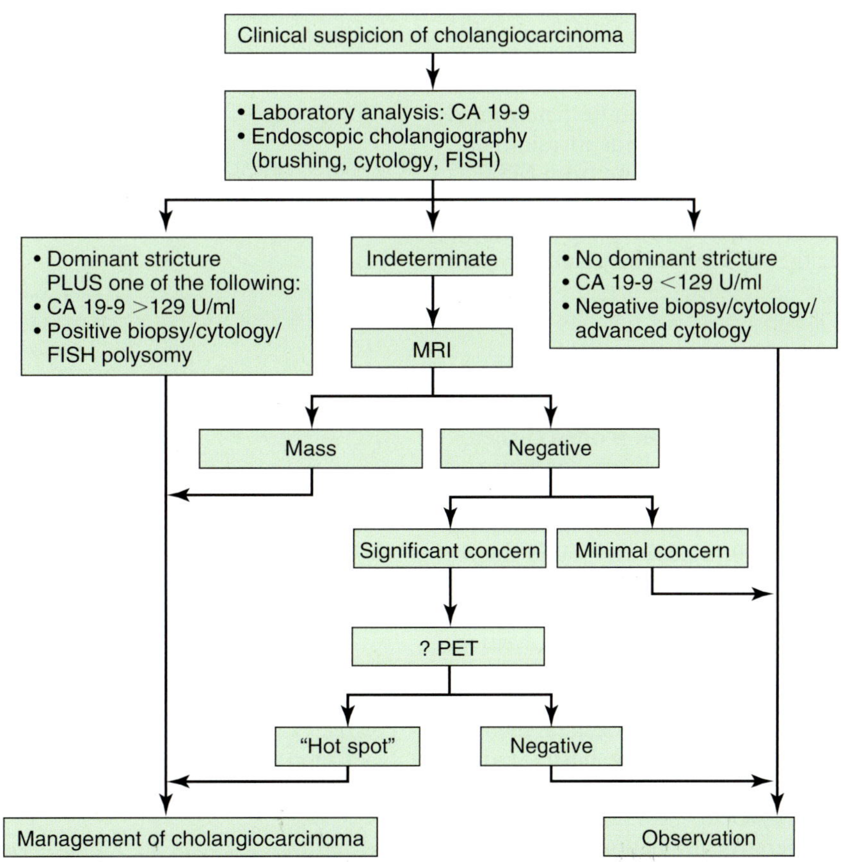

Figure 10-5 Flow chart for diagnosis of hilar cholangiocarcinoma. *Used with permission from Blechacz B, Komuta M, Roskams T, Gores GJ: Clinical diagnosis and staging of cholangiocarcinoma, Nat Rev Gastroenterol Hepatol 8:512–522, 2011.*

metastasis not recognized by CT or MRI.[76-78] Typically, PET scan is not employed as much for ECC as with ICC.

Directly accessing the bile duct can be performed either by ERCP or PTC and can provide valuable information on the biliary anatomy. Both modalities allow for direct imaging of the biliary tree, biliary drainage, and biopsy. Cholangioscopy has been increasingly utilized to directly visualize the biliary tree, thereby allowing for the identification of bile duct abnormalities, mucosal ulcerations, polyps, nodules, or other anomalies in addition to the identification of strictures with cholangiography.[79] One study showed that the use of direct cholangioscopy in addition to ERCP increased diagnostic accuracy and sensitivity.[80] Biopsy to obtain diagnostic tissue specimens has good specificity, but low sensitivity.[25] Tissue diagnosis is not required for patient management and one should proceed with the diagnosis of a probable malignancy in the proper clinical setting in the presence of a malignant-appearing stricture. Direct access and drainage of the biliary tree can also relieve the symptoms of jaundice and lower the bilirubin levels. This is important as elevated bilirubin levels prior to surgery may be associated with decreased rates of hepatic regeneration after resection and increased postoperative mortality.[81]

STAGING

Similar to ICC, there is also a lack of consensus on an optimal staging system for hilar cholangiocarcinoma. The Bismuth-Corlette classification provides an anatomic description of the tumor location and longitudinal extension in the biliary tree. This classification is probably the most common manner in which surgeons describe hilar lesions. With regard to postoperative prognosis, the most widely utilized systems are the MSKCC and the AJCC/TNM staging systems. The MSKCC system proposed a T score that is based on a number of factors: the location and extent of bile duct involvement (as determined by the Bismuth-Corlette system), portal venous invasion, and hepatic lobar atrophy (Table 10-3).[82] The group from MSKCC has shown that this T score is associated with resectability and survival. Despite this, the most widely used staging system for hilar cholangiocarcinoma is the AJCC or TNM staging system (Table 10-4).[55]

SURGICAL TREATMENT

The mainstay of curative therapy for hilar cholangiocarcinoma remains surgical resection. However, resection is often challenging because of advanced disease at the time of presentation and the proximity of the tumor to important vascular and biliary structures. Ito and colleagues published a review of resection for hilar cholangiocarcinoma from 1990 to 2008 and found the resectability rate to range from 28% to 95%, with a median of 70%.[83] Typically, hilar cholangiocarcinoma lesions are deemed locally unresectable if there is bilateral biliary duct involvement to the secondary radicles, main portal vein or hepatic artery encasement or occlusion, hepatic lobe atrophy with contralateral encasement or occlusion of portal vein or contralateral involvement of secondary biliary radicles, secondary biliary radicle involvement with contralateral portal vein branch encasement or occlusion.[82] Of note, even among patients with tumors seemingly resectable based on the preoperative evaluation, the ultimate determination of resectability can only be made during surgical

TABLE 10-3 MSKCC T Stage Criteria

Stage	Criteria
T1	Tumor involving biliary confluence ± unilateral extension to second-order biliary radicles
T2	Tumor involving biliary confluence ± unilateral extension to second-order biliary radicles and *ipsilateral* portal vein involvement ± *ipsilateral* hepatic lobar atrophy
T3	Tumor involving biliary confluence ± unilateral extension to second-order biliary radicles; or unilateral extension to second-order biliary radicles with *contralateral* portal vein involvement; or unilateral extension to second-order biliary radicles with *contralateral* hepatic lobar atrophy; or main or bilateral portal vein involvement

Used with permission from Jarnagin WR, Fong Y, DeMatteo RP, et al: Staging, resectability, and outcome in 225 patients with hilar cholangiocarcinoma, *Ann Surg* 234:507–517, 2001.

TABLE 10-4 AJCC TNM Staging for Hilar Cholangiocarcinoma

TNM Classification	
Tx	Primary tumor cannot be assessed
T0	No evidence of primary tumor
Tis	Carincoma in situ
T1	Tumor confined to the bile duct, with extension up to the muscle layer or fibrous tissue
T2a	Tumor invades beyond the wall of the bile duct to surrounding adipose tissue
T2b	Tumor invades adjacent hepatic parenchyma
T3	Tumor invades unilateral branches of the portal vein or hepatic artery
T4	Tumor invades main portal vein or its branches bilaterally, the common hepatic artery, the second-order biliary radicals bilaterally, or unilateral second-order biliary radicals with contralateral portal vein or hepatic artery involement.
Nx	Regional lymph nodes cannot be assessed
N0	No regional lymph node metastasis
N1	Regional lymph node metastasis
N2	Metastasis to periaortic, pericaval, superior mesenteric artery, and/or celiac artery lymph nodes
M0	No distant metastasis
M1	Distant metastasis
Stage groupings	
Stage 0	Tis N0 M0
Stage I	T1 N0 M0
Stage II	T2a-b N0 M0
Stage IIIA	T3 N0 M0
Stage IIIB	T1-3 N1 M0
Stage IVA	T4 N0-1 M0
Stage IVB	Any T N2 M0, Any T Any N M1

Used with permission from Edge SB, Compton CC: The American Joint Committee on Cancer: the 7th edition of the AJCC Cancer Staging Manual and the future of TNM, *Ann Surg Oncol* 17: 1471–1474, 2010.

exploration, and a subset of patients will be found to be unresectable at the time of surgery.[84]

The addition of hepatic resection to extrahepatic bile duct resection for hilar cholangiocarcinoma is critical and has resulted in increased rates of negative surgical margins.[39,85] As such, standard surgical therapy for hilar cholangiocarcinoma should include combined hepatic and bile duct resection.[39] In a select group of patients, portal vein embolization may be needed to increase the size of the future liver remnant (FLR) before hepatic resection is considered. Typically, if the FLR is less than 20%–30%, the risk of complications, liver insufficiency, and mortality increase.[86,87] For patients with underlying liver dysfunction, such as steatosis or fibrosis, the remnant liver must be even larger, ranging from 30% to 40% of the original volume. In these situations, portal vein embolization should be used to allow induction of hypertrophy of the contralateral liver, increasing the liver remnant by as much as 8%–16%.[88] Embolization of either the right or left portal vein is typically done using embolic materials such as cyanoacrylate, polyvinyl alcohol, coils, or gelatin microspheres.

At the time of surgery, portal vein resection and caudate lobe resection are two strategies that may increase the likelihood of an R0 resection rate. Although Neuhaus and colleagues[89] advocated routine portal vein resection, most surgeons will only resect the portal vein when there is local tumor involvement of the vein. In contrast, resection of the caudate lobe, or segment 1, should be routine as this is associated with decreased local recurrence and improve survival, likely because of removal of ducts draining directly into the caudate from the hepatic hilum.[90,91] Lymph node metastases are found in approximately 30% to 50% of hilar cholangiocarcinoma cases, and therefore routine lymphadenectomies should be performed.[92]

It is important to note that the morbidity and mortality associated with surgery for hilar cholangiocarcinoma is higher than for other types of hepatic resection. Specifically, the reported morbidity and mortality rates range from 14% to 75% and 0% to 18% respectively.[39] Some of the additional morbidity and mortality may be associated with the increased risk of liver insufficiency in these patients, many of whom require major hepatic resections in the setting of cholestasis.[84]

Following surgery for hilar cholangiocarcinoma, the 5-year survival rate is approximately 20%–40%.[39,85,93-95] Patients with R0 resection show a significantly prolonged survival versus those who underwent an R1 or R2 resection.[82,84,95-100] In fact, few patients who underwent an R2 resection survive to 5 years, and therefore this needs to be avoided.[82,101] Lymph node status is also an important prognostic factor. In one study of 137 patients, 5-year survival was 38% versus 10% among patients without and with nodal disease, respectively.[102] Other factors that have been shown to adversely affect survival include gallbladder invasion, adenosquamous histologic type, male gender, preoperative serum albumin <3 g/dL, and total bilirubin >10 mg/dL.[84,94]

Orthotopic liver transplantation as a feasible treatment option for hilar cholangiocarcinoma continues to be an area of debate. Although initial results were disappointing, with high recurrence and mortality rates,[103,104] more recent protocols that employ better patient selection as well as preoperative radiation and chemotherapy have noted improved survival among patients undergoing liver transplantation for hilar cholangiocarcinoma.[105] The Mayo Clinic has been at the forefront of transplantation for hilar cholangiocarcinoma and have proposed both patient selection (Table 10-5) and exclusion (Table 10-6) criteria.[106] In general, the Mayo protocol consists of external beam radiation and 5-FU followed by brachytherapy and capecitabine prior to liver transplantation.[106] The reported 5-year survival for all patients undergoing neoadjuvant therapy and subsequent transplantation ranges from 55% to 71%.[107]

LOCOREGIONAL THERAPY

As with ICC, the role of adjuvant radiotherapy is unclear. Usually, external beam radiotherapy, brachytherapy, or stereotactic radiotherapy is employed in case of positive surgical margins. Several retrospective studies have shown a survival benefit in patients with positive (and, in some cases, negative) surgical margins.[108-112] However, other studies have not noted a survival benefit of adjuvant radiotherapy.[109,113] As such, although it is unclear whether routine adjuvant radiotherapy is beneficial, it should be strongly considered in the setting of positive surgical margins.

Another potential locoregional treatment is photodynamic therapy, which is an ablative technique utilizing a photosensitizing drug administered systemically and allowed to collect in the area of the tumor. Following administration of the drug, the

TABLE 10-5 Mayo Clinic Criteria for Neoadjuvant Therapy and Liver Transplantation

Diagnosis of Cholangiocarcinoma
Transcatheter biopsy or brush cytology
CA 19-9 >100 mg/mL and/or a mass on cross-sectional imaging for a malignant appearing stricture on cholangiography
Unresectable tumor above cystic duct
Pancreatoduodenectomy for microscopic involvement of common bile duct
Resectable cholangiocarcinoma arising in PSC
Radial tumor diameter ≤3cm
Absence of intra- and extrahepatic metastases
Candidate for liver transplantation

Abbreviation: PSC, primary sclerosing cholangitis

Used with permission from Rosen CB, Heimbach JK, Gores GJ: Liver transplantation for cholangiocarcinoma, *Transplant Int* 23:692–697, 2010.

TABLE 10-6 Exclusion Criteria for Liver Transplantation for Hilar Cholangiocarcinoma

Intrahepatic cholangiocarcinoma
Uncontrolled infection
Prior radiation or chemotherapy
Prior biliary resection or attempted resection
Intrahepatic metastases
Evidence of extrahepatic disease
History of other malignancy within 5 years
Transperitoneal biopsy (including percutaneous and EUS-guided FNA)

Abbreviations: EUS, endoscopic ultrasound; FNA, fine-needle aspiration

Used with permission from Rosen CB, Heimbach JK, Gores GJ: Liver transplantation for cholangiocarcinoma, *Transplant Int* 23:692–697, 2010.

use of a laser light causes a reaction that forms oxygen cytotoxic radicals, causing cell death in and around the tumor. Photodynamic therapy may be a possible mode of neoadjuvant therapy. One study showed that photodynamic therapy administration in the area of tumor growth increased the likelihood of R0 resection as well as survival rate.[114] However, the sample size was small ($n = 7$), which renders the results difficult to interpret and inconclusive.

SYSTEMIC THERAPY

The role of systemic therapy for hilar cholangiocarcinoma in the adjuvant setting is also ill defined. Many regimens have been used, including oxaliplatin and 5-FU, gemcitabine, and gemcitabine plus capecitabine. One study of 42 patients reported an association between the use of gemcitabine in the adjuvant therapy regimen and prolonged survival,[115] with a 5-year survival of 57% compared to 23% in the group with no adjuvant therapy. As noted, given the data from the ABC-02 trial, standard systemic therapy for unresectable hilar cholangiocarcinoma should include the combination of gemcitabine plus cisplatin.[67] The use of adjuvant combined therapy should be strongly considered among those patients with resected disease who have lymph node metastasis.

Evidence from retrospective studies also suggests a potential benefit in patients receiving adjuvant chemoradiation.[58,95,111,112,116,117] However, prospective data are lacking and although chemoradiation should probably be routinely utilized in patients with positive margins, the benefit is less clear among R0 patients.

PALLIATIVE CONSIDERATIONS

Palliation in hilar cholangiocarcinoma centers on relief of symptoms and maximization of quality of life rather than prolonging survival. Approximately 25%–50% of the liver usually needs to be drained to relieve symptomatic jaundice and pruritus.[118] Symptoms caused by biliary obstruction can be treated with surgical bypass or nonoperative stenting procedures. In general, biliary-enteric bypass should only be performed when the patient is found to be unresectable intraoperatively. In patients with unresectable disease that is discovered preoperatively, palliation of symptoms usually can be achieved through endoscopic or percutaneous stenting. The stent material is also an important consideration. Plastic stents are less costly and easier to insert and remove, but are narrower and more prone to occluding.[119] As a result, plastic stents may be most useful preoperatively or for temporary stenting. Metal stents require less reintervention because of their larger diameter and decreased likelihood of migration, as well as having a longer patency.[120]

Radiation therapy for inoperable hilar cholangiocarcinoma has also been shown to be a safe and effective palliative procedure.[121,122] An MSKCC study showed that biliary drainage plus external beam radiotherapy allowed patients to improve their quality of life.[123] In the setting of unresectable disease, two small randomized controlled trials have also shown promising results of photodynamic therapy.[124,125]

Conclusion

Cholangiocarcinoma remains difficult to diagnose and treat. Surgical resection remains the best chance for a cure. For both ICC and ECC, resection requires hepatic resection and lymphadenectomy; hilar cholangiocarcinoma also requires concomitant extrahepatic bile duct resection. Prognosis following resection remains modest, with lymph node and margin status strongly associated with long-term survival. As such, adjuvant therapies such as chemotherapy and radiotherapy should be considered, especially in these high-risk cohorts. Considering the guarded prognosis of resected patients, as well as the high rates of unresectability at diagnosis, more effective systemic therapies and adjuvant therapy regimens are sorely needed to improve the outcome of patients with cholangiocarcinoma.

REFERENCES

The complete reference list is available online at www.expertconsult.com.

11

Percutaneous Management of Cholangiocarcinoma

JAMIL MUASHER | WAEL E. A. SAAD

KEY POINTS

- In general, the higher the cholangiocarcinoma (type 3 and type 4) and the more multifocal the disease/obstruction, the more likely the patient is to require percutaneous therapy/drainage rather than endoscopic drainage.
- The two chief indications for preoperative biliary drainage are (1) the presence of preoperative cholangitis and (2) estimated FLR <30%. The goal of percutaneous biliary drainage is hepatic reserve optimization by improving coagulopathy and resolving any hepatorenal syndrome, thereby improving surgical outcome.
- The disadvantages of performing drainage prior to resection include introduction of polymicrobial organisms to the biliary tree.
- Ultimately, the possible advantages of covered stents should also be weighed against their increased expense, especially in light of the fact that many patients will not outlive a bare metal stent. This may explain why recent randomized trials (bare stents vs. covered stents) have not shown a clear and significant patency advantage of covered stents when compared to bare stents.
- A randomized trial of photodynamic therapy versus conventional biliary drainage demonstrated a survival benefit so significant (98 vs. 493 days, $P < 0.0001$) that the trial was terminated early.
- Transarterial catheter therapy (whether chemoemboliza-tion or radioembolization) have shown promising initial results in the management of cholangiocarcinoma.
- Percutaneous tumor ablation is feasible, with good results; however, its role in the overall management of cholangiocarcinoma is yet to be determined.

Introduction

Cholangiocarcinoma is the second most common primary liver malignancy, after hepatocellular carcinoma, and its incidence appears to be increasing.[1] Approximately 2000 cases are reported annually in the United States. Nearly two thirds of cases occur in patients aged 50–70, with a male predominance.[2] The presenting symptoms of cholangiocarcinoma include jaundice, weight loss, pruritis, pain, and liver failure. Because symptoms typically occur late in the disease, staging at diagnosis tends to be advanced and prognosis for the disease is poor overall, with certain subgroups having extremely poor survival. Overall, patients with biliary duct malignancies have a reported median survival of 3–10 months.[3] It should also be noted that gallbladder carcinoma, central intrahepatic metastasis, and metastatic lymphadenopathy may also result in malignant biliary obstruction, which may present similar to cholangiocarcinoma. Although this chapter attempts to primarily reflect the scientific literature on cholangiocarcinoma, some of the principles will also apply to these other etiologies of biliary obstruction. Moreover, on review of the literature, all etiologies of malignant biliary obstruction are commonly amalgamated and, as a result, it is difficult to ascertain outcomes that are specific to cholangiocarcinoma.

The current chapter focuses on the percutaneous biliary drainage and management of cholangiocarcinoma. Cholangiocarcinomas are a heterogenous group of tumors in terms of their size, location, symptoms, and survival (Table 11-1). The complexity of this multifaceted subject, with its numerous variables, is compounded by the fact that varying techniques and methods are often amalgamated from an outcomes standpoint (Table 11-1). This goes as far as amalgamating the outcomes of endoscopic and percutaneous management together, and thus in many studies it is commonly difficult to ascertain specific outcomes of percutaneous management overall, let alone evaluate outcomes that are specific to particular percutaneous techniques/stent. In this chapter, we will first discuss biliary drainage for cholangiocarcinoma in terms of its indications, technique, and method of drainage (endoscopic vs. percutaneous). We will also discuss the various types and configurations of biliary catheters and stents available, and the rationale for their use. In addition, the impact of the obstructing lesion (distal vs. hilar, right vs. left) on the treatment approach will be discussed (Table 11-1). The preliminary results of covered versus bare stents will also be discussed along with locoregional transluminal therapies.

Management Overview

Cholangiocarcinomas are a heterogenous group of tumors in terms of their size, location, symptoms, and survival. Figure 11-1 demonstrates the terminology of cholangiocarcinoma based on location. Management needs to be individually tailored for each patient. In terms of location, multiple classification schemes exist. Cholangiocarcinoma may be described as proximal/distal or, using the Bismuth-Corlette classification system as types 1, 2, 3a, 3b and 4 according to their intrahepatic/hilar/extrahepatic distribution (Figure 11-2). Type 1 lesions generally have the best prognosis, while type 4 lesions have the poorest prognosis.[4]

Overall, patients with biliary duct malignancies have a reported median survival of 3–10 months, particularly when the presenting symptoms are associated with biliary obstruction, which is usually the case.[3] Medical therapy is very limited for cholangiocarcinoma and no standard chemotherapy regimen

TABLE 11-1 Complexity and Variability in Evaluating Cholangiocarcinoma From the Literature

Variables in Describing and Managing Cholangiocarcinoma	
Indications	Preoperative vs. palliative management
Location of Cholangiocarcinoma	Hilar vs. distal cholangiocarcinoma (Figure 11-1)
Modality of management	Endoscopic vs. percutaneous management
Laterality of approach	Right-sided vs. left-sided PTC and percutaneous biliary drainage
Degree of drainage	Unilobar vs. bilobar hepatic biliary drainage
Endoprosthesis (stents)	Plastic vs. metallic endoprosthesis (stents)
	Covered metallic vs. bare metallic stents
	Y-configured vs. T-configured metallic stents

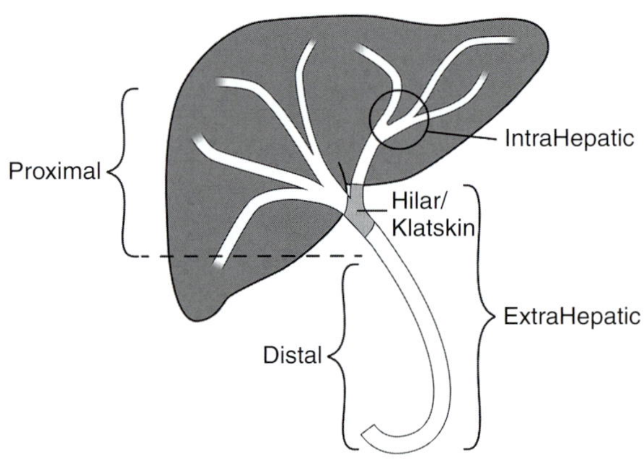

Figure 11-1 Terminology associated with the location of cholangiocarcinoma. Hilar cholangiocarcinoma (Klatskin tumor) is further classified according to the Bismuth-Colette classification (see Figure 11-2).

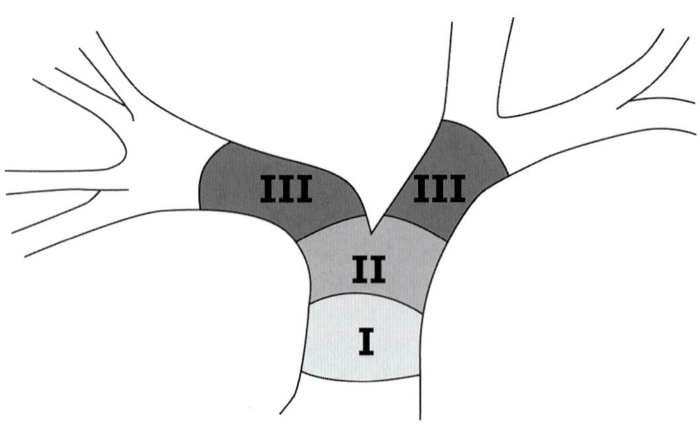

Figure 11-2 Bismuth classification. Bismuth-Corlette Type I: Tumor is in the common hepatic duct and does not involve the confluence of the right and left main biliary ducts. Bismuth-Corlette Type II: Tumor is at the confluence of the right and left main biliary ducts. Bismuth-Corlette Type III: Tumor is at the confluence of the right and left main biliary ducts and extends to one of the second-order confluences: either right or left. Bismuth-Corlette Type IV (not drawn): Tumor is at the confluence of the right and left main biliary ducts and extends to both of the second-order confluences: right and left.

exists, because of minimal survival benefit. Radiation therapy is controversial because of limited efficacy and increased risk of complications (cholangitis, gastroduodenitis, and increased hospitalization). Decompressive surgery is the traditional treatment for obstructing cholangiocarcinoma. The majority of surgeries are performed for palliation, with less than 30% of patients with cholangiocarcinoma having a chance for a curative resection.[5] Moreover, many patients at the time of presentation are not surgical candidates, with up to 70%–80% of patients being nonsurgical candidates.[1] As a result, most nonsurgical patients are managed by minimally invasive means (endoscopic or percutaneous biliary drainage). These minimally invasive approaches are now considered standard of care for many patients along with systemic or new loco-regional therapies.

ENDOSCOPIC VERSUS PERCUTANEOUS BILIARY DRAINAGE

Studies have shown that the method of biliary drainage has no impact on survival.[6] However, endoscopic retrograde cholangiopancreatography (ERCP)–guided internal biliary drainage is often the preferred method of drainage and is generally thought to be less invasive than percutaneous drainage, because it does not require creation of an invasive transhepatic/transcapsular (Glisson capsule) tract. As a result, ERCP is the most definitely preferred procedure in patients with severe coagulopathy or ascites. However, there are several scenarios in which endoscopic drainage may fail or may not be feasible. In terms of disease location, ERCP generally can adequately drain the liver when a distal lesion is present, but may be more problematic in hilar lesions or in cases with multiple strictures. In general, the higher the cholangiocarcinoma (type 3 and type 4) and the more multifocal the disease/obstruction, the more likely the patient is to require percutaneous therapy/drainage rather than endoscopic drainage.

Additionally, previous upper gastrointestinal tract surgery (Bilroth II or gastric bypass, to name two) may make endoscopic stent placement difficult or impossible. In these cases, percutaneous drainage may succeed where endoscopic drainage has failed. In cases of proximal lesions or in patients with multiple strictures (numerous intrahepatic isolated biliary segments), percutaneous drainage may be superior because it can specifically target the area of abnormality or biliary tract dilation. However, it is important to note that cholangiocarcinomas with more advanced Bismuth class (corresponding to more diffuse involvement) tend to have fewer dilated intrahepatic ducts on imaging studies and that hilar cholangiocarcinoma accounts for 40%–60% of all cholangiocarcinomas.[7]

Percutanous Transhepatic Management

Patients undergoing percutaneous transhepatic cholangiography (PTC) for purely diagnostic purposes is largely a thing of the past and the vast majority of patients are now diagnosed on the basis of noninvasive imaging such as magnetic resonance cholangiopancreatography (MRCP), computed tomography (CT), or ultrasonography prior to any minimally invasive procedure (ERCP or PTC) (please see Preprocedural Imaging section). Percutaneous transhepatic management can be classified into (1) PTC and percutaneous transhepatic biliary drainage, (2) internalization of drainage by stent placement, and (3) new loco-regional therapies such as brachytherapy and photodynamic therapy.

INITIAL PTC AND PERCUTANEOUS DRAINAGE

Preoperative Versus Palliative Biliary Drainage

Percutaneous biliary drainage is typically indicated in one of two broad-based scenarios, preoperative (for surgical candidates) or palliative (in patients who will not have surgery). Surgery for cholangiocarcinoma can be performed with either the goal of a curative resection or for palliative decompression. In either of these scenarios, preoperative drainage can be entertained. Complete surgical resection, often necessitating major hepatic resection, remains the only possibility for cure in patients with cholangiocarcinoma. The role of orthotopic liver transplantation in this population is not well defined at present.[8] As many as 90% of patients with cholangiocarcinoma are not candidates for curative resection. For patients who are not surgical candidates or who do not elect to undergo surgery, percutaneous biliary drainage may be performed as a palliative measure.

Currently, performing the drainage procedure prior to surgery is controversial and has been debated for years. As a result, practice varies between institutions. Many Asian centers have advocated preoperative drainage routinely, while Western centers have tended to be more conservative.[9] The advantages of preoperative drainage include resolution of any preexisting cholangitis and optimization of the hepatic reserve.[8,9] The goal of hepatic reserve optimization is to improve coagulopathy and to resolve any hepatorenal syndrome, thereby improving the patient's surgical outcome. The disadvantages of performing drainage prior to resection include introduction of polymicrobial organisms to the biliary tree.[10,11] Another potential disadvantage is increased morbidity both from the drainage procedure itself and from the associated increase in hospital stay. Moreover, a percutaneous biliary drainage catheter may hinder the ability to assess the full extent of the tumor both on preoperative imaging and intraoperatively.

In terms of hepatic reserve, the concept of future liver remnant (FLR) is important to understand. Future liver remnant, as the name implies, is defined as the difference between the total liver volume and the volume of resected liver. The FLR cannot be truly known until after the surgery; however, it can be accurately predicted preoperatively on CT or magnetic resonance imaging (MRI) using volumetric analysis.[8,9] If the FLR is expected to be less than 30%, patients tend to have worse surgical outcomes. Therefore, optimization of the hepatic reserve becomes more important in this group as it will improve the liver's capacity for postoperative hypertrophy.[8,9] Two studies demonstrated that without percutaneous biliary drainage, postoperative hepatic dysfunction with an FLR less than 30% and greater than 30% was 24% vs. 0%, respectively. Similarly, the postoperative death with an FLR less than 30% and greater than 30% was 19% versus 5%, respectively.[8,9]

Therefore, the two chief indications for preoperative biliary drainage are (1) the presence of preoperative cholangitis and (2) estimated FLR <30%. These indications apply to both curative and palliative resections. These indications should be weighed against the significant risk of introducing polymicrobial infection from the procedure. Incidence of cholangitis following percutaneous drainage is reported at 20%–60%. Review of five Level 1 clinical trials demonstrates that 65% of patients who received preoperative drainage had biliary aspirates positive for polymicrobial organisms compared to 8% of patients who did not receive preoperative drainage.[10,11] In terms of preoperative management, it is important to obtain high-quality abdominal imaging prior to drainage in order to avoid the catheter compromising the preoperative imaging.

Indications

Patients undergoing PTC for purely diagnostic purposes is largely a thing of the past. Drainage for simply the relief of asymptomatic obstruction or visualization of dilated/obstructed biliary radicals is not an indication for PTC and subsequent percutaneous biliary drainage.[12,13] The clinical indications for PTC and subsequent biliary drainage is pruritis (particularly refractory to medical therapy), cholangitis, biliary sepsis, and hyperbilirubinemia in patients who will undergo systemic chemotherapy with agents that require hepatic metabolism and/or biliary excretion.[12,13] In a study by Robson and coworkers, the proportions of patients with the primary indication of pain/pruritis, jaundice precluding chemotherapy, and cholangitis were 18%, 53%, and 10%, respectively.[13] These chemotherapeutic agents include 5-flourouracil (5-FU), irinotecan, and gemcitabine. The degree of reduction in serum bilirubin is the chief indicator of successful drainage.[14] The target total bilirubin after percutaneous drainage for the administration of chemotherapeutic regimens is usually less than 2 mg/dL.[13,14]

Preprocedural Workup and Clinical Evaluation

Preprocedure workup should include a detailed history (assessing indications and contraindications), physical examination, laboratory data, and noninvasive imaging. Because of the risk of bleeding from the procedure, coagulation parameters and platelets should be optimized. There are no set coagulation parameters; however, an international normalized ratio (INR) of less than 1.5 and a platelet count greater than 50,000–75,000/mm^3 are common thresholds.[15] The presence of preprocedure cholangitis should be carefully assessed for, as percutaneous drainage may worsen/disseminate any underlying infection. Prophylactic antibiotics are recommended.[16] Common prophylactic antibiotics used include intravenous piperacillin and tazobactam combination or intravenous ceftriaxone. Preprocedural sedation and/or anesthesia evaluation is also performed, as PTC with subsequent drainage can be performed under moderate sedation, deep sedation, or general anesthesia.

Preprocedural Imaging Evaluation from a Technical Safety Standpoint

Preprocedural imaging is vital for planning of effective percutaneous transhepatic biliary drainage.[12] Preprocedural imaging is used to evaluate for intrahepatic anatomy and pathology such as portal vein thrombosis, hepatic segmental atrophy and hypertrophy, intrahepatic masses and tumors, and obviously, levels of biliary obstruction, degree of biliary obstruction, and isolated biliary segments. Preprocedural imaging is also required for evaluating extrahepatic anatomy and pathology such as ascites, bowel, subcostal access routes, and chest anomalies. Bowel and distorted hepatic anatomy is particularly prevalent in chronic obstruction, prior therapy, and prior hepatic resections.

Ultrasonography is effective in determining the degree of biliary dilation and the level of biliary obstruction.[12] However, its effectiveness varies with operators and there is considerable interoperator variability. More importantly, it may overlook or underestimate extrahepatic anatomic aspects such as bowel and it may not reliably and accurately assess intrahepatic tumors that may need to be avoided. MRI is very effective for determining affected segments and determining intrahepatic tumors and extrahepatic structures. However, it is not effective in identifying calcifications and metal objects such as surgical clips and prior stents (metal or plastic) that are used as landmarks during PTC by experienced operators.[12] Thus, it is particularly less suitable in patients with recurrence who commonly have complicated obstructions and prior stents. Moreover, the quality of MRI may vary from one patient to another depending on body habitus, patient cooperation, and respiratory artifacts. CT, especially contrast-enhanced CT, is the most reliable, most available, and most reproducible imaging modality when it comes to prebiliary drainage planning. It shows the pertinent intra- and extrahepatic anatomy and pathology as well as dense landmarks such as calcifications, stents, and clips. It also identifies the most dilated biliary segments, degree of dilation, and isolated segments. In the authors' opinion, as in the case with prior authors, the most ideal imaging modality for preoperative planning is CT.[12] Needless to say, ultrasonography is a more important imaging modality for image guidance for drain placement (see below) but less important for predrainage planning.

Preprocedural Imaging Evaluation from a Drainage Efficacy Standpoint

Drainage efficacy depends on the indication of drainage (intended/desired clinical endpoint). If the primary clinical indication is cholangitis with or without biliary sepsis or pruritis (a biliary stagnation issue leading to systemic dissemination of bile/bacterial infection), then the target biliary segments should be the most dilated segments regardless of hepatic parenchymal volume and portal vein thrombosis (see next section). In this respect, all cross-sectional imaging modalities (including ultrasonography) are effective in preoperatively identifying the most dilated biliary segment(s). Obviously, no operator can safely say which biliary segment is the source of infection; however, targeting the most dilated segments is "statistically" prudent. The most dilated segments are probably the most chronically obstructed and have the largest stagnant biliary volume; both of which are higher probabilities of the presence of infected bile. It should be mentioned that cholangitis with or without biliary sepsis is not a frequent presenting symptom/indication in a "virgin biliary system" that has not been instrumented.[12] Moreover, it is not uncommon to find contamination of isolated biliary segments that are not drained (by endoscopy or percutaneously) but are adjacent to drained biliary segments.[12] These adjacent undrained isolated biliary segments are a source of recurrent cholangitis and possibly sepsis that translates into increased patient morbidity. This should be avoided at all costs and it emphasizes the strict adherence to the clinical indications of endoscopic and/or percutaneous biliary drainage.

If the primary indication is hyperbilirubinemia (a biliary stagnation issue leading to poor function) with or without the need to optimize hepatic function, then the target biliary/hepatic segments are not necessarily those with the most dilated biliary radicals. The ideal target hepatic segments for drainage are the largest functional hepatic segments exhibiting biliary obstruction and displaying patent portal venous supply and not replaced by tumor (the size of the healthy and portal-perfused parenchymal and not the size/degree of dilation of the biliary radicals). The patency of the portal venous supply is paramount because the portal vein provides the trophic blood supply of the liver.[12,17] Portal vein occlusion, by thrombosis and/or tumor invasion, particularly when accompanied by same-segment(s) biliary obstruction leads to hepatic parenchymal atrophy.[17]

PTC and Percutaneous Drainage Technique

PTC and subsequent percutaneous biliary drainage can usually be performed with the patient undergoing moderate sedation. This can be complemented with intercostal nerve blocks. Less than 10% of cases require deep sedation or general anesthesia. However, some operators/institutions routinely utilize deep sedation or general anesthesia. Anecdotally, patients undergoing PTC under general anesthesia may have a larger incidence of pleural complications because respiratory splinting in patients undergoing PTC with moderate sedation may reduce the extent of the cephalad (downward) extent of the pleural reflections (this applies to right-sided PTC only). Regardless of the degree of sedation/anesthesia, all patients should be well hydrated and have adequate venous access in case aggressive fluid resuscitation is required. This is because it is not uncommon to have worsening cholangitis and/or biliary sepsis during or after percutaneous biliary drainage.[18]

The approach of the biliary tract (target biliary segment) should be governed by indications and imaging findings and planning (see above). If all things are considered, a right-sided (right midaxillary) versus left-sided (subxiphoid/epigastric) approach varies between operators from a preference standpoint (Figure 11-3). This choice almost always occurs in cases with central extrahepatic biliary obstruction and has become less commonly encountered by interventional radiologists because many of these cases are drained endoscopically. The advantages and disadvantages of left-sided and right-sided approaches are listed in Table 11-2.

PTC and percutaneous biliary drainage is commonly performed using fluoroscopic guidance.[12,19,20] Grayscale ultrasound guidance can be used for real-time bile duct access followed by fluoroscopic guidance for catheter wire manipulation and drain placement. Ultrasound guidance is commonly used for left-sided approaches (Figure 11-3, *E* and *F*); however, it can be used for right-sided approaches as well (Figure 11-4). Very detailed technical aspects are beyond the scope of this chapter and could be reviewed in technical articles in "Techniques of Vascular Interventional Radiology: Biliary Interventions—Part 1," *Tech Vasc Interv Radiol.* 2008;11(1):14-50.[12,19,20]

Local anesthesia should be generously administered because of the likely need for multiple needle passes. The two primary initial imaging guidance modalities for biliary access are (1) fluoroscopic guidance, (2) ultrasound and fluoroscopic guidance.[9-20] For the fluoroscopic method, a site is marked on the right lateral abdomen in the midaxillary line usually at the 10th or 11th intercostal space just above the rib(s) to avoid the intercostal neurovascular bundle[20] (see Figure 11-3, *A*). The goal of the initial access site is to avoid pleural puncture, which could lead to biliary drainage into the right pleural space.[20] After a small skin incision is made, a 22-gauge Chiba needle (which can accept an 0.018-in. guide wire) is advanced into the liver usually toward the 9th or 10th costovertebral junction (see Figure 11-3, *A*).[20] The stylet is then removed and the needle is slowly withdrawn while injecting small amounts of contrast to opacify the biliary tree.

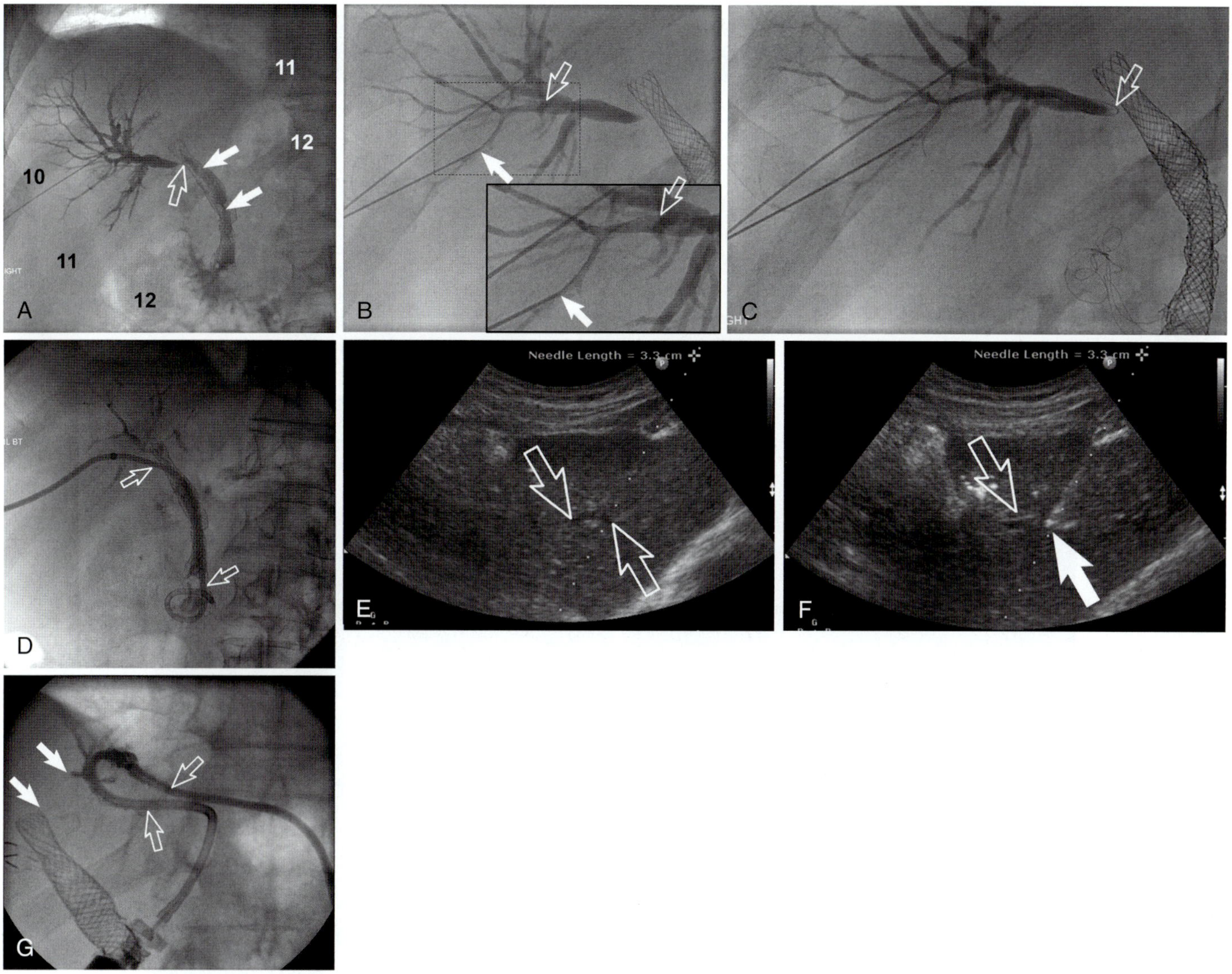

Figure 11-3 Recurrent cholangiocarcinoma with right-sided fluoroscope-guided access and left-sided ultrasound-guided access and left-sided U-tube external drain placement and a right-sided internal–external biliary drain. (A) Fluoroscope-guided percutaneous transhepatic cholangiography (PTC) in a patient with a prior metallic stent and recurrent biliary obstruction. The PTC is performed under fluoroscopic guidance from the right side (right midaxillary) from the 9th intercostal space above the 10th rib (*black 10*) using a 22-gauge needle. The needle is pointed to just above the 11th costovertebral junction/joint (*white 11*). The black numbers are the counted posterior right ribs and the white numbers are the costovertebral joints/junction. There is occlusion of the right posterior biliary duct outside the stent (*hollow white arrow*/overgrowth) and inside the metallic stent (*solid white arrows*/ingrowth). (B) A second 22-gauge needle has been advanced into a more peripheral branch (*solid white arrow*). A 0.018-in. guide wire has been advanced through the needle and has buckled (*hollow white arrow*) within the biliary system. The advantage of the 0.018-in. guide wire is that it can buckle inside the biliary tract and achieve wire purchase. (C) The 0.018-in. guide wire has been advanced further through the needle leading with its buckled portion (*hollow white arrow*), which has reached the area of obstruction. The disadvantage of the 0.018-in. guide wire is that it may shear off at the beveled needle tip as well as provide a flimsy wire support for the upsizing transitional dilator. (D) After access to the small bowel adjacent to the old metallic stent, an 8-French internal–external biliary drain (*hollow arrows*) was placed outside (adjacent) to the metallic stent. A metallic stent was subsequently placed (not shown, see Figure 11-3, *G*). (E) Subsequently (a month later), the patient had cholangitis and a decision was made to drain the left biliary system. Grayscale image demonstrates a dilated left biliary system (between *hollow arrows*). (F) Grayscale image demonstrating ultrasonography guided 21-guage needle access (*solid arrow*) in the dilated left biliary system (*hollow arrow*). (G) Fluoroscopic image demonstrating a left-sided U-tube (U-configured external biliary drain). The operator resorted to this because the left main biliary duct (between *solid arrows*) could not be traversed. The U-tube enters and exits the left-sided biliary system at the hollow arrows.

It is critical to not overinject contrast as this will lead to obscuration of the liver and biliary anatomy. Bile ducts can usually be differentiated from hepatic arteries, portal veins, and hepatic veins because contrast will tend to remain stagnant rather than washing out. Moreover, there are structural and anatomic feature differences between the three vessels.[20] Once the Chiba needle (Cook Corp, Bloomington, IN) is confirmed to be within a biliary duct, a limited cholangiogram is obtained. The cholangiogram should be limited to confirm biliary access and to opacify and confirm the target biliary radicals based on the preprocedural imaging planning (see above). Too much contrast may lead to compression of the biliary tree and bacterial vascular escape, which may translate to worsening cholangitis and biliary sepsis.

TABLE 11-2 Right-Sided Versus Left-Sided Percutaneous Transhepatic Cholangiogram (PTC) and Percutaneous Biliary Drainage (PBD)

	Right-sided PTC / PBD	Right-sided PTC / PBD
Advantages	Usually more peripheral duct access Usually a greater hepatic territory drained Favorable angles for metallic stent placement More convenient for operator and less radiation exposure to operator	More convenient for patient (less painful) More convenient for patient care of drain (better self-care) Less morbidity with ascites Less pleural complications
Disadvantages	More painful to patient Higher pleural complications Poor self-care Higher morbidity in the presence of ascites	Usually less hepatic territory drained Usually more central access Less favorable angles for stent placement More radiation to operator hands

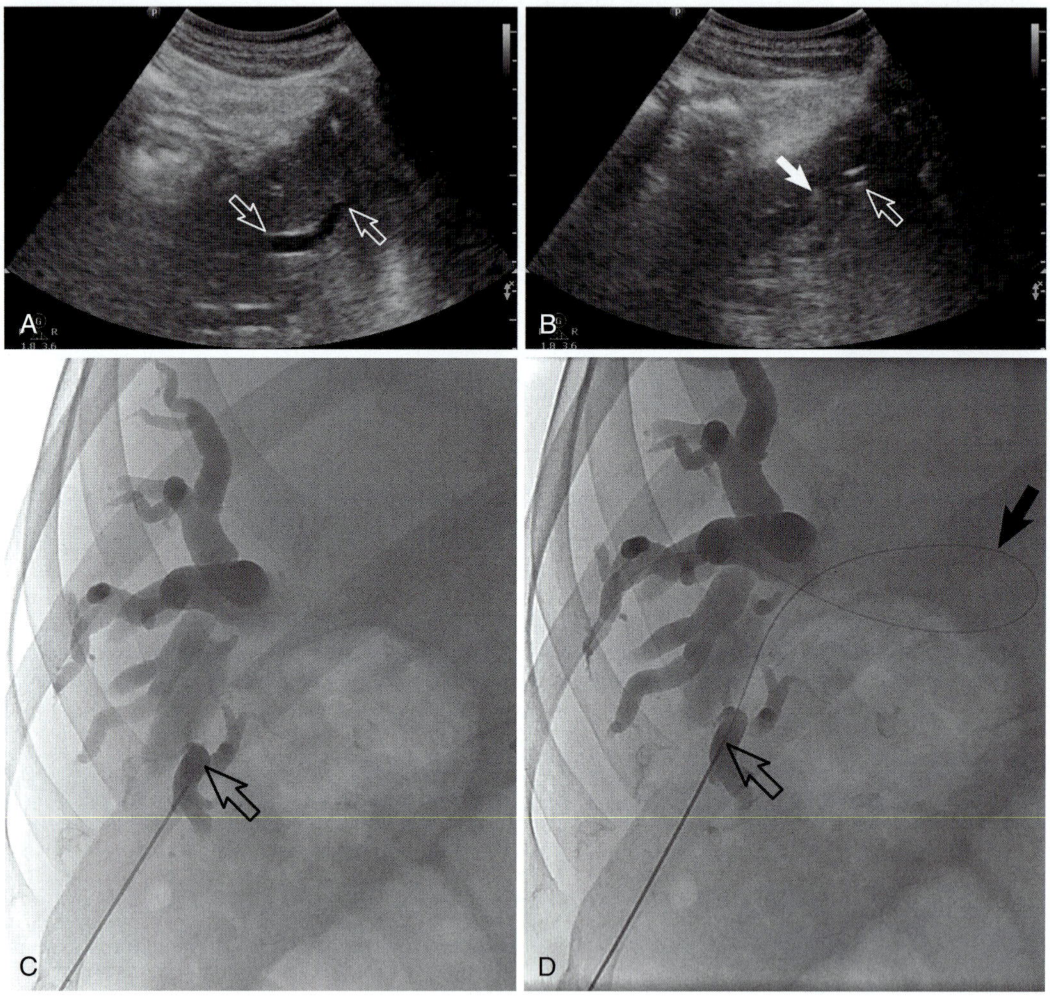

Figure 11-4 Ultrasound-guided right-sided subcostal approach. (A) Grayscale image demonstrates a dilated right biliary system (between *hollow arrows*). The transducer is placed in a subcostal location. (B) Grayscale image demonstrating ultrasound-guided 21-guage needle access (*solid arrow*) in the dilated left biliary system (*hollow arrow*). (C) Fluoroscopic image after ultrasound needle access (*hollow arrow*) and injection of contrast in the right biliary ducts. (D) A 0.018-in. guide wire has been advanced through the needle (*hollow arrow*) and has buckled (*solid arrow*) within the dilated right-sided biliary system.

If the initial needle access is not ideal, a second Chiba needle (intended to be the definitive biliary drainage access) is used to target an appropriate third- or fourth-order (more peripheral) bile duct. The rationale for accessing a peripheral bile duct is to decrease the risk of vascular injury, as the larger vessels are located close to the hilum.[20] Oblique views are helpful in targeting the second needle access sites. Under fluoroscopy, a characteristic pop may be seen as the needle deforms/effaces and ultimately punctures the bile duct.[20] Once the needle is within the duct (which can be confirmed with contrast injection), a 0.018 wire is then advanced into the biliary tree (see Figure 11-3, *B* and *C*). Hydrophilic wires may be useful because of their steerability and ability to buckle within the biliary tree (see Figure 11-3, *B* and *C*).[20] Although there is an increased risk of wire shearing with hydrophilic wires, a retained wire fragment in the liver does not carry the consequences it would in the vascular system.[20] The ideal intended definitive access (1) should be in the target biliary segment planned by preoperative imaging, (2) should enter the target biliary segment from a peripheral biliary branch, and (3) should take into consideration angulation issues for more central drainage and interventions (stent placement).[20]

Once the definitive biliary access is obtained with adequate 0.018-in. guide-wire access, a telescoped transitional dilator (tapered to 0.018 in. and allows a 0.035-in. wire placement) is then placed over the 0.018-in. wire and used to upsize the guide-wire platform to a 0.035-in. guide wire. At this point, depending on the patient's symptoms and degree of hemodynamic stability, the operator may elect to leave an external biliary drainage catheter connected to bag drainage. A particular type of an external drain is a U-tube (see Figure 11-3, *G*). A U-configured tube is the most secure tube from a dislodgment standpoint. If the patient is hemodynamically stable, the operator should attempt to advance the 0.035-in. wire into the small bowel and place an internal/external biliary drainage catheter. If this is unsuccessful, the patient can be brought back within the next 48–72 hours for internalization, after cholangitis/biliary sepsis has resolved. For the internalization procedure, hydrophilic steerable guide-wires are often useful for crossing the occlusion. It is essential when placing the multi-side-hole drainage catheter to confirm that side holes are present above and below the obstruction. Additional side holes may need to be placed. It is also important to make sure that the most proximal side hole (closest to the hepatic capsule access point) is within the biliary tree and not the raw transhepatic biliary tract. If this is overlooked, bile may leak along the tract and into the peritoneum or a portal venous bleed may occur.[20]

Invasive Cholangiography (Direct CT Cholangiography)

A rarely described imaging technique is direct CT cholangiography or transhepatic contrast-enhanced CT cholangiography.[21-23] This is performed by direct injection of diluted contrast (1 part ionic contrast to 5–7 parts saline, 1 part gadolinium to 1–2 parts saline) into the biliary drain and obtaining CT images (either cone-beam CT in the angiography suite or in a CT scanner). Postimaging processing includes three-dimensional reformats and maximum-intensity projections (MIPs) as well as minimal-intensity projections (MinIPs).[21] This technique can be important for identifying poorly dilated isolated biliary segments and it can provide imaging details for identifying the subtle extent of cholangiocarcinoma with "pinching" (subtle stenosis) of biliary radicals (Figure 11-5).[20-23] Obviously, the most common application for this technique is in hilar and centrally located intrahepatic cholangiocarcinoma.[20-23]

Technical and Clinical Outcomes of Percutaneous Drainage

Percutaneous drainage is a highly effective procedure in the palliative setting, with reported technical success rates of 95%–100% and clinical success rates of 70%–80%.[13,18] In one study, 57% of patients had a significant reduction in their serum bilirubin following drainage, with 44% experiencing a reduction to less than 2 mg/dL. The average period for bilirubin to drop to less than 2 mg/dL was 2.8 weeks.[13] Pruritis was reported to improve at 1 and up to 4 weeks.[13] Interestingly, quality of life (QoL) parameters did not improve following percutaneous biliary drainage.[13] Minor complications of drainage occur in up to 31% of patients and are listed, with the most common being pain, catheter leaks, and fever.[13,18] Major complications occur in up to 7.3% of patients and are listed, with the most common being cholangitis. Of note, while transient hemobilia is a relatively common finding following percutaneous drainage, less than 2% of patients will experience significant bleeding that requires transfusion (considered a major complication).[13,18] Procedure-related mortality is reported at 0%–2.6%. However, mortality at 30 and 60 days is reported to be at 2.3%–11% and 28%, respectively.[13,18] In terms of long-term complications, catheter dysfunction is frequent and is seen in up to 47% of patients, with 8%–17% of patients experiencing catheter dislodgement.[13,18] These data underline the importance of patient education and of prompt tube evaluation by a physician whenever problems are suspected.

Tsai et al. demonstrated predictors of high biliary output following percutaneous drainage, including higher serum albumin, absence of liver metastases, and lower Bismuth classification.[14] Tumor size and degree of biliary dilation were not found to be related to biliary output. Interestingly, in the same study, a high biliary output from a drainage catheter (defined as 300 mL/day) was not associated with more rapid reduction of serum bilirubin. In terms of drop in serum bilirubin, the significant factors were serum albumin, bilirubin, and prothrombin time, which were closer to normal values. Bismuth classification, tumor size, and presence of liver metastases were not found to correlate with drop in serum bilirubin.[1,14] Relief of the biliary obstruction, in addition to providing symptom relief, is also correlated with improved survival overall. Patients with serum bilirubin >4 mg/dL after percutaneous biliary stent placement are reported to have poorer outcomes. Advanced age and Bismuth IV lesions also represent poor prognostic factors.[3] Tsai et al. found that in 74 patients with hilar lesions and unresectable cancers, biliary drainage was not associated with a survival benefit.[14] Indar et al. found that prestenting serum bilirubin had a correlation with survival.[24] It is important to note that regardless of therapy, most of the patients who are nonsurgical candidates will die of cholangitis/biliary sepsis and/or liver failure.[24]

INTERNALIZATION OF BILIARY DRAINAGE (STENT PLACEMENT)

Indication for Stent Placement

For most patients, the ultimate goal of the percutaneous drainage procedure is usually to either place a definitive internal/external drainage catheter or to provide an access portal for internal metallic stent placement. The only clinical scenario for metal stent placement is palliation. Metallic stents should not be used as a preoperative drainage tool. The rationale for stent internalization in both cases is to limit the amount of fluid and electrolyte loss from external drainage as well as to improve quality of life (reduce patient morbidity). With an internal/external stent, catheter position becomes more critical and catheter malfunction may become more frequent, putting the patient at risk for recurrent episodes of cholangitis, as well increased number of procedures and tube manipulations.

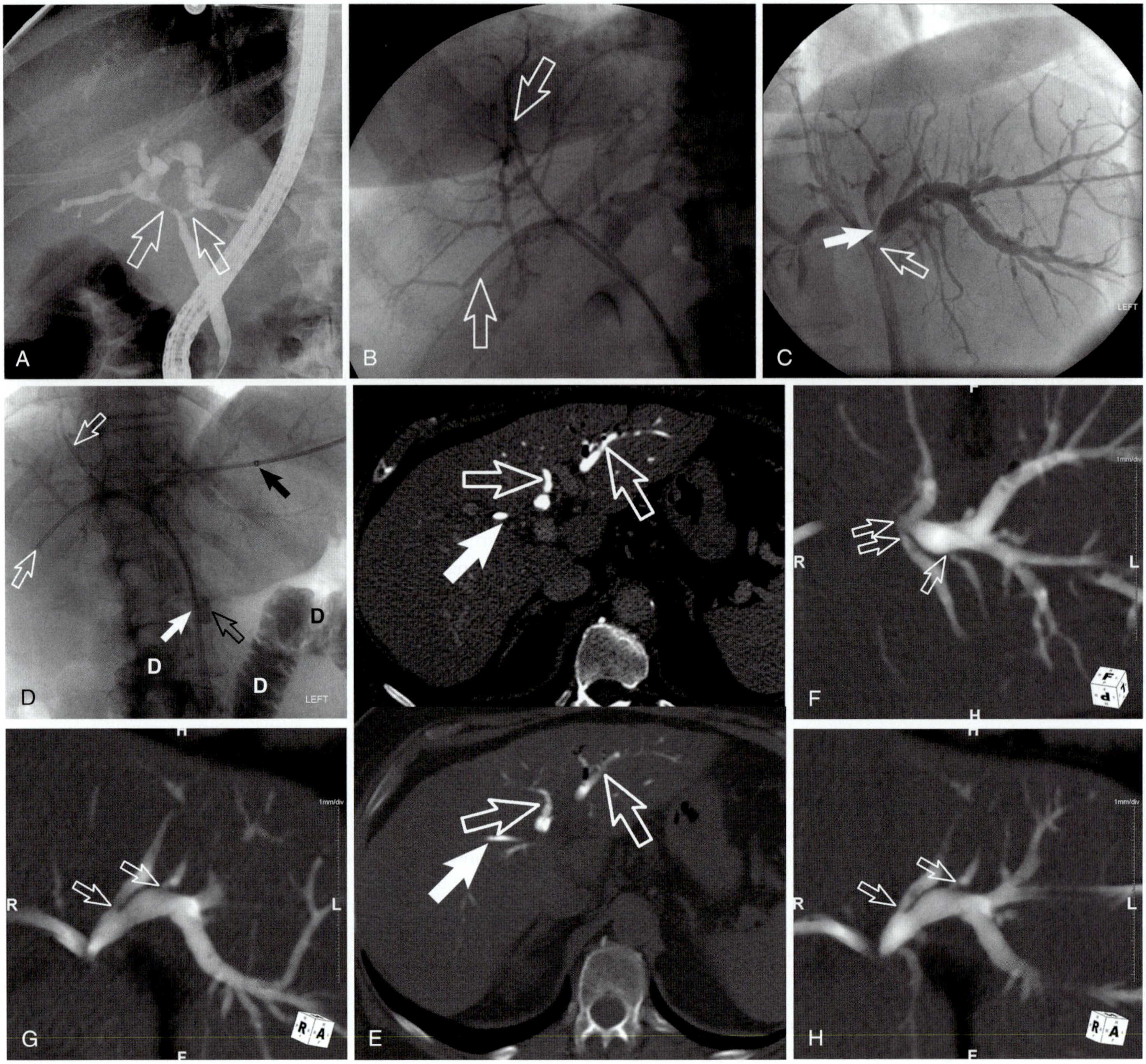

Figure 11-5 Left-sided percutaneous biliary drain and direct CT cholangiography. (A) Endoscopic retrograde cholangiopancreatography (ERCP) fluoroscopic image demonstrating dominant strictures (*hollow arrows*) in the right main and left main biliary ducts at their confluence. (B) Fluoroscopic image after successful ERCP plastic stent placement in the right posterior and right anterior ducts (*hollow arrows*). The ERCP operator failed to place a plastic stent in the left biliary duct. (C) Left-sided percutaneous transhepatic cholangiogram (PTC) demonstrating the dominant stricture in the left main biliary duct (*hollow arrow*). In addition, a secondary stricture is seen in the segment IV duct (*solid arrow*). (D) Fluoroscopic image during the preparation for direct transhepatic computed tomographic (CT) cholangiography. Notice that the biliary ducts are filled with diluted contrast (1 part contrast to 4–5 parts saline). Because there are ERCP plastic stents (*hollow white arrows*) that go down the common bile duct, it is difficult to retain contrast within the biliary system. To retain the diluted contrast within the biliary system and prevent it from emptying into the duodenum (D), a balloon occlusion catheter is advanced through the percutaneous left-sided sheath (*solid black arrow*) and is inflated (*hollow black arrow*) in the common bile duct adjacent to the two plastic ERCP stents (*solid white arrow*) in the common bile duct. At this point, a dedicated spiral CT is obtained. Intravenous contrast can also be administered to delineate the hepatic vasculature (hepatic artery and portal vein branches). This was not performed in this study (see Figures 11-5, *E–H*). (E) Two axial CT images with varying windowing are demonstrated. These are a sample of the source images (raw data) that forms the reformatted images in Figure 11-5, *F–H*). The plastic ERCP stent is seen (*solid white arrows*) and the diluted contrast is seen in the left biliary system *(hollow white arrow)*. (F–H) Three reformatted CT images with varying rotational projections are demonstrated. The images show considerable three-dimensional details demonstrating numerous "pinch-offs"/narrowings (*hollow arrows*) in the second- and third-order branches of the left biliary ducts. With these images, the patient was considered to be nonoperable.

The rationale behind stent placement is that stents improve the patient's quality of life by limiting their need for an external appliance. Additionally, stents are less prone to dislodgement and malfunction when compared with percutaneous drainage catheters. The benefits of stent placement should be weighted against their potential shortcoming compared to drainage catheters. Stents offer no backup route for biliary drainage if they should be obstructed in the future. Therefore, the decision to place a stent should be carefully considered and not all patients will require stent placement. Again, metallic stents should be palliation only. Moreover, most operators do not place metal stents (without transhepatic access) unless the life expectancy of the patient does not exceed 6–9 months. Even when the life expectancy of the patient is within 6–9 months, the patient should be counseled that if biliary obstruction occurs, he or she may have to undergo another PTC and biliary drain placement that may be more difficult than the initial PTC and drain placement.

The two primary stent options are plastic removable stents (typically placed by gastroenterologists using endoscopy but can be placed percutaneously) and self-expanding metallic biliary stents (which can be placed by either gastroenterologists or interventional radiologists).

Plastic vs. Metal Stents

In the opinion of the authors, this is a moot point from a percutaneous transhepatic (interventional radiology) standpoint. Internalization in the setting of malignancy should be metallic stents and for palliation. This is because metal stents have consistently shown improved patency over plastic stents (see next section). The debate may still have importance for endoscopists. This is reflected in that most of the debate concerning stent selection has taken place in the gastroenterology endoscopic literature.

Metallic stents have been shown to be superior to plastic stents in terms of patency, quality-of-life, and complication rates.[3,25] Metallic stents have high technical and clinical success rates, >95% and 88%–97%, respectively. Retrospective studies demonstrate an average primary patency of 5.6–6.9 months, with an average secondary patency of 8.1 months. Patient survival in this cohort, meanwhile, is 3.1–8.7 months.[24-29] The take-home point here is that for many (though not all) patients, the patency of a metallic stent will exceed the patient's life span, and this point must be kept in mind when discussing treatment options with patients and their families in order to choose the appropriate stent.

Raju et al. demonstrated average patency of 5.6 months for metallic stents, in a group of patients who had a median survival of 9.1 months.[25] Plastic stents demonstrated a much shorter primary patency of 1.9 months, leading to an average reintervention rate of 4.6 per patient, compared to metallic stents that had a reintervention rate of 1.5 per patient.[25] Khan et al. proposed that in patients with less than 3–6 months' life expectancy, plastic stents are more cost-effective and associated with lower morbidity.[27] In patients with more than 3–6 months' life expectancy, a metallic stent was recommended because of the higher reintervention rates associated with plastic stents in that period.[27] Metallic stent patency is far better in distal lesions than hilar lesions. Predictors of poor survival in patients who receive metallic stents is a postprocedural bilirubin level that remains above 4 mg/dL (>3.5 times mortality) and/or Bismuth IV lesion (>4.5 times mortality).[3]

Unilobar vs. Bilobar and Hilar vs. Distal Tumors

For hepatic functional palliation, 25%–50% of the hepatic parenchyma needs to be drained. Therefore, many authors advocate unilobar drainage, as bilobar drainage has not been shown to have superior results and carries a higher complication rate.[3,27,30-32] Placement of more than one stent is highly controversial, as each additional stent placed increases the potential for complications. With that said, we believe that in some cases, multiple drainage catheters are necessary. In a Bismuth-Corlette Type I (distal) cholangiocarcinoma, one drainage catheter is often sufficient. In Bismuth-Corlette Type II and III (both of which involve the hilum), two drainage catheters may be necessary to obtain satisfactory drainage.

Conversely, Bulajic et al., studying 49 patients with Bismuth-Corlette Type II (hilar) tumors, demonstrated that bilateral drainage resulted in lower serum bilirubin levels at 7 days compared to unilateral drainage.[4] The incidence of early complications was similar between the two groups; however, late complications were more frequent in the bilateral group. Survival, however, did not differ between the two groups, with only 18% of patients alive at 1 year. It can be therefore inferred that bilateral drainage may provide better symptomatic control in hilar tumors than unilateral drainage even if it does not prolong survival.[4,33] In Bismuth-Corlette Type IV (multifocal or diffuse involvement), more than two may be necessary on occasion.[33] Few authors advocate placing more than three drainage catheters, and the current authors concur with this. However, more than three percutaneous biliary drains have been described in up to 7% of patients[33] with only 54% requiring one percutaneous biliary drain (39% requiring two to three drains).[33]

Y- vs. T-configured Stents

For metallic stent placement (internalization) in patients requiring multiple bilobar drainage to achieve sufficient drainage, two primary metallic stent configurations have been described. These are the Y-configured stents (Figure 11-6, *A*) and T-configured stents. A Y-configured stent placement relies on bilateral percutaneous biliary access or, rarely, a unilateral metal stent placement by endoscopy and a contralateral metal stent placement placed percutaneously. The common ("kissing part," where the two stents run parallel) inferior limb of the Y configuration is typically central in the common hepatic duct or (if commonly extended) common biliary duct. A T-configured stent placement only requires one percutaneous biliary access whereby the crossbar of the T crosses from right to left (if the access is from the right) or from left to right (if the access is from the right). The central stent is then placed in the common hepatic duct or common bile duct. The "kissing part" of the T-configured stent placement (where the two stents run parallel) is intrahepatic and on the side of the percutaneous access. The advantage of the T-configured stent placement is that it only requires one percutaneous access or can be performed in cases of bilateral percutaneous access where only one side can be internalized. Conversely, the Y-configured stent placement requires bilateral percutaneous placement and bilateral internalization of the percutaneous biliary drains. However, the inability to internalize the second biliary drain should be a thing of the past given the described techniques on internalizing the second biliary access utilizing the internalized biliary access.[34,35] This includes the Forced Buckle Technique described by Saad.[34]

Obviously, the anatomic, pathologic, and clinical applications of T- and Y-configured stents apply to Bismuth-Corlette Type II, III, and IV and not Type I (see Figure 11-2). The majority of studies have shown no significant difference between Y and T configurations of multiple stents.[3,27,30-32] In Bismuth-Corlette Type IV lesions, Y configuration has been shown to have higher patency.[36] Moreover, recurrent disease due to stent overgrowth (see below) may be better (easier to manage) in Y-configured stents compared to T-configured stents (an anecdote of the authors).

Covered Metal Stents vs. Bare Metal Stents

Bare-metal stents can narrow and ultimately occlude after placement at an average of 6 to 7 months after placement.[24-29] Occlusion can be due to tissue ingrowth through the interstices of the bare metal stent (cancer ingrowth) (Figure 11-6, *B*), and/or it can be due to occlusion at the ends of the stent (cancer overgrowth), which can cause narrowing and ultimately obstruction of the stent (Figure 11-6, *B*). This is the most common cause of metallic stent failure leading to reintervention. Covered stents have been proposed as an improvement since they, in theory, do not experience ingrowth at the interstices of the stent, and therefore have improved patency compared to bare metal stents.[37,38] However, covered stents have the disadvantage of obstructing biliary duct branches intrahepatically in hilar and intrahepatic lesions and the cystic duct in extrahepatic lesions.[26,27] To reduce this risk, fenestrations in the covered lining (e-PTFE: expanded poly-tetrafluoroethylene) are placed in certain types of stents (Figure 11-6, *C*).[26,27] Despite this, some operators believe that bare metal stents should be employed in hilar or other complex lesions, in order to avoid "jailing" biliary branches. There is also a concern for migration of a covered

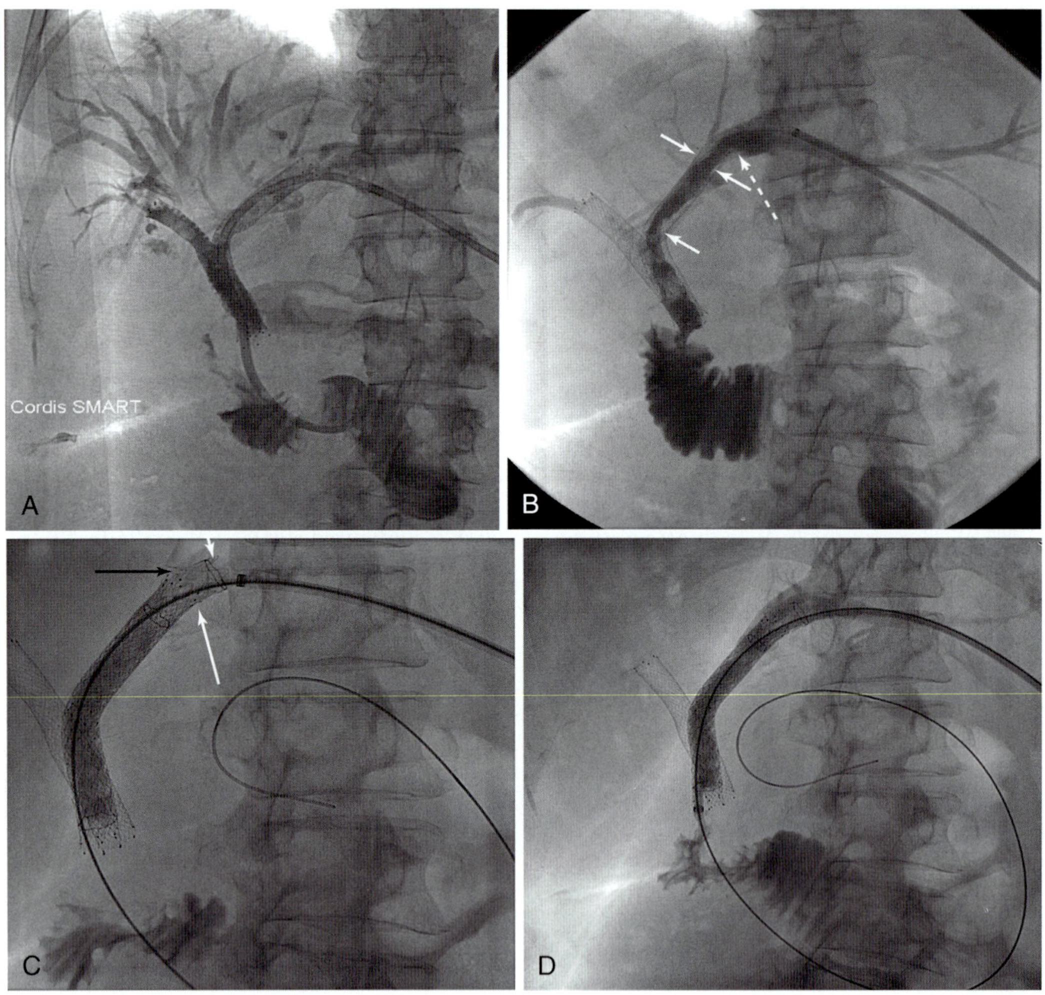

Figure 11-6 Patient with cholangiocarcinoma biliary obstruction recurrence after prior bare stent placement managed with covered stent placement. (A) Cholangiogram through a left-sided percutaneous biliary drain demonstrating biliary occlusion. (B) Detailed magnified cholangiogram through a left-sided percutaneous biliary drain demonstrating occlusion of the previously placed left-sided bare stent. The occlusion is due to cancer ingrowth (*uninterrupted white arrows*) through the interstices of the bare stent as well as overgrowth (*interrupted white arrows*) extending beyond the ends of the bare stent. (C) An e-PTFE (expanded polytetrafluoroethylene) covered stent has been advanced through the old left-sided bare stent and has been deployed. The covered stent is a Viabhil (Gore & Assoc., Flagstaff, AZ) which, in this case, has side holes (*black arrow*). The covered stent has been extended slightly (between *white arrows*) inwards. (D) Completion cholangiogram demonstrating patency of the newly placed left-sided covered stent.

stent, which is not seen with bare metal stents.[26,27] Ultimately, the possible advantages of covered stents should also be weighed against their increased expense, especially in light of the fact that many patients will not outlive a bare metal stent. This may explain why recent randomized trials (bare stents vs. covered stents) have not shown a clear and significant patency advantage of covered stents when compared to bare stents (because the patients do not survive long enough to show the potential patency advantage of covered stents.[37,38] The average occlusion time from stent placement for bare stents versus covered stents is 52–133 days versus 74–180 days, respectively ($P = 0.046–0.800$).[37,38]

ENDOLUMINAL BILIARY TUMOR THERAPY

Endoluminal biliary tumor therapy includes brachytherapy and photodynamic therapy (PDT). A relatively new direction in minimally invasive treatment of cholangiocarcinoma is endoluminal tumor ablation or debulking. Photodynamic therapy (PDT) refers to administration of a photosensitizer that accumulates in tumor tissue. This photosensitizer is nontoxic in the dark but becomes toxic when exposed to low-level light.[39] The treatment is well tolerated and, as opposed to palliative decompression, has been shown to have a survival benefit. The mechanism of tissue damage is the generation of singlet molecule oxygen (O_2) which causes both direct and indirect photodamage resulting in tumor thrombosis and death.[39] PDT is typically performed via an endoscopic approach; however, in cases where endoscopic therapy has failed or is impossible, the treatment can be performed from a percutaneous access. PDT is usually repeated at 3-month intervals and can be performed in the same setting as endoscopic stent or percutaneous drain replacement.[2] Periprocedural antibiotics are recommended.[2] PDT is a two-step procedure, with the first step involving the deployment of the diffuser probe (carrying the photosensitizer) within the area to be treated. The second step involves the photoactivation of the photosensitizer. Predilation of the stricture with a balloon may be necessary to facilitate diffuser probe placement.[2] Multiple photosensitizers are available; however, the most studied, and only U.S. Food and Drug Administration–approved, photosensitizer is porfimer sodium. The diode laser system (InGaAIP Laser Diode; Diomed Inc., Andover, MA), which is used for probe deployment and photoactivation, can be introduced through a 10-French sheath.[2] In 2003, Ortner et al. conducted a randomized trial which demonstrated a survival benefit so significant (98 vs. 493 days, $P < 0.0001$) that the trial was terminated early.[39] Although no multicenter randomized controlled trial exists, several additional single-center studies have supported these initial findings.[2]

LOCOREGIONAL TUMOR THERAPY

There has been increased interest in recent years for the application of locoregional therapies (typically used in treatment of hepatocellular carcinoma or liver metastases) to nonresectable cholangiocarcinoma. These treatment modalities include transarterial chemoembolization (TACE), radioembolization with Y90 microspheres, and percutaneous tumor ablation. A recent meta-analysis revealed that patients who received locoregional therapy for unresectable cholangiocarcinoma had a median survival of 15.6 months, compared to the reported survival following palliative chemotherapy of 5–11 months.[40]

Transarterial Chemoembolization

A single-institution study in 2005 included 17 patients over a 9-year period who underwent transarterial chemoembolization for unresectable cholangiocarcinoma. Exclusion criteria included Child-Pugh class C, large ascites, and liver failure. The majority of patients received a combination of lipiodol, cisplatin, doxorubicin hydrochloride, and mitomycin-C, based on TACE protocols for hepatocellular carcinoma (HCC). Most patients experienced either no side effects or short-term embolization syndrome symptoms (including nausea, vomiting, transient abdominal pain, and diarrhea). One patient died within 30 days of the procedure and the authors suggested that his underlying cirrhosis was a major factor and perhaps should have excluded him from TACE. Median survival in these patients was 23 months.[41] A more recent study involved 62 patients at two institutions treated with transarterial chemotherapy (cisplatin/doxorubicin/mitomycin-C), ethiodol and PVA, with many patients receiving multiple treatments. Median survival was reported to be 20 months, with few major complications.[42]

Yttrium-90

A pilot study in 2008 involved 24 patients with unresectable cholangiocarcinoma who were treated with Y90 radioactive microspheres at a single institution. Median survival in patients without portal vein thrombosis was 31.8 months, while those patients with portal vein thrombosis at the time of treatment had a median survival of 5.7 months. The most frequent side effects were fatigue and transient abdominal pain with no evidence of pulmonary or gastrointestinal toxicity in any of the patients.[43] A study of 40 patients treated with Y90 particles reported a 5% incidence of radiation hepatitis and 5% incidence of obstructive jaundice following therapy.[44] Figure 11-7 demonstrates pre- and post-Y-90 therapy CT images of an intrahepatic cholangiocarcinoma.

Percutaneous Tumor Ablation

The largest series of patients treated with percutaneous tumor ablation was published in 2012 and included 17 patients at a single institution over an 11-year period. A range of tumors from 2.1 to 6.8 cm were treated with a median diameter of 4.4 cm. Exclusion criteria included Child-Pugh class C, tumors >7 cm, diffuse disease, and portal vein thrombosis. Early tumor necrosis was reported to be 96.2%. Median survival in this study was 33 months, which again suggests a significant survival benefit compared to standard of care chemotherapy. Tumor differentiation was found to be the only variable with a significant impact on survival (Figure 11-8).[45]

Conclusion

In summary, cholangiocarcinoma tends to be very advanced at the time of diagnosis and is associated with poor survival. Medical, surgical, and radiation therapies are limited, making endoscopic and percutaneous procedures standard of care for many patients with the disease. In patients in whom endoscopy has failed, percutaneous drainage by an interventional radiologist is an important palliative therapy and occasionally

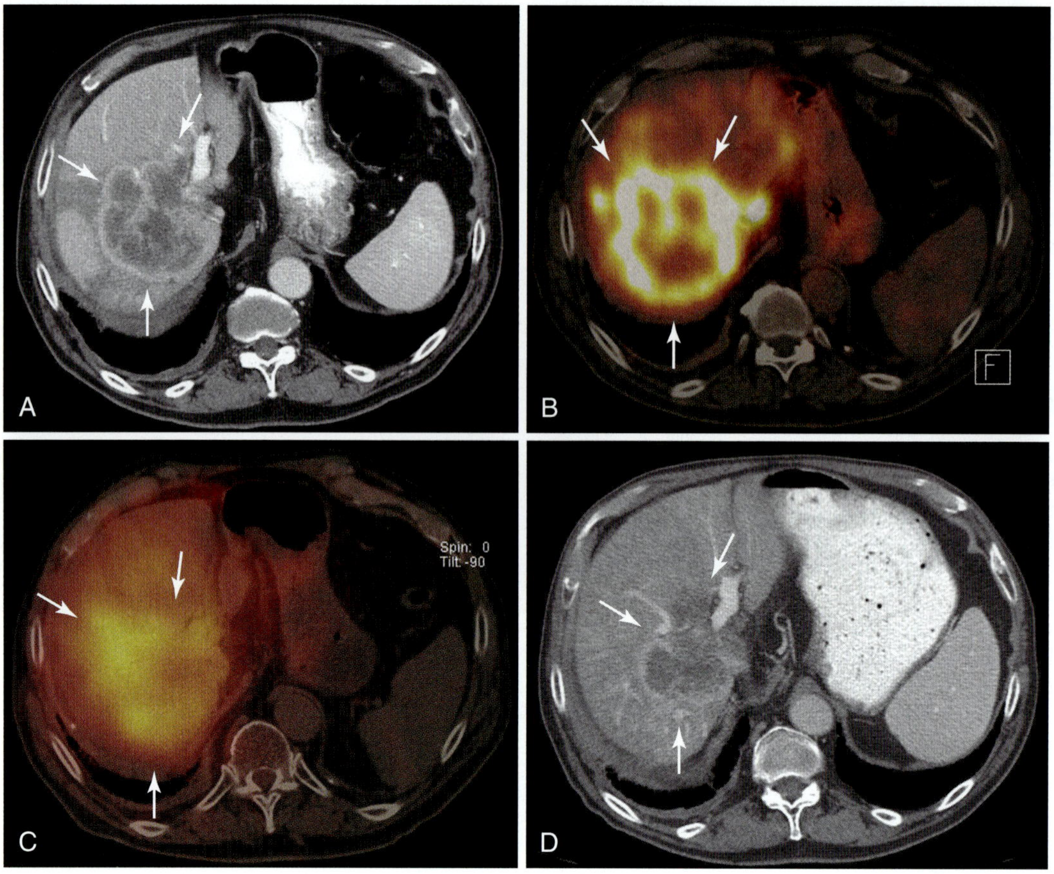

Figure 11-7 Transcatheter yttrium-90 radioiembolization for cholangiocarcinoma. (A) Contrast-enhanced computed tomographic (CT) images demonstrating a large right-hepatic lobe intrahepatic cholangiocarcinoma (between *white arrows*). (B) Fused CT and single-photon emission CT (SPECT) technetium macroaggregated albumin (MAA) scan demonstrating avid radiotracer uptake by the intrahepatic cholangiocarcinoma (between *white arrows*). (C) Fused SPECT scan after Y-90 treatment demonstrating diffuse uptake by the intrahepatic cholangiocarcinoma (between *white arrows*). (D) 6-month follow-up contrast-enhanced CT images demonstrating good tumor response.

a presurgical prelude/preparatory therapy. In the preoperative/resectable group of patients, the indications for percutaneous biliary drainage includes cholangitis and predicted FLR of less than 30%. In the palliative/nonresectable group, the indications for percutaneous biliary drainage includes the presence of cholangitis, pruritis, or the need for reducing the total bilirubin to less than 2 mg/dL in patients who may receive chemotherapy. It is important to note that survival does not improve with palliative decompression.

Multiple treatment options are available after external drainage has been established with a biliary drainage catheter. These include internal/external biliary catheter drainage, plastic stent, metallic self-expanding stent, and photodynamic therapy.

Initial results, in terms of survival benefit, of locoregional therapies have been promising. Side-effect profile for the different locoregional therapies appears similar to what has been reported for HCC and metastatic liver disease.

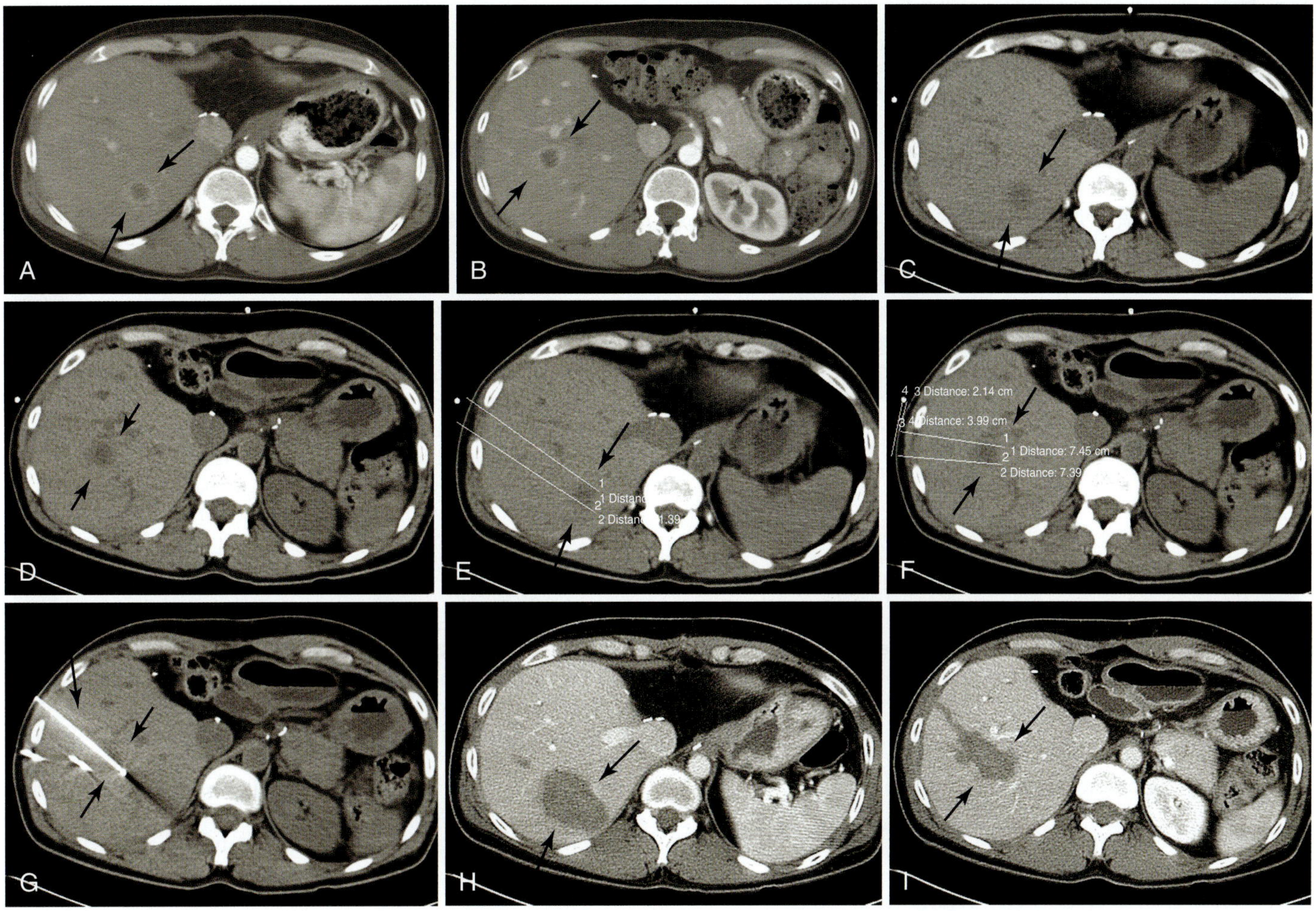

Figure 11-8 Radiofrequency Ablation (RFA). Forty-three-year-old female with known intrahepatic cholangiocarcinoma who underwent left hepatectomy, caudate lobectomy, wedge resection segment 6, lymphadenectomy, and cholecystectomy presents with two sites of recurrence in the hepatic remnant. (A and B) Pre-RFA intravenous (IV) contrast-enhancing CT demonstrates enhancing lesions representing the patient's recurrent disease in the liver remnant. (C and D) Therapy planning non–IV contrast-enhanced CT demonstrates the corresponding lesions to be well identified as low attenuation areas in the right lobe. (E and F) Figure demonstrates the calculation of the intended trajectory of the RFA probes. (G) Unipolar radiofrequency probe in lesions. (H and I) Intraprocedural post-RFA IV contrast-enhanced CT scan demonstrates lack of enhancement in the region of the ablation zones encompassing the location of the previous lesions.

Much of the data limitation is simply owed to the fact that cholangiocarcinoma is relatively rare, particularly in the Western world. Patient selection in particular requires more investigation. Several phase 2 trials are currently ongoing. The treatment choice needs to be tailored to each individual patient based on their symptoms, biliary anatomy, expected survival, and functional status. Care of these patients requires a multidisciplinary approach, including surgeons, oncologists, gastroenterologists, and interventional radiologists.

REFERENCES

The complete reference list is available online at www.expertconsult.com.

12

The Multidisciplinary Management of Liver Metastases in Colorectal Cancer

HARPREET S. WASAN | DUNCAN SPALDING | PAUL TAIT

KEY POINTS

- The treatment of colorectal cancer, metastatic to liver, should be optimally managed within the context of a multidisciplinary team to improve patient-centered outcomes.
- Treatment intent should be categorized as "curative," "potentially curative," "noncurative for active therapy" (the majority) and "noncurative for palliation" of symptoms (best supportive care).
- Increasing options for combined modality approaches require a treatment pathway and strategy, both at the outset (first presentation), and repeatedly if necessary as the clinical course progresses.
- Access to new modalities and evolving treatments will advance the effectiveness of the team

Introduction: Multidisciplinary Team Approach

The diagnosis, staging, and treatment of colorectal cancer (CRC), as well as the management of potential medical and psychological complications, requires a multidisciplinary or team approach. Throughout a patient's cancer journey, the central tenet for the team is providing continuous optimal care from all aspects, of a typically incurable condition. Evidence-based medicine provides changing guidelines for the benefit, almost exclusively, of a single intervention in the context of controlled clinical trials, where patients fit very selective, often rigorous, criteria. However, the *real-life* challenges are significantly more complex and more commonplace as the whole colorectal cancer patient population encompasses a broader and more multifaceted spectrum and invariably need multiple interventions at various levels of evidence. In reality the impact of potential toxicities of sequential treatments and impact on quality of life are rarely disclosed within the published literature. The challenge is therefore for each patient to be analyzed systematically by the colorectal multidisciplinary team, and then to use a contemporaneous evidenced-based approach to justify and facilitate a sequence of clinical interventions. Patients should be made aware and be offered choices, where options are available, as there is often a limited impact of treatments on quantity of life and the potential effects on the quality of life. An independent patient-linked advocate, which is usually an "advanced nurse practitioner" (ANP) or a "clinical nurse specialist' (CNS), helps immensely, in what is a terrifying situation for patients and their families.

The role of complex liver interventions and surgery for colorectal liver metastases is discussed later in this chapter and is one of the specific areas where the prospective planned management of colorectal cancer patients is changing rapidly. It may have a major, potentially curative, impact on some patients and may also contribute to prolonging survival in as many as 20% of patients presenting with, or relapsing with, metastatic disease.

Epidemiology and Staging

Colorectal cancer is the second leading cause of cancer deaths in developed nations. There are approximately 1,000,000 cases per year globally with more than half a million deaths. There is a wide geographical global incidence range, with most Western countries at 20–40 per 100,000 population. Colorectal cancer is the third most common cancer in the United States, with more than 100,000 cases of colorectal cancer diagnosed. Colon cancer affects both sexes with approximately equal frequency; however, tumors in the rectum appear more commonly in men at a ratio of 1.5:1 to women. Colorectal cancer incidence is gradually decreasing in western countries. The probability of developing colorectal cancer rises sharply with age, with 83% of all cases arising in people who are 60 years or older and median age at diagnosis over 70 years. The lifetime risk for men of colorectal cancer is estimated to be 1 in 18, and 1 in 20 for women.[1]

The overall survival (mortality) is stage-specific, with the 5-year overall mortality decreasing incrementally over the last 30 years. This is due to the synergy between individual advances in diagnostics, surgery, and oncology. The overall 5-year survival of all CRC cases in Western countries ranges from 52% to 65%. A total of 80%–85% of patients with colon cancer have some symptoms at the time of diagnosis. At disease presentation, around 55% of people have advanced cancer that has either spread to lymph nodes or other organs, or is so locally advanced that surgery is unlikely to be curative (stage III or IV or Dukes' C or D). More advanced stages of local and distant spread correlate inversely with survival; however, positive anomalies have now appeared, because of improvements in advanced colorectal cancer management. The first example is with the advent of adjuvant chemotherapy, in that the prognostic outcomes of substages of II and III now overlap: Stage IIa and stage IIIa have similar survival rates, with stage IIb (T4N0) actually having significantly worse outcomes compared to stage IIIa.

The second example is more recent, and is almost certainly attributable to successful liver surgery for limited CRC metastases. The prognostic outcomes of substages of III and IV now also overlap in that the worse subsets of stage III and best of stage IV (limited surgically operable metastases) have similar survival rates. The staging systems are thus only tools in assessment but increasingly are understood to be one of many factors that influence outcomes. Increasingly, patient-related clinical factors and biolog parameters, including chemosensitivity and genetic profiles, often outweigh the impact of staging both adversely and favorably, in ways that we as yet cannot predicate.

Tissue diagnosis is mandatory in all cases, unless the patient is not fit for any treatment interventions. Modern centers now add immediate genetic testing for somatic mutations, as these have major implications for systemic treatment options, both from a predictive and prognostic point of view. At a minimum, KRAS and BRAF testing should be done at the outset, in all metastatic cases. Many centers have moved to multigene testing systems, as small subsets of cancers have "druggable" mutations with targeted therapies that are already available.

A strong family history or multiple recurrent polyps should invoke potential discussions about family, genetic, and mutation testing with qualified geneticists and counselors. A detailed discussion on this subject is beyond the scope of this chapter.

Staging is mandatory prior to discussion on treatment planning. A minimum of a modern high-quality computed tomography (CT) scan of chest/abdomen and pelvis should be performed in a patient with confirmed cancer. The focus of the radiology should be to look specifically at common sites and patterns of spread of colon cancer: (in descending order) liver, peritoneum, lung and distant lymph nodes. Note that in contrast to the other common adenocarcinomas (i.e., breast, lung, and prostate), bone, spinal cord and brain, and CRC metastases are uncommon and occur in less than 5% of metastatic patients at presentation.

Additional radiologic tests are extremely useful in rectal cancer for planning management. An MRI of the pelvis in rectal tumors is used to assess whether primary surgical curative removal is potentially feasible and whether any neoadjuvant chemoradiotherapy is warranted to try and improve local control and overall outcomes. Modern evidence suggests that MRI is better than CT for local staging of primary rectal cancer, particularly in assessing unresectable disease (or "threatened margins") and identification of cancer-positive lymph nodes. There is, however, wide variability between results reported in different studies and, which highlights the need for dedicated and trained site-specific radiologists to minimize the false-negative and false-positive rates of determining involved lymph nodes. In a phase II prospective series (MERCURY) of 712 patients, the correlation between MRI and pathologic staging after surgery alone was 0.92, with an observed agreement of 84% (kappa 0.49, 95% CI: 0.35–0.61) between the MERCURY assessment of prognosis and pathology findings after primary surgery.

In situations where liver or lung surgery (metastatectomy) is contemplated, dual, triple, or even quadruple imaging modalities are often necessary. Liver MRI, liver ultrasonography (preferably with contrast enhancement with microbubbles) and ^{18}F-fluorodeoxyglucose positron emission tomography (^{18}F-FDG-PET) scanning are often complimentary to a CT. ^{18}F-FDG-PET is particularly useful in detecting occult extrahepatic disease. Because of the difficulty in localizing structures with an ^{18}F-FDG-PET, this investigation is always performed in conjunction with a separate CT contrast-enhanced scan, despite dual-modality combination advances (CT-PET, which do not have the same specificity or sensitivity for liver imaging).

Although blood tests are frequently nonspecific, they can impart useful information for treatment planning and prognostication. For example, a low serum albumin, high alkaline phosphatase, and high lactate dehydrogenase (LDH) level and possibly high neutrophil and platelet counts are poor prognostic factors. In advanced disease, the liver and renal function can significantly alter the choice or doses of chemotherapeutic agents or interventional therapy that can be offered safely.

Specific tumor markers for colorectal cancer have become commonplace through their clinical utility. About two-thirds of CRC are associated with an elevated serum CEA (carcinoembryonic antigen). This and the serum CA19.9 antigen can be very useful tools in monitoring treatment response in conjunction with other modalities such as radiology. In isolation, they have low specificity and so always need validation with imaging to confirm their trend. A crucial learning point is that tumor markers are not validated to confirm changes in treatment pathway decisions and are not allowable in regulatory clinical trials as valid end points of response or progression.

Systemic Chemotherapy

In deciding treatment options, the primary question is whether the patient has a technically or potentially curable malignancy. The secondary and equally important point is whether it is clinically appropriate for the patient to be subject to this potentially curative approach.

The only clear level 1, curative modality is resection. All other modalities of treatment can add or accentuate the benefit of resection, but are rarely curative in their own right. Resection of the primary colonic or rectal tumor is the principal first-line treatment in the majority of colorectal cancer patients. However, in the context of advanced metastatic disease, it is noncurative and predominantly performed for palliation of symptoms alone. In more recent practice, and with the improvement of systemic chemotherapy tumor response rates, the frequency of the first intervention being primary colorectal surgery is decreasing and is as low as 60% now in contemporaneous clinical studies. When curative resection is not possible, patients may benefit from palliative resection, which is becoming increasingly minimally invasive, and more alternatives such as endoluminal stenting to relieve partial or subacute obstruction are now available as means to expedite the systemic treatment.

Indeed, a risk of attempting primary surgery first is significant delay in starting treatment in metastatic disease, which is the usual cause of constitutional deterioration in advanced patients and ultimately responsible for deaths.

High-quality surgery is thus crucial to patients' survival, and the surgical outcomes are the platform of overall success of the MDT. Hence, specialist colorectal cancer surgeons should be able to demonstrate low tumor involvement at the margins of the excised cancer specimens, low rates of surgical complications, and high survival rates among their patients. If surgery is not the planned primary modality, a rediscussion at various time points, should ensue, as to whether there is an appropriate treatment window, and where it can be integrated without significant disturbance to the systemic objectives. There is mounting retrospective evidence that, even in systemic disease, a strategy to remove the primary tumor adds to the improved survival of that patient. Another major advantage of early removal of the primary tumor is the accurate locoregional tumor staging, especially the identification of involved lymph nodes and presence of lymphovascular invasion or T4 local disease. These features are crucial for patient prognosis and thus management for two reasons. First, residual involved lymph nodes after surgery can precipitate local recurrence (especially in rectal cancer). Second, decision making on the need for adjuvant chemotherapy depends on the pathologic stage of the cancer. Chemotherapy offers proven survival benefit (level 1 evidence) for those with stage III tumors. There is some evidence for benefits also in high-risk stage II tumors with features of lymphovascular invasion, emergency presentations with obstruction or perforation, poorly differentiated and T4N0 tumors. Three variables contribute to the yield of lymph nodes: the aggressiveness of surgery, the diligence of the pathologist in searching the specimen, and the anatomy of the patient and the tumor. Evidence shows that when more nodes are pathologically examined (at least 12), tumors are significantly more likely to be classified as node-positive.[2] The implication for patients with limited colorectal liver metastases is that this may influence the timing and sequence of when to integrate systemic chemotherapy. A heavily node-positive pathology (in relation to the primary site) implies that the attempted adjuvant eradication of extrahepatic micrometastatic disease weighs just as heavily in the decision-making process as eradication of the liver metastases, and both concepts need to be integrated in the MDT planning process.

Over the last 35 years, 5-fluorouracil (5-FU)–based adjuvant therapy has become the mainstay of treatment for patients with Dukes C or stage III colon cancer. The standard treatment has been a course of 5-fluorouracil and folinic acid (FUFA), given intravenously (IV) over 6 months. Pooled data from seven randomized controlled trials in patients with stage II or III colon cancer suggest that 5-FU/FA regimens increase disease-free survival at 5 years from 55% to 67% and overall survival from 64% to 71% when compared to surgical resection alone. The potential benefits and risks of chemotherapy should be discussed with patients for whom it is judged appropriate, so that they can make an informed choice. Adjuvant chemotherapy should be scheduled to begin within 6–8 weeks postsurgery. The MOSAIC study was the first trial to show a statistically significant disease-free survival benefit for a treatment regimen other than 5-FU for stage III colon cancer in the adjuvant setting. At 4 years, there was a 25% reduction in the risk of disease recurrence in these patients for the combination oxaliplatin/5-FU/FA compared with 5-FU/FA alone ($P = 0.002$).[3] The place of chemotherapy in the treatment of patients with Dukes stage B cancer must be a matter for discussion between patients and their oncologists, as the benefits in some groups are small. The QUASAR1 trial and MOSAIC both showed statistically significant risk reductions in those treated compared to the control arms of no-treatment (best supportive care) and the addition of oxaliplatin to 5-FU, respectively. The survival benefit for patients with rectal cancer is believed to be similar, although the evidence is much weaker, and often confounded by the need to give chemoradiotherapy.

Distinctive Considerations for Metastatic Rectal Cancer

The decision-making process for primary rectal cancer with metastases, especially if the primary is locally advanced, as is usually the case, is more complex as the overall disease-free survival outcomes are worse, the surgery potentially more complex, "disfiguring" (e.g., requiring a stoma), and functional bladder, sexual, and bowel outcomes have a high impact on the quality of the (frequently limited) remaining life of the patient. On the other hand, local rectal recurrences can lead to serious morbidity (severe pain, fistulae, and obstruction leading to death). Total mesorectal excision (TME) is a technique that involves meticulous mobilization, followed by either colo-anal anastomosis or completion as an abdominoperineal anorectal excision, is the standard of surgery for cancers of the middle and distal thirds of the rectum. TME is associated with about half the rate of local recurrence, compared with previous techniques in the lower two-thirds of the rectum. In rectal cancer, because of the high risk, and associated morbidity, of local recurrence, radiotherapy can play an important part in the overall management of the patient to specifically reduce this risk.

Pelvic radiotherapy in primary rectal cancer is now considered as a standard primary modality treatment option. This can be as adjuvant or (increasingly) neoadjuvant, prior to surgery. In the advanced metastatic patient, its role has to be carefully planned as it is often integrated with systemic chemotherapy approaches, to aim to control both distant metastases and locoregional disease simultaneously.

In the Swedish randomized preoperative radiotherapy controlled trial, patients in the treatment arm assessed their bowel movement as "excellent," compared with 32% of 87 patients who had had surgery alone. Seven percent of the irradiated group, but none of the controls, rated their bowel function as "bad." Nearly 50% of those in the irradiated group had to use fecal incontinence pads, compared with 22% in the control group. Other problems, such as urgency of defecation and loss of skin on the perineum, were also significantly more troublesome in irradiated patients.

Advances in Chemotherapy for Metastatic Colorectal Cancer

After over 40 years of frustratingly slow progress, with only 5-FU (usually given with leucovorin/folinic acid; LV), as the mainstay of treatment for metastatic colorectal cancer (mCRC), the last 10 years have been remarkable because of the realization of four new active agents of different biologic mechanisms of action, which have incrementally improved response rates and overall survival over and above 5-FU and best supportive care (BSC) alone. In 2012 alone, two further active agents were identified as part of the potential chemotherapy armament in the routine "standard of care," with level-one evidence. Thus, the median overall survival in incurable mCRC has improved from 9 to 12 months with 5-FU/LV monotherapy in the 1980s to near 22–24 months currently. The number of patients living 5 years (with or without disease) in stage IV has also gradually increased to around 10%.

The chemotherapeutic agents, irinotecan and oxaliplatin, now form part of the "doublet" chemotherapy approach (with 5-FU/LV) in the majority of patients worldwide. Two targeted biologic agents that are more cancer specific, with less conventional toxicity profiles, are also used additionally (although limited in some countries because of their high cost). These are an anti–vascular endothelial growth factor (anti-VEGF) monoclonal antibody (mAb), bevacizumab, and the human epidermal growth factor receptor (HER-1 or EGFR) targeted mAb, cetuximab. In addition, patient convenience is also improving as the fluoropyrimidines that previously could only be given intravenously (5-FU/LV) can now also be delivered orally.

However, as the number of agents and survival increase, choosing the most effective treatment strategy is becoming increasingly complex, uncertain, and progressively expensive. As more lines of therapy are being offered in palliative situations, and as monotherapy has moved to combinations and, more recently, to sequential combination therapy, cumulative toxicity profiles will influence choice, progressively more in palliative situations. Conversely, aggressive sequential approaches, also involving surgical or ablative metastasectomies in liver and lung, or locoregional approaches are desirable where cure may be attainable in individual presentations of mCRC.

The key chronologic developments in chemotherapy for mCRC based on randomized clinical trials contributing to the current general paradigms of treatment are summarized here:

1. FU administered as a continuous intravenous (IV) infusion led to a significantly higher response rate and a better toxicity profile than bolus IV FU (Mayo protocol) (22% vs. 14%, respectively; OR = 0.55; $P = 0.0002$), although the median survival times were similar (infusional FU 12.1 months vs. bolus FU 11.3 months; HR = 0.88; $P = 0.04$). These conclusions are from a pooled analysis incorporating data from six randomized trials.[4]
2. FU activity is enhanced with the biochemical modulator folinic acid (leucovorin [LV]) confirmed by a meta-analysis of 3300 patients randomized in 19 trials (response rates 21% vs. 11%, respectively; $P < 0.0001$).[5]
3. Irinotecan, a topoisomerase I inhibitor, *alone* and in combination with FU/LV has survival benefit. Infusional FU combinations are significantly safer with higher efficacy, with diarrhea being the main adverse effect.[6]
4. Oxaliplatin is a cisplatin derivative, with significant activity *only* in combination with FU/LV. Phase III studies consistently show higher response rates, longer median progression-free survival (PFS), time to progression, and survival than those observed with FU/LV alone, but survival differences are not consistently statistically significant. There is a dose-dependent, mostly reversible, sensory neuropathy as a cumulative dose-limiting toxicity (increasing from about 800 mg/m^2).[7]
5. Comparing first-line combination superiority between oxaliplatin and irinotecan is highly complex, and overall all the trials essentially show equivalence for survival. They reconfirm that bolus FU combinations have more toxicity, and that combining oxaliplatin and irinotecan together is not worthwhile without infusional FU. The largest trial (UK FOCUS study) gives confidence to clinicians who are familiar in detail with all the published evidence, that there are numerous choices in the chemotherapeutic options for all patients. Thus careful selection of individual treatment pathways for patients, based on the combined aims, comorbidty, and toxicity profile of the regimens, is achievable without compromising potential patient benefits.[8] Trials sequencing the drugs in different ways again conclude that overall survival is no different, as long as patients have access to all three compounds at some stage. This was shown in a meta-analysis of seven phase III trials.[9]
6. The oral fluoropyrimidines capecitabine, UFT-tegafur, and S1 are established as being equivalent to IV 5-FU. The data for oral combinations with irinotecan and oxaliplatin is standard, although the toxicity profiles are different.
7. Tumors cannot grow beyond 1–2 mm without the formation of a blood supply or angiogenesis. This also allows a pathway for tumor cells to seed into the systemic circulation and establish further metastases. The transition, or switch, of a tumor to an angiogenic phenotype is caused by an increase in proangiogenic factors, including VEGF, basic fibroblast growth factor (bFGF), and transforming growth factor beta (TGF-β). VEGF is highly upregulated in most human tumors, including colorectal cancer. This has been correlated with increased tumor invasion, microvessel density, disease recurrence, and a poor prognosis.[10] Bevacizumab in combination with chemotherapy in the first- and second-line settings in patients with mCRC has significant activity. More than 900 patients were randomized to one of three treatments with *bolus* 5-FU: IFL/placebo, IFL/bevacizumab, or FU/LV/bevacizumab. The addition of bevacizumab to IFL resulted in a significantly increased response rate, duration of response, PFS, and improved overall survival by almost 5 months (20.3 months vs. 15.6 months; $P < 0.001$). For the subgroup of patients who received second-line therapy with oxaliplatin-containing regimens, overall survival times were 25.1 months and 22.2 months for the IFL/bevacizumab and IFL/placebo arms, respectively.[11] There is now second-line survival benefit data with oxaliplatin-5-FU-bevacizumab combinations. Chemotherapy with bevacizumab is generally well tolerated, with no overlapping toxicities. Adverse events include bleeding, thrombosis, proteinuria, and hypertension, which are generally manageable. However, a low percentage of patients (~2%) have serious gastrointestinal events, including bowel perforation. There also has to be caution with regard to healing following VEGF inhibitors (and chemotherapy), especially in complex multidisciplinary pathways requiring liver, vascular, or surgical intervention.
8. The HER-1/EGFR signaling pathway is thought to play a pivotal role in tumor growth and progression of colorectal and other cancers where overexpression is correlated with disease progression, poor prognosis, and reduced sensitivity to chemotherapy. EGFR belongs to the HER family of receptors. These receptors are transmembrane glycoproteins, with an extracellular ligand-binding domain, and an intracellular tyrosine-kinase (TK) domain. Ligands that bind to the HER-1/EGFR extracellular domain induce receptor homo- or heterodimerization with other HER-1/EGFR receptor or family members. This results in activation of the receptor's TK activity, initiating a downstream-signaling cascade that ultimately leads to tumor cell proliferation, migration, inhibition of apoptosis, and angiogenesis. Demonstrable activity with cetuximab plus irinotecan in patients with irinotecan-refractory CRC showed response rates of around 23%, leading to its licensing. Unfortunately, responses did not correlate with the degree of EGFR expression as predicted by preclinical studies. First-line randomized trials with cetuximab combinations with irinotecan (FOLFIRI regimen in the CRYSTAL study) have now established this as a standard of care, and more importantly the clinical–translational work arising has led to the first definitive biomarker of nonresponse to EGFR inhibitors in mCRC. Thus, mutation detection within the important oncogene KRAS leads to resistance to the effects of cetuximab and panitumumab. In liver metastases, the KRAS wild-type

(no mutation detectable) subgroup have the highest recorded objective (RECIST) response rates in randomized phase III studies, making triplet combinations with EGFR inhibitors a very attractive, if not the de facto, option in neoadjuvant therapy for potentially operable metastatic disease (i.e., down-sizing of inoperable liver metastases to operable; see also below). Cetuximab's most common grade 3 or 4 adverse events are hypersensitivity, asthenia, fatigue, malaise, or lethargy. More curiously, an acne-like rash typically associated with HER-1/EGFR inhibition is also observed. Panitumumab is an equivalent humanized version of cetuximab with different scheduling.

9. Two new agents with broader antiangiogenesis activity have recently (2012) gained registration, after positive results from large-scale (phase 3) randomized studies. Regorafenib, an oral multikinase inhibitor has shown a significant survival advantage, after failure of all known chemotherapy drugs (i.e., in the salvage setting), compared to BSC in the CORRECT trial. Similarly, and more impressively, the phase 3 "VELOUR" study of Aflibercept and FOLFIRI, in second line (after failure of an oxaliplatin regimen), also showed a significant survival advantage, even in patients showing resistance to prior bevacizumab exposure. Aflibercept is formed from the fusion protein of key domains from human VEGF receptors 1 and 2 with human IgG Fc1 and blocks all human VEGF-A isoforms, VEGF-B, and placental growth factor (PlGF-2), indeed at such high affinity that it binds VEGF-A and PlGF more tightly as compared to the native receptors. Mechanistically aflibercept is a VEGF-trap, as opposed to a pure VEGF ligand inhibitor such as bevacizumab.
10. Although, "quadruplet' regimens are being tested, it is unlikely that the increasing and often severe toxicity of these combinations will allow significant dose delivery or intensity, and so benefit will be limited. The randomized trials with these regimens are yet to report, so cannot be recommended at this stage in routine care. Thus, the majority of patients will receive a doublet or triplet as the first-line standard of care.

An understanding of the principles of systemic chemotherapy and rapidly evolving standards of care generated from Level 1 evidence (adequately powered randomized phase III multicenter trials) is very important in the context of a starting framework in the MDT discussion of mCRC, especially if multiple interventions are planned to be integrated, as certain sequences of treatment may be better tolerated as well as being more efficacious.

Potentially Curative Liver Surgery in Stage IV Disease

Despite major and rapid advances in the palliative systemic treatment of colorectal metastatic disease and median survivals for stage IV disease now averaging 2 to 2.3 years (from 6 to 9 months only 20 years ago), there is still disappointment that even with the newer biologic targeted agents, the complete pathologic response rates and so cure rates from chemotherapy alone remain exceedingly low. Disease (chemotherapy) resistance to the available systemic agents invariably occurs within 6–9 months of exposure. The 5-year overall survival of all patients with stage IV disease remains at 7%.[12,13] The challenge is thus to develop multidisciplinary treatment pathways, for appropriate patients, that increase the probability of 5-year survival and ultimately "cure" rates.

In colorectal cancer, there is a relatively predictable pattern of systemic metastases development (for unclear reasons) in a subset of patients. This is unlike the patterns seen in the other common cancers where metastases represent widespread and disseminated incurable disease. Thus (after locoregional primary colorectal nodal involvement), CRC metastatic disease usually develops first in the liver. Twenty percent to 25% of patients have clinically detectable liver metastases at the time of the initial diagnosis and a further 40%–50% of patients develop liver metastases within 3 years of primary surgery. When the metastatic deposits *appear* confined only to the liver with modern imaging techniques (as they do in about one-third of all mCRC liver metastases patients), in about 30%–40% of *these* patients, the metastases can be completely resected by expert liver surgeons. Within this group, 20%–25% of patients are eventually cured (survive to 10 years without recurrent disease) and an *additional* 10% remain as longer-term survivors at 5 years (i.e., up to 35%), despite disease recurrence. This leads to the enthralling prospect for our patients that a combination of different MDT specialist approaches can be utilized for major overall and disease-free survival gains for individual patients.[14,15]

This process has been made significantly easier by the low morbidity and mortality (less than 1% currently) of liver surgery in mCRC that have been demonstrated from major liver centers around the world. Furthermore, the surgical techniques and approaches, including locally ablative therapies and support from complex interventional hepatic radiology, have made the technicality of almost all liver surgery feasible. Resections extending to almost 85% of liver volumes, staged resections over 2–3 procedures over a few months, and even vascular reconstruction techniques are rapidly pushing the limits of what is possible to new ever-expanding frontiers.

Thus, expert liver surgery offers the *possibility* of long-term cancer-free survival. About 8%–15% of all mCRC patients are potential candidates for liver resection, of which one-third are long-term survivors. Over the last 10 years, this proportion has risen rapidly as chemotherapeutic advances (as outlined above) have converted a further subset of mCRC patients into resectable or operable categories, having initially presented as unresectable disease. This subset is frequently referred to as "potentially operable." With increasing response rates to systemic therapies now approaching 60%–70% for modern chemotherapeutic regimens, if well managed and screened regularly by the specialist or extended MDT, with a liver focus, can select out such patients by this neoadjuvant or preoperative approach. Indeed, the challenge now, paradoxically, is to select the appropriate patients who are deemed to potentially benefit from liver surgery rather than choosing patients who are technically possible to resect. Thus, the target of the MDT discussion of liver surgical selection is clinical benefit rather than technically feasible or safe.

Chemotherapy can induce steatosis, fibrosis, and functional liver derangements that need to be considered in the overall management planning in such scenarios. Chemotherapy, even at a minimum of 3 months' exposure with oxaliplatin regimens such as FOLFOX, does increase liver morbidity post hepatic resection. We now have randomized clinical trial data to clearly define this (as well as definitive outcomes in operable liver metastases,[16] as discussed below.

There is now increasing data to support that limited (less than 3) extrahepatic metastases in the lung and possibly, and more rarely, isolated in the peritoneum may also still lead to cure in about one-third of patients. Thus, the surgical or ablative control of liver metastases *may* still be desirable, even if there is limited extrahepatic disease, as this may exploit further the synergies of local and systemic therapies.

Inoperable Liver Metastases: Debulking Strategies and the Concept of "Organ"-Directed Approaches

The approach of treating metastases with systemic therapies is palliative in intent in the majority, whereas surgical resection of limited metastases can be curative. Unfortunately, less than 5% of all metastatic patients eventually fall into the latter category (even if this is not apparent at the outset), as the majority of these relapse eventually. The disappointment has been that even with the newer biologic agents, the complete response rates and so cure rates from chemotherapy alone remain exceedingly rare. The 5-year overall survival of all patients with stage IV disease remains at 7%.[8] The challenge is thus to develop treatment pathways that increase the probability of 5-year control or preferably disease-free survival.

The liver is a vital organ and as already discussed, is the most frequent site of colorectal metastases; it leads to organ-specific morbidity, which often translates to dominant global symptoms in terminal care, impacting both quality and quantity of life. Progress in therapies having overall impact on the patient can thus be organ directed. Rapid advances in medical technologies are enabling this and allowing evidence from trials to support this concept. More extraordinarily, focusing on one organ can often achieve better response outcomes that can translate to a bridge to curative outcomes—the ultimate goal of cancer research. Improved outcomes with such a multimodality approach have already been demonstrated in rectal cancer with radiotherapy and better surgical and imaging technologies. In principle, other metastatic sites such as liver, lung, and peritoneum are developing similar paradigms.

Response rates to systemic chemotherapy over the last 20 years have been gradually improving, as new active agents developed, but the proportional gains in terms of overall survival benefits (of the order of months) and percentage of complete responders have been disappointing. However, liver-specific response rates have major relevance, if advantage can be taken with other interventional modalities at the time of maximum chemotherapy response. This has been retrospectively and comparatively demonstrated in many phase III trials. Traditionally the other modality has been liver surgery, but other nonoperative modalities are increasingly being used, expanding the possible patient cohorts and selection criteria. Biologically this has rationale, as residual disease postchemotherapy will contain resistant populations that other modalities eradicate (i.e., potentially eliminate the putative cancer stem or key propagating cells).

There is good evidence from clinical trials that:

1. A synergistic approach with systemic chemotherapy and liver surgery in *operable* liver metastases (1–4 deposits) can improve disease-free survival outcomes.
2. In a subset of patients, chemotherapy can downstage *inoperable* liver metastases, enabling potentially curative surgery with similar outcomes to *operable* liver metastases.
3. Liver-directed chemotherapy infused via the portal vein (PVI) or hepatic artery (HAI) improves overall survival. A meta-analysis of six HAI trials has shown benefit in terms of improved response rates as compared to the equivalent systemic chemotherapy and improved statistically significant overall survival advantage (14.5 vs. 10.1 months, $P = 0.0009$). However, many centers have methodologic and practical problems with HA or PV infusion, making it less popular as other parallel developments occurred in both systemic therapy and liver resection techniques. The evidence base, however, does still support the principle of potential benefits of organ-directed strategies.
4. Synergistic approach with systemic chemotherapy and palliative liver ablative techniques such as radiofrequency ablation (RFA), traditionally considered noncurative, may improve disease-free survival outcomes or may be good surrogates to formal liver surgery, where the clinical situation dictates.

Thus, there is good clinical evidence that liver-focused approaches, in a multimodal context, can significantly and incrementally benefit selected patients. Research in the technologies, delivery, potential synergies, and multimodal integration is rapidly offering new possibilities.

The Concept of Local vs. Locoregional Modalities

Despite rapid imaging advances, the best cross-sectional technologies (CT and MRI) have a maximum liver resolution in the order of millimeters. This equates to approximately 10^7 cancer cells, which even with newer functional imaging technologies such as PET only improves by one order of magnitude at best. Thus, retrospective analysis of the timing and patterns of relapse observed after attempted curative resections of colorectal liver metastases can define the nonvisible micro-metastatic disease burden probability for each situation, allowing the development of suitable patient selection criteria. The information from the EORTC Intergroup 40983 randomized controlled phase III trial is the unbiased benchmark (criterion standard) in the best prognostic groups. It demonstrates that in the presence of 1–4 visible potentially curable metastases at presentation, 50% or more of patients will have relapsed within 18 months of curative liver surgery, many within the liver. By 3 years, only one-fourth to one-third of patients remain disease free.[1] Thus, by definition of long-term follow-up, the vast majority of patients (~70%) have "invisible" micrometastatic disease, even when selected for curative surgery with less than four liver metastases. This data highlights that the major strategic approach to curing liver-confined metastases should be whole organ-directed (local and regional) versus imaging-directed (local) approaches. Alternatively, it confirms that the majority of patients will need a multimodal sequenced approach with other systemic or locoregional strategies, if we are to improve longer-term outcomes further.

LOCAL VS. LOCOREGIONAL LIVER THERAPIES

"Local" approaches are image-guidance-based approaches and, as an extension, are directly complementary to liver surgical approaches in principle. They aim to eradicate any imagable metastases after staging and attempt to do this via nonresective means. The aim is to reduce the morbidity of the liver resection, that is, without open surgery, reduce hospital stay (improve recovery and quality of life), and at the same time potentially allow temporally repetitive multiple interventions. They may also increase the time that patients are off cytotoxic chemotherapy ("holiday"), especially if they are used to consolidate an initial chemotherapy response, as it is uncommon to see complete visual (radiologic complete response) disappearance of lesions. They are not liver restricted and can often target lesions in the lung, adrenal, skin, kidneys, and even bone. Their main limitation is that that by definition, they cannot target nonradiologically visible lesions (i.e., 5–8 mm or less or micrometastatic disease, which, by definition, is difficult to clearly visualize). Furthermore, the true evidence of benefit to patients, in terms of randomized controlled trials is lacking, with quality of life and morbidity outcomes often poorly documented. They also often have the same restrictions of liver surgery in terms of the anatomy and amount of functional liver reserve that must remain. Nevertheless, with good patient selection, some patients do benefit. On the contrary, patients with rapidly (within 3 months) progressive chemoresistant disease rarely benefit.

On the other hand, locoregional approaches are non–image-guided or whole-organ-based approaches and a natural extension of the previous HAI and PVI chemotherapy approaches, which became feasible as the liver has a dual blood supply. They are based on the principle that liver tumors including metastases obtain their cancer neovasculature predominately through the hepatic artery (70%–85% of blood flow), whereas the portal vein supplies the majority of normal (noncancerous) liver parenchyma. This creates an "Achilles heel" that can be potentially be clinically exploited by targeting the arterial supply. Locoregional therapies aim to eradicate metastases *irrespective* of whether they can be visualized by any imaging techniques, on the basis that the majority of patients who have visual metastases will also have micrometastases. This is irrefutable and shown by the high and rapid liver recurrence rates even in liver operable, potentially curable, mCRC, where there are *less than four* metastases.[1] A higher number of visible metastases, coupled with the pathologic knowledge that even with complete radiologic respons to chemotherapy, 97% of such sites will still have histologically detectable microscopic metastatic disease implies that locoregional approaches should have a higher impact in the medium- to longer-term outlook for cure. Locoregional approaches, therefore, expand the potential cohorts of patients that are suitable for additional interventions, although are currently still considered noncurative.

These approaches are liver restricted and may not be transposable to other organs because of anatomic, physiologic, or safety constraints. The specific benefit to patients in terms of randomized controlled trials are ongoing, with the most advanced clinical trials data available from hepatic arterial radioembolization.

HEPATIC ARTERIAL RADIOEMBOLIZATION AS A PLATFORM TO BUILD THE TRIAL SYNERGIES WITH CHEMOTHERAPY STANDARDS OF CARE

Chemoradiotherapy is an integral component of the multidisciplinary approach for the management of localized rectal cancer. However, a key limitation of external beam radiation in the treatment of liver tumors is the tolerance of normal liver parenchyma to doses higher than 35 Gy, which is unfortunately below that required to eradicate most tumors (for mCRC, this is estimated at ≥70 Gy for monotherapy or ≥50 Gy with concurrent chemotherapy as a radiosensitizer). Hence, the concept of a more targeted vascular approach using radioembolization (also termed selective internal radiation therapy, or SIRT) began to develop more than 50 years ago. Technical problems hindered the adoption of this approach until the development of the current generation of products now in use for more than 15 years. Both resin and glass microspheres containing yttrium-90 (^{90}Y) as the therapeutic isotope are used. The resin microspheres (SIR-Spheres™) have the largest clinical evidence database in CRC (at least 30 trials reported to date). These have shown that radioembolization using ^{90}Y microspheres is associated with very high response rates in the first-line setting (>80%) in combination with concurrent, standard systemic 5-FU and oxaliplatin. Randomized studies have suggested a survival benefit beyond first-line chemotherapy, and all reported series have shown activity in chemorefractory ("salvage") patients. In salvage, where no other treatment options remain, there are compelling data that significant palliative benefits can be achieved in one-third of patients selected for liver-predominant metastases, with good performance and liver functional status. A randomized control multicenter Belgian trial, testing the value of adding SIRT in the salvage setting, confirmed that despite the late stage of disease and potential crossover of radioembolization, that intervening early (in combination with infusional 5-FU chemotherapy) with ^{90}Y demonstrated a significant benefit. Remarkably, this trial showed, for the first time, the potential value overall on primary efficacy parameters compared to an organ-directed approach, in that even in patients who relapsed outside the liver (as their first site of relapse after ^{90}Y), treating the liver appeared to confer a survival benefit.

The quantitative benefits of radioembolization appear to be greatest when this intervention is used earlier in the colorectal treatment paradigm as well as in combination with concurrent chemotherapy. Two pivotal adequately powered randomized phase III controlled trials (FOXFIRE and SIRFLOX) are examining the role of ^{90}Y resin microspheres in combination with chemotherapy for the first-line treatment of colorectal hepatic metastases (integrated with the contemporaneous chemotherapy standards of care).

The short-term toxicities appear manageable, with the most serious ones being a 1%–3% risk of radiation hepatitis and 2%–5% risk of a radiation gastroduodenal ulcer, which is self-limiting in most cases. Little is known about the long-term effects on the liver parenchyma that will be tested in the ongoing trials. To date, there are no obvious concerns, especially as the treatment in hepatocellular carcinoma, with associated severe cirrhosis appears to be remarkably safe and well tolerated by the cirrhotic liver.

The Y90 SIRT clinical trials program shows how even with multidisciplinary complex interventions, clinical evidence that can benchmark our progress in a nonbiased way can eventually be established and used as a platform for further developments.

Summary and Future

Advances in systemic chemotherapy and biologic agents have improved noncurative, median survivals incrementally in metastatic disease over the last 20 years. However, to effect even higher cure rates in a subset of patients (survival ≥5 years), there remains dependency on selection for liver surgical excision of residual metastases, as the complete pathologic, and thus durable, response rates of chemotherapy alone remain imperceptible. The keys are thus to have improved patient (clinical) and molecular selection, combined with expanding the populations suitable for integrated combination modalities including liver surgery, leading to complete eradication of organ-confined metastases. Rapid technology developments with reducing morbidities are making this an increasing reality.

The expertise of the multidisciplinary team, with a patient-centered focus, allows interpretation and implementation of a significant cumulative evidence base, to achieve the best treatment pathway and outcomes for each individual. It follows from concurrent clinical trials, to thus allow informed decisions about safety, efficacy, and quality of life, for better long-term qualitative and quantitative outcomes. There is increasing evidence that these multitude of technologies can be synergistic as opposed to additive, if selected and tested properly. The application of an innovative multidisciplinary approach that integrates advanced approaches (such as radioembolization and local ablative therapies) should ultimately allow the benefits of curative hepatic resection to be extended to a broader group of patients.

There may also be significant quantitative palliative benefits, hitherto ignored, if the novel concept of "Vital organ" salvage develops an evidence base. That is, targeting metastases early in the treatment pathway in specific organs such as the liver may have an overall higher impact on the patient than generally controlling systemic metastatic disease in other sites.

Current multidisciplinary approaches should be truly cross-specialty in *effect*, with integrated treatment options discussed on a regular basis from the outset. Not, as was often the case, being single technology or single specialty dependent, or only discussing other options at the salvage (end) of the treatment pathway, when unfortunately, no realistic treatment options exist and the patient cohorts are significantly smaller and less functionally able or likely to benefit.

REFERENCES

The complete reference list is available online at www.expertconsult.com.

13

Surgical Management of Hepatic Metastases

JUNICHI SHINDOH | GIUSEPPE ZIMMITTI | JEAN-NICOLAS VAUTHEY

KEY POINTS

- Precise assessment of disease progression and adequate selection of initial therapeutic options should be performed through a multidisciplinary approach in the treatment of liver metastases.
- Selected patients with colorectal liver metastases are candidates for curative hepatic resection with 5-year survival up to 58%.
- Number, size, and bilobar distribution of liver metastases do not limit the indication of surgery when R0 resection is feasible.
- Surgical resection should be deferred in patients with significant progression of metastatic disease during treatment with optimal preoperative chemotherapy until achieving disease control with second-line systemic chemotherapy or regional therapies.
- Minimal requirement of standardized future liver remnant is dependent on the status of the underlying liver (>20% in normal liver, >30% in damaged liver, and >40% in cirrhosis).
- Selected patients with advanced liver metastases benefit from reversed approach (resection of metastases prior to primary lesion) or staged hepatectomies.
- Radiologic complete response to chemotherapy does not signify complete pathologic response. Therefore, surgical resection should include all the original sites of metastases.
- Surgical resection of metastases from neuroendocrine tumor reduces symptoms and prolongs survival even after cytoreduction surgery. However, multidisciplinary approach is usually required in advanced disease.
- Significance of surgical resection of metastases of noncolorectal and nonneuroendocrine origin is still unclear.

Introduction

The liver is the most common site of hematogenous metastases from various malignancies, particularly those originating from the gastrointestinal tract. Although the patients having liver metastases are classified as stage 4 in TNM (tumor, node, metastasis) classifications, favorable long-term outcomes have been reported when curative resections are feasible especially in the patients with colorectal liver metastases (CLMs)[1,2] or neuroendocrine tumors (NETs).[3,4]

With recent advancements in chemotherapy and growing use of portal vein embolization (PVE), resectability of CLM has dramatically increased, and long-term survival after resection of CLM has significantly improved.[2] The practical keys in initial clinical management of patients with CLM are (1) precise assessment of extension of disease and (2) adequate selection of therapeutic options. Surgical resection is potentially the most curative therapeutic strategy for liver metastases. However, to select the patients who would truly have prognostic advantages from surgery, a multidisciplinary approach by surgeons, medical oncologist, radiologist, and pathologist is essential (Figure 13-1).

Colorectal Liver Metastases

Colorectal cancer is the second leading cause of cancer-related death in the United States. The 20%–25% of patients are found to have synchronous CLM,[5,6] and 35%–55% of patients develop CLM during the course of the disease.[7] However, the 5-year survival after curative resection of CLM has been reported to be up to 58%,[8-10] whereas median survival of CLM without any treatment is approximately 6 months.[6] Therefore, adequate assessment and preoperative management are important to select the patient with resectable or potentially resectable CLM.

PREOPERATIVE ASSESSMENT

Assessment of Oncological Resectability

In pretreatment assessment of oncological status of CLM, liver dynamic computed tomography (CT) is a standard imaging modality with an adequate sensitivity and specificity.[11] Magnetic resonance imaging (MRI) and positron emission tomography (PET) can be added in selected cases to improve the diagnostic accuracy, especially for diagnosis of indeterminate lesions, detection of local recurrence, or screening of extrahepatic disease. However, the choice of imaging modalities should be based on the local expertise and the balance between the costs and benefits.

Previously, four or more tumors, size >5 cm, bilateral disease, and narrow surgical margin <1 cm were reported to be negative prognostic factors,[12-14] and accordingly, they have been considered as contraindications for liver resection. In the era of effective systemic therapy and PVE, however, the oncologic criteria for liver resection is shifting toward complete resection of all viable disease because favorable outcomes would be expected in a selected patient amenable to curative resection even with extrahepatic diseases.[15-17] Also, a multicenter study of 557 patients has reported that width of surgical margin does not affect the overall survival if negative margin can be obtained (Figure 13-2).[10] Therefore, large number, size, and bilobar distribution of tumor are no longer absolute contraindications for hepatic resection as long as R0 resections are feasible (Table 13-1).[18]

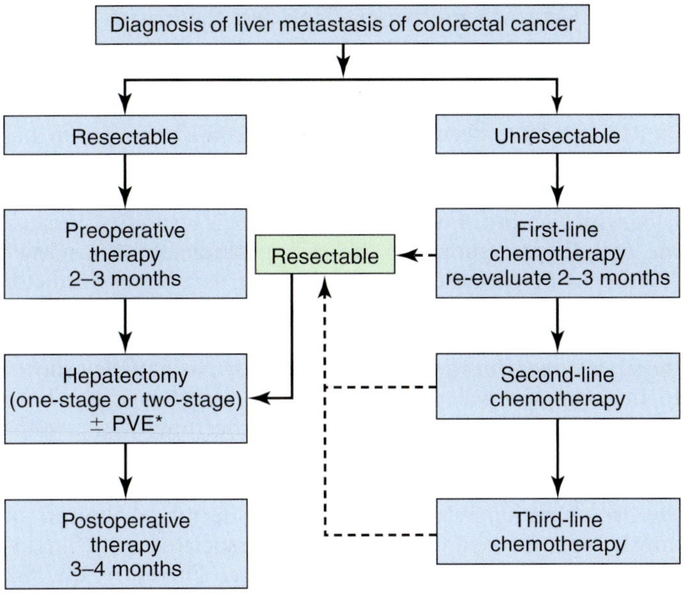

Figure 13-1 Treatment algorithm for colorectal liver metastases (CLMs). Patients with initially resectable tumors go straight to surgery or have preoperative therapy first. In initially unresectable cases, multidisciplinary management should be initiated, and potentially resectable patients should be selected under an appropriate therapeutic management. *(With permission from Kopetz S, Vauthey JN: Perioperative chemotherapy for resectable hepatic metastases,* Lancet *371(9617): 963–965, 2008.)*

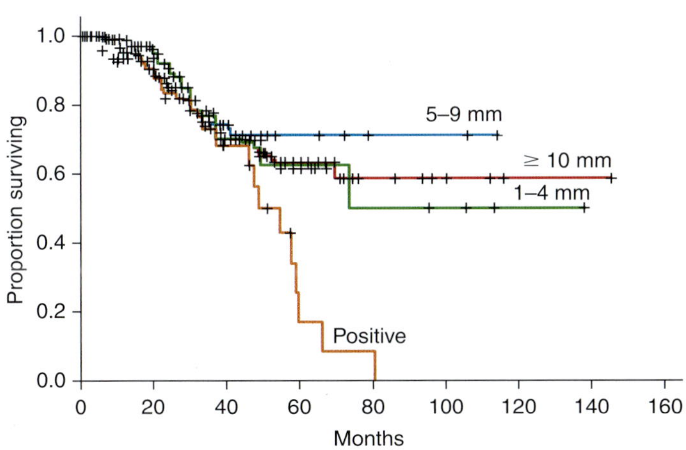

Figure 13-2 Width of surgical margin and overall survival *(With permission from Pawlik TM, Scoggins CR, Zorzi D, et al: Effect of surgical margin status on survival and site of recurrence after hepatic resection for colorectal metastases,* Ann Surg *241(5):715–724, 2005.)*

Assessment of Technical Resectability

Technical resectability is determined by the balance between the feasibility of curative resection (R0 resection) and preservation of adequate inflow–outflow pathways for the liver remnant. Technical feasibility of liver resection basically depends on the distribution of tumors and vascular anatomy. Because the metabolic performance of the liver is highly dependent on both intact inflows (i.e., arterial and portal flows) and adequate outflows (i.e., venous flow and biliary drainage), patency of these four vessels is essential to expect a full performance of the future liver remnant (FLR).

TABLE 13-1 Changing Paradigm of Indications of Liver Resection in Patients with Colorectal Liver Metastases

	Conventional Criteria	Current Consensus
ONCOLOGIC CRITERIA		
Number	≤3	No limitation if R0 resection is feasible
Size	≤5 cm	No limitation if R0 resection is feasible
Distribution	Unilateral distribution	No limitation if R0 resection is feasible
Extrahepatic disease	Contraindication	If curatively resectable or long-term control can be expected
TECHNICAL CRITERIA		
Surgical margin	≥1 cm	Microscopic R0 resection
Future liver remnant (FLR)	Anticipated ability to preserve adequate FLR volume with intact blood flow and biliary drainage	Anticipated ability to preserve adequate FLR volume (>20% in normal liver, >30% in extensively treated liver)[a] with intact blood flow and biliary drainage

[a]Zorzi, et al.[20]

Currently, functional reserve of the liver is estimated by both static and dynamic measurements. The most reliable static variable is the FLR volume. Because absolute volume of FLR against standardized liver volume (SLV) (i.e., sFLR: standardized FLR) has strong correlation with the rates of postoperative morbidity and mortality (Figure 13-3),[18,19] minimal requirements of sFLR has currently been set at >20% in normal liver, >30% in damaged liver after extensive treatment, and >40% in cirrhotic liver (Figure 13-4).[20] These cutoff values offer a good practical decision making in patients requiring major hepatectomy. Dynamic measurements such as degree of hypertrophy,[18] indocyanine green clearance test,[21] or hepatic scintigraphy[22] have also been reported to be a sensitive variable to evaluate functional reserve of the liver. Because FLR volume itself is not correlated with functional reserve, dynamic measurements should be integrated to estimate the total functional reserve of FLR in individual patients.

PREOPERATIVE MANAGEMENT

Neoadjuvant Chemotherapy

Recent advancements in chemotherapeutic agents and delivery have changed the treatment of CLM dramatically. With introduction of oxaliplatin and irinotecan, the response rate of CLM has reached more than 50% and the conversion rates from unresectable to resectable metastases has been reported to be up to 38%.[23,24] Moreover, molecular target agents such as bevacizumab has further augmented these responses upward of 80%.[25,26] When patients are treated with preoperative systemic therapy, they benefit by observing the biological behavior of the tumor. Progression in the form of development of new lesions (growth in more than three existing liver metastases and/or the development of multiple new lesions) during treatment with optimal preoperative chemotherapy is strongly associated with

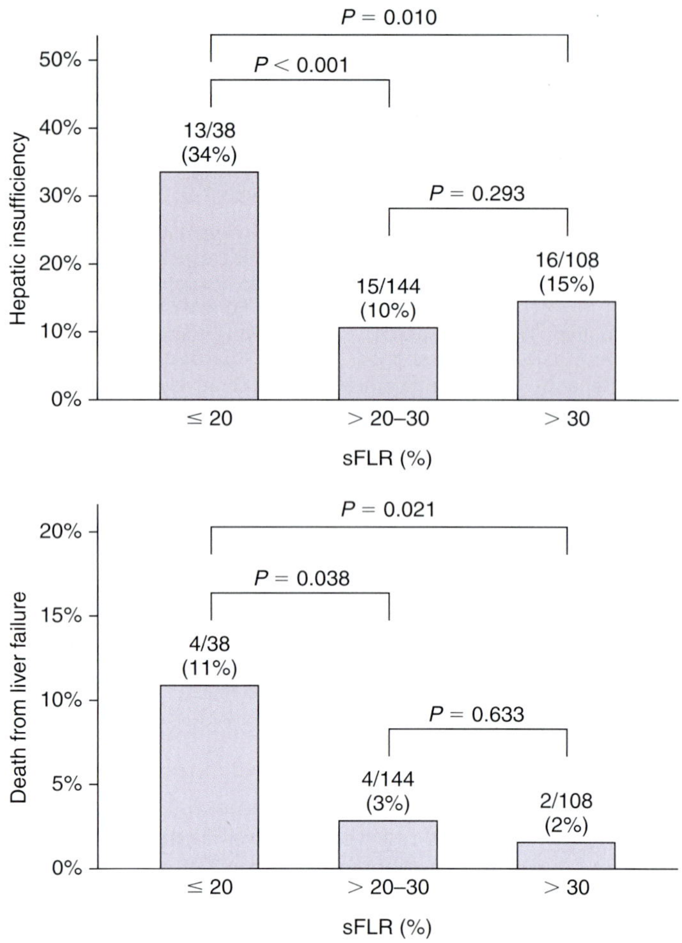

Figure 13-3 Posthepatectomy liver insufficiency and mortality rates based on standardized future liver remnant (sFLR). *(Adapted with permission from Kishi Y, Abdalla EK, Chun YS, et al: Three hundred and one consecutive extended right hepatectomies: evaluation of outcome based on systematic liver volumetry,* Ann Surg *250(4):540–548, 2009.)*

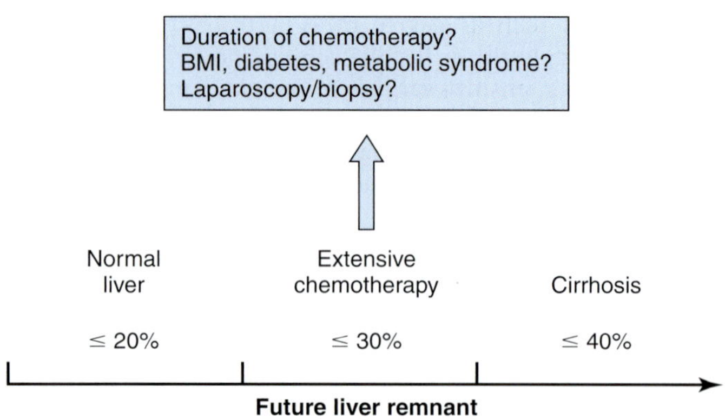

Figure 13-4 Criteria for minimal requirement of standardized future liver remnant (sFLR). *(With permission from Zorzi D, Laurent A, Pawlik TM, Lauwers GY, Vauthey JN, Abdalla EK: Chemotherapy-associated hepatotoxicity and surgery for colorectal liver metastases,* Br J Surg *94(3):274–286, 2007.)*

poor hepatectomy outcomes.[27] Therefore, surgical resection should be deferred until achieving disease control with second-line systemic or regional therapies.

Conventionally, the Response Evaluation Criteria in Solid Tumors (RECIST)[28,29] have been utilized to assess the response rate of CLM to chemotherapy. However, there is an inconsistency between this unidimensional measurement and pathologic response,[30] and also better predictive value of dynamic changes in tumor size compared to the established cutoff value in RECIST have been reported.[31,32] Recently, our group has reported a new morphologic criterion to assess the response to chemotherapy (Figure 13-5).[33] These criteria are well correlated with viability of tumor cells (pathologic response). Because the pathologic response is the strong predictor of survival[34] (Figure 13-6), morphologic classification is a better predictor of surgical outcomes after neoadjuvant chemotherapy.

Despite the oncologic advantages of preoperative chemotherapy, longer duration of chemotherapy has not been shown to improve survival over shorter courses,[35] but it has been associated with liver toxicity,[36] posthepatectomy liver insufficiency, and mortality.[37,38] In the recent EORTC (European Organization for Research and Treatment of Cancer) trial,[39] the use of perioperative chemotherapy decreased the rate of nontherapeutic laparotomy but was associated with an increase in posthepatectomy complications. Therefore, the risk and benefit should be balanced in preoperative chemotherapy.

Portal Vein Embolization

PVE is a safe, minimally invasive procedure that leads to an atrophy in the side of the liver to be resected and compensatory hypertrophy of FLR.[40-42] Our previous studies have shown that sFLR >20% is a minimal requirement in patients with a normal underlying liver and the extended right hepatectomy can be performed safely in patients who have achieved an sFLR >20% after PVE for insufficient initial FLR.[19,43] Based on the criteria according to baseline status of liver parenchyma (see Figure 13-4), PVE should be considered if a patient is found to have insufficient volume in pretreatment measurement of FLR.

To maximize the regeneration of FLR in PVE, optimal selection of embolic materials[44] and concurrent embolization of segment 4 portal vein[45,46] has been recommended. Our previous work comparing right PVE with and without segment 4 embolization revealed significant difference in volume increase rates in segment 2+3 (median, 26% vs. 54%; $P = .021$) (Figure 13-7).

Contraindications of PVE include portal hypertension, tumor extension to the FLR or portal vein, coagulopathy that cannot be corrected, biliary dilation in the FLR, and renal failure.

SURGICAL APPROACH

Basic Concepts

The surgical strategy for CLM is determined by its safety and oncological efficacy. When the tumor burden is limited with anatomically favorable distribution, a one-stage surgery involving one or more simultaneous partial to lobar liver resection is safe and effective.[12,47-50] Type of liver resection (anatomic resection vs. nonanatomic resection) has no significant impact on the outcome in patients with CLM.[51,52]

Also, width of surgical margin does not affect the overall survival if R0 resection is feasible.[10] For the cases with extensive bilobar metastases, several strategies are still available in selected patients. With the use of preoperative chemotherapy and PVE, these patients would benefit from surgical resection. Therefore, surgery should actively be considered in possibly resectable patients through a multidisciplinary approach.

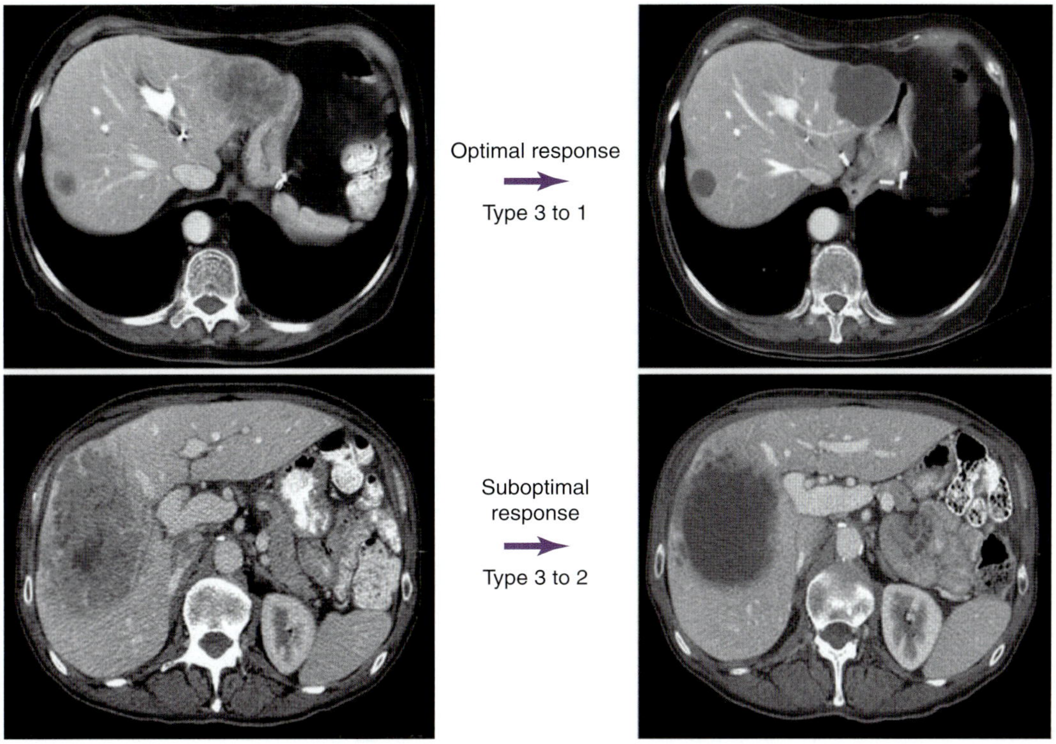

Figure 13-5 Morphologic response after systemic chemotherapy. Optimal morphologic response (i.e., type 1 response: homogenous hypoattenuation with clear margin) predicts well both tumor viability and survival. *(Adapted with permission from Chun YS, Vauthey JN, Boonsirikamchai P, et al: Association of computed tomography morphologic criteria with pathologic response and survival in patients treated with bevacizumab for colorectal liver metastases,* JAMA *302(21):2338–2344, 2009.)*

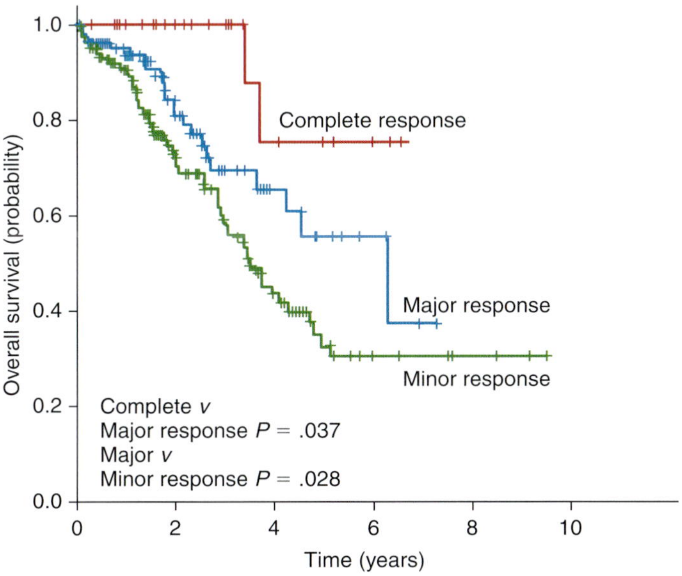

Figure 13-6 Survival stratified by pathologic response to systemic chemotherapy. *(With permission from Blazer DG III, Kishi Y, Maru DM, et al: Pathologic response to preoperative chemotherapy: a new outcome end point after resection of hepatic colorectal metastases,* J Clin Oncol *26(33):5344–5351, 2008.)*

Strategy for Synchronous Metastases

In patients with synchronous presentation of CLM at the diagnosis of colorectal cancer, liver resection was conventionally performed after resection of primary lesion followed by adjuvant chemotherapy (Classic approach). A combination strategy, with simultaneous resection of the primary lesion and CLM (Combined approach) has also been used to avoid delaying surgical resection of metastatic disease. However, this strategy is associated with an increased risk of postoperative complications when major liver resection is combined with the resection of primary lesion.[53–55] A "Reverse approach" is another option that has been proposed recently, where liver resection precedes resection of the primary tumor.[56] A study that compared these three different surgical approaches revealed no difference among these groups in survival rates[57] (Figure 13-8). Therefore, the optimal approach should be selected according to the status of both the primary lesion (symptoms, invasiveness, node status, etc.) and CLM.

Staged Liver Resection

In patients having bilateral CLM who are initially identified as unresectable, staged surgery may provide survival benefit if all the tumor burdens can be curatively resected after chemotherapy.[58,59] Two-stage resection (TSR) is indicated for patients with advanced bilateral CLM who responded to chemotherapy and in whom limited resection can clear the less affected side of the liver before a planned extended contralateral liver resection. In majority of the cases, patients undergo first-stage limited resection of the left lobe, followed by right PVE with segment 4 embolization, and extended right hepatectomy is completed after sFLR meets the volume criteria. A previous study from the M.D. Anderson Cancer Center reported that 72.3% (47/65) of the patients among planned TSR completed TSR, and 5-year survival in these patients was 51% compared to 15% in the cases treated with chemotherapy (P = .005) (Figure 13-9).

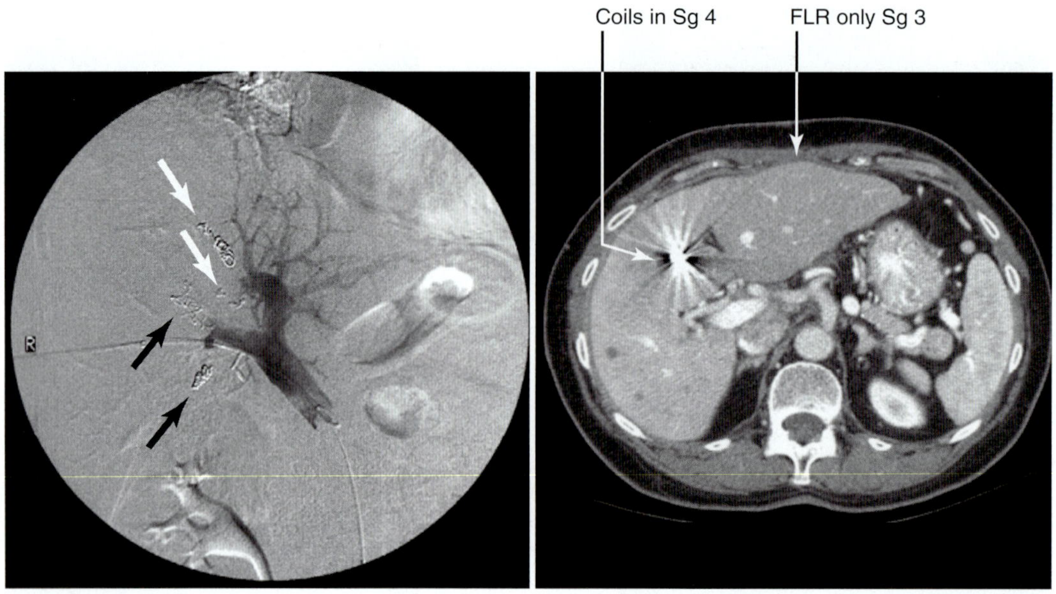

Figure 13-7 Right portal vein embolization extending to segment 4 prior to extended right hepatectomy. *(With permission from Kishi Y, Madoff DC, Abdalla EK, et al: Is embolization of segment 4 portal veins before extended right hepatectomy justified?* Surgery *144(5):744–751, 2008.)*

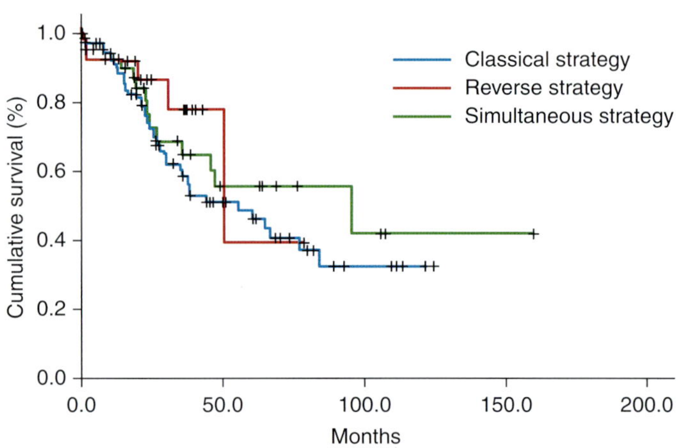

Figure 13-8 Overall survival treated for synchronous colorectal liver metastases. *(With permission from Brouquet A, Mortenson MM, Vauthey JN, et al. Surgical strategies for synchronous colorectal liver metastases in 156 consecutive patients: classic, combined or reverse strategy?* J Am Coll Surg. *2010;210(6):934-941.)*

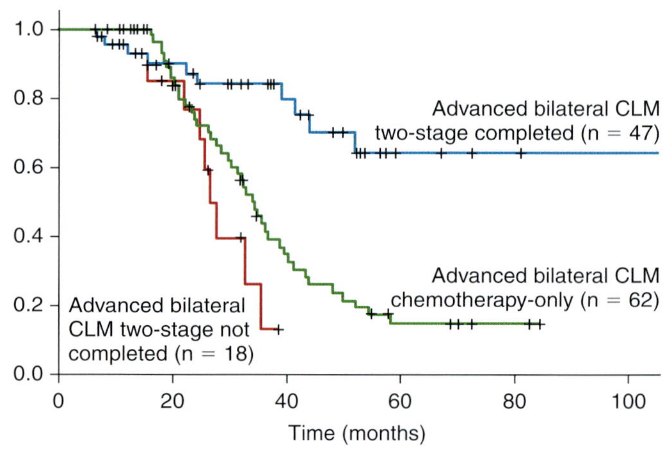

Figure 13-9 Overall survival in patients with advanced bilateral colorectal liver metastasis after two-stage resection (TSR). *(With permission from Brouquet A, Mortenson MM, Vauthey JN, et al: Surgical strategies for synchronous colorectal liver metastases in 156 consecutive patients: classic, combined or reverse strategy?* J Am Coll Surg *210(6): 934–941, 2010.)*

Management of the Disappearing Metastases

With the introduction of recent new chemotherapeutic and targeted agents, response rates of CLM to chemotherapy have dramatically increased. The incidence of disappearing lesions (complete radiologic response) after extensive chemotherapy has been reported, ranging from 5% to 38%.[30,60-64] Although favorable survival would be expected in such patients, disappearing lesion is becoming a new issue in the treatment for CLM because the natural history of patients with complete radiologic response is still unclear.[30] A complete radiologic response does not signify a complete pathologic response as residual microscopic disease can be expected in up to 80% of patients with resected disappearing liver metastases after preoperative systemic chemotherapy.[30,61-64] Therefore, surgical resection of CLM should include all original sites of the disease. In patients with metastases at risk of disappearing or missing lesion at surgery, placement of a fiduciary marker in interventional radiology prior to chemotherapy should be considered.[65]

POSTOPERATIVE MANAGEMENT AND OUTCOME

Short-Term Outcome

With adequate criteria to assess the hepatic functional reserve and PVE, hepatic resection can be performed safely with mortality rates of less than 5%, and even close to 0% in experienced centers.[66] Although postoperative complications tend to increase in patients pretreated with chemotherapy,[35,39,67] optimal criteria of sFLR[20] and evaluation of dynamic variables[18,21,22] reflecting hepatic functional reserve allows safe major hepatectomy.

Follow-Up and Long-Term Outcome

Patients undergoing hepatic resection should be carefully observed to allow for early detection of recurrence. Scheduled evaluation including tumor markers (CEA and CA 19-9), liver function test, pelvic and abdominal CT, chest radiography, and colonoscopy should be continued with adequate intervals for at least 5 years after surgery.

Selected patients should undergo repeated resection for recurrent lesions. Adam et al.[68] showed 5-year survival rates of 32% after the third hepatectomy, with no increase in postoperative morbidity or mortality. Overall 5-year survival is now reported to be as high as 58% in single and multiinstitutional studies. The common prognostic factors are margin status (R1 status), size and number of lesions, and presence or absence of extrahepatic disease.[10,69,70]

CASE PRESENTATION

A 60-year-old man who was diagnosed with asymptomatic sigmoid colon cancer having synchronous metastases to the liver was referred to our institution. Initial liver dynamic CT revealed two liver metastases measuring 4.1 cm in segment 4 and 5.8 cm in segment 6, respectively (Figure 13-10). Segment 4 tumor involved the middle hepatic vein and was also very

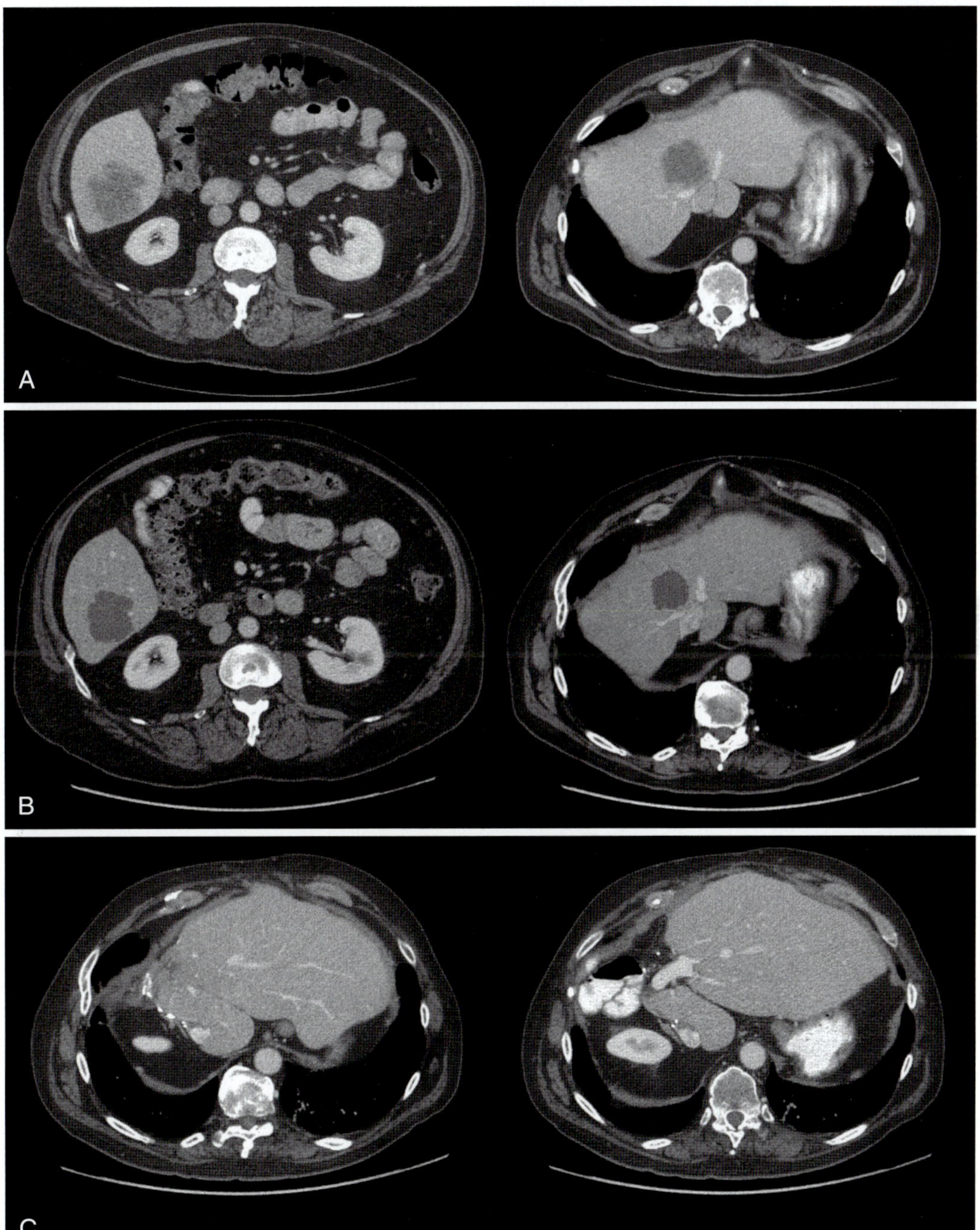

Figure 13-10 (A) Before chemotherapy. (B) After 6 cycles of chemotherapy with FOLFOX + bevacizumab. (C). After liver resection.

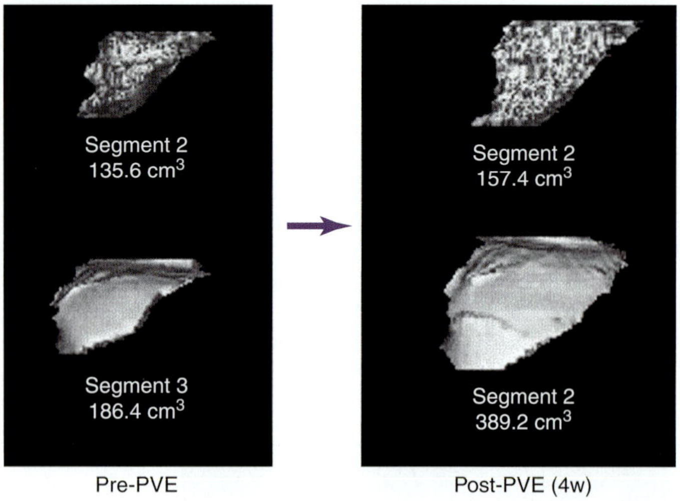

Figure 13-11 *Left*: Pre–portal vein embolization (PVE) (future liver remnant [FLR] 321 mL; standardized future liver remnant [sFLR] 9%). *Right*: Post-PVE (FLR 546ml; sFLR 33%)

close to the left hepatic vein. Therefore, right trisectionectomy was considered to be a curative surgical option. Although he was serologically positive for hepatitis C, liver function tests were normal and no clinical evidence suggesting active hepatitis or cirrhosis was identified. However, three-dimensional volumetry revealed that sFLR was 9%. Therefore, he was initially treated with systemic chemotherapy.

After 6 cycles of FOLFOX + bevacizumab, CT revealed good responses in liver lesions both in size and morphology (see Figure 13-10). There was also no evidence of progression of extrahepatic metastases. Therefore, right PVE combining with embolization of segment 4 portal vein embolization were performed. Four weeks after the PVE, sufficient growth in FLR was observed in up to 33% (Figure 13-11). Considering the advanced oncologic status in the liver and the risk of simultaneous surgery for both primary lesion and metastasis, he underwent right trisectionectomy first, leaving the primary lesion (Reversed Approach). Postoperative course was uneventful. Pathologic specimen revealed <5% viable tumor and negative surgical margin (4 mm).

Two months later, based on the fact that no intrahepatic recurrence and extrahepatic disease was found, we moved on to the resection of the primary lesion, and sigmoid resection was performed without any complications. Final pathologic stage was T2, N1 (two positive nodes out of eight). Adjuvant chemotherapy was administered for another six cycles with FOLFOX + bevacizumab. After 22 months, recurrence in pelvic node was detected and systemic chemotherapy was started. However, the patient is still alive with good control of recurrent lesion at 30 months after surgery.

Resection of Noncolorectal Liver Metastases

NEUROENDOCRINE LIVER METASTASES

NETs are indolent growing and metastasize primarily to the liver. Because nonfunctioning NET is the most common subtype, patients with high tumor burden can remain asymptomatic for years, whereas others with minimal lesions can suffer various symptoms caused by excessive production of hormones by the tumor.

The best treatment for patients with liver metastases of NETs remains controversial. However, resection of functioning NETs reduces symptoms and prolongs survival. It has been reported that almost 100% of patients can get amelioration and 70%–80% of them have complete relief after resection of liver metastases.[71,72] Although curative resection rate is relatively low, survival rate of patients undergoing liver resection is relatively high, reaching up to 91% at 3 years[3] and 61% at 5 years.[4,73] Cytoreduction of more than 90% of tumor volume is also reported to improve survival compared to other treatment options such as transarterial embolization or systemic chemotherapy.[71,74]

More evidence is needed to define the ideal treatment for NET liver metastases. However, this type of neoplasm is basically incurable in most of the cases with advanced stage. Therefore, a multidisciplinary approach including surgery, transarterial embolization, systemic chemotherapy, and radiation is needed.

NONCOLORECTAL, NONNEUROENDOCRINE LIVER METASTASES

In contrast to the considerable evidence for long-term survival after resection of CLM or NETs, prognostic contribution of surgery to the other types of liver metastases is unclear. There are a few single-institution studies reporting surgical outcomes of liver metastases from melanoma, sarcoma, and gynecologic, gastric, and pancreatic cancers. However, no sufficient data are available to make a recommendation at present.

Conclusions

With advancements in chemotherapy, PVE, and surgical approaches, resectability and long-term outcomes have been dramatically improved, especially in CLM and NETs. In the treatment of hepatic metastases, multidisciplinary approaches are essential to optimize the therapeutic strategy and select the patient who would benefit from surgical resection. Preoperative chemotherapy and PVE play a central role in testing oncologically high-risk groups and selecting patients anticipated to have prognostic advantages by extended hepatectomies.

REFERENCES

The complete reference list is available online at www.expertconsult.com.

14

Interventional Radiology in the Management of Colorectal Cancer Liver Metastases

CONSTANTINOS T. SOFOCLEOUS | PANAGIOTIS A. SIDERAS | ELENA N. PETRE

Colon Cancer—An Overview

Colorectal cancer (CRC) is the fourth most frequently diagnosed cancer, the second leading cause of cancer-related death in the United States, and recent studies estimate that 100,000 new cases of colon cancer and 40,000 of rectal cancer will occur annually. During the same time, 50,000 people will die from CRC. Within the past 30 years, the incidence of CRC has decreased from 60.5 to 46.4 per 100,000 people. Similarly CRC-related mortality has decreased by 35% in the past 15 years.[1]

Approximately 20% of colon cancer cases are associated with familial clustering.[2] Genetic susceptibility to colorectal cancer includes inherited syndromes such as Lynch syndrome (hereditary nonpolyposis colorectal cancer/HNPCC) and familial adenomatous polyposis (FAP). Colorectal cancer is one of the most common solid tumors and is responsible for approximately 10% of cancer-related death in the Western world.[3] Treatment of primary colorectal cancer with surgical resection, combined with chemotherapy and radiotherapy, may be effective in many patients. About 10%–25% of patients present with synchronous liver metastases at the time of primary diagnosis and another 20%–25% of patients developed metachronous liver metastases. Surgical resection of distant CRC metastases may result in long-term survival and even cure in a subset of selected patients.[3] The 5-year survival rates after resection of all detectable liver metastases can reach up to 40%. However, only 25% of the patients with colorectal liver metastases are candidates for liver resection, whereas the majority remain unresectable.[4] Chemotherapy and newer therapies can extend patient survival of patients with unresectable colorectal liver metastases.[5] Several image-guided procedures have evolved within the past 10 years that allow the management of liver metastases in nonresectable patients and those that have recurred after resection. These local therapies include local tumor ablation, hepatic arterial chemotherapy (HAC), selective internal radiation therapy (SIRT), as well as traditional arterial chemoembolization (TACE) and the more recent use of irinotecan-loaded drug-eluting beads (DEBIRI-TACE). To date, TACE and SIRT have been mostly used in patients who have failed several prior chemotherapy regimens (salvage therapies). Small randomized controlled trials showed that the addition of SIRT or DEBIRI to systemic chemotherapy result in longer disease-free and overall patient survival when compared to chemotherapy only.

In this chapter, we will elaborate on appropriate image-guided local therapies based on disease distribution and patterns. The chapter will review the indications and results of image-guided percutaneous local tumor ablation and intraarterial therapies in the management of colon cancer liver metastases (CLM).

Introduction

The natural history of CLM varies significantly based on the pattern of disease distribution.[1] As described in a surgical review of the mid-1980s, solitary CLM, if left untreated, had survival rates of about 70% and 45% at 1 and 2 years, respectively. If the disease was widespread in one lobe or two lobes, that is, multiple unilobar or bilobar lesions, 1- and 2-year survival rates varied from 65% to 30% and 40% to 15%, respectively. Survival rates at 3 and 5 years were significantly decreased for either solitary CLM or multiple unilobar and bilobar disease to 5% or less.[6] Thirty years later, in 2011, survival rates have dramatically improved to higher than 60% at 2 years and 35% at 5 years. This improvement is attributed to the availability of new chemotherapeutic agents along with improved imaging for early tumor detection as well as aggressive surgical debulking and locoregional therapies including image-guided interventions.[5]

National Comprehensive Cancer Network (NCCN) guidelines emphasize the value of systemic chemotherapy in the management of CLM.[5] Although NCCN guidelines indicate the value of surgery (or ablation) for well-selected patients, they do not endorse the widespread use of intraarterial locoregional therapies largely because of their lower level of evidence (mostly level 3, small numbers of level 2, and sparse numbers of level 1 studies). This discordance between NCCN guidelines and the 2002 FDA approval in particular for SIRT with resin microspheres for CLM stems from the fact that with the exception of a handful of small randomized controlled trials showing better progression-free survivals for the patients using SIRT in addition to chemotherapy to date, there is no large randomized controlled study conducted for loco-regional therapies to document a statistically significant overall survival benefit.

Ablation in the Treatment of Colorectal Metastases

Ablative technologies involve the delivery of tumoricidal energy directly within the tumor in order to destroy the target tumor and a surrounding margin of normal liver while minimizing the impact on the rest of the nonaffected liver. Advantages include less physiological stress, since ablative therapies do not require open surgery but can be applied percutaneously under imaging guidance or laparoscopically.

These advantages allow the treatment of patients unfit or unwilling to undergo major abdominal surgery and those who are poor candidates for general anesthesia. Ablative therapies minimize the destruction of healthy liver tissue as compared to hepatic resection.[7] This is an important parameter for patients with low volume of healthy functioning parenchyma such as those with underlying cirrhosis or steatohepatitis from prolonged chemotherapy exposure as well as those that have previously undergone extensive liver resection. Image-guided ablation has also been used as a salvage therapy for recurrences after prior hepatectomy.[8,9] The "test of time" approach using percutaneous ablation was proposed by Livraghi et al. in 2003 to allow the biology of the disease to express itself and to maintain quality of life in patients with liver metastases from colorectal cancer waiting for surgery.[10] The concept is that many patients may be able to avoid unnecessary surgery by undergoing ablation of liver metastases while waiting for hepatic metastasectomy. In summary, this approach allows the disease to express its biology. Patients with indolent disease and a successful ablation as well as those with very aggressive and prolific disease who develop nonresectable metastases during follow-up after ablation are spared unnecessary and morbid resection. This concept offers an interesting management approach with the use of the least morbid therapy (ablation) first, in a setting that benefits the patient and monitors for progression of disease.[10] As such, this approach could be used if there was ever an attempt to undertake a randomized controlled trial between ablation and resection for CLM.

The most common indications for image-guided ablation are:

1. Limited number (arguably less than four) and size (arguably less than 5 cm in largest diameter) of hepatic metastases in patients that cannot undergo or refuse surgery.
2. The ideal tumor for percutaneous ablation is a solitary lesion with largest diameter up to 3 cm. There is no absolute number of tumor eligibility but most series agree that patients with more than four simultaneous liver metastases are not good candidates for image-guided percutaneous ablation.
3. A tumor size up to 5 cm may be acceptable for ablation although multiple overlapping ablation will be required to achieve complete ablation with a sufficient surrounding margin (ideally a 1-cm margin all around the tumor should be created).

Contraindications:

1. No safe access of the ablation needle to the tumor despite protective maneuvers such as hydrodissection.
2. Uncorrectable coagulopathy.
3. A relative contraindication is the inability of a patient to undergo general anesthesia.

Ablation Modalities

RADIOFREQUENCY ABLATION

Radiofrequency ablation (RFA) involves the administration of energy with a frequency of <900 kHz into tissue via needle electrodes. Transmission of current through tissue causes ionic agitation, resulting in temperature elevation to lethal levels over 60°C and cellular death by coagulation necrosis. One limitation of this technique is tissue desiccation when temperature reaches 100°C, resulting in high tissue impedance, limiting the amount of energy that can be delivered in the tumor, preventing expansion of the lethal temperature within tissue and thus the volume of tissue that is exposed to temperatures high enough to cause cell death. Another well-established and important limitation of thermal ablation and in particular radiofrequency ablation is heat dissipation when applied near blood vessels. This phenomenon called the "heat sink effect" occurs when ablating tumors near blood vessels and is the result of cooling by the flowing blood at the nearby tumor edge. This compromises the effect of RFA when treating tumors larger than 3 mm in size near vessels, resulting in a relatively high rate of local tumor progression.[11] The highest success rates of ablation are achieved in patients with solitary CLM or patients with a small number of metastases <3 cm in largest diameter.[7] As with surgical resection, the aim of RFA is to achieve a clear margin around the target tumor. In recent publications, it was clearly shown that the size of ablation margin correlates with local tumor progression.[12-15] A margin of at least 5 mm as demonstrated 4–8 weeks after ablation was associated with best local tumor control and lower local tumor progression rates.[12] It has also been indicated that a 1-cm margin should be the gold standard for ablation whenever safe and ideally it should be demonstrated by imaging immediately after ablation.[12] Table 14-1 summarizes series of RFA in the management of CLM.[7,8,16-38]

CRYOBLATION

Cryoablation utilizes the administration of liquid nitrogen or argon to a probe tip, causing rapid cooling of tissue and the formation of intracellular ice crystals. Subsequent damage to the adjacent microvasculature disrupts tissue perfusion, leading to ischemia. Tissue death occurs by freezing at temperatures reaching −40°C.[39] Tissue death can be achieved by repetitive cooling–thawing cycles. One of the advantages of this procedure is the formation of visible ice-balls that can be detected by various imaging modalities and correlates with the tumor-ablation margins. Similarly to RFA, the major limitation of cryoablation is the heat sink effect as explained before that can lead to high recurrence rates.[40] Reports of cryoshock when early-generation devices were used in the treatment of liver metastases have impacted the widespread use of this modality in the treatment of liver tumors.[41] Reported median 5-year survival after cryoablation of liver tumors ranges between 22 and 24 months.[39] When using cryoablation with surgery and specifically when cryotherapy was applied to the resection margins in order to extend the depth of the resection, a 26%–44% 5-year survival was reported.[42] Table 14-2 summarizes study series using cryoablation in the treatment of CLM.[43-56]

MICROWAVE ABLATION

Microwave utilizes high-frequency waves in the range of 900 MHz and 2.4 GHz. These high-frequency waves cause water molecules to oscillate, creating friction, causing heat and tissue destruction by coagulation necrosis similar to RFA.[57] The theoretical advantage of this therapy over RFA is that it is less prone to heat-sink phenomenon, there is more controlled tissue ablation because microwave ablation (MWA) is not affected by charring of tissue, and it can achieve similar or larger areas of ablation faster than RFA. MWA and cryoablation unlike RFA do not require any grounding pads to be placed on the patient's body. Table 14-3 summarizes the results of series using MWA for the treatment of CLM.[58-62]

RESULTS

The precise role of ablation in the management of CLM may vary based on institutional and local preferences. There is, however, an overall recognition that this modality may offer good

TABLE 14-1 Results of Series Using Radiofrequency Ablation for the Treatment of CLM

Author	Mean Number of Metastases	Modality	1-Year Survival (%)	3-Year Survival (%)	5-Year Survival (%)	Median Survival (Months)
De Baere et al[16]	1.8	Percutaneous RFA	81			
Solbiati et al[17]	1.6	Percutaneous RFA		33		30
Stippel et al[18]	5.6	Intraoperative RFA				18
Cheng et al[19]	2.3	Laparoscopic RFA				25.4
Pawlik et al[20]	3.0	Resection + Percutaneous RFA				37.3
Abdalla et al[21]		Resection + RFA		43		
Berber et al[22]	3.2	Percutaneous RFA				28.9
Ellias et al[23]	2.4	Resection + RFA + hemo	92	47		36
Gillams et al[7]	4.1	Percutaneous RFA	91	28	25	38
Hildebrand et al[24]	3.5	Percutaneous RFA	92	42		28
Amersi et al [25]	3.3	Percutaneous RFA				29.7
Lermite et al[26]	2.0	Percutaneous RFA	90	54		
Abritabile et al[27]	3.1	Percutaneous RFA	88	57		4
Suppiah et al[28]	1.9	Percutaneous RFA	75	7		23.2
Siperstein et al[29]	2.8	Percutaneous RFA		20.2	18.4	24
Sorensen et al[30]	3.3	Percutaneous RFA	87	46		32
Terraz et al[31]	1.8	Percutaneous RFA	84			
Berber et al[32]	1.0	Laparoscopic RFA		20.6	30	20.5
Veltri et al[33]	1.6	Percutaneous RFA	79	38	22	31.5
Park et al[34]	1.2	Percutaneous RFA				36
Gleisner et al[35]	2.0	Resection + RFA	92.3	51.1	28.3	38.1
Lee et al[36]		RFA			46.5	40
Knudsen et al[37]		Percutaneous RFA		26	34	
Hur et al[38]		RFA		60	25.5	
Sofocleous et al[8]	1.4	Percutaneous RFA	91	41		31

TABLE 14-2 Results of Series Using Cryoablation for the Treatment of CLM

References	No. of Patients	Mean No. of Metastases	Follow- Up (Months)	1-Year Survival (%)	3-Year Survival (%)	5-Year Survival (%)	Median Survival
Korpan et al[43]	63	NA	60	NA	60	44	NA
Finlay et al[44]	75	2	NA	NA	80	NA	29
Gruenberger et al[45]	86	2	39	NA	83	NA	32
Sheen et al[46]	41	NA	NA	83	68	NA	32
Rivoire et al[47]	24	2.9	23	92	58	NA	39
Yan et al[48]	172	4.2	NA	89	41	19	28
Kerkar et al[49]	56	NA	54	NA	43	22	30
Brooks et al[50]	86	4	18	85	43	19	33
Seifert et al[51]	55	2.4	24	NA	NA	26	29
Chen et al[52]	61	3.38	16	87	NA	36	26
Niu et al[53]	124	4.1	NA	84	43	24	29
Paganini et al[54]	49	5.1	39.3	87	43	23	31
Bageacu et al[55]	53	2.6	NA	86	33	NA	NA
Kornprat et al[56]	20	1.7	21.1	NA	NA	NA	NA

TABLE 14-3 Results of Series Using Microwave Ablation for the Treatment of CLM

Author series	Mean No. of Metastases	1-Year Survival (%)	2-Year Survival (%)	3-Year Survival (%)	4-Year Survival (%)	5-Year Survival (%)	Median Survival (Months)
Seki et al[58]]	1.0						24.2
Shibata et al[59]	4.1	71		57		14	27
Liang et al[60]	2.0	91.4	60	46.4		29	20.5
Tanaka et al[61]	2.2	80		51		17	28
Ogata et al[62]	4.0					32	43

local control and for small tumors that can be ablated completely with clear margins, it may be able to provide results similar to those of surgery. In a systemic review of 36 series, the 1-, 3-, and 5-year survival rates for patients treated with RFA alone varied between 75%–93%, 7%–60%, and 18%–63%, respectively. Median survival ranged from 4 to 40 months and local recurrence rate ranged from 8% to 38%.[63] In general, it appears that smaller numbers of tumors, smaller size of treated tumors, absence of extrahepatic disease, and no involvement of the lymph nodes at initial excision as well as longer time between initial diagnosis to the development of liver metastasis correlate with best outcomes.[8,64]

IMAGING FOLLOW-UP OF ABLATION THERAPIES

Different approaches in measuring response rates developed, including the World Health Organization (WHO) criteria, the Response Evaluation Criteria in Solid Tumors (RECIST) and the Positron Emission Evaluation Response Evaluation Criteria in Solid Tumors (PERCIST).[65-67]

A well-recognized limitation of existing criteria for tumor response to treatment applies when evaluating response to any locoregional treatment. This is in particular the case for ablated tumor where the ablation zone is by definition larger than the target tumor. For the proper evaluation of response to treatment and the early detection of local tumor progression a postablation scan at 4–8 weeks is considered the new baseline for future comparisons. By definition, the ablation defect is larger than the treated tumor and any future comparisons to detect local tumor progression are made to this scan. Subsequent scans at 2–4 months are recommended to detect local, near local, and distant disease progression. The natural evolution of an ablation defect is depicted in Figure 14-1. Despite the use of positron emission tomography–computed tomography (CT) and implementation of the new PERCIST criteria[65-67] assessment of treatment response with ablation modalities still remains suboptimal. It would be useful if a new set of criteria could be implemented similarly to the proposed modified RECIST (mRECIST) criteria, recently described for the evaluation of treatment response of hepatocellular carcinoma.[68,69] Having said that, the concept of measuring viable tumor response in hepatocellular carcinoma by showing a significant change in tumor enhancement during the arterial phase of dynamic CT or magnetic resonance imaging (MRI) may be also applied for CLM. Although the enhancement pattern of CLM is different from that of HCC, a response to treatment and measurement of enhancing residual tumor versus nonenhancing treated CLM could be achieved by measuring Hounsfield units in the zone of ablation necrosis or in the territory of the targeted arterial distribution.

Arterially Directed Therapies

The concept of intraarterially directed liver therapies is based on the dual vascular supply to the liver where tumors are primarily fed by branches of the hepatic artery and normal parenchyma by the portal vein. The most common techniques of intraarterial therapies for CLM include hepatic arterial chemotherapy (HAC), transarterial chemoembolization (TACE), and systemic internal radiation therapy with yttrium-90-impregnated microspheres (SIRT). Two more therapies are available, namely, intraportal drug delivery and isolated liver perfusion, but these are still under preliminary evaluations; hence, they will not be discussed at present.

Such treatments have been used mostly as salvage therapies, after standard chemotherapy regimens fail. Interestingly, when used as adjunct with the chemotherapy agent that failed previously, response rates were high. These therapies have also been used as induction therapies in order to obtain a response and downstage a nonsurgical candidate to surgical thus improving the rates of cure.[70] In the following section, a brief description of these techniques will be given along with an overview of results in regards to overall response, patient survival and tumor free survival.

HEPATIC ARTERIAL CHEMOTHERAPY

This technique provides higher drug concentration in metastatic tumor deposits while minimizing the systemic effects of the chemotherapeutic agent. The advantage of this route is proportional

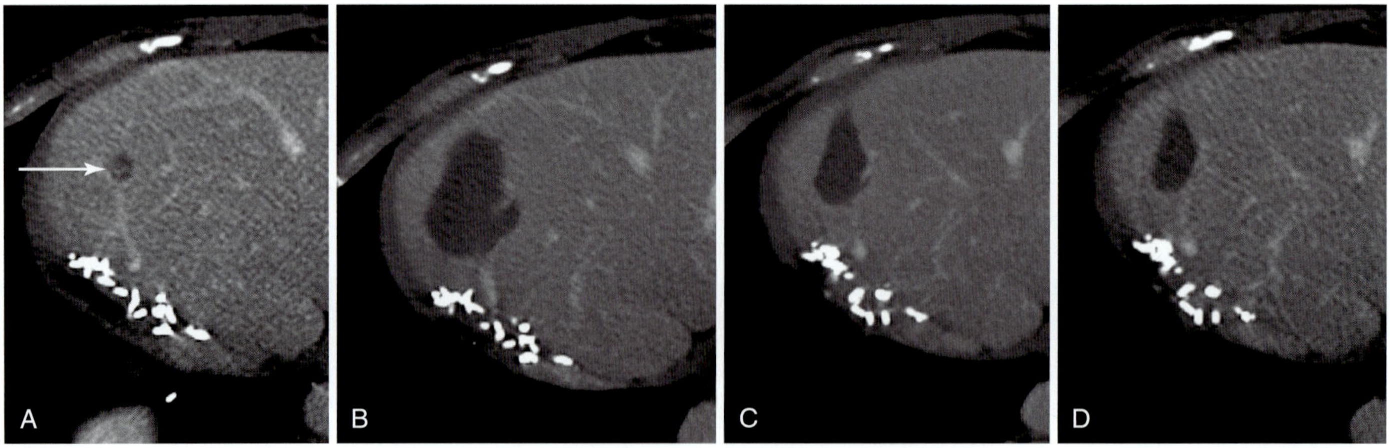

Figure 14-1 (A) 40-year-old female with a solitary liver metastasis after a partial hepatectomy. This new lesion was treated with radiofrequency ablation (not shown). (B) The ablation defect is larger than the ablated tumor as seen on the 4-week postablation CT scan, confirming successful treatment with good margins. (C) 12-month follow-up CT scan shows the ablation defect has decreased. (D) The ablation defect continued to decrease as seen on this follow-up CT scan at 32 months after treatment.

to the first pass extraction of the drug by the liver. HAC requires the percutaneous[71] or surgical[72] placement of a permanent intra-arterial catheter linked to a port. During surgical implantation of the device, the surgeon skeletonizes the hepatic arteries around the tip of the catheter placed at the origin of the gastroduodenal artery. This is done to prevent any extrahepatic delivery of the chemotherapeutic agent in the gastrointestinal tract. When no resection is anticipated, the device can be placed through minimal invasive techniques, replacing largely the need for open surgery or repeated catheterizations. After surgical ligation of arterial branches during HAC device placement, interventional radiologists may perform coil embolization of small arteries that can cause extrahepatic perfusion from undetected or recanalized branches.[73] This ensures remodeling of flow before the insertion of the indwelling catheter, so that there is only hepatopedal flow from the point where chemotherapy is released in a distribution that covers all the intrahepatic metastases and prevents the extrahepatic delivery of cytotoxic agents. Arteries that do not feed the liver, such as the right gastric and gastroduodenal, are routinely coil-embolized to avoid extrahepatic drug perfusion that might lead to gastrointestinal toxicity due to gastritis or formation of gastroduodenal ulceration.[74] This can occur when a small branch was not detected or recanalized after surgical ligation or coil embolization.

A Tc-99 macroalbumin aggregate (MAA) study after hepatic arterial pump placement is routinely performed to indicate that there is only hepatopedal flow without extrahepatic accumulation of tracer. In the event of extrahepatic accumulation of tracer, angiographic embolization may still correct the flow and salvage the intraarterial pump/catheter for safe chemotherapy administration.[73,75]

TRANSARTERIAL CHEMOEMBOLIZATION

There are several different techniques under the acronym TACE. The most common procedure has been the intraarterial injection of chemotherapy emulsified with Lipiodol Ultra-Fluid (LUF; Lab. Guerbet, Aulnay, France) followed by injection of embolic material. Lipiodol was first injected into the hepatic arteries in the early 1980s because of its capacity to target and remain fixed in tumors. LUF was first used as a diagnostic tool for the evaluation of disseminated hepatocellular carcinoma and then emulsified with various drugs for the treatment of liver tumors.[76] The emulsion produces oil drops in the arterial flow, and these drops have a propensity to go through the largest arteries (which are the tumor feeders) without entering the small ones due to surfactant properties of the oil drops.[77] Embolization after chemo-lipiodol increases the efficacy of treatment by providing additional ischemia to the highly hypervascularized tumor usually targeted with this treatment. Such embolization has been reported to induce failure of the transmembrane pump, thus increasing drug retention inside the cells.[78] More recently, gelatin spheres loaded with doxorubicin (drug-eluting beads [DEBs]) have been used for TACE in HCC. The use of DEBs which can be loaded with irinotecan (DEBIRI) was reported for the first time in 2006 for the treatment of CLM in clinical practice.[79] In the pre-DEBIRI era, several regimens have been used to deliver TACE. In one regimen, cisplatin, doxorubicin, mitomycin C, Ethiodol, and polyvinyl alcohol was used resulting in an overall response rate (ORR) of 43%, median survival of 33 months from initial diagnosis, 27 months from the time of liver metastases, and 9 months from the start of chemoembolization. This study suggested a possible improvement over historic reported survival time for systemic therapies alone.[80]

Another regimen using mitomycin C alone (52.5%), mitomycin C with gemcitabine (33%), or mitomycin C and irinotecan (14.5%) resulted in an ORR of 63%.[81] With the invention of DEBs and specifically DEBIRI for CLM, there is the advantage of reduced systemic delivery and thus toxicity of chemotherapy. DEBIRI administration resulted in a 75% reduction of the systemic plasma level when compared with direct intraarterial irinotecan only administration.[82]

Approximately 30% of TACE sessions are associated with adverse events during or after the treatment. Factors predictive of adverse events and significantly longer hospital length of stay are lack of pretreatment with hepatic arterial lidocaine ($P = 0.005$), more than three treatments ($P = 0.05$), achievement of complete stasis ($P = 0.04$), treatment with >100 mg DEBIRI in a single session treatment ($P = 0.03$), and initial bilirubin > 2.0 g/dL with >50% liver involvement ($P = 0.05$).[83] Table 14-4 summarizes the results of chemoembolization series for the treatment of CLM.[79-81,83-86]

TABLE 14-4 Results of Series Using Chemoembolization for the Treatment of CLM

Publication	No. of Metastases	Response Rate (SD, CR, PR)	PFS TTP (Months)	Downstaged	Survival: Median Months	Survival: 1-Year	Survival: 2-Year	Survival: 4-Year
Albert et al[80,*]]	121	43%	3	NA	9			
Vogl et al[81,*]	463	63		NA	14	62%	28%	
Martin et al[115,†]	55	66%	11	10%	19			
Aliberti et al[79,†]	82	78%		20%	25			
Fiorentini et al[84,†]	36	80%	7	22%	22		56%	15%
Telez et al[85,‡]	30	75%			8.6			
Wasser et al[86,‡]	21		5.8		13.8			

*TACE
†DEBIRI
‡other TACE
CR, complete response; PR, partial response; PFS, progression-free survival; SD, stable disease; TTP, time to progression.

RADIOEMBOLIZATION

Currently, two different Yttrium-90-microsphere (Y-90) products with a mean diameter of 20–35 μm are available: Theraspheres (Theragenics Corporation, Buford, GA) are glass microspheres and Sirspheres (Sirtex Sirspheres Pty Ltd, Lane Cove, Australia) are resin microspheres. Resin microspheres is the only device that has FDA approval for use in the treatment of CLM. Radioembolization delivers targeted radiation therapy to unresectable liver metastases by the injection of β-emitting isotope Y-90, which is bound to nondegradable microspheres into the arterial supply of the liver. These microspheres are unable to pass through the capillaries and are therefore trapped in the tumor. Y-90 is a pure β-emitter with a half-life of 64.1 hours (2.5 days) and tissue penetration of 2.5–11 mm, thus allowing immediate release of the patient after treatment without the risk of radiation exposure to others. The selective administration of Y-90 in the hepatic arterial branches feeding the tumors allow the delivery of high ionizing radiation doses to the tumor with tolerable exposure to the liver parenchyma.[87]

Indications for radioembolization include unresectable CLM, in patients without or minimal extrahepatic disease and life expectancy of at least 3 months. Selected patients must have an acceptable hepatic reserve as reflected by a bilirubin level lower than 2.0 mg/dL.

Once the patient is selected for radioembolization, the hepatic arterial supply must be determined and aberrant arteries identified and embolized. Similarly, arterial branches such as the right gastric and the gastroduodenal are embolized to prevent extrahepatic delivery of the Y-90 beads in the gastrointestinal tract. Once vessels are embolized and there is only hepatopedal flow from the desired point of future Y-90 injection, a simulation of the treatment is undertaken. This is performed with the injection of technetium-99 (^{99m}Tc) MAA in the hepatic artery exactly where the future Y-90 injection is anticipated.[88] Immediately after the injection of the ^{99m}Tc-MAA, the patient is transported to the nuclear medicine department, where a liver–lung scintigram is obtained. This study is performed to identify possible shunts from liver to lungs (Figure 14-2) or to the gastrointestinal system (Figure 14-3).

Identification of a noncorrectable lung shunt over 20% is considered an absolute contraindication for Y-90 administration to prevent radiation-induced pneumonitis. Shunts of 10%–20% (see Figure 14-2) require dose adjustment for safe delivery of the Y-90 without affecting the lungs.[88] Identification of gastrointestinal uptake (see Figure 14-3) may require repeat arteriography and embolization of the responsible arterial branch and sometimes modification of the planned treatment and repeat the ^{99m}Tc-MAA scintigram prior to Y-90 therapy to avoid toxicity. Radioembolization has mostly been used for the treatment of chemorefractory CLM.

In this setting, overall response of 17%–35% and stable disease rates of 24%–61% has been recorded.[89] Median survival after radioembolization in the salvage setting ranged from 6.7 to 17 months.[90] Table 14-5 represents overall survival after SIRT treatment in heavily pretreated patients with CLM.[89,91-94] The effects of radioembolization could be seen when it was used as a salvage monotherapy after complete chemotherapy failure. Radioembolization alone in this case showed an overall response of 24%, a progression-free survival of 3.7 months, and 1-, and 2-year survival rates of 50.4% and 19.6%, respectively.[95]

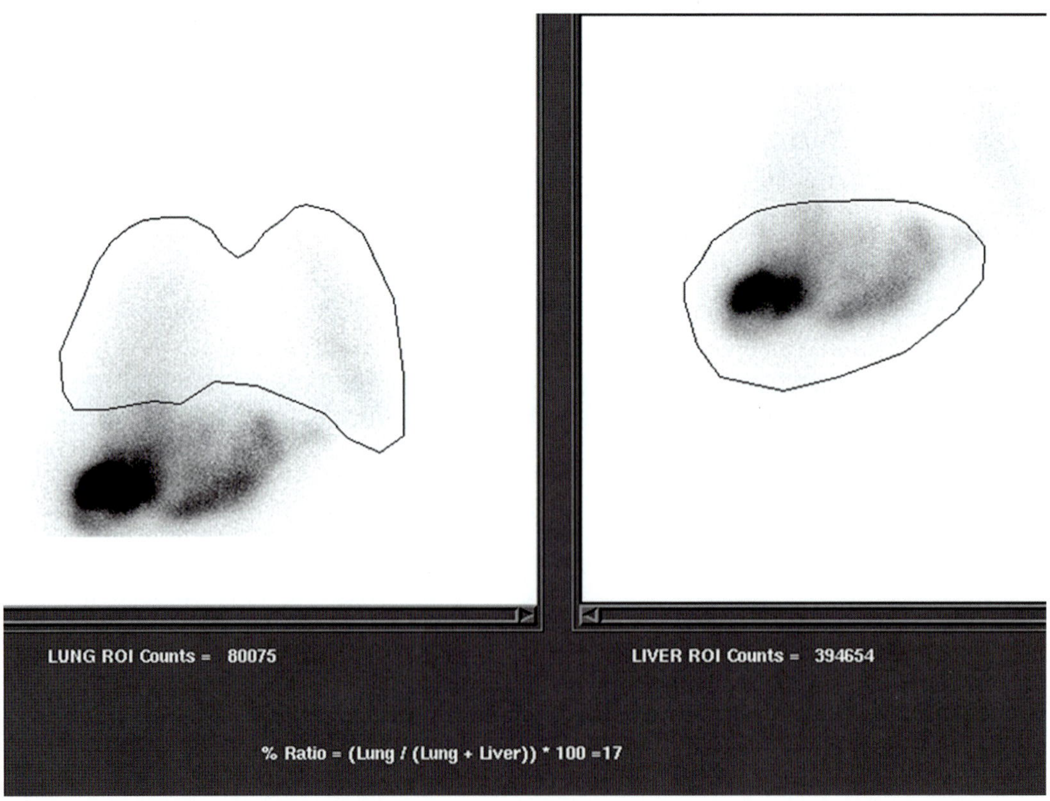

Figure 14-2 Hepatopulmonary shunting of 17% identified during scintigraphy using ^{99m}Tc-labeled MAA before radioembolization. This requires dose adjustment to prevent radiation-induced pneumonitis.

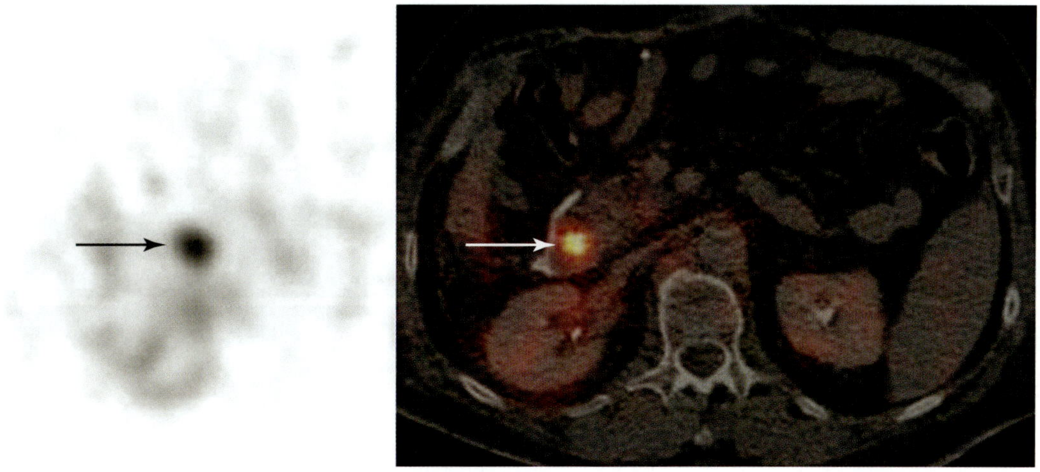

Figure 14-3 Gastrointestinal (duodenal) accumulation of ^{99m}Tc-labeled MAA during scintigraphy (*arrows*). This requires repeat mapping for identification and embolization of the vessel responsible for the extrahepatic perfusion and/or new plan for Y-90 administration. This must be done in order to safely deliver the Y-90 microspheres, without resulting in gastrointestinal toxicity as a result of nontarget radiation gastroenteritis or ulcers.

However, the best oncologic outcomes were recorded when radioembolization was used together with systemic chemotherapy. This is attributed to tumor radiosensitization by prior chemotherapy that maximizes response to radioembolization.[96] Figure 14-4 portrays an example of radiologic response in a patient treated with concomitant second-line chemotherapy.

Table 14-6 represents median overall patient survival after combination treatment of chemotherapy and SIRT.[97-101]

To date, there are only few small studies that compared SIRT with chemotherapy to chemotherapy alone. All of these studies showed that there is longer median progression-free survival; however, none has reached statistically significant prolongation of patient survival. The study by Gray et al.[98] was the first randomized controlled trial where Y-90 was administered via an intrahepatic arterial pump in combination with intraarterial floxuridine (FUDR) and compared to patients who received only the intrahepatic FUDR. The study demonstrated a significantly longer PFS in the group that received SIRTX with intrahepatic chemotherapy (15.9. months) when compared to the group treated with intrahepatic chemotherapy only (9.7 months). This difference was sufficient evidence for the FDA to approve SIRTX as a therapy for CLM at which point the study was terminated. The same study was accompanied with a prolonged survival in the combination group when compared to the intrahepatic chemotherapy only group; however, this difference did not reach statistical significance at the time of study discontinuation.

Discussion

Several factors have been correlated with survival in patients with unresectable CLM, and among them is the extent of liver involvement.[102] This suggests that liver-directed therapies could increase life expectancy while decreasing toxicity and mortality. In many cases, the liver is the only or the dominant site of

TABLE 14-5 Results of Series Using SIRT for the Treatment of CLM

		Response (%)		
Study/Series	No. of Patients	By CT	By PET	Median Overall Survival After Y-90 Treatment (Months)
Lewandowski et al[91,*]	27	35	88	9.3
Kennedy et al[89]	208	35		10.5†
Jakobs et al[92]	36	17	91	10.5
Mulcahy et al[93,*]	72	40	77	14.5
Cianni et al[94]	41	46		11.6

Note: Disease control rates include patients with complete response, partial response, or stable disease.
*Treated with Theraspheres.
†In responders (vs. 4.5 months in nonresponders).

TABLE 14-6 Results of Series Using Combination of Chemotherapy and SIRT for the Treatment of CLM

Authors/ Series	Number of Patients	Study Design	Median Overall Survival (Months)
van Hazel et al[97]	21	5-FU/LV with/ without Y-90	29.4
Gray et al[98]	74	Floxuridine HAC with/without Y-90	17
Hendlisz et al[99]	46	5-FU with or without Y-90	10
van Hazel et al[100]	25	5-FU/LV with/ without Y-90	12.2
Kosmider et al[101]	19	5-FU/LV or FOLFOX plus Y-90	37.8

CLM, colorectal metastases; 5-FU, 5-fluorouracil; FOLFOX = folinic acid, fluorouracil, and oxaliplatin [systemic chemotherapy regimen]; HAC, hepatic arterial chemotherapy; LV, leucovorin.

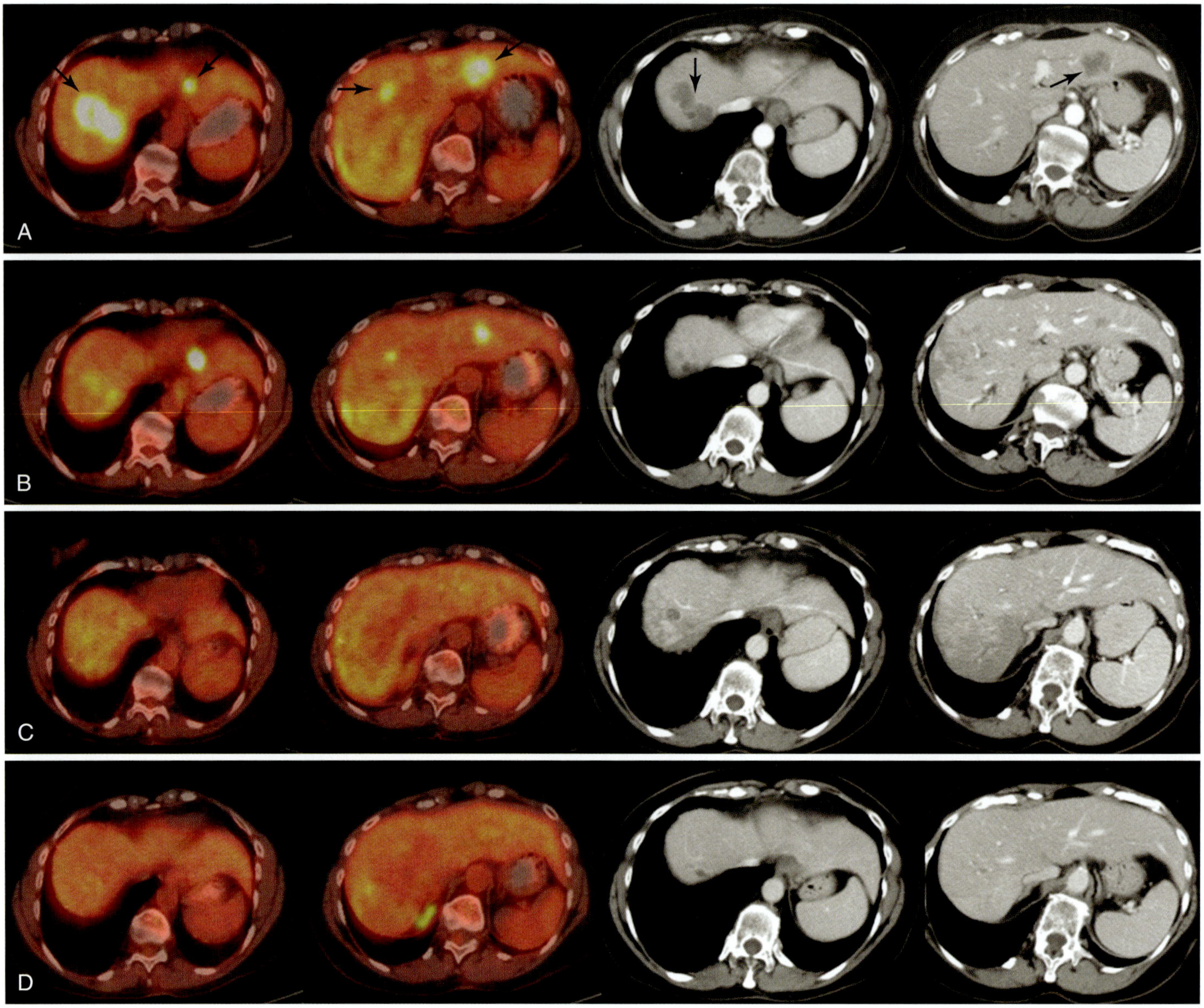

Figure 14-4 Fused PET/CT and PV phase CT images of a patient with metastatic colorectal cancer who underwent Y-90 radioembolization. (A, first row) Preprocedure imaging showing multifocal liver metastases (*arrows*). (B, second row) Four-week follow-up imaging shows decrease in size and FDG activity of hepatic metastases. (C, third row) Three-month and (D, fourth row) 6-month follow-up imaging shows further decrease in size and eventual resolution of FDG activity of treated liver metastases. It appears that radiologic response to Y-90 radioembolization may be better appreciated in scans obtained 3 months or more since treatment. PET/CT may give an earlier indication of response to this therapy.

disease. This, along with the dual vascular supply to liver, makes this organ ideal for arterially directed therapies to destroy the tumor while minimizing the toxic effect on uninvolved liver supplied by the portal vein.

Since the application of ablative therapies, an increased number of CLM have been controlled successfully with image-guided percutaneous ablation in selected nonresectable patients with limited number of small tumors.[7-9,64] Ablation has been accepted as an efficient therapy for local tumor control, especially for patients who cannot undergo resection or have tumor recurrence after surgery.[8]

When considering that image-guided ablation series included the patients that were not eligible for, or in whom the disease recurred after, surgery, the reported median survival of 36 months and 1-, 3-, and 5-year survival rates of 86%, 80%, and 24% compare well to the surgical historic data for CLM.[103] Similarly to surgery patients with favorable profile[104,105] such as those without extrahepatic disease, patients with less than five liver lesions, each smaller than 5 cm in the largest diameter reached significantly higher 5-year survival rates of 30% after RFA.[7] A relevant modification of the previously described clinical risk score (CRS)[104,105] was designed for patients undergoing salvage ablation to treat posthepatectomy recurrences.[8] Tumor size greater than 3 cm, lymph nodal infiltration at the time of resection, a disease-free interval from primary diagnosis to liver metastasis under 12 months, and more than one lesion were considered risk factors. Patients accumulating more than 2 of these factors were considered high risk and had worse outcomes than those with 0–2 factors (overall survival of 74% for CRS of 0–2 vs. 42% for CRS of 3–4 at 2 years; $P = 0.03$). Similarly, the local tumor progression-free survival was better for the low-risk patients (66% for CRS of 0–2 vs. 22% for CRS of 3–4 at 1 year after a single ablation; $P < 0.01$). Although there has not yet been a randomized controlled trial to compare surgery versus RFA for the treatment of CLM, small retrospective studies comparing the two modalities demonstrated comparable outcome for small lesions in similar small groups of patients.[38,106]

Using ablation for CLM within the test-of-time approach as proposed by Livraghi et al.[10] allows the treatment of surgical patients who subsequently are closely monitored with imaging for the early detection of progression. In this study, 58% of patients were spared unnecessary and morbid surgery either because they were completely treated by ablation alone or because they developed multifocal disease during the waiting period, rendering them unresectable. The subset of patients with local only progression was treated with repeat ablation or resection. This approach allows the disease to declare its true nature with regard to its ability to progress that is important and can be employed if and when a randomized controlled trial between surgery and local ablation is ever possible. Complete ablation or A_0 ablation as determined by imaging can be discrepant with residual microscopic disease remaining undetected at the site of the ablation defect.[107] This is because unlike surgery, marginal analysis and tissue sampling from the ablation zone is not routinely performed. This may also in part explain the relatively higher rates of progression after RFA when compared to surgery. This is supported by studies that analyzed the tissue extracted on the electrode after liver tumor RFA[108,109] that correlated the identification of residual prolific[110] or viable tumor cells[111] with local tumor progression[110,111] as well as overall patient survival.[112] These studies certainly support the incorporation of tissue sampling routinely after liver tumor ablation similarly to surgery. The identification of residual tumor at the ablation zone before its radiologic detection may allow for additional locoregional or systemic treatment that can improve oncologic outcomes after CLM ablation.

Recent publications have shown that similarly to surgery,[113] local tumor control depends on appropriate technique and creation of sufficient margins around the target tumor.[12-15] These data suggest that curative ablation should not be offered unless the creation of sufficient margins around the tumor is feasible.

Arterially directed therapies such as HAC, TACE, and SIRT take advantage of the unique dual vascular supply of the liver. They all deliver cytotoxic drugs or agents via the arterial tree to the tumor aiming to maximize their tumoricidal effect while minimizing the toxicity to the rest of the organ and the systemic circulation. All of these therapies can be used as an adjunct to systemic chemotherapy in an attempt to downsize unresectable liver metastases to resection in the hopes of a definite cure for selected patients with liver only diseases.[80] In particular, HAC and SIRT have reported a fraction of treated patients being downstaged to resection. Both HAC and SIRT have also been associated with best oncologic outcomes when combined with earlier lines of systemic chemotherapy.[98]

Earlier series of TACE with several chemotherapeutic agents indicated that chemoembolization may offer some benefit in the control of CLM in particular for those patients who progressed through prior lines of systemic chemotherapy.[79,80]

The recent development of DEBIRI directly in the CLM is very interesting and shows initial promise. A very recent randomized controlled trial by Fiorentini et al. demonstrated that DEBIRI in combination with FOLFIRI offered a statistically significant prolongation of the progression-free survival and more importantly the overall survival of patients with CLM.[84] This study sets the stage for more similar trials to prove the value of arterially directed therapies for nonresectable CLMs and those unsuitable for ablation.

SIRT with impregnated Y-90 beads is another new therapy that essentially delivers very high doses of radiation directly in the tumor via the arterial tree. Several series have shown the efficacy of this treatment that is now accepted in the salvage setting when systemic chemotherapy has failed to control CLM.[91,95]

Similarly to DEBIRI, several series have indicated that SIRT in combination with different systemic regimens prolongs the progression-free survival (statistically significant data) and may prolong survival (no statistical significance has been reached yet).[97-99,101]

All these data show that currently there are several intraarterial therapies for the patient with CLM that cannot be resected or ablated. The selection of the best therapy for each patient remains controversial and certainly requires multidisciplinary discussion and cooperation. SIRT has the advantage of a limited recovery time allowing the patient to be discharged the same day.

It carries a risk, however, for radiation-induced liver disease that can occur up to 4 months after therapy.[114] In addition, SIRT requires a preparatory arteriogram for proper preparation and detailed dose calculation that is not required by TACE.

On the other hand, TACE with or without DEBIRI is associated with postembolization syndrome requiring a short stay in the hospital for supportive care. One point that should be kept in mind is that one type of therapy does not preclude the use of another treatment. Therefore, if local progression is documented at short time after one arterially directed therapy, one might consider the use of a different arterially directed treatment.

This manuscript was undertaken with the intention to give an overview of the interventional therapies available for the treatment of CLM. As such, we performed a relatively concise description and discussion of the most commonly used image-guided, interventional treatments and have provided most of the relevant references. We would like to close by stating that we, like many others in the field, aspire that Interventional Oncology may have reached the point to be considered the fourth pillar in oncology along with medical, surgical, and radiation oncology. This is in particular the case when it comes to the management of CLM.

REFERENCES

The complete reference list is available online at www.expertconsult.com.

15

Gastroenteropancreatic Neuroendocrine Tumors

RAVI MURTHY | SANJAY GUPTA | ALEXANDRIA T. PHAN | JAMES C. YAO

KEY POINTS

- Incidence and prevalence of GEP-NET is increasing.
- Recently approved systemic targeted therapeutic agents and local therapies have rekindled interest in NET management.
- Multidisciplinary centers employing a myriad of tumor therapies including strategies of image-guided techniques are poised to play a significant role in the management of these complex patients.

Introduction

The neuroendocrine system exists in two phenotypes, either as (1) discreet organoid aggregates (pituitary, adrenal, parathyroid) or as (2) disseminated, nonuniform distribution of cells, This latter group has been assigned the term *diffuse neuroendocrine system* (DNES; e.g., enterochromaffin cells in the gut mucosa, Merkel cells in the dermis). Collectively, the neuroendocrine system forms the largest group of hormone-producing cells in the body.

Neuroendocrine neoplasms/tumors (NET) once considered "rare" have been steadily increasing in incidence and prevalence over the past 3 decades. In fact, over the last 32 years (1973–2005), the incidence has increased 520% translating to an annual increase of 5.8%.[1,2] In 2011, it is estimated that approximately 18,000 cases and 8200 deaths will occur from NET in the United States alone (not just GEP-NET).[3] Analysis of the SEER database encompassing the period 2003–2007 reveals that NET incidence and prevalence was 5.76/100,000 and 35/100,000, respectively, in 2004, These increases may represent a reflection of the increasing awareness and diagnostic capabilities over the same time period.

DNES NETs occur most frequently in the lung and gastro-entero-pancreatic (GEP) regions. NETs currently represent 2% of all cancers and GEP-NETs represent the second most prevalent gastrointestinal neoplasm after colorectal cancer.[4] GEP-NETs are most common in the small intestine (30.8%), followed by rectum (26.3%), colon (17.6%), pancreas (12.1%), stomach (8.9%), and appendix (5.7%) (Figure 15-1).

When compared to GE-NETs, pancreatic NETs (P-NETs) possess different patterns of underlying genetic defects that lead to malignant transformation. For GE-NETs, the cell of origin is believed to be the enterochromaffin cell, whereas for P-NETs it appears to be pluripotent cells in the pancreatic duct epithelium.[5] This fundamental difference combined with differing natural histories, management, response to therapy(s), clinical course, and worse prognosis than GE-NETs leads many investigators to consider P-NETs as a distinct tumor entity.[1] P-NETs account for less than 2% of all pancreatic cancers, with 50%–90% of these tumors being nonfunctional, meaning they are not associated with any hormone-related clinical syndrome, the so-called non-syndromic.[6] The prevalence of these occult NETs is corroborated by the higher incidence of P-NET at autopsy studies ranging from 0.8% to 10%.[7,8] The incidence of P-NET from the SEER database was 0.22/100,000.[9]

The clinical manifestations of this relatively uncommon disease are protean and nonspecific, thereby leading to alternative diagnoses and the average lag between first symptoms and diagnosis of NET of about 7 years.[2] It is therefore understandable that 60%–80% have metastases at presentation, with the liver being the most common distant metastatic site.[10] An important consequence of metastases, the "carcinoid syndrome" (diarrhea, abdominal pain, sweating, flushing, bronchospasm, tachycardia, and fibrotic heart disease), develops in 7%–10% with GE-NET and 35%–50% of those with hepatic metastases[11] (Table 15-1). Pancreatic neuroendocrine tumors can also be associated with clinical syndromes associated with hormone release[12-16] (Table 15-2). There has been a gradual increase of the incidence or reporting of stomach and rectal NETs and a decrease in that of appendicular NETs.[1,17] The increasing burden of disease coupled with new therapies have increased the awareness of this disease and rekindled interest in exploring the benefits of intervention in GEP-NETs.

DEFINITION

Neuroendocrine tumors consist of a heterogeneous group of cells that have both phenotypical and biochemical characteristics of neural and endocrine cells and the potential for malignancy. These bicameral cells must satisfy three criteria to qualify as being of neuroendocrine origin: (1) absence of axons, (2) production of neurotransmitter/neuromodulator hormones, and (3) membrane-bound vesicles from which these hormones are released by a process of regulated exocytosis in response to external stimuli.[18] The substances that can be considered to arise from neural tissue are chromogranins A, B, and C; neuron-specific enolase; and neural cell adhesion molecule CD56[19,20] and biogenic amines.[21]

BACKGROUND

The recognition that single or clusters of hormone-producing chromium-staining cells were present in the intestine was described in 1868 by Heidenhain[22] and later confirmed by Kulchitsky, The first case of intestinal NET was recorded by Langhans[23] and also in an autopsy in two patients by Lubarsch.[24] Ransom described a patient with ileal cancers

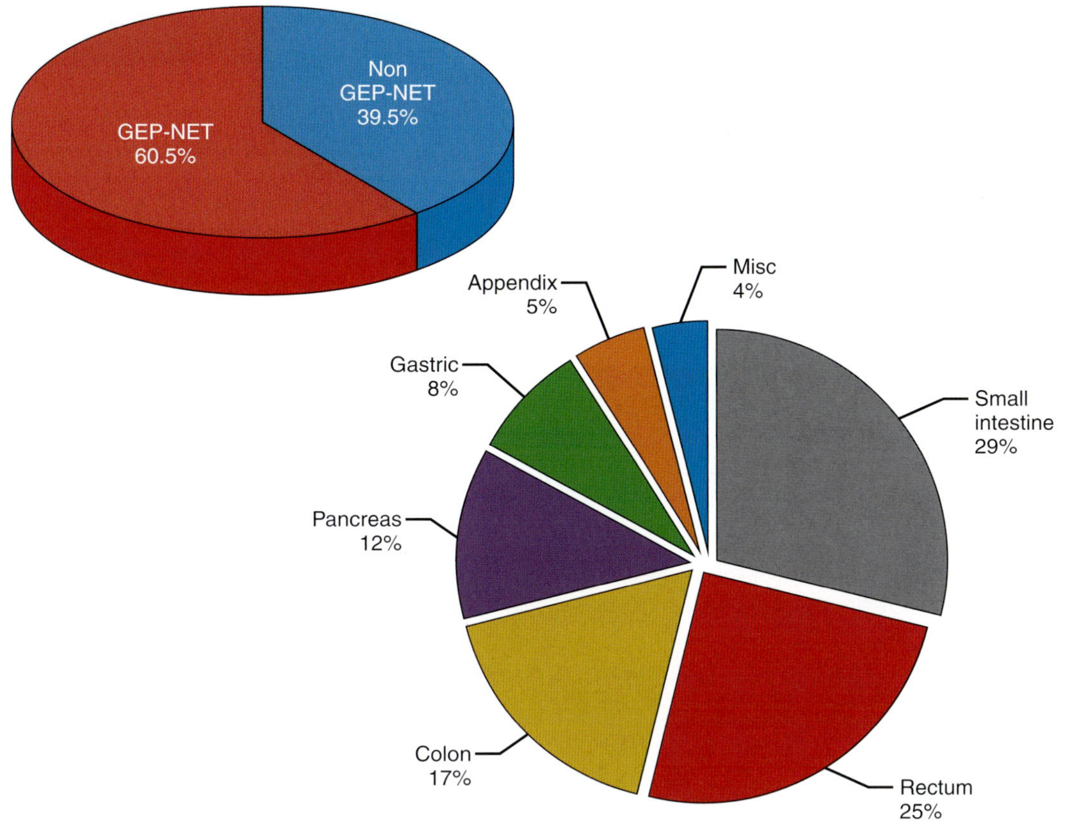

Figure 15-1 Neuroendocrine neoplasms, Surveillance Epidemiology and End Results (SEER) 1973–2007. GEP neuroendocrine neoplasms constitute 2% of all malignancies. *(Adapted from Modlin, et al.: The archaic distinction between functioning and nonfunctioning neuroendocrine neoplasms is no longer clinically relevant,* Langerbecks Arch Surg *396:1145–1156, 2011.)*

TABLE 15-1 Gastro-Enteric NET Clinical Entities

Location	Dominant Location	Syndrome	Clinical Caveats
Stomach	Fundus	No	80% Type 1-ECL cell origin. F>>M. Associated Chronic atrophic gastritis. Multifocal polyps <1cm. Benign.
	Fundus	Zollinger Ellison	6% Type 2 - ECL cell origin. Associated with MEN-1.
	Antrum	No	29% Type 3 - Poorly differentiated. Metachronous Gastric AdenoCA 5-10%. M>F, 5th decade, Metachronous metastases.
Duodenum & Proximal Jejunum	Proximal Duodenum	Zollinger Ellison	G Cell origin. 70% of all Gastrinomas occur in duodenum; 90% occur in 1st & 2nd portion → 50% of Duodenal Gastrinoma are associated with ZES → 20–30% of these are associated with MEN-1.
	Ampullary Periampullary	Somatostatinoma	D cell origin. 14–43% associated with NF1
	Periampullary	No	Triphasic lineage. Gangliocytic Paraganglioma. Rare
Distal Jejunum & Ileum	Ileocecal valve region	Seritonoma	EC cell origin. Multicentric NET 30%. Metachronous Colorectal Cancer 39%. Mesenteric fibrosis → Bowel or Venous Obstruction Carcinoid syndrome if 1) Liver metastases 2) Porto-systemic venous drainage
Appendix	Tip >> Base	Seritonoma	EC cell origin. Goblet cell type more aggressive.
Colorectal	Rectum>Ascending > Cecum> Sigmoid	Rare	L Cell origin. Higher incidence Synch/Metachronous Non-NET CA. Rectal NET 80%<0.6cm median. Rectum 50%, Ascending 22%, Cecum 11% , Sigmoid 10.5%.

with extensive metastases who experienced diarrhea and dyspnea after eating possibly was the first description of the carcinoid syndrome.[25] The eponym of "karkinoide tumoren," or "carcinoid," was coined by Oberndorfer in 1907[26] after recognizing this as a discrete disease entity. Nicholls described the first pancreatic islet cell tumor in 1902.[27] In the early 20th century, special silver stains were used by Masson and Gossett[28,29] to demonstrate the argentaffin and argyrophilic properties of these tumors that appeared to have a neural origin. They suggested that the cell of origin was the

TABLE 15-2 **Pancreatic NET Clinical Entities**

	Tumor	Average Size cm	Typical Phenotype "Sporadic" Type Distribution	Clinical Caveats
α	Glucagonoma	3–7	Solitary Large/Tail	Uncommon. 60% Metachronous metastases. 5 yr Survival 50–60%. 8–13% Syndrome of "4D's"[1]
β	Insulinoma	0.5-2	Solitary 85% / Uniform	Commonest PNET. 4–7% Associated with MEN-1. 90% Benign, 5 yr Survival 97% Whipple's Triad[4] Pre-resection localization mandatory.
δ	Somatostatinoma	Large	Solitary Large / Head	Rare; <5%. 70–92% Metachronous metastases. 5 yr Survival 60–75%. Non-specific Syndrome[5]
G	Gastrinoma	2	Solitary / Head	2nd most common PNET. 50% Metachronous metastases. Zollinger-Ellison Syndrome[6]. 90% in "Gastrinoma Triangle"[2]. Enucleation Rx
VIP	VIPoma	Large	Solitary Large / Tail	Rare; 3–8%. 5% Associated with MEN-1. Verner-Morrison Syndrome[3]

1 – Diabetes, dermatitis, Deep Vein Thrombosis, Depression[3]
2 – Triangle created by the 3 angles —1. Pancreas body/neck 2. 2nd/3rd portion of duodenum 3. Cystic & Common bile duct
3 – Profuse watery diarrhea. Water, sodium, chloride, potassium loss.[5]
4 – Hypoglycemia symptoms. Low plasma glucose. Symptom resolution with glucose adminstration.[6]
5 – Diabetes, malabsorption, steatorrhea, cholelithiasis, anemia, achlorhydria[8]
6 – Triad-peptic ulcer, gastric acid hypersecretion & non-β cell pancreas tumor[9]

enterochromaffin cell, previously described by Kulchitshy in 1897, from the crypts of Leiberkuhn.[28,30] The concept that the DNES was composed of these argentaffin-positive and argyrophilic-clear cells was introduced by Feyrter in 1938.[31] Many of these cells have the capacity for the uptake and decarboxylation of precursors of biogenic amines and were referred to as "APUD" (amine precursor uptake and decarboxylation)[32] and were initially hypothesized to arise from the neural crest; this theory was subsequently disproved.[33] In 1953, Lembeck described the production of serotonin in carcinoid tumors[34] and in 1955 Page demonstrated the association of increased urinary 5-hydroxyindoleacetic acid (5-HIAA) in carcinoid syndrome.[35] The malignant carcinoid syndrome was described originally by Cassidy in 1934,[36] and one of the first detailed descriptions of the carcinoid syndrome was described in a patient who was dying from a clinical syndrome that included flushing, diarrhea, edema, wheezing, and right-sided heart failure.[37] Pathology demonstrated the presence of fibrotic subendocardial plaques In 1953, enterochromaffin cell secretion of serotonin was confirmed.[38]

CARCINOID SYNDROME

Carcinoid heart disease occurs in up to 50%–60% of patients with the carcinoid syndrome.[39] This system complex represents the clinical manifestation of serotonin, and tachykinin release that occurs in 20% of G1/2 NETs of the jejunum and ileum. Specific signs and symptoms in descending order of frequency are dry flushing with or without palpitations (70%), diarrhea (50%), intermittent abdominal pain (40%), lacrimation, and rhinorrhea. Wheezing and pellagra are uncommon. More recent reports have suggested that the incidence of carcinoid heart disease has declined, perhaps because of the introduction of somatostatin analogs and other antitumor therapies designed to reduce the tumor load and the production of vasoactive products.[40]

CARCINOID CRISIS

This GE-NET–associated entity has been characterized as profound flushing, bronchospasm, tachycardia, and rapidly fluctuating blood pressure, These paroxysms are usually precipitated by anaesthesia induction, handling of tumor, embolization, or radiofrequency ablation (RFA). To counterbalance these events, short-acting octreotide is used as a constant infusion of 50 μg/hour initiated 12 hours before and given 24–48 after intervention.[41] Short-acting 100–500 μg octreotide administered intravenously (IV) is followed by continuous infusion. These events can occur in nonsyndromic patients also; therefore, prophylactic octreotide is recommended in these patients as well.

CLASSIFICATION

The biologic complexity, functional diversity, low incidence, and nonuniform distribution of these cells have resulted in NET being recategorized on multiple occasions as new information has become available over the last 3 decades. Early attempts were made based on their histologic, biochemical, and clinical characteristics that paralleled their embryologic origin into foregut, midgut, and hindgut "carcinoid tumors."[42] Those approaches failed to provide prognostic and therefore therapy guidance. To better predict biologic behavior, the WHO introduced a classification for GE-NET[43] in 2000 and in 2004 for PNEN[44] that allowed for prognostic stratification and adjusted treatment[45,46] along with a standardized diagnostic procedure[20]; this has been validated for P-NET and foregut NET. The American Joint Committee on Cancer (AJCC)/International Union Against Cancer (UICC) tumor–node–metastasis (TNM) classification differs from the European Neuroendocrine Tumor Society (ENETS) system.[47,48] In the second half of 2010, a revised version of the WHO classification appeared for GEP-NETs.[49] From a prognostic standpoint, the division between functional and nonfunctional tumors has no clinical significance.[50] Nonfunctioning tumors typically present as larger masses detected by the appearance of an abdominal mass, pain, weight loss, or obstructive jaundice.

HEREDITARY SYNDROMES

Four autosomal dominant disorders are known to be associated with GEP-NETs (Table 15-3). Collectively, they account for less than 1% of all GEP-NETS. Their importance lies in the fact that they usually manifest at ages 2 decades earlier compared to the sporadic variety. Patients often have multiple synchronous G1/2 foci and have a family history. Nearly all patients harbor occult NETs at autopsy.[51] The multifocality poses contradictions while attempting to resect the disease and as such many are considered unresectable at diagnosis. Medical management and family screening are paramount in theses cases.

TABLE 15-3 Hereditary Syndromes

Hereditary Syndrome	Tumor	Percent Association	Incidence Million per year
MEN-1[56,140,141]	Insulinoma	5	1-2
	Gastrinoma	25–40	1-2
	Glucagonoma	10	0.1
	VIPoma	5	0.1
	Somatostatinoma	45	<0.1
	"Non-Syndromic"	20	1-2
VHL[56]	"Non-Syndromic" Islet or Ductal	10–17%	-
NF-1[56]	Insulinoma	<10%	-
Tuberous Sclerosis[56]	Somatostatinoma	<1%	-

Grade and Stage

Determining the cellular characteristics of NET is central to determining an appropriate therapeutic approach. There are about 17 different types of neuroendocrine cells of the DNES residing in the GEP system.[4] Each cell secretes a dominant chemical (Figure 15-2). GEP-NETs are distributed asymmetrically and are clustered at the gastric fundus, proximal duodenum, papilla of Vater, terminal ileum, tip of appendix, lower rectum[52] (Figure 15-3).

Tumors should be classified according to the recent WHO 2010 classification, which has been based on the recently validated concept that all NETs have malignant potential. Grading is based on morphologic criteria seen on light microscopy with conventional staining (mitoses and necrosis) and proliferative activity performed via immunohistochemistry (Ki-67) (Table 15-4).

Staging is in accordance with AJCC/UICC TNM 7th edition and ENETS criteria for stomach, pancreas, and appendix (Table 15-5). NETs may have mixed adenocarcinoma elements. The rate of proliferation can be quantified by counting the number of mitoses per field and the percentage of

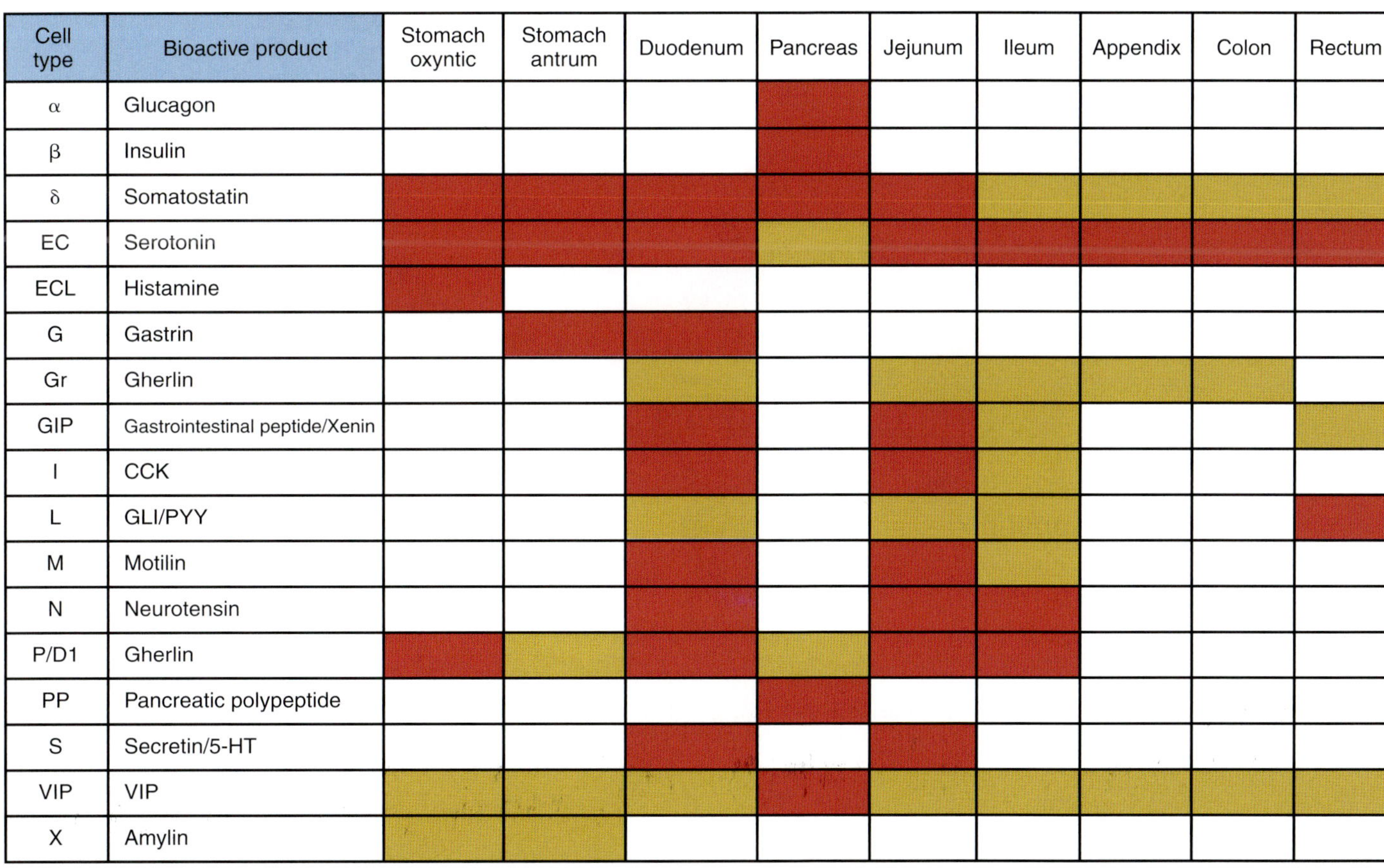

Figure 15-2 GEP-NET cell types, products and distribution. Red: abundant; yellow: present; white: sparse/absent. *(From Schimmack, et al.: The diversity and commonalities of gastroenteropancreatic neuroendocrine tumors [table 1],* Langenbecks Arch Surg *396:273–298, 2001.)*

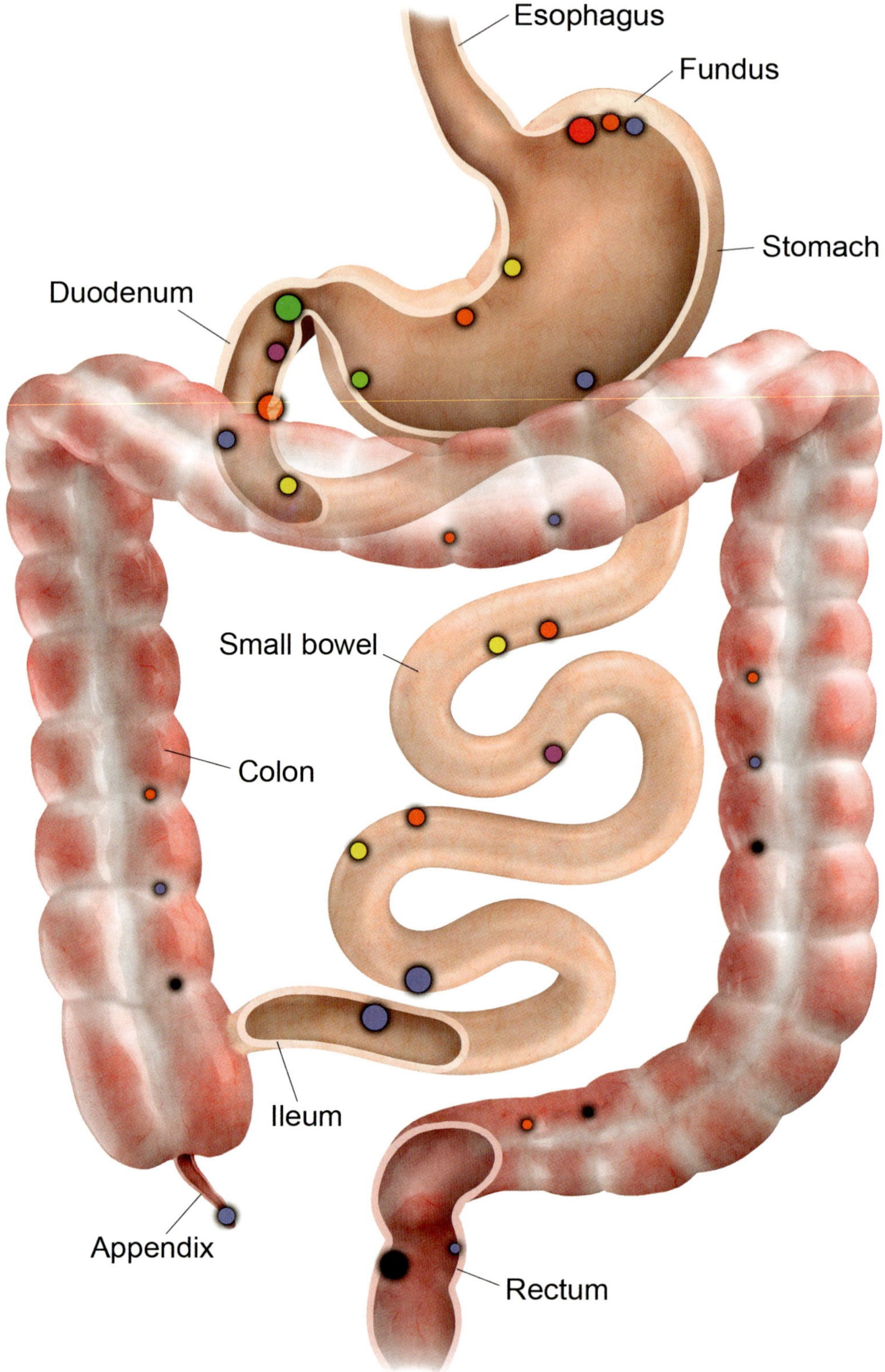

Figure 15-3 Relative distribution and proportion of GE-NET. Red: ECL; green: G cell; orange: D cell; blue: EC cell; black: L cell; yellow: PD1 cell; purple: S cell. Relative diameter of circle directly proportional to the incidence of type.

TABLE 15-4 WHO 2010 Grading System

Differentiation	Grade	Mitotic count	Ki-67 Index	ENETS/WHO
Well	Low (G1)	< 2 / 10 HPF	< 3%	NET Grade 1
	Intermediate (G2)	2–20 / 10 HPF	3%–20%	NET Grade 2
Poor	High (G3)	> 20 / 10 HPF	> 20%	NET Grade 3

Note: Mitotic index: counted in 10 high-power fields (10 HPF = 2 mm^2 in 40 fields at 400×), Ki 67: percent positive in 2000 cells in area of highest nuclear labeling.

TABLE 15-5 Staging of GEP NET

	Stage	TNM	T	Definition
Pancreas NET	Stage 0	Tis N0 M0	TX	Primary Tumor can not be assessed
			T0	No evidence of primary tumor
			Tis	Carcinoma in-situ
	Stage IA	T1 N0 M0	T1	Limited to pancreas, ≤ 2cm greatest dimension
	Stage IB	T2 N0 M0		
	Stage IIA	T3 N0 M0		
		T1 N1 M0		
	Stage IIB	T2 N1 M0	T2	Limited to pancreas, > 2cm greatest dimension
		T3 N1 M0		
	Stage III	T4 Any N M0	T3	Extends beyond pancreas, without involvement of celiac axis or superior mesenteric artery
	Stage IV	Any T Any N M1	T4	Involves celiac axis or the superior mesenteric artery

	Stage	TNM	T					
GE NET	Stage 0	Tis* N0 M0	TX	Primary Tumor cannot be assessed				
			T0	No evidence of primary tumor				
			Tis	**Stomach** - Carcinoma in-situ/dysplasia (<0.5mm), intra-mucosal				
	Stage I	T1 N0 M0		**Stomach**	**Small Intestine**	**Colon**		**Ampullary**
			T1	≤ 1cm	≤ 1cm	A < 1cm	B 1-2cm	≤ 1cm
				And Lamina propria ***Or*** submucosa invasion				
	Stage IIA	T2 N0 M0	T2	> 1cm	> 1cm	> 2cm		> 1cm
				Or Muscularis propria invasion				
	Stage IIB	T3 N0 M0						
				Stomach	**Jejunum or Ileum**	**Duodenum**	**Colon**	Invasion of Pancreas, non peritonealized tissues ***or*** Retro-peritoneum
	Stage IIIA	T4 N0 M0			Subserosal Invasion			
			T3	N/A	***And*** No penetration of overlying serosa ***or*** Non-peritoneal invasion	***And*** Invasion of Pancreas, Non-peritonealized tissues ***or*** Retro-peritoneum	***Or*** into non-peritonealized pericolic ***or*** perirectal tissues	
	Stage IIIB	AnyT N1 M0						
	Stage IV	Any T Any N M1	T4	Visceral peritoneum ***or*** other organs invasion				

	Stage	TNM	T	Definition
Appendix NET	Stage I	T1 N0 M0	TX	Primary Tumor can not be assessed
			T0	No evidence of primary tumor
			T1A	≤ 1cm greatest dimension
			T1B	≥ 1cm but < 2cm in greatest dimension
	Stage II	T2, T3 N0 M0	T2	≥ 2cm but < 4cm ***Or*** extends to cecum
		T4 N0 M0		
	Stage IIIA	AnyT N1 M0	T3	> 4cm ***Or*** extends to ileum
	Stage IV	Any T Any N M1	T4	Invades adjacent organs or structures

From *AJCC Cancer Staging Handbook*, ed 7, New York, 2010, Springer.

cells that stain positive with Ki-67 antibody, which is the cardinal feature of tumor grading[53] and has 5-year survival prognostication.[54,55] Difficulty sometimes arises in distinguishing benign from malignant behavior, and the presence of adjacent organ invasion, distant metastases, and lymph node involvement often are used to determine malignancy.

BIOCHEMISTRY

Different granules store individual peptide hormones; however, several peptides of amines may colocalize in the same granule. These secretory products allow for both serologic diagnosis, prognosis, and follow-up. The absence of a marker does not indicate absence of tumor.

Chromogranin A (CgA) is a water-soluble acidic glycoprotein stored in the secretory granules of neuroendocrine cells and can be used as a tumor marker regardless of hormone-related symptoms.[56] CgA is sensitive but nonspecific and can be elevated in some other cancers. CgA levels have been found to correlate with tumor burden and may be used to monitor treatment.[57] A CgA level reduction of >80% is predictive of symptom relief and disease control following surgery. CgA may not be elevated in insulinoma, and measurement of C peptide or proinsulin is helpful in this instance. Fasting serial blood glucose analysis is the gold standard diagnostic tool. CgA and gastrin are elevated in gastrinoma and an EGD with biopsy is usually needed to differentiate gastrinoma from atrophic gastritis. Rectal tumors do not secrete CgA.

Pancreatic polypeptide is found in high concentrations in 50%–80% of P-NETs and >30% of GE-NETs. Measurement of serotonin in plasma has been problematic, and the breakdown product 5-HIAA has been used, that is, as a 24-hour collection of urinary 5-HIAA; overnight 5-HIAA may be as sensitive.[58] False-positive results may be encountered with the ingestion of tryptophan-containing foods.

IMAGING

Endoscopy is the investigation of choice for suspected gastric, duodenal, and colorectal NETs. Endoscopic ultrasonography (EUS) can assess the depth of invasion and guide biopsy.[59,60] Computed tomography (CT) is most useful when suspicion for small bowel NET exists.[61,62] CT may not detect the primary disease, but it is useful for assessment of mesenteric disease, lymphadenopathy, and liver disease; CT enteroclysis is more sensitive for detection of bowel lesions of 85% and 97%, respectively.[63] Capsule endoscopy is usually reserved when other techniques have failed because it is often unable to determine the location of the pathology.[64]

Functional P-NETs are usually picked up earlier than nonfunctional ones. Resection may be curative, so accurate localization is important using a combination of imaging techniques. Multidetector CT may detect 94% of all insulomas and when combined with EUS this approaches 100%. Magnetic resonance imaging (MRI) is equivalent to CT for pancreatic lesions. EUS is very useful for demonstrating multiplicity in multiple endocrine neoplasia type 1 (MEN-1) and von Hippel-Lindau syndrome (VHL) and in deciding changes to disease management, for example, enucleation versus pancreaticoduodenectomy.[65-67] Intraoperative ultrasonography is a useful adjunct to intraoperative palpation of the gland and assessment of the liver.[68] Intraarterial calcium stimulation with hepatic venous sampling may be useful for localizing occult gastrinomas and insulinomas.[69-71]

Seventy percent to 90% of GEP-NETs express somatostatin receptors (SSTR) with dominant 2 and 5 subtypes. Somatostatin receptor scintigraphy (SRS) based on utilization of indium 111 diethylene triamine-penta-acetic acid (DTPA)-D-Phe-octreotide (^{111}In pentetreotide; Octreoscan Mallinckrodt Medical BV, Petten, Netherlands) is superior to standard imaging modalities in the detection of primary tumors and their metastases, with a median detection rate of 89%.[72] SRS is indicated when the primary lesion has not been detected by other cross-sectional imaging methods or to assist with staging.[73] It is also indicated when contemplating therapeutic SRS or somatostatin analogue therapy. In a study designed to understand the relative contribution when MRI, CT, and SRS SPECT-CT are done sequentially compared to the gold standard of surgery or liver biopsy. MRI detected 190 liver metastases missed by SRS and 69 missed by spiral CT. Therefore, MRI is the single most useful method in assessing hepatic metastatic tumor burden from NETs.[74]

THERAPY

General principles of therapy are to attempt curative intent resection whenever possible, but given the natural history of the disease, therapy is mostly palliative (Figure 15-4). Maintaining quality

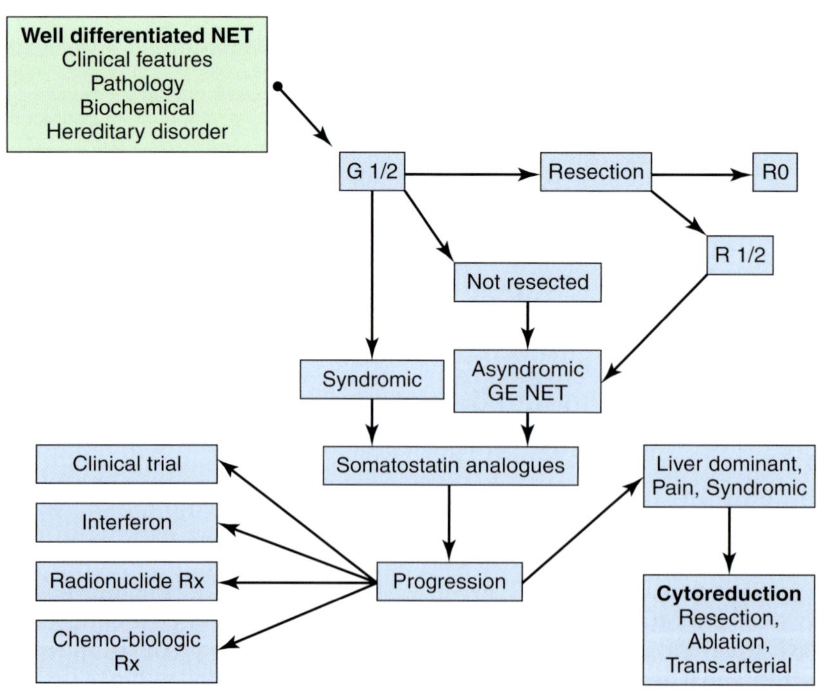

Figure 15-4 General schema of the management of NET.

of life in these circumstances becomes paramount and optimal management requires a multidisciplinary approach. In general, when the tumor size is less than 2 cm (exception appendix <1 cm), the disease is considered to have a high chance of cure after resection because the likelihood of metastases is low. However, about 46%–93% of patients with NET will have hepatic metastases at the time of diagnosis[75] and more than half of them will have 50% of their liver replaced.[76] Therefore, in GEP-NET resection is only possible in 10% of patients.[77] In this circumstance, the 5-year survival is 0%–20%[78,79] compared to the typical postresection 5-year survival of 60%–80%[80,81] Noncurative, resection should be undertaken only if the debulking is more than 90%.[82] In fact, the Cochrane database concluded that resection was the mainstay of survival-prolonging treatment.[83] For GE-NETs, no proven systemic adjuvant therapy has been identified. However, some believe cytoreduction should be performed whenever possible even if complete resection may not be achievable.[77,84-87] Survival may also be influenced by the presence of high disease burden or hormone-related symptoms[77,78,88] as disease recurrence occurs in the majority.[89,90] Some authors also suggest that the addition of long-acting somatostatin can prolong symptom-free survival.[91]

If midgut GE-NET is localized, resection is indicated.[92] It is important to inspect the gut because 30% may be multicentric. According to ENETS consensus guidelines, resection should still be considered reasonable to prevent the development of intestinal obstruction or desmoplastic reaction or compression of the mesenteric vein.[93] Studies have shown survival benefit with radical resection of mesenteric metastases in the presence of liver metastases[86] and palliation of symptoms after removal of mesenteric tumor burden. In some studies of symptomatic liver metastases, a survival benefit may be noted if >80% of the primary tumor and hepatic metastases can be resected.[82,88] However, the majority of patients will develop recurrent disease.[77] Liver transplantation is still considered experimental.[94]

SYSTEMIC THERAPY

G1/2 midgut NETs should receive somatostatin analogues (SSA) even in the absence of symptoms.[95] SSAs are the only proven hormonal management at present. SSTRs are found in 75%–95% of NETs and are less common in G3 NETs and somatostatinomas. SSAs bind principally to subtypes 2 and 5.[96] Biochemical effects have been noted in 30%–70% of patients and symptomatic control in the 60%–80%. The standard therapeutic dose is octreotide LAR 10–30 mg every 4 weeks or lanreotide (Somatuline Autogel) 60–120 mg every 4 weeks.[97] Patients often develop tachyphylaxis to octreotide, and in that circumstance pasireotide has shown to be an effective salvage option. In a phase 3 randomized trial of octreotide LAR versus placebo (PROMID trial) for midgut NETs, the progression-free survival favored the treatment arm (14.3 months vs., 6 months for placebo).[61] SSAs have also shown effectiveness for P-NET.[64] When clinical or radiologic progression occurs, midgut NET should receive radionuclide therapy (if functional imaging positive) or interferon alpha or liver-directed therapy if liver dominant. G1/2 P-NET should receive chemotherapy as first-line choice.[98,99] Streptozotocin combinations should be used for G1/2 P-NET when there is rapid clinical or radiologic progression. Streptomycin has a better response than doxorubicin.[100] Sunitinib maleate is an oral tyrosine kinase that inhibits downstream from key drivers of angiogenesis, including vascular endothelial growth factor (VEGF) 2/3, platelet-derived growth factor (PDGF), and c-kit. In the registration phase 3 clinical trial in well-differentiated progressive P-NET, the improvement in progression-free survival was significantly improved at 11.4 m versus 5.5 m. Objective response rate was 9.3%.[101]

Genetic abnormalities in the mTOR pathway are critical to the development of NETs. In a phase 3 study evaluating the mTOR inhibitor everolimus in G1/2 P-NETs, the response rate was noted to be 9.6% with a significant improvement in progression-free survival of 11.0 versus 4.6 months.[102] Both these agents are now US Food and Drug Administration approved for use in this setting. A brief summary of recent management-altering trials is presented in Table 15-6.

IN SITU LOCAL THERAPY

Indications are adjunct intraoperative ablation with surgical resection, inoperable candidates, palliation of symptoms, treatment

TABLE 15-6 Pivotal Systemic Therapy Trials

Agent	Year	Phase	Response	End Point	Significance
GE NET Rx					
placebo *vs.* octreotide	2009	3	2.4% BOTH	TTP 14.3M *vs.* 6M	Benefit of octreotide in symptomatic mid gut net
octreotide + everolimus vs. placebo	2011	3	2.3 vs. 1.9%	PFS 16.4 *vs.* 11.3 M	Benefit of everolimus in Bowel nen
PANCREATIC NET					
Agent	**Year**	**Phase**	**Response**	**End Point**	
sunitinib *vs.* placebo	2011	3	9.3%	PFS 11.4M vs. 5.5M	1st Line Rx
everolimus *vs.* everolimus+ octreotide	2010	2	9.6% *vs.* 4.4%	PFS 9.7M vs. 16.7M	Benefit of Everolimus in patients receiving standard of care therapy
everolimus vs. placebo	2011	3	5% *vs.* 2%	PFS 11M vs. 4.6M	1st Line Rx

This table illustrates the momentum in the Oncology community in treating NET since 2005 (i.e, modern era). The highlighted area are the trials that made a clear difference in NET management.

TABLE 15-7 Embolotherapy for GE NET

Author	Year	G1/G2	Total	Embolotherapy	CR+PR	Symptom Benefit %	↓Tumor Marker %	Med Surv months	% 5 yr Survival
Hanssen[136]	1991	nr	36	Particle + IFN	60	100	NR	NR	75
Hajarizadeh[137,138]	1992	6	8	5FU HAI + Cis/MitoC/Dox + Particle	50	100	NR	NR	NR
Ruszniewski[(61)]	1993	14	18	Dox + Particle	33	73	57	NR	NR
Therasse[139]	1993	13	20	Chemo*+Particle	33	100	91	22.5	NR
Moertel[107]	1994	nr	23	Particle	56	NR	82	27	NR
Moertel[107]	1994	nr	42	IV Chemo + Particle	75	NR	83	49	NR
Diaco[140]	1995	7	10	5FU HAI + Cis/MitoC/Dox + Particles	60	100	nr	53	nr
Wangberg[141]	1996	nr	40	Particle	43	NR	100	NR	56
Eriksson[114]	1998	29	29	Particle	52	NR	38	80	60
Kim[134]	1999	9	16	Cis/Dox + Particle	25	NR	75		NR
Dominguez[135]	2000	8	15	STZ+Particle	50	60	50	NR	NR
Schell[142]	2002	24	24	Particle	79	64	nr	nr	71
Roche[137]	2003	12	14	Dox+Particle	43	90	NR	NR	83
Loewe[138]	2003	23	23	Liquid	73	NR	62	69	65.4
Gupta[109]	2005	69	69	Particle or Chemo+ Particle[¥]	66.7	NR	NR	33.8	26.6
Ho[86]	2007	18	35	Particle or Cis/MitoC/Dox + Particle	23	78	NR	@20	32
Sward[139]	2009	nr	107	Particle	nr	71	>50	56	nr

TABLE 15-8 Embolotherapy for PNET

Author	Year	Total	Embolotherapy	CR + PR	Symptom Benefit %	Tumor Marker Response %	Median Survival (months)	% 5-year Survival
Ajani[132]	1988	22	STZ/5FU + Particle	50	NR	90		NR
Mavligit [133]	1993	5	STZ+Particle	57	75	57	NR	NR
Moertel[107]	1994	17	Particle or Chemo+ Particle[¥]	35.2	NR	NR	23.2	13.7
Moertel[107]	1994	29	Particle	60	NR	NR	33.7	NR
Eriksson[114]	1998	12	Cisplatinum/Vinblastine+Particle	80	NR	NR	NR	NR
Kim[134]	1999	14	Particle	43	NR	69	9	NR
Dominguez[135]	2000	7	IV Chemo + Particle	78	NR	87	35	NR
Gupta[109]	2005	54	Particle	50	NR	42	20	NR
Ho[86]	2007	15	Particle or Cis/MitoC/Dox + Particle	18	75	NR	30	35

of recurrent disease to decrease tumor burden, and lowering of hormone levels, The combination of dual afferent nutrient supply to the liver, hypervascularity of metastases, regenerative capabilities of hepatocytes, and preferential afferent hepatic arterial supply to metastases make it possible to occlude the arterial supply to tumors without significant damage to healthy liver.[103-106] Considering the rate of recurrence and nonresectability, most patients are considered candidates for these in situ therapies, The first report of transarterial embolization (TAE) for carcinoid syndrome was by Allison in 1977.[107] The benefit of addition of chemotherapy to the embolic admixture or with concomitant systemic administration (transarterial chemoembolization [TACE]) remains controversial.[108,109] However, some authors suggest that the addition of chemotherapy may add benefit to P-NET and overall NET therapy.[110] A recent small prospective randomized study comparing 14 TAE with 12 TACE in midgut NET cases demonstrated no difference in 2-year progression-free survival.[111] It is also unclear if patients with a high volume of tumor burden will have any meaningful benefit.[112] Tumor response rates vary depending on the system used but ranges vary between 7.7% and 100%, with most studies demonstrating an imaging response rate of 50%. Symptomatic responses have also been variable (50%–100%) but not reported by most studies. Median duration of response extends up to 18 months[113] and median survival durations are quoted between 9 and 86 months, with most papers citing an average of 3 years.[114] Some authors suggest that delayed or late embolization may be as effective as early embolization[115] and that repeat TACE may be beneficial[116] (Tables 15-7 and 15-8, Figure 15-5).

Portal vein thrombosis or underlying hepatic insufficiency and other relative exclusion criteria require extreme caution and highly selective embolization.[117,118] TACE may have mortality of 5% with a median symptom palliation of 13 months.[118] Biliary enteric bypass is a contraindication because of a high incidence of infectious complications.[119]

RADIOEMBOLOTHERAPY

Given the serious adverse-event profile of the newly approved biologic agents for NET, the ability to add an outpatient liver-directed therapy with a low acute adverse-event profile is appealing. Yttrium-90 microspheres are delivered transarterially

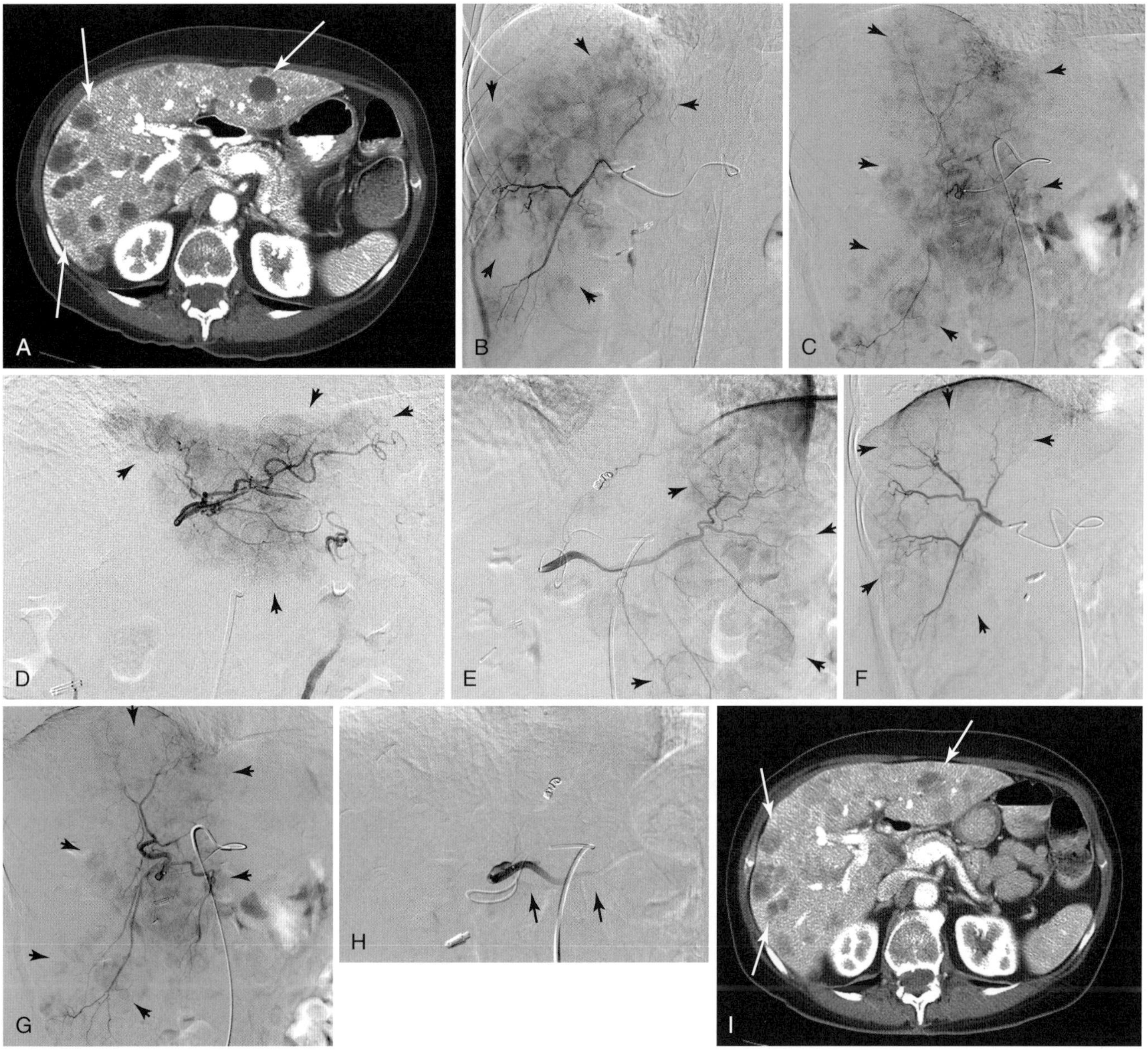

Figure 15-5 Fifty-nine-year-old woman with well-differentiated metastatic ileal NET. Flushing responsive to octreotide LAR but refractory intermittent diarrhea. Embolization requested for extensive hepatic tumor burden with progression. (A) IV contrast–enhanced CT; preembolotherapy. Numerous bilobar low-attenuation foci consistent with known NET hepatic metastases (*white arrows*). (B–E) Preembolotherapy arteriogram. Performed in four different territories separated by 2–3 weeks each. Right anterior, right posterior, segment 2, and segment 3 left hepatic/gastrohepatic trunk territories demonstrate numerous bilobar hypervascular foci consistent with known NET metastases (*black arrowheads*). (F–H) Postembolotherapy arteriogram. Embolization was performed with 100–300-μm spherical polyvinyl alcohol (Contour SE, Boston Scientific Corporation, Natick, MA) and 100-μm polyzene microspheres (Embozene, Celonova Biosciences, San Antonio, TX). Decreased hepatic artery arborizing after embolotherapy. (I) IV contrast–enhanced CT; postembolotherapy, NET metastases are less pronounced. Symptomatic improvement.

and they "embolize" within the vascular plexus of tumors, The first description by Simon et al, in 1968[120] used 15-μm carbonized spheres. Since then, two products are currently commercially available and approved for use in humans: TheraSphere (Nordion, Kanata, Canada; Glass microspheres) and SIR-spheres (SIRTEX Medical, Wilmington, MA). Their application for NETs represents an off-label application of an approved device. The initial results suggest equivalency in efficacy to TACE/TAE in this setting (Table 15-9, Figure 15-6).

Drug-eluting beads (DEBs)/microspheres have shown benefit in the treatment of hepatocellular cancer and colorectal cancer. The addition of doxorubicin to DEBs combines the benefits of calibrated embolotherapy with chemotherapy. Immediate benefits include ease of use and fixed delivery of drug, with encouraging response rates and reversible biliary toxicity.[121-123] Some authors have compared DEBOX to Y90 microspheres.[122] Isolated hepatic perfusion eliminates systemic side effects but is still not commercially available.[124]

TABLE 15-9 Radioembolotherapy for NET

Author	Year	GEP NET	Total Patients	Embolotherapy	Study Design	Median Activity/ Treatment	CR + PR	Symptom Response%	Tumor Marker Response%	Median Survival (months)	5-year Survival (months)
McStay[141]	2005	21	23	90Y-DOTA- Lanreotide +/- Particles	Observation	1	16	61	60	15	nr
Granberg[142]	2007	3	3	Resin 90Y	Observation	1	100	nr	67	nr	nr
King[143]	2008	23	34	IV 5FU+90Y Resin	Phase 4	1.99	50	55	nr	@36	nr
Kennedy[144]	2008	133	148	Resin 90Y	Observation	1.14	63.2	nr	nr	70	nr
Rhee[145]	2008	22	22	Glass 90Y	Observation	nr	54	nr	nr	22	nr
Rhee[145]	2008	20	20	Resin 90Y	Observation	nr	50	nr	nr	28	nr
Kalinowski[146]	2009	8	9	Resin 90Y	Phase 4	2.1	66	nr	nr		
Cao[147]	2009	40	58	Resin 90Y +/- IV 5FU	Observation	1.8	37	nr	nr	36	nr
Saxena[148]	2010	39	48	IV 5FU+90Y Resin	Phase 2	1.94	54	nr	nr	35	nr
Memon[149]	2011	21	40	Glass 90Y	Observation	1.98	64	84	nr	34.4	nr
Rajekar[150]	2011	nr	14	Resin 90Y +/- IA 5FU	Observation	nr	nr	100	71	25	42%
Paprottka[151]	2012	37	42	Resin 90Y	Observation	1.63	22.5	95	54.8	nr	nr

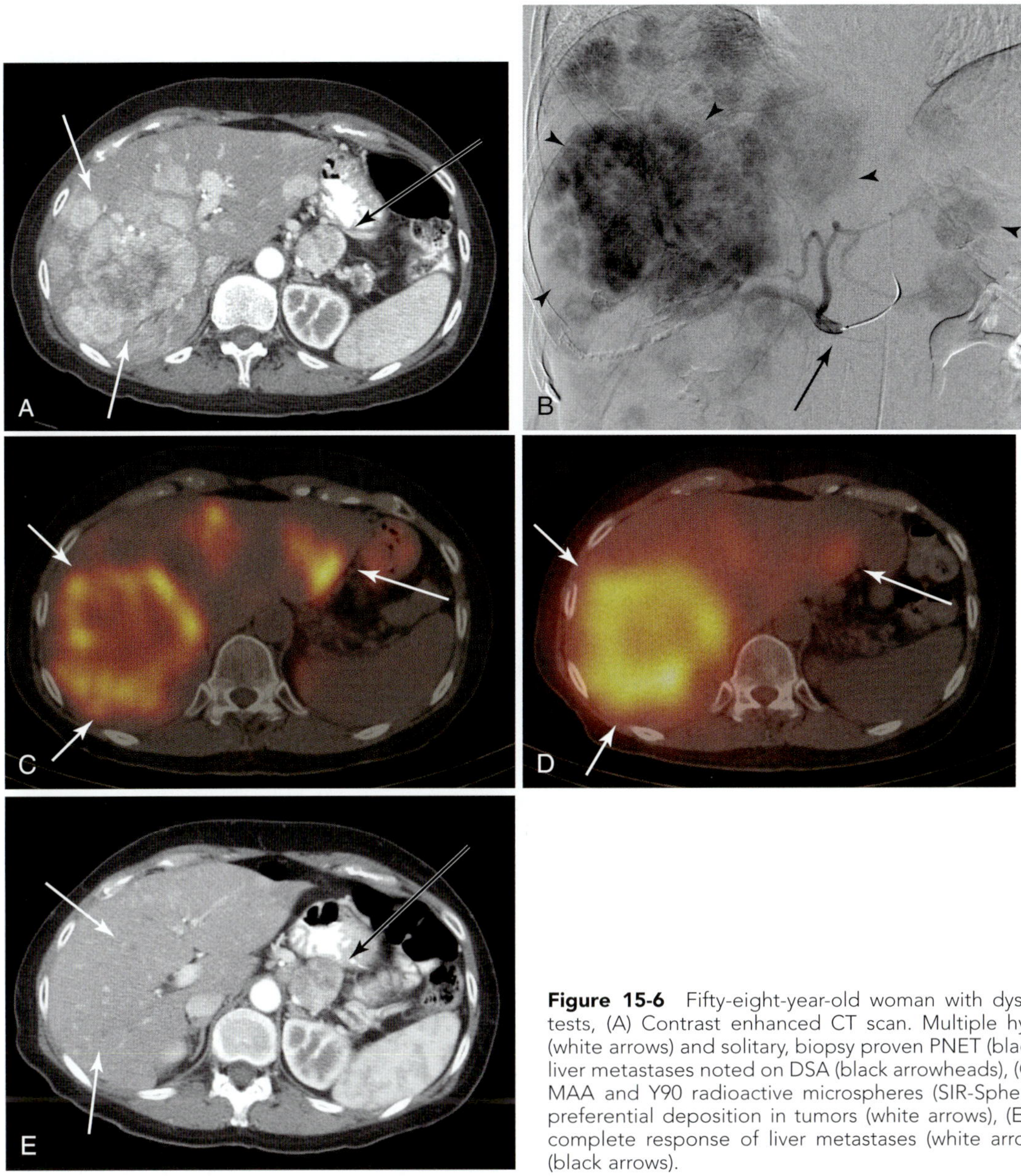

Figure 15-6 Fifty-eight-year-old woman with dyspepsia and abnormal liver function tests, (A) Contrast enhanced CT scan. Multiple hypervascular metastatic liver lesions (white arrows) and solitary, biopsy proven PNET (black arrows), (B) Multiple hypervascular liver metastases noted on DSA (black arrowheads), (C and D) Axial SPECT-CT post Tc99m MAA and Y90 radioactive microspheres (SIR-Spheres, Wilmington, MA) demonstrates preferential deposition in tumors (white arrows), (E) Contrast enhanced CT scan. Near complete response of liver metastases (white arrows) with unchanged primary PNET (black arrows).

THERMAL ABLATION

Because resection of up to 90% of tumor is known to provide survival benefits, aggressive ablation of hepatic metastases should provide similar benefits.[113] Ablation is best suited for lesions less than 3 cm. Some authors believe that open RFA is better than closed.[125,126] In a large laparoscopic RFA series of 54 NET patients, the 30-day morbidity was 5% and mortality 0%. Median duration of symptom control was 11 months. In this series, the median tumor size was 2.3 cm and median survival was 3.9 years.[127] Symptom responses after RFA have been documented[128] and may also be used after failure of embolization.[129] Alcohol ablation can be performed in structures adjacent to other vital structures or blood vessels, ducts, or when approaching small, indistinct metastases. Cryotherapy has also been proven to be effective.[130] Microwave may be better when larger tumors are noted.[131]

RADIONUCLIDE THERAPIES

Somatostatin receptor scintigraphy has also allowed the specific targeting of NET cells with radiation. SRS analogues are combined with high-energy β radiation-emitting radionuclides that are preferentially deposited in tumors when injected systemically. Patient selection remains paramount with promising initial results (Table 15-10).

TABLE 15-10 Summary of Peptide Radionuclide Receptor Therapy for NET

Agent	Author	Year	Patients	Progression inclusion	CR+PR	PD	Outcome
Y90-DOTA-TOC							
	Otte[155]	1999	18	NR	6	11	NR
	Waldherr[156]	2001	37	81	27	11	TTP >26
	Waldherr[156]	2002	37	100	22	8	NR
	Paganelli[157]	2002	87	76	28	20	TTP 14
	Bodei[155]	2003	20	NR	30	20	TTP 10
	Valkema[156]	2006	58	76	9	24	TTP 29
	Forrer[158]	2006	116	93	26	11	NR
	Cwikla[158]	2010	60	100	23	0	PFS 17
Y90-DOTA-TATE							
	Buschnell[156]	2010	90	100	4	12	PFS 16
Lu 177-DOTA-TATE							
	Kwekkeboom[157]	2008	310	43	30	20	PFS 33

Conclusion

Incidence and prevalence of GEP-NET is increasing, Following decades of stagnation, new effective systemic targeted therapeutic agents are creating an optimistic milieu for NET management. Best outcomes are from multidisciplinary centers. IO techniques will play a larger role in the future, and integration of systemic and local therapies may provide the optimal outcome in the management of these complex patients.

REFERENCES

The complete reference list is available online at www.expertconsult.com.

16

Interventional Oncology Management of Noncolorectal and Nonneuroendocrine Hepatic Metastatic Disease

MOHAMED MANSOUR | SANJAY GUPTA

KEY POINTS

- Liver metastasis is a major cause of mortality and morbidity in patients with cancers of various origins and presents a therapeutic challenge because only a few patients are candidates for surgical resection, and systemic chemotherapy offers limited benefit.
- Locoregional therapies have been shown to be safe and effective in selected patients with liver metastases from melanomas, breast cancer, and other gastrointestinal tumors.

Introduction

The liver is a common site for metastases from various malignancies. In addition to colorectal cancers and neuroendocrine tumors, other cancers that frequently metastasize to liver include melanoma, especially uveal melanoma, breast cancer, and gastrointestinal stromal tumors (GISTs). Metastasis to the liver is common in patients with melanoma. Approximately 30% of patients with ocular melanomas develop systemic metastases, and hepatic metastases are seen in 95% of such patients.[1] Hepatic metastases can be seen in 14%–20% of patients with metastatic cutaneous melanomas.[2] Breast cancer has a tendency to metastasize to the liver, with approximately 25% of patients with metastatic breast carcinoma developing hepatic involvement during the course of their disease.[3,4] GISTs are rare but are the most common mesenchymal neoplasms of the gastrointestinal tract. The liver is the most common site of metastasis from GISTs, with a reported incidence of 55%–72% in patients with recurrence.[5,6]

The presence of hepatic metastases is associated with a poor prognosis and is a major cause of morbidity and mortality in patients with malignant tumors of different origins. The presence of hepatic metastases in patients with ocular melanoma is associated with median survival rates of only 6–8 months, and the 1-year survival is approximately 1015%.[7,8] For patients with breast cancer metastatic to the liver, median overall survival from the beginning of therapy ranges from 4 to 14 months, and the survival of untreated patients is 0.5–4 months.

Treatment options for patients with liver metastases are limited. Surgery is the only therapy that offers the possibility of cure for patients with liver metastases. Several studies have shown that surgical resection may prolong survival time of patients; however, only a small percentage of patients (10%–15% in various studies) are suitable for curative resection.[9-11] Systemic chemotherapy, immunotherapy, and hormone therapy are considered mainstays in the treatment of patients with inoperable liver metastases but offer only limited benefit, and trials using systemic therapies have shown disappointing results. Systemic chemotherapy alone or in combination with immunotherapy yields response rates of less than 20% in patients with liver metastases from ocular or cutaneous melanomas, with median response durations of 5–7 months.[2,7,12] Although systemic treatment can prolong survival of patients with metastatic breast cancer, the mean survival is dismal, ranging from 4 to 17 months.[4,13] For GIST, imatinib is a tyrosine kinase inhibitor (TKI) that has been shown to produce a partial tumor response or tumor stabilization in 70%–85% of patients with advanced disease.[14,15] With imatinib therapy, the median progression-free survival is in the range of 20–24 months, and the estimated median overall survival duration exceeds 36 months. Unfortunately, approximately 15% of patients have tumors that show no response to this drug, and in a proportion of patients whose tumors do respond, resistance to the drug develops after an average of 2 years of treatment.[14,15] For these reasons, local or regional liver-directed treatment options that include ablative therapies and transcatheter intraarterial therapies play a major role in the management of patients with unresectable liver metastases. In this chapter, we will review the current role of these treatment options in patients with liver metastases.

Transcatheter Intraarterial Tumor Therapies

The Society of Interventional Radiology defines "image-guided transcatheter tumor therapy" as the intravascular delivery of therapeutic agents via selective catheter placement with imaging guidance.[16] Various agents such as chemotherapeutic agents, embolic particles, and radioactive materials can be injected via feeding vessels into tumor(s) in an attempt to achieve tumor cell death by enabling more focused delivery or by deposition of higher concentrations within the tumor.

HEPATIC ARTERIAL CHEMOINFUSION

Direct hepatic arterial infusion of chemotherapy offers pharmacokinetic advantage over systemic administration.[17] Enhanced first-pass extraction of chemotherapy by cancer cells permits relatively high doses of chemotherapy to be delivered with fewer significant systemic side effects. The increased intratumoral drug concentration can potentially lead to an increased therapeutic response.[18]

Hepatic arterial chemoinfusion is generally administered through implantable catheters that are inserted into the hepatic artery and connected to a subcutaneous port to allow easy and repetitive infusion of chemotherapy. This can be done with either surgical laparotomy or percutaneous insertion using minimally invasive interventional techniques.[19,20] Various percutaneous access routes, such as subclavian, hypogastric, femoral, and brachial arteries, have been described for placement of arterial catheters and subcutaneous ports.[21,22] Alternatively, temporary catheters can be placed multiple times for repeated cycles of chemotherapy.

Safe and optimal drug distribution to liver tumors requires arterial redistribution methods to convert multiple hepatic arteries into a single vascular supply and to reduce extrahepatic cytotoxic side effects.[22] In patients with multiple hepatic arteries, all hepatic arteries except the one to be used for chemotherapy infusion are embolized proximally with coils or liquid embolic agents.[23] This results in the opening of intrahepatic arterial collaterals that allows drug delivery to the entire liver through a single hepatic artery catheter. To prevent nontarget infusion of cytotoxic agents to extrahepatic organs, arteries such as the gastroduodenal artery, the right gastric artery, the accessory left gastric artery, and the replaced posterior superior pancreaticoduodenal artery must be embolized, if they share a common origin with the hepatic artery to be used for infusion of chemotherapy. A number of novel techniques can be used to secure the catheter tip in the hepatic arteries.[24]

Hepatic artery infusion chemotherapy treatment has been for patients with metastatic uveal melanoma (Table 16-1). Cantore et al.[25] reported an overall response rate of 38% and a median survival of 15 months in a series of 8 patients with uveal melanoma metastatic to the liver treated with HAI using a carboplatin-based chemotherapy. Leyvraz et al.[26] reported the use of hepatic arterial infusion in a phase 2 trial of 30 patients treated with intraarterial fotemustine through an implanted hepatic artery catheter. They noted an objective response rate of 40% (four complete responses [CRs] and eight partial responses [PRs]), a median duration of response of 11 months, and a median overall survival of 14 months. A subsequent multicenter study involving 101 patients treated with hepatic arterial infusion of fotemustine reported an objective response rate of 36% (15 CRs and 21 PRs); median overall survival for the whole group was 15 months, with a 1-year survival rate of 67%.[27] Siegel et al.[28] used hepatic arterial infusion of fotemustine to treat 30 patients with metastatic cutaneous or uveal melanomas and found no significant difference in response rates between cutaneous and uveal melanoma patients. In the study by Becker et al.,[29] patients treated with hepatic arterial infusion of fotemustine had a higher response rate than those treated with systemic chemotherapy (22% and 8%, respectively); however, the median survival durations were similar in the two treatment groups (12.1 and 11.5 months, respectively).

Hepatic arterial infusion chemotherapy is also an attractive alternative to systemic approaches for breast cancer patients who have unresectable liver metastasis and no or minimal extrahepatic tumor burden (see Table 16-1). In a pilot study involving 26 patients with breast carcinoma metastatic to the liver and refractory to prior chemotherapy treated with sequential hepatic arterial infusion of vinblastine, Fraschini et al.[30] reported a partial response in 9 and a minor response in 4 of the 25 patients evaluable for response. In another study, 34 patients with metastatic breast carcinoma were treated with hepatic arterial infusion of cisplatin and vinblastine; partial response was observed in 33% of evaluable patients. Fraschini et al.[31] reported a partial response in 11 (33%) and a minor response in 8 (24%) of the 33 patients evaluable for response. Median time to progression for responding patients was 31 weeks (range, 6+ to 74 weeks), and median survival was 11 months (range, 5–19 months). However, many patients developed adverse events, and seven failures were related to treatment

TABLE 16-1 Hepatic Arterial Chemoinfusion

Author, year	Tumor type	Number of patients	Chemotherapy used	Response	Overall survival
Cantore et al., 1994[25]	Melanoma (uveal)	8	Carboplatin	PR, 3; PD, 5	Median, 15 months
Leyvraz et al., 1997[26]	Melanoma (uveal)	30	Fotemustine	CR, 4; PR, 8; SD, 15	Median, 14 months
Becker et al., 2002[29]	Melanoma (uveal)	23	Fotemustine; subcutaneous interleukin 2 and interferon $alpha_2$	22%	Median, 12 months
Peters et al., 2006[27]	Melanoma (uveal)	101	Fotemustine	CR, 15; PR, 21; SD, 48	Median, 15 months; 1-year, 67%
Siegel et al., 2007[28]	Melanoma (uveal or cutaneous)	36	Fotemustine	PR, 9; SD, 10, PD, 11	Median,14 months
Fraschini et al., 1987[30]	Breast	26	Vinblastine	PR, 9	Median, 11 months
Fraschini et al., 1988[31]	Breast	34	Cisplatin, vinblastine	PR, 11	Median, 11 months
Arai et al., 1994[32]	Breast	56	Doxorubicin, 5-fluorouracil, mitomycin	81%	Median, 12.5 months
Ikeda et al., 1999[33]	Breast	26	Doxorubicin, 5-fluorouracil	63%	Median, 25.3 months
Camacho et al., 2007[34]	Breast	10	Paclitaxel	PR, 3; SD, 5, PD, 2	N/A
Tsimberidou et al., 2010[35]	Breast	8	Cisplatinum and systemic liposomal doxorubicin	PR, 3; SD, 5	Median, 8.5 months

CR, complete response; NR, not recorded; PD, progressive disease; PR, partial response; SD, stable disease intolerance or major toxicity. Arai et al.[32] reported a response rate of 81% and a median survival of 12.5 months in a study involving 56 patients with unresectable liver metastases from breast cancer treated by repeated hepatic arterial infusion chemotherapy. In a phase 1/2 study of continuous intraarterial infusion chemotherapy using doxorubicin and 5-fluorouracil in 26 patients with metastatic breast cancer, the median duration of response was 5.8 months (range, 1–23+) and median survival was 25.3 months (range, 6.2–54.7+).[33] In a more recent study, Camacho et al.[34] used repeated hepatic arterial infusion of paclitaxel to treat 10 patients with breast carcinoma and dominant liver metastases. Fifty-six courses of paclitaxel were delivered. No procedure-related complications were observed. Three patients (30%) attained partial responses that lasted for 6, 7, and 48 months; 4 other patients had stable disease for 5–9 months. One patient underwent liver resection after receiving hepatic arterial infusions of paclitaxel and remained disease free for 48 months. Hepatic arterial chemoinfusion can also be combined with systemic treatment in patients with both hepatic and extrahepatic metastatic disease. A recently reported phase 1 clinical trial of hepatic arterial infusion of cisplatin in combination with intravenous liposomal doxorubicin in patients with advanced cancer and dominant liver involvement included 11 patients with breast cancer.[35] The regimen was well tolerated, and partial response was observed in 3 of the 11 breast cancer patients.

HEPATIC ARTERY EMBOLIZATION AND CHEMOEMBOLIZATION

Liver metastases derive 90% of their blood supply from the hepatic artery.[36] This feature, combined with the facts that the liver has a dual-blood supply and a healthy liver receives 80% of its blood supply from the portal vein, provides a good rationale for using either hepatic arterial embolization or chemoembolization to treat these metastases.[37] Chemoembolization involves infusion of a mixture of chemotherapeutic agents with or without iodized oil into the hepatic arteries supplying the tumor, followed by embolization with particles.[16] The purpose of embolization is to prevent washout of the drug from the tumor and to induce ischemic necrosis. The resulting tumor drug concentrations are reported to be 10–25 times higher than those achieved by infusion alone and the dwell time of the agents is markedly prolonged.[38]

A preliminary arteriography of the celiac axis and superior mesenteric artery is performed to evaluate the arterial supply to the liver and to ensure the patency of the portal vein. After the initial diagnostic arteriogram, the selected hepatic artery is catheterized with a 5-F catheter or a coaxially advanced microcatheter. Currently, there is no consensus on the best chemoembolization protocol in terms of patient selection criteria, choice of the embolic agents used, choice and dose of the anticancer agents, the embolization end points, and time interval between treatments.[39]

In patients with bilobar disease, embolization of the whole liver in a single treatment session is generally avoided because of the risk of prolonged postembolization syndrome or liver failure. Only one lobe of the liver is subjected to embolization during each treatment session; generally, the hepatic lobe with the greatest tumor burden is treated first. To avoid liver failure in patients with extensive (>75% liver parenchyma replaced with tumor) liver involvement, only a small portion of the liver lobe is subjected to embolization during each session. Additional hepatic artery chemoembolization procedures are performed with the goal of treating the entire liver.

The timing of subsequent chemoembolization procedures is generally determined by the patient's physical condition, tumor status, response to initial embolization, and ability to tolerate the procedure. Extensive liver involvement and mildly abnormal liver functions (serum albumin level <3 g/dL, aspartate transaminase level >100 U/L, lactate dehydrogenase level >425 IU/mL, and serum bilirubin level >2 mg/dL) indicate an increased risk of liver failure after chemoembolization. If several of these factors are combined, the risk of liver failure may be unacceptable.

Chemoembolization has become an accepted locoregional therapy for uveal melanoma metastatic to the liver (Table 16-2). Studies have shown some survival benefit in patients with metastatic uveal melanoma who had responses to chemoembolization. The use of chemoembolization for liver metastases of uveal melanoma was first reported by Carrasco et al,[40] who reported tumor regressions in two patients after one or two chemoembolization sessions using polyvinyl sponge material and cisplatin. A study at the University of Texas M.D. Anderson Cancer Center involving 30 patients with uveal melanoma metastatic to the liver treated with chemoembolization using cisplatin and polyvinyl alcohol particles reported a response rate of 46% and a median overall survival of 11 months.[41] A more recent study by the same group involving a larger number of patients (n = 64) reported a response rate of 36% for first-line and 25% for subsequent chemoembolization treatments, and a median survival of 14.5 months in responding patients.[42] In fact, more recent studies have shown even lower radiologic response rates, ranging from 0% to 25%.[43-46]

In another report, Huppert et al.[47] performed 34 chemoembolization procedures with cisplatin or carboplatin in 14 patients with uveal melanoma metastatic to the liver. Partial response was seen in eight patients (57%) and stable disease in four patients (29%). Median time to progression was 8.5 months (range, 5–35 months). Median survival after first chemoembolization was 14.5 months in responders compared with 10 months in nonresponders. Patients with less than 25% liver involvement had a higher incidence of PR (86% vs. 29%) and a longer median survival (17 vs. 11 months; $P = 0.02$) compared with those patients with more than 25% liver involvement.

In a phase 2 trial involving 29 patients, Patel et al.[44] used 1,3-bis(2-chloroethyl)-1-nitrosourea (BCNU) in combination with ethiodized oil (lipiodol) followed by embolization with gelatin sponge particles. Among 24 evaluable patients, one patient achieved a CR, four patients achieved a PR, and 13 patients had stable disease (SD). Median overall survival of the entire intent-to-treat group of patients was 5.2 months (range, 0.1–27.6 months); median overall survival was 21.9 months (range, 7.4–27.6 months) for patients with CR or PR, 8.7 months (range, 2.9–14.4 months) for those with SD, and 3.3 months (range, 1.6–5.6) for those with progressive disease. Patients who had less than 20% of liver replaced with tumor had a better survival than those with 20%–50% tumor in the liver (median, 19.0 vs. 5.6 months, respectively).

Vogl et al.[46] used the super-selective chemoembolization technique in 12 uveal melanoma patients with solitary ($n = 6$) or oligonodular hepatic metastases ($n = 6$). The embolization consisted of infusion of a maximum of 10 mg/m^2 mitomycin C and a maximum of 15 mL of iodized oil, followed by embolization

TABLE 16-2 Hepatic Arterial Embolization and Chemoembolization

Author, year	Tumor type	Number of patients	Chemoembolization regimen	Response	Liver- PFS/TTP	Overall survival
Mavligit et al., 1988[41]	Melanoma (uveal)	30	Cisplatin; PVA	CR, 1; PR, 13; SD, 7; PD, 9	NR	Median, 11 months
Bedikian et al., 1995[42]	Melanoma (uveal)	44	Cisplatin ± other drugs; PVA	Response rate, 36%	NR	14.5
Huppert et al., 2009	Melanoma (uveal)	14	Cisplatin/carboplatin; PVA	PR, 8; SD, 4; PD, 2	Median TTP, 8.5 months	Median, 11.5 months
Patel et al., 2010[47]	Melanoma (uveal)	30	BCNU; Gelfoam	24 evaluable patients - CR, 1; PR, 4; SD, 13; PD, 6	Median TTP, 6.7 months (patients with CR,PR, SD)	Median, 5.2 months
Sharma et al., 2008[45]	Melanoma (uveal and cutaneous)	20	Cisplatin, doxorubicin, mitomycin; ethiodized oil, PVA or Gelfoam	PR, 0; SD, 13; PD, 7	Median PFS, 185 days	Median, 271 days
Vogl et al., 2007[46]	Melanoma (uveal)	12	Mitomycin C; lipiodol, and resorbable microspheres	PR, 3; SD, 5; PD, 4	NR	Mean, 19.5 months
Gupta et al., 2010[48]	Melanoma (uveal)	125	Cisplatin ± other drugs; PVA or Gelfoam	105 evaluable patients—PR, 12; MR, 17; SD, 68; PD, 8	Median PFS, 3.8 months	Median, 6.7 months
Fiorentini et al., 2009[50]	Melanoma (uveal)	10	Drug-eluting beads (irinotecan)	PR, 10	NR	Median, 6.5 months
Ahrar et al., 2011[51]	Melanoma (cutaneous)	42	Cisplatin ± other drugs; PVA or Gelfoam	36 evaluable patients; PR, 5; MR, 9; SD, 17; PD, 5	Median TTP, 6 months	Median, 7.7 months
Brown et al., 2011[49]	Melanoma (uveal)	6	Drug-eluting beads (Doxorubicin)	Response rate, 100%	NR	Median, 12.3 months
Maluccio et al., 2006[52]	Sarcomas (16 GIST)	24	PVA or trisacryl microspheres	Response rate, 60%	NR	Median, 24 months
Mavligit et al., 1995[54]	GIST	14	Cisplatin, vinblastine; PVA	Response rate, 70%	NR	Median, 12 months
Rajan et al., 2001[55]	Sarcomas (11 GIST)	16	Cisplatin, doxorubicin, mitomycin C; ethiodized oil and PVA	Response rate, 13%	NR	Median, 13 months
Kobayashi et al., 2006[56]	GIST	85	Cisplatin; PVA or Gelfoam	PR, 13%; SD, 69%	Median PFS, 8.2 months	Median, 17.2 months
Giroux et al., 2004[58]	Breast	8	Cisplatin, doxorubicin, mitomycin; ethiodized oil with PVA	Response, 5; SD, 1; PD, 2	NR	Mean, 6 months
Li et al., 2005[61]	Breast	28	5-FUDR, cisplatin, doxorubicin; ethiodized oil or Gelfoam	PR, 10; SD, 13; PD, 5	NR	Median, 28 months
Vogl et al., 2010[60]	Breast	208	Mitomycin C only , Mitomycin C with gemcitabine , gemcitabine only; ethiodized oil and starch microspheres	PR, 27; SD, 105; PD, 76	NR	Median, 18.5 months; Mean, 30.7 months
Martin et al., 2011[62]	Breast	40	Drug-eluting beads (doxorubicin)	Response rate, 50%	Median PFS, 26 months	Median, 47 months

BCNU, 1,3-bis (2-chloroethyl)-1-nitrosourea; CR, complete response; GIST, gastrointestinal stromal tumor; MR, minimal response; NR, not recorded; PD, progressive disease; PFS, progression-free survival; PR, partial response; PVA, polyvinyl alcohol; SD, stable disease; TTP, time to progression.

with 200–450 mg of resorbable microspheres. Three patients achieved a PR and five had SD without significant side effects. The median survival rates of patients with SD and PR after chemoembolization were significantly longer at 15.7 months and 21.0 months, respectively, whereas patients with progressive disease survived only 8.3 months ($P = 0.01$). Vogl et al.[46] also found that retention of ethiodized oil in the tumors after chemoembolization is a predictive marker for good radiologic response. In their series, the patients who showed significant accumulation of ethiodized oil in their hepatic metastases achieved CR or PR, whereas patients with a lower degree of ethiodized oil enhancement had progressive disease.

Sharma et al.[45] treated 21 patients with chemoembolization using a mixture of 50 mg of cisplatin, 50 mg of doxorubicin, and 10 mg of mitomycin C emulsified with ethiodized oil followed by embolization with either absorbable gelatin sponge or 300–500 μm polyvinyl alcohol (PVA) particles. Of 20 evaluable patients, there were 13 with SD but no patients with CR or PR. The median overall survival of patients was 271 days. In their study, the angiographic pattern of liver metastasis was strongly predictive of survival after chemoembolization. Patients with lesions that had a nodular angiographic appearance had longer overall survival than patients with lesions that had an infiltrative appearance (median overall survival, 750 vs. 109 days; $P = 0.0002$).

In a recently published study, we reported our institution's experience with chemoembolization in 125 patients with uveal melanoma metastatic to the liver.[48] We found an overall response rate of 28.6%, which was not significantly different from that reported in most previous studies. Of 105 patients in whom radiologic responses could be evaluated, 12 (11%) had partial responses, 17 (16%) had minor responses, 68 (65%) had stable disease, and 8 (8%) had progressive disease (Figure 16-1). The median overall survival and progression-free survival were 6.7 and 3.8 months, respectively. Multivariate analysis showed that >75% liver involvement and high lactate dehydrogenase levels were associated with short overall survival. Patients who had radiologic responses to chemoembolization had a longer median overall survival duration than did patients who did not (15.8 vs. 6.1 months; $P = 0.0005$). Patients with >75% liver involvement had a median overall survival duration of only 2.4 months.

In recent years, drug-eluting beads have been used for chemoembolization in an effort to deliver a more accurate dose of drugs to liver tumors over a more prolonged period. Drug-eluting beads are biocompatible, hydrophilic, nonresorbable hydrogel microspheres that are available in various sizes and capable of loading chemotherapeutic medications, including doxorubicin and irinotecan. In a recent study, 6 patients with unresectable hepatic metastases from melanoma underwent chemoembolization using drug-eluting beads loaded with doxorubicin.[49] Over a median follow-up of 12 months, response rates of 100%, 83%, and 60% were observed at 3, 6, and 9 months, respectively. Median overall survival after initial treatment was 12.3 months.

In another study, Fiorentini et al.[50] performed chemoembolization with drug-eluting beads loaded with irinotecan (100 mg) in 10 patients with uveal melanoma metastatic to the liver. In this phase 2 trial, three patients had a major response with evidence of metastasis reduction of 90%, three patients had a reduction of 80%, and four patients experienced reductions between 70% and 60%. The median survival was 6.5 months (range, 4–9 months). These authors found that the degree of liver involvement was related to the radiologic response. Three patients with less than 25% liver involvement obtained nearly complete reduction of metastases. Three patients with multiple metastases occupying up to 75% of the liver had less evidence of response. A phase 2 clinical trial for metastatic uveal melanoma using doxorubicin-eluting beads is ongoing in the United States.

Although chemoembolization has become an accepted locoregional therapy for patients with uveal melanoma metastases to the liver, there is little information on patients' outcomes after chemoembolization therapy for cutaneous melanoma metastases in the liver. In a recent report from our institution involving 42 patients with cutaneous melanoma metastatic to liver who underwent chemoembolization, radiologic response was seen in 38.9% and disease stabilization in 47.2% patients.[51] The median overall survival and time to progression of liver disease were 7.7 and 6 months, respectively. Patient's age, lactate dehydrogenase levels, type of treatment, number of extrahepatic metastatic sites, and response to therapy were found to be significant predictors of overall survival after chemoembolization. Although the response rates were low, the beneficial effect of chemoembolization for such patients is suggested by the fact that those patients who achieved a radiologic response after chemoembolization had a survival benefit relative to those who did not achieve a radiologic response (14.08 months vs. 7.4 and 8.5 months, respectively; $P = 0.031$). Future studies are needed to develop novel strategies, including the use of new chemotherapeutic agents, to improve the response rates for chemoembolization in patients with liver metastases from cutaneous melanomas.

Hepatic arterial embolization or chemoembolization has been used in the treatment of liver-dominant metastatic GIST

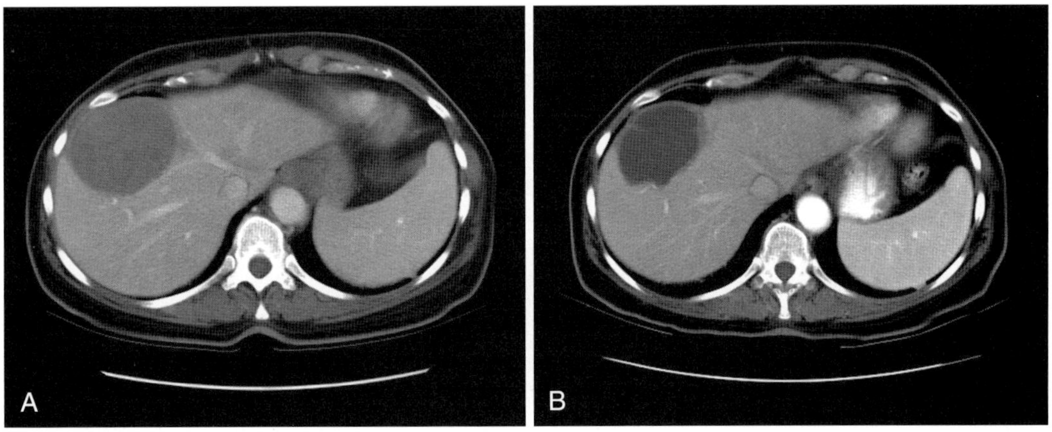

Figure 16-1 Patient with liver metastases from ocular melanoma treated with chemoembolization using cisplatin and PVA particles. (A) Preembolization contrast-enhanced CT scan shows tumor in right liver. (B) Contrast-enhanced CT scan obtained after two sessions of chemoembolization shows tumor necrosis.

and other sarcomas (see Table 16-2). Maluccio et al.[52] reported a series of 24 patients who had metastatic sarcoma treated with bland HAE, including 16 patients with GIST. The embolization was performed with PVA microspheres (Cook Inc., Bloomington, IN) or trisacryl microspheres (Embosphere, Wayland, MA). No chemotherapy or iodized oil was used in combination with the embolic material. The overall survival rates for the 24 patients were 62% at 1 year, 41% at 2 years, and 29% at 3 years, with an overall median survival of 24 months. The seven patients who remained alive for more than 4 years after the initial embolization had metastatic GIST. Four studies have investigated the use of chemoembolization for locoregional therapy of liver-dominant metastatic GIST. In the initial report in 1991, Mavligit et al.[53] reported tumor regression in two patients with gastrointestinal leiomyosarcoma after chemoembolization with cisplatin and PVA followed by hepatic arterial infusion of vinblastine. Later, in 1995, Mavligit et al.[54] published a study that considered 14 patients with gastrointestinal leiomyosarcoma metastatic to the liver treated with chemoembolization using the combination of cisplatin and PVA followed by arterial infusion of vinblastine. The authors reported a 70% radiologic response rate with an overall median survival of 12 months after an average of two procedures. In 2001, Rajan et al.[55] published their experience with chemoembolization for the treatment of 16 patients with metastatic sarcomas, including 11 GISTs. These authors used a combination of cisplatin, doxorubicin, mitomycin C, iodized oil, and PVA. They found that 13% of the patient population had radiologic response and 69% had stable disease. The overall survival from time of embolization was 67% at 1 year, 50% at 2 years, and 40% at 3 years, with a median survival time of 13 months.

The largest published series to date of patients with metastatic GIST, from Kobayashi et al.[56] in 2006, reported on 85 patients with metastatic GIST treated with chemoembolization using cisplatin and PVA or Gelfoam particles followed in some patients by hepatic arterial infusion of vinblastine. Among these patients, 14% showed a partial response and 74% had stable disease (Figure 16-2). The overall survival rates in this group were 62% at 1 year, 32% at 2 years, and 20% at 3 years, with a median survival duration of 17.2 months. Patients who had more than five liver metastases and received only one chemoembolization treatment had shorter progression-free survival than did patients with fewer metastases or those who received two or more TACE sessions. Extensive liver involvement, presence of extrahepatic metastases, and progression of liver disease after chemoembolization were associated with poor overall survival. Concomitant use of imatinib prolonged survival time.

Because imatinib is now the first-line treatment for metastatic GIST, transcatheter hepatic arterial embolization and chemoembolization are viable alternatives for patients whose disease has failed to respond to imatinib therapy. This failure is usually a result of the tumor's drug resistance. It is important to mention that sunitinib, the TKI used as second-line therapy for imatinib-resistant GISTs, has no effect on certain imatinib-refractory GISTs having a specific set of gene mutations, such as platelet-derived growth factor A-D842V. Hepatic arterial embolization or chemoembolization causes destruction of local tumor, irrespective of the mechanism of resistance. At our institution, we performed hepatic arterial embolization or chemoembolization in 14 patients with imatinib-resistant GIST with progressive liver metastasis.[57] On the basis of RECIST, one patient demonstrated a partial response and 12 patients had stable disease. In a multidisciplinary approach, hepatic arterial embolization or chemoembolization can be offered to patients with GIST and liver-dominant metastasis who have primary or acquired resistance to imatinib and are not surgical candidates. These treatments are particularly suitable for patients who exhibit an initial response to imatinib in all lesions but later develop progression of focal disease in the liver.

Although chemoembolization is not a commonly used method for treatment of patients with metastatic breast cancer, a few reports have shown that it is safe and can induce response in some of these patients (see Table 16-2). Giroux et al.[58] reported some tumor regression in five patients and symptom relief in 50% of eight patients with liver metastasis from breast cancer, after treatment with chemoembolization. Bujis et al.[59] used chemoembolization to treat 114 patients with liver metastasis from breast cancer. In their study, the mean tumor size decreased by 18% after treatment and the median patient survival was 25 months. Vogl et al.[60] performed chemoembolization treatments in 208 patients with breast cancer and liver metastases. The chemotherapy protocol consisted of mitomycin C only ($n = 76$), mitomycin C with gemcitabine ($n = 111$), and

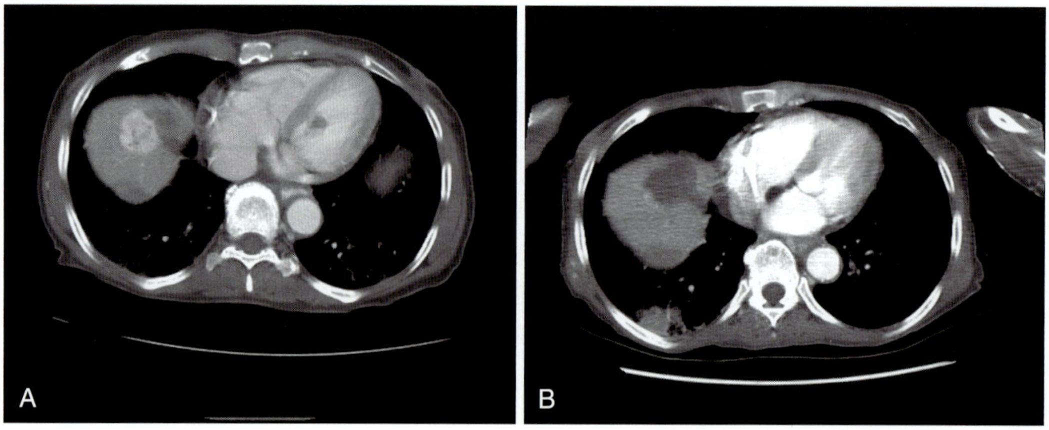

Figure 16-2 Patient with hepatic metastasis from gastrointestinal stromal tumor. (A) Contrast-enhanced CT demonstrates an enhancing mass in the right liver. (B). Contrast-enhanced CT scan obtained after chemoembolization demonstrates a decrease in the density and lack of enhancement of the mass.

gemcitabine only ($n = 21$). Embolization was performed with lipiodol and starch microspheres. Partial response was seen in 27 patients (13.0%), stable disease in 105 patients (50.5%), and progressive disease in 76 patients (36.5%). The 1-, 2-, and 3-year survival rates after chemoembolization were 69%, 40%, and 33%, respectively. Median and mean survival times from the start of chemoembolization were 18.5 and 30.7 months. Patients treated with a combination of mitomycin C and gemcitabine had longer survival times than patients treated with single drugs. In another study, Li et al.[61] reported a 35.7% radiologic response in 48 breast cancer patients treated with chemoembolization using fluorouracil or 5-FUDR, cisplatin, and doxorubicin as the chemotherapeutic agents. The 1-, 2- and 3-year survival rates were 63%, 30%, and 13%, respectively. In a recent multicenter, prospective, open, noncontrolled repeat treatment registry study reported by Martin et al.,[62] 40 patients with unresectable liver metastasis from breast cancer underwent 75 chemoembolization treatments with doxorubicin-loaded drug-eluting beads. The treatment was well tolerated, with 13 minor adverse events seen in eight patients. The objective response rates at 3, 6, and 12 months were 58%, 50%, and 50%, respectively. The median hepatic progression-free survival and overall survival durations were 26 months and 47 months, respectively. The authors concluded that chemoembolization with doxorubicin-loaded drug-eluting beads is a safe and effective local therapy with very high response rates in patients with breast cancer metastatic to the liver. These results, although in a small patient population, suggest that chemoembolization is a viable treatment option and should be considered in patients with liver-dominant unresectable metastatic disease from breast cancer, especially after failure of standard systemic chemotherapy.

IMMUNOEMBOLIZATION

In a novel approach, Sato et al.[63] used an immunologic stimulant, granulocyte–macrophage colony-stimulating factor (GM-CSF), instead of standard chemotherapeutic agents for the chemoembolization procedure. The procedure, called immunoembolization, is aimed at (1) inducing tumor necrosis by the ischemic effects of embolization; (2) stimulating antigen-presenting cells such as dendritic cells and Kupffer cells by GM-CSF, facilitating antigen uptake; and (3) possibly enhancing systemic immunity against tumor cells. In a phase 1 clinical trial of immunoembolization with GM-CSF involving 31 uveal melanoma patients with less than 50% involvement of the liver, no treatment-related deaths or life-threatening events were observed up to and including the 2,000-μg dose level of GM-CSF. CR was noted in 2 patients, PR in 8 patients, and SD in 10 patients.[63] The median overall survival in intent-to-treat patients was 14.4 months. Multivariate analyses indicated that female sex, high doses of GM-CSF (>1,500 μg), and radiologic response (CR and PR) were correlated with longer overall survival. Yamamato et al.[64] compared the results of immunoembolization with their institution's historical control of patients who were treated with chemoembolization using BCNU. They found that compared with patients who received chemoembolization, patients who received immunoembolization had significantly better overall survival (20.4 vs. 9.8 months, $P = 0.005$) and progression-free survival in systemic (extrahepatic) sites (12.4 vs. 4.8 months, $P = 0.001$). The authors concluded that treatment with high-dose immunoembolization prolonged survival of patients with uveal melanoma who underwent embolization of hepatic metastases and possibly delayed progression of extrahepatic metastases. On the basis of these encouraging results, a randomized phase 2 clinical trial is ongoing, in which uveal melanoma patients with hepatic metastasis receive embolization of the hepatic artery with or without 2,000 μg of GM-CSF.

^{90}Y MICROSPHERE RADIOEMBOLIZATION

Hepatic arterial radioembolization with yttrium-90 (^{90}Y) microspheres is an emerging technique for treatment of patients with unresectable metastatic liver tumors. Two FDA-approved ^{90}Y microsphere products are available for clinical use: TheraSphere® (MDS Nordion Inc., Kanata, Ontario, Canada) and SIR-Spheres® (SIRTeX Medical Ltd., Sydney, New South Wales, Australia). Hepatic arterial administration of these ^{90}Y microspheres results in preferential distribution of the microspheres into the tumor vasculature, allowing the delivery of high doses of radiation to the tumor, while relatively sparing the normal liver. Radioembolization allows delivery of radiation doses as high as 150 Gy without development of the clinical complications seen with external beam therapy.

Diagnostic angiography is initially performed to evaluate the hepatic arterial anatomy and to determine the pulmonary shunt fraction, via technetium-99 macroaggregated albumin (^{99m}Tc-MAA) infusion. Nontargeted embolization to the pulmonary parenchyma can result in radiation-induced injury. Nontargeted delivery of radioactive microspheres to organs such as the stomach, duodenum, and pancreas is avoided by performing selective embolization of all extrahepatic arteries before the treatment. Radioembolization is generally associated with a lower incidence of postembolization syndrome compared with standard HACE, allowing for treatment planning on an outpatient basis.

Over the past few years, a number of studies using radioembolization have shown promising results in patients with hepatocellular carcinoma or metastatic disease from colorectal cancer and neuroendocrine cancer. However, there is limited literature on the use of radioembolization for the treatment of patients with liver metastases from other cancers.

In a study by Sato et al.[65] involving 137 patients with hepatic metastatic disease who were treated with radioembolization, median survival in patients with noncolorectal and nonneuroendocrine tumors (207 days) was lower than that for patients with colorectal (457 days) and neuroendocrine tumors (776 days).

Kennedy et al.[66] treated 11 patients with metastatic melanoma with 12 radioembolization treatments at five centers. No treatment-related deaths or radiation-induced liver disease was reported. At 3 months' follow-up, CR was seen in one patient, PR in six patients, SD in one, and progressive disease in one patient. In another more recent study by Gonsalves et al.,[67] 32 ocular melanoma patients with hepatic metastases were treated with radioembolization. The median overall survival and progression-free survival were 10.0 months and 4.7 months, respectively. Patients who had a pretreatment tumor burden less than 25% had longer median overall survival (10.5 vs. 3.9 months, $P = 0.0003$) and progression-free survival (6.4 vs. 3.0 months, $P = 0.03$) than patients who had a pretreatment tumor burden of 25% or greater. Patients who had a complete response ($n = 1$), partial response ($n = 1$), or stable disease

($n = 18$) had longer median overall survival (14.7 vs. 4.9 months, $P = 0.0006$) and progression-free survival (7.9 vs. 3.1 months, $P < 0.0001$) than did patients with tumor progression ($n = 12$). A phase 2 clinical trial to prospectively investigate the safety and efficacy of radioembolization using 90Y SIR-Spheres (Sirtex Medical, Wilmington, MA) in uveal melanoma patients with hepatic metastases is ongoing. These early results suggest that radioembolization is a safe and effective salvage therapy for patients with limited metastasis of uveal melanoma.

Radioembolization also has been used in patients with breast cancer that is chemotherapy refractory. Coldwell et al.[68] observed a computed tomographic imaging partial response in 47% and a positron emission tomographic response in 95% of 44 patients with unresectable liver metastases from breast cancer that were refractory to multiple treatment regimens and were treated with radioembolization. In the study by Bangash et al.,[69] 27 female patients with progressing liver metastases on standard of care polychemotherapy were treated with standard lobar radioembolization with yttrium (^{90}Y) microspheres. At 90-day follow-up, computed tomography showed complete and partial responses in 9 (39.1%) patients, stable disease in 12 (52.1%) patients, and progressive disease in 2 (8.8%) patients. Positive tumor response on positron emission tomography was noted in 17 (63%) patients. Median survival for Eastern Cooperation Oncology Group 0 versus 1, 2, or 3 patients was 6.8 months and 2.6 months, respectively, and for patients with tumor burden <25% versus >25% was 9.4 and 2.0 months, respectively ($P = .46$). In another report, by Jacobs et al.,[70] 30 patients who had been previously treated with polychemotherapy regimens underwent radioembolization in a single-session, whole-liver treatment. Follow-up at a median of 4.2 months demonstrated partial response, stable disease, and progressive disease in 61%, 35%, and 4% of patients, respectively. The median overall survival was 11.7 months. The median survivals were 23.6 months for responders and 5.7 months for nonresponders, and the median survivals were 9.6 months for patients with extrahepatic disease and 16 months for those without extrahepatic disease. These early results, although from a small number of patients, seem promising and suggest that radioembolization can achieve tumor regression in patients with highly treatment-refractory liver metastases from breast cancer.

ISOLATED HEPATIC PERFUSION

Isolated hepatic perfusion is a procedure that involves isolation of the vascular supply to the liver, hepatic arterial delivery of a chemotherapeutic agent at high doses, and a veno-venous bypass circuit for hemofiltration.[7] This can be accomplished surgically via an exploratory laparotomy to expose and isolate the inferior vena cava, porta hepatis, gastroduodenal artery, and perihepatic collaterals. Alternatively, percutaneous hepatic perfusion can be performed with the help of a fenestrated multilumen double-balloon catheter (Delcath Systems, Stamford, CT) and two biocompatible hemoperfusion filters.[71] The double-balloon catheter is inserted percutaneously via the femoral vein, and the balloons are inflated to occlude the inferior vena cava above and below the hepatic veins. The chemotherapeutic agent is infused via a percutaneously placed hepatic artery catheter. The venous outflow is extracted through the fenestrations in the double-balloon catheter, filtered through the bypass circuit, and returned to the patient via a catheter placed in the internal jugular vein.

Response rates of 33.3%–62% and survival durations of 9.9–12.1 months have been reported in studies using surgical isolated hepatic perfusion with melphalan in patients with uveal melanoma metastatic to the liver.[72-75] Pingpank et al.[76] used percutaneous hepatic perfusion with melphalan to treat 10 patients with metastatic uveal melanoma; they reported 2 CRs and 3 PRs, with 3 of the 5 responses lasting 1 year or longer. Results from a multicenter randomized phase 3 trial comparing percutaneous hepatic perfusion and the best available treatment for patients with hepatic metastases from metastatic ocular or cutaneous melanoma showed improved response rates (34.1% vs. 2.0%; $P = 0.001$) and longer medial hepatic progression-free survival (245 vs. 49 days; $P = 0.001$) for patients receiving percutaneous hepatic perfusion compared with those receiving standard of care treatment.[77]

Percutaneous Ablative Therapies

The Society of Interventional Radiology defines image-guided tumor ablation as the direct application of chemical or thermal methods to a specific tumor (or tumors) in an attempt to achieve eradication or substantial tumor destruction.[78] Chemical tumor ablation involves direct intratumoral injection of ethanol or acetic acid to induce coagulative necrosis. Thermal ablation uses thermal energy sources with either heat (e.g., radiofrequency ablation, laser ablation, microwave ablation) or cold (cryoablation) to induce tumor cell death. The heating thermal techniques raise the tissue temperature to between 60°C and 100°C, resulting in coagulative necrosis of tumor cells. Cryoablation uses repetitive freezing and thawing of tissue to produce necrosis.

Percutaneous thermal ablative therapies offer a less invasive alternative to surgery in the locoregional treatment of liver metastases. Of the several technologies used for the local thermal ablation of tumor tissue, RFA is the most widely used for the ablation of liver tumors. Although the use of local ablative treatments has become an established treatment option for patients with colorectal liver metastases, the literature on the use of these methods for liver metastases from other cancers is limited.

In the study by Yun et al.,[79] 25 patients with 40 hepatic metastases (tumor size, 0.5–5.0 cm) from noncolorectal origins (stomach, biliary, breast, pancreas, kidney, and skin) were treated with RFA. The median intrahepatic disease-free interval was 10.1 months. The 1-, 3-, and 5-year overall survival rates after RFA were 86%, 39%, and 19%, respectively. The authors concluded that RFA showed intermediate therapeutic effectiveness for the treatment of liver metastases of noncolorectal origin.

Some recent studies have suggested that percutaneous RFA can be effective in the treatment of liver metastases from breast cancer. Livraghi et al.[80] reported their experience with 24 patients with 64 breast cancer liver metastases treated with RFA. A single lesion was treated in 16 patients, and multiple lesions were treated in eight patients. Complete necrosis was achieved in 59 (92%) of the 64 lesions. Ten of these 24 patients developed new liver metastases during follow-up; 23 patients were alive at the end of the study (median follow-up, 19 months). Another study by Jakobs et al.[81] involving 43 patients in whom RFA was performed reported a median survival time of 58.6 months from the date of RFA. In a recent report by Meloni et al.,[82] RFA was used to treat 87 breast cancer liver metastases in 52 female patients; 45 of these patients had been unsuccessfully treated with multiple lines of chemotherapy. All these patients had either liver-only disease or else the extrahepatic disease was stable with systemic therapy, and they had fewer than five hepatic tumors with maximum tumor diameter up to 5 cm. Complete tumor necrosis was achieved in 97% of tumors. Median survival duration and 5-year survival rate from the time of first RFA were 29.9 months and 27%, respectively. Patients with tumors 2.5 cm in diameter or larger had a worse prognosis (hazard ratio, 2.1) than did patients with smaller tumors. No treatment-related deaths or major complications were encountered, and the minor complication rate was 4%. These authors concluded that survival rates after RFA in selected patients with breast cancer liver metastases, notably patients with disease confined to the liver or with stable extrahepatic metastases, were comparable to those reported after surgery.

Other local thermal ablative therapies have also been used to treat patients with liver metastases from breast cancer. Mack et al.[83] treated 578 liver metastases from breast cancer in 232 female patients with magnetic resonance-guided laser ablation and achieved 3- and 5-year survival rates of 66% and 38%, respectively, from the time of treatment. Abe et al.[84] used microwave ablation to treat eight patients with liver metastasis from breast cancer. Five of the eight patients were alive at the end of the study (at a mean follow-up duration of 25.9 months), although all of them had new metastases.

The literature on the use of ablative therapies in sarcomas metastatic to the liver is limited. In the study by Dileo et al.,[85] nine patients with GIST presenting with a solitary or limited number of hepatic lesions were successfully treated with percutaneous RFA. These patients had received imatinib for a median of 25 months before the ablation therapy. At a median follow-up of 5.8 months, disease remained stable in four patients. In another study, Hasegawa et al.[86] reported on a series of three patients who had advanced GIST with focal liver progression successfully treated with RFA. Those patients remained progression free at 8, 15, and 16 months after ablation. RFA is a therapeutic option for patients with GIST who develop focal progression of liver disease during imatinib therapy and who are not candidates for surgical resection.

Conclusions

Image-guided locoregional transcatheter and ablative therapies play an important role in the management of patients with unresectable liver metastases from various cancers. Their minimally invasive nature, along with decreased systemic toxicity and high local effectiveness, makes these therapies an attractive therapeutic option for these patients, who have few viable alternatives. Several studies have shown the safety and efficacy of these locoregional therapies in selected patients with liver metastases from melanomas, breast cancer, gastrointestinal tumors, and other cancers. However, given the lack of randomized trials comparing the efficacy of various locoregional treatments, there is no consensus regarding the ideal approach for treating such patients, and the choice of treatment generally depends on the availability of treatment modalities and the experience at individual institutions.

REFERENCES

The complete reference list is available online at www.expertconsult.com.

PART 3

Genitourinary and Gynecologic Oncology

DANIEL J. A. MARGOLIS

17

Percutaneous Management of Renal Tumors

TIMOTHY D. McCLURE

KEY POINTS

- Imaging plays an important role in diagnosis
- Thermal ablation is becoming a treatment option for select patients with small tumors
  - techniques include radiofrequency and cryoablation
  - long-term follow-up with imaging is necessary
- Embolization can be used in the treatment of angiomyolipomas, and in select patients with renal cell carcinoma

Introduction

Imaging has evolved to play a significant and integral role in both the diagnosis and treatment of renal tumors. Over the past decade, image-guided procedures have increasingly been used in the management of renal tumors including angiography and embolization, targeted biopsy, and thermal ablation. The use of thermal ablation to treat renal tumors has increased, particularly in older patients with small (T1a) tumors.[1] This chapter first reviews both benign and malignant renal tumor imaging characteristics and then focuses on their percutaneous management of renal tumors. A brief review of the surgical options is included to give a multidisciplinary understanding to the management of renal tumors.

Renal Tumors

There has been an increase in the incidence of renal cell carcinoma over the past several decades, with an estimated number of 58,240 new cases being diagnosed in 2010.[2,3] This is in part due to the increased use of cross-sectional scans; however, this cannot be fully explained by imaging use alone.[2,4] The classic triad presentation of abdominal pain, mass, and hematuria is no longer typical, with the majority of tumors now being found incidentally. These tumors are typically lower grade and smaller when compared to those identified because of symptoms.[5]

The imaging characteristics of renal tumors can, for the most part, predict the histology of the visualized renal lesion. Benign renal tumors include oncocytoma and angiomyolipoma. Although oncocytomas may have the classic appearance of a central stellate scar and a "spoke and wheel" on angiography, they rarely present this way. The majority of oncocytomas are extremely difficult to differentiate from clear cell renal carcinoma both on imaging and with biopsy. Unlike oncocytomas, angiomyolipomas can be reliably diagnosed on imaging, by identifying the presence of macroscopic fat. Sporadic cases of angiomyolipoma tend to occur in women in their fifth decade, whereas cases associated with tuberous sclerosis complex are likely to be multiple and occur in patients 2 decades earlier.

Malignant tumors include primary renal tumors, transitional cell carcinoma of the collecting system, and more rarely, lymphoma and collecting duct carcinoma. Primary renal tumors can be further divided according to the Heidelberg Classification into clear cell, medullary, chromophobe, and papillary carcinoma. Pathologic subtypes largely determine prognosis. Clear cell renal carcinoma generally has a worse prognosis, with a 10-year cancer specific survival rate of 60%, versus 80% for both chromophobe and papillary types.[6] Pathologic subtypes also suggest a patient's response to chemotherapy with clear cell subtypes responding favorably to tyrosine kinase inhibitors.[7] The classification of these tumors is important as these different subtypes portend different prognosis, and can often be suggested by imaging studies based on enhancement characteristics.[8,9]

Ultrasonography, computed tomography (CT), and magnetic resonance (MR) are the main imaging modalities for the assessment of renal lesions. Ultrasound's use is limited to the diagnosis of simple cysts, which demonstrate a well-circumscribed anechoic lesion within the renal parenchyma. CT and MRI diagnosis depend on enhancement and fat detection to characterize renal lesions. A lesion that contains gross fat, less than −20 HU on CT or by chemical characteristics on MRI, is diagnostic of renal angiomyolipoma.[10] The vast majority of enhancing renal masses are renal cell carcinoma, unless they are less than 3 cm, in which case 25% are benign.[11] The enhancement pattern of these lesions helps classify them as clear cell, chromophobe, or papillary renal carcinoma. This difference is best seen in the corticomedullary (late arterial) phase, with clear cell subtypes enhancing avidly, chromophobe subtypes enhancing intermediately, and papillary subtypes enhancing poorly.[9] In fact, using an 84% change in enhancement when comparing the lesion to the cortex in the corticomedullary phase can reliably differentiate clear cell from papillary renal cell carcinomas.

TREATMENT OPTIONS (FOR MALIGNANCY)

Surgery

The historic standard of reference in the management of renal cancer is the radical nephrectomy first described by Robson. This includes resection of the entire kidney, Gerota's fascia, ipsilateral adrenal gland, and lymph nodes from the crus of the diaphragm to the aortic bifurcation.[12] The past two decades have seen a dramatic change in the management of renal tumors: initially with partial nephrectomy (removing only the tumor), then with laparoscopic nephrectomy, and finally with laparoscopic partial nephrectomy.[13] These innovations in surgical technique have lead to improved convalescence, preservation of renal function, and overall survival, without compromising oncologic outcomes when compared to radical nephrectomy for tumors less than 4 cm.[14,15] Focally ablative techniques, which are truly minimally invasive and offer excellent renal preservation, are becoming viable treatment options in the appropriate patient population. Cryoablation of renal tumors was first reported in 1995 and radiofrequency ablation of a renal tumor was subsequently reported in 1999.[16,17] Since this time, there has been a trend toward nephron sparing techniques with a decrease in radical nephrectomies and increase in partial nephrectomy and ablative therapies.[18] The indications for focal ablation are described in a dedicated section.

Targeted Renal Biopsy

Biopsy can play an important role in patient management of patients with metastatic disease (e.g., melanoma, lymphoma, lung cancer, or breast cancer). When performing a biopsy in a lesion for which ablation is planned, it is important to perform the biopsy prior to the ablation as the underlying tumor pathology impacts patients' prognosis and postablative samples will only demonstrate postablative histologic changes, not initial pathology. Needle biopsy has a detection rate for malignancy of 80%–92% and a sensitivity of 83%–100%.[19] The biopsy is generally performed immediately before the ablation. The biopsy sample is optimally taken with a 17/18-gauge coaxial system after the probes have been placed. The reason for this is, when using ultrasound guidance of needle placement, the sampling process can introduce artifacts, making imaging with ultrasound difficult for subsequent probe placement. A 17/18-gauge system is used because an 18-gauge needle core biopsy has been shown to provide adequate sample for tissue diagnosis.[20] After samples have been taken, the ablation is performed, and the coaxial biopsy system is removed at the termination of the procedure, just prior to probe removal (Figure 17-1). The risk of track seeding is extremely rare, with only a single case report of tract seeding.[21]

Active Surveillance

Bosniak first suggested active surveillance in lesions less than 3 cm, as approximately 25% of these tumors are benign.[22] Other authors have reiterated this finding and suggested active surveillance in the proper patient population.[23] A large meta-analysis of observed renal masses found that the overall growth rate is 0.28 cm/year for small renal masses and that the chance of metastasis is less than 1%.[24] However, having no or low measurable growth in renal lesions does not completely reassure against malignancy.[25] Given that there is a real and significant risk for malignancy, active surveillance is generally reserved for lesions of less than 1 cm diameter in patients with significant comorbidities and limited life expectancy.[19] For patients in whom active surveillance is chosen, the patients are observed with imaging and surgery or ablation will occur when lesion growth rate is greater than 0.5 cm/year.[19,26]

Radiofrequency Ablation

The setup for radiofrequency ablation includes an electrical generator, a needle electrode, and grounding pad. There are three radiofrequency ablation devices that are currently U.S. Food and Drug Administration approved in the United States—Starburst probe (Angiodynamics, Latham, NY), LeVeen Probe (Boston Scientific, Natick MA), and Cool-Tip (Covidien, Boulder, CO)—and their probe sizes range from 14 to 17 gauge. The RFA generator produces a high-frequency alternating current with a wavelength of 460–500 kHz and a power setting of 150–200 W. A fluctuating current produces ion agitation and frictional heat deposition at the tip of the needle and causes an increase in temperature.[27] This increase in temperature leads to coagulation necrosis—cell membrane and cytoplasm damage and protein degeneration. Cell death occurs at temperatures higher than 45°C. Complete tumor necrosis occurs at temperatures of 60°–100°C. Current, and thus energy delivery to the target tissue, is inversely proportional to the square of the distance from the electrode.[28] The maximum zone of ablation of a 17-gauge needle electrode is approximately 1.6 cm.[29] To increase the ablation zone, there has been development of multi-tined electrodes, cluster arrangement of multiple electrodes, pulsing electrical current, internal cooling of the electrode, and interstitial saline infusion of electrodes. These have been developed to decrease the risk of vaporization and charring, thereby allowing the spread of heat and subsequently increasing the zone of ablation.

Cryoablation

Cryoablation is based on the Joule-Thomson effect that converts argon gas to cold low-pressure liquid. The cryoablation system is composed of gas distribution apparatus, needle-like cyroprobes, and a thermocouple. Two cryoablation devices are available: ICerod (Oncura, Plymouth Meeting, PA) and Cyrocare device (Endocare, Irvine, CA).

Cell death occurs directly by cytotoxic effects from ice crystallization and indirectly by ischemia associated with local microvascular occlusion leading to coagulative necrosis at temperatures between −19.4°C and −40°C.[30] Histologic pathology shows vascular congestion, nuclear pyknosis, mitochondrial damage, and coagulative necrosis.[31] The temperature at the edge of the ice ball is 0°C, which is nonlethal; therefore, the ice ball must extend 3.1 mm beyond the tumor margin. Double freeze–thaw cycles can be used to increase the size of the ice ball.[32]

Embolization

Embolization of renal tumors was first described in the 1970s and is used for three main indications. Embolization is used in the management of large renal tumors with caval thrombus to help decrease overall tumor size, improve surgical technique by inducing edema (which helps surgical dissection), and decrease perioperative blood loss.[33] Embolization has also been shown to improve survival in patients with unresectable renal cancer, with one study demonstrating a 1-year survival rate of 29% in patients undergoing embolization versus 13% in nonembolized patients.[34] Some authors also argue that embolization may improve paraneoplastic syndromes and hematuria. The combination of both embolization and RFA to treat renal cell cancer by decreasing the vascular heat sink affect has been shown to be feasible by improving the efficacy of RFA.[35] Embolization is performed using three embolic agents: liquids such as absolute ethanol, particles such as microspheres, and metallic coils. The interventionalist's selection of embolic agent depends on the vascular composition of the tumor and kidney. Initially reported complication rates were as high as 10%, but this has decreased significantly with more recent groups reporting complication rates as low as 0%.[34,36] Almost all patients will experience some form of postembolization syndrome, which includes flank pain, fever, nausea, and vomiting within the first 24–96 hours.

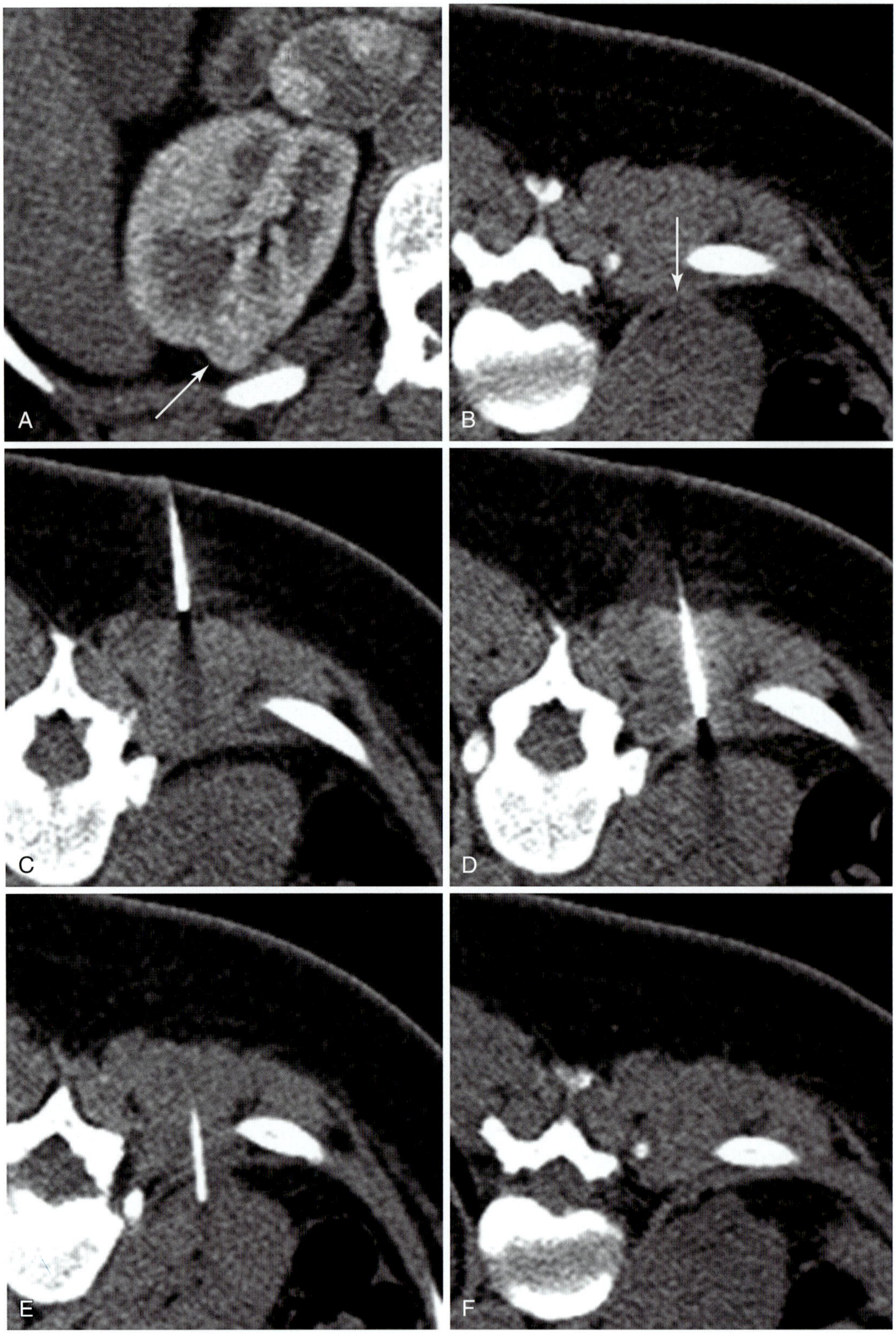

Figure 17-1 CT-guided biopsy of incidentally found enhancing lesion in the right kidney (*arrow*) (A). Body habitus limited safe ultrasound-guided biopsy, and therefore a CT-guided biopsy was performed. The patient was placed in the prone position (B). Using intermittent CT guidance, a 19-gauge coaxial biopsy needle was advanced to the mass and multiple 20-gauge biopsies were performed (C–E). After the biopsy system was removed and manual compression was applied, there was no evidence of any complication (F).

The postembolization syndrome is self-limiting. Renal embolization has demonstrated utility in the preoperative management of large resectable tumors and in the management of unresectable disease. The combination of RFA and tumor embolization is feasible to help reduce heat sink effects, resulting in larger zones of ablation.

TREATMENT CONSIDERATIONS

Initial Workup

The initial evaluation of a patient with a renal mass should include contrast-enhanced cross-sectional imaging (CT or MRI) and a chest x-ray. Both an interventional oncologist and urologist should be consulted prior to tumor ablation if this is a consideration. Laboratory analysis should include complete blood count (CBC), coagulation profile including international normalized ratio (INR), partial thromboplastin time (PTT), and a chemistry panel. A bone scan can be ordered if there is concern for bony metastatic disease as evidenced by bone pain, elevated calcium, or an elevated alkaline phosphatase level. Neurologic symptoms reported by a patient warrant a contrast-enhanced brain scan to rule out metastatic disease. This workup determines the TNM staging, which is important as it correlates with patient prognosis and, therefore, management considerations. Survival at 5 years is 95% with stage I disease, 88% with stage II, 59% with stage III, and 20% with stage IV.[37]

Indications For Nonsurgical Management

General indications are less than 10-year but greater than 1-year life expectancy, multiple renal tumors, solitary kidney, limited renal function, and comorbid conditions precluding surgery. Special considerations should be applied to patients with genetic predisposition to renal cell carcinoma (RCC), including von Hippel-Lindau (VHL), hereditary papillary RCC (HPRCC), and Birt-Hogg-Dubé syndrome. In this cohort of patients, lesions greater than 3 cm have been historically treated surgically[38]. However, focal thermal ablation may be optimal in the management of these patients in order to preserve renal function.

The American Urologic Association's recommendation on the management of Stage I tumors (renal lesions confined to the kidney ≤7 cm) with regard to thermal ablation is that it should be considered in patients with T1a lesions (renal lesions confined to the kidney ≤4 cm) with major comorbidities and increased surgical risk.[26]

A comprehensive discussion on the oncologic efficacy for informed consent is discussed after the section on technique.

Contraindications

Healthy patients who do not have increased surgical risk or major comorbidities should be counseled on the limited long-term data that is available regarding thermal ablation. Generally speaking, lesions >4 cm (T1b) should be advised to undergo surgical management.[39] Bleeding diatheses (including platelets fewer than 70,000/μL and INR greater than 1.5) and inability to remain in position for an extended period of time are established contraindications.

TECHNIQUE

Anesthesia

The choice of general anesthesia, monitored anesthesia care, or conscious sedation is variable and depends largely on both the interventionalist and patient. General anesthesia provides excellent control over patient breathing, allowing for better control in assessing difficult-to-target lesions. When considering the type of anesthesia, radiofrequency ablation is generally considered to be more painful than cryoablation.

Patient Positioning

The goal is to achieve an acceptable window for needle placement that avoids critical structures. Positioning is largely operator dependent. however, lesion location tends to predict patient positioning. Upper-pole lesions are best approached with an ipsilateral decubitus position that allows the bowel to fall dependently out of position, minimizes respiratory motion effects on the kidney, and brings the ipsilateral lung down, thereby decreasing the risk of entering the lung and pleural space. Lower-pole tumors are best approached with the patient in the prone position (Figure 17-2). The pleural space extends to the 10th rib, so care must be taken when approaching a lesion intercostally so as to avoid the pleural space and lung. Anterior and lateral lesions can be accessed with the patient in the supine position; however, the liver, spleen, and colon can obstruct access. Anterior lesions can also be approached in the oblique position, with the ipsilateral side up 30°, which allows the bowel to fall dependently out of position.

Probe Placement

Contrast-enhanced imaging prior to ablation is integral for ablation planning. When ablating left renal tumors, attention to the large bowel, small bowel, spleen, pancreas, and adrenal gland is important. When ablating a right-sided renal tumor, one must pay close attention to the location of the liver, duodenum, large bowel, gallbladder, and adrenal gland. Once the location of the lesion to be ablated is identified, the need for organ displacement is determined. Lesions that will be within 5 mm of an adjacent organ should undergo organ displacement to protect them during the ablation. If the location of the tumor is within 5 mm of the collecting system and ureter, pyeloperfusion should be performed. This is commonly seen in both central- and lower-pole lesions.

Any cross-sectional modality can be used for probe placement: ultrasonography, MRI, and CT. Probe placement and subsequent ablation has been done entirely with ultrasound, with comparable results to CT- and CT/ultrasound-guided ablation.[40] A limitation with ultrasound is that both the formation of an ice ball with cryoablation and air bubbles with RFA reflects sound waves, thus limiting full evaluation of the tumor when the ablation is ongoing.

When treating large tumors with a single electrode, the probe may be repositioned to ablate the tumor in totality.[41]

Cryoablation allows multiple probes to be used at the same time. A single cryoprobe will produce a 2-cm ice ball. Because a 3.1-mm margin of tissue is generally needed, 2- to 3-cm tumors are usually treated with two to three probes. Multiple freeze–thaw cycles involving a 15-minute freeze and a 10-minute thaw can be used with temperatures reaching −130°C.

Lesion Position

The location of tumor is an important predictor of successful ablation. Classifying tumors as either *exophytic*, *central*, or *mixed* can help predict outcomes with regards to treatment and complications. *Exophytic* tumors are defined as tumors that

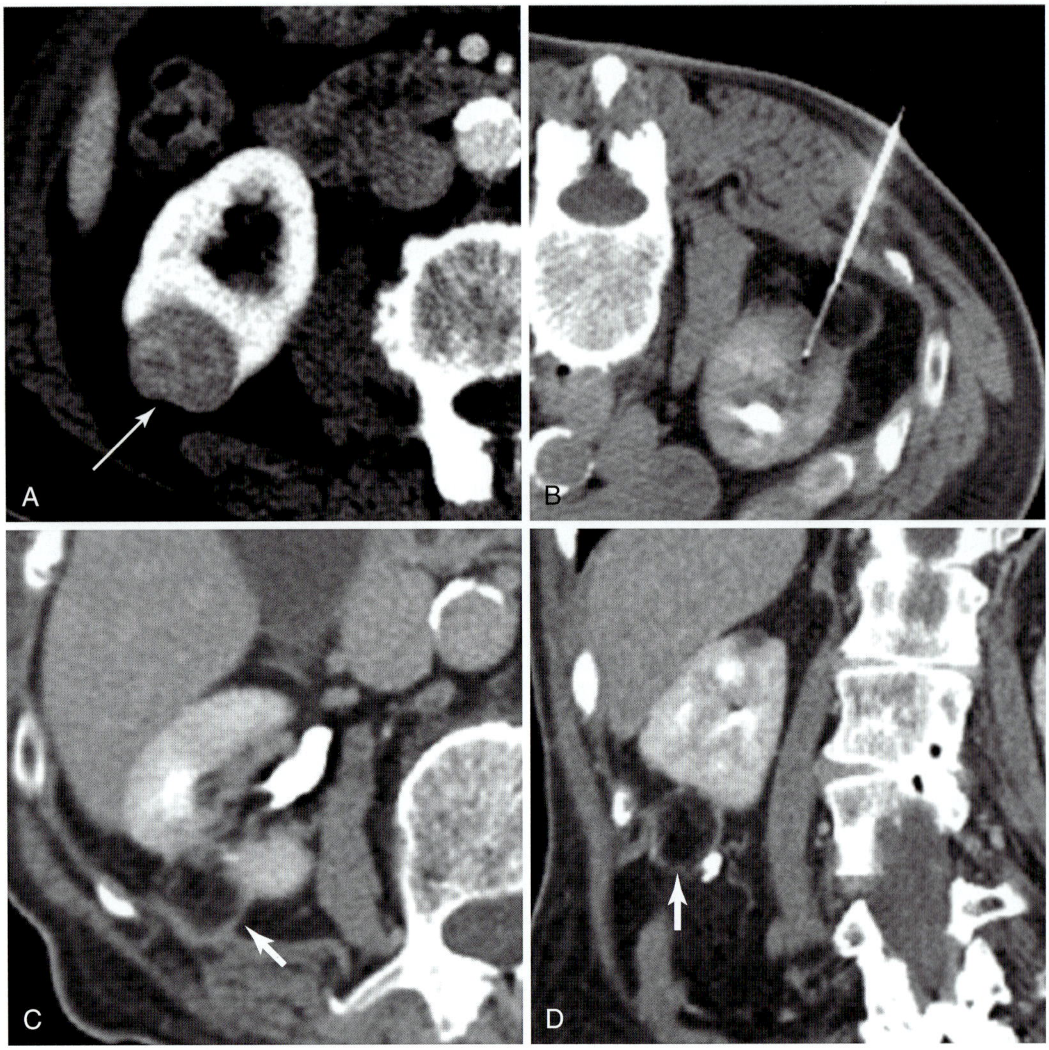

Figure 17-2 Right lower-pole enhancing mass, which was biopsy-proven renal cell carcinoma. Axial image showing the preablation lesion in the right kidney (*thin arrow*, A). After positioning the patient in the prone position, ultrasound and CT were used to guide placement of the radiofrequency probe and a successful ablation was performed (B). Five-year follow-up CT demonstrated no enhancement within the ablation defect (*thick arrow*): axial (C) and coronal (D) planes.

have at least 25% of the tumor diameter in contact with the perinephric fat, *central* tumors are defined as lesions that extend into the renal sinus, and *mixed* tumors have tumor in both the renal sinus and perinephric fat. Exophytic tumors usually have a higher rate of primary success, probably because their distance from the central vessels reduces the overall heat-sink effect.[29] Central tumors are more likely to have not only a lower rate of primary success (heat-sink effect) but also a higher risk for complications compared with exophytic tumors.[42] Tumor size also predicts success with tumors greater than 4 cm having increased rates of recurrence.[39]

Hydrodissection

Hydrodissection with sterile water or 5% dextrose (D5W) has been shown to be effective in protecting surrounding organs during thermal ablation.[43] Carbon dioxide and air have also been used for this purpose.[44] Hydrodissection with fluid usually will require continuous fluid instillation during the ablation. Normal saline or other electrolyte-based, electrically conductive solutions should be avoided when using radiofrequency ablation. If D5W is used for a diabetic patient, serum glucose levels should be monitored.

Hydrodissection is performed when a lesion is within 5 mm of the organ of concern. A 5-Fr sheath needle is placed under ultrasound guidance, and CT or MRI can then be performed to ensure appropriate position (Figure 17-3). Once in place, a nonelectrolyte-based solution is instilled. Hydrodissection is monitored with repeat cross-sectional imaging.

Organ Displacement

Another method of moving the ablation zone away from adjacent structures is to use the ablation needle to shift the kidney. The mobility of the kidney within the retroperitoneum allows for organ displacement when the ablation probe is in place. Once the treatment lesion is identified and a probe placed within the lesion, torque can be applied to move the kidney. Image guidance should be used when performing this technique.[45]

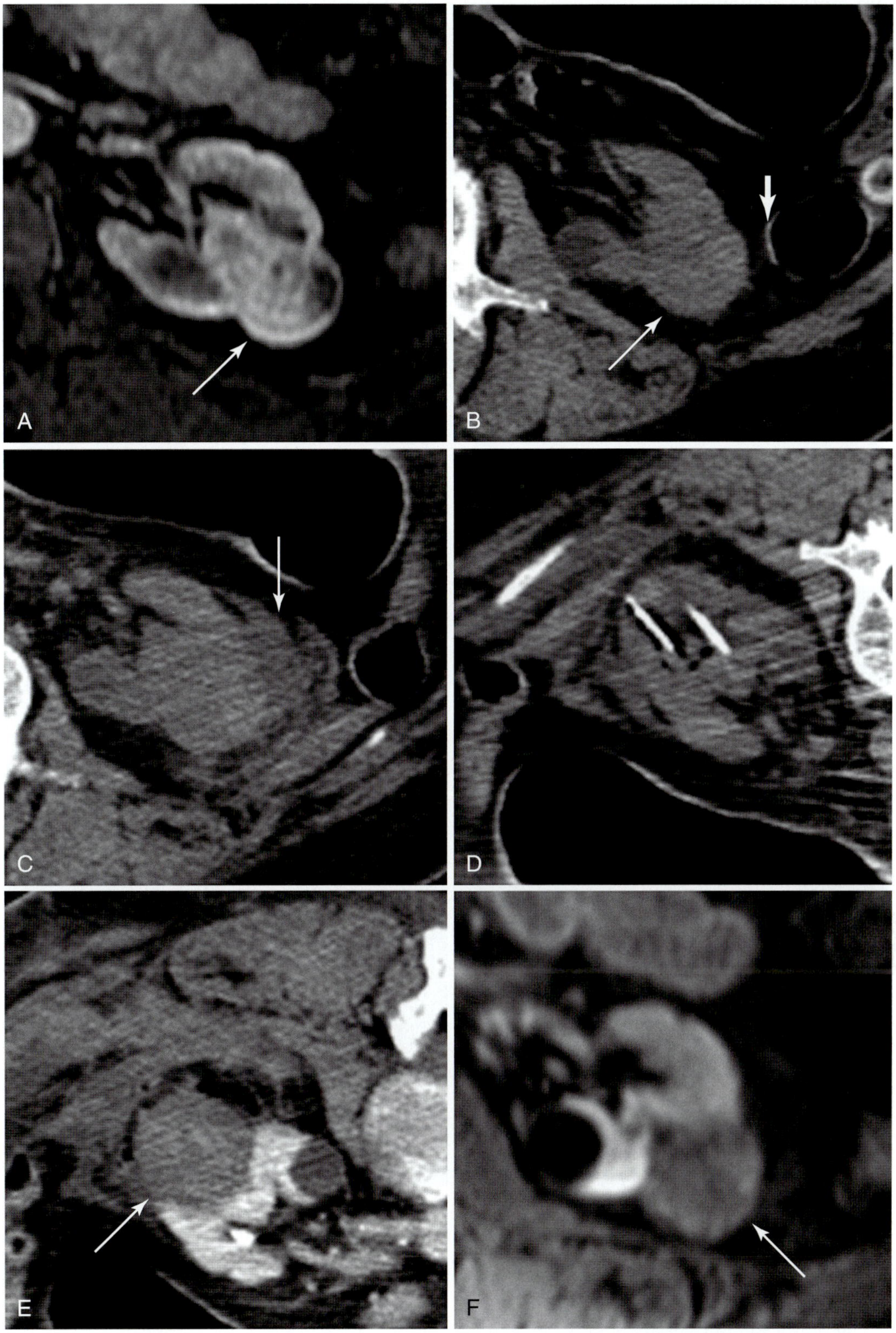

Figure 17-3 Incidentally found 2.9-cm exophytic enhancing mass (*thin arrow*) that was less than 5 mm from adjacent descending colon (A). The patient was placed in a prone position that confirmed proximity of the descending colon (*thick arrow*, B). Hydrodissection was performed after a 5-Fr sheath needle was placed under ultrasound guidance into the lateral perinephric space between the kidney and descending colon. One liter was instilled by gravity into the left perinephric space, which displaced the descending colon approximately 30 mm from the target lesion (*long arrow*, C). Successful ablation was performed after biopsy and placement of three electrodes (D). Immediate postablation contrast-enhanced CT demonstrated a nonenhancing ablation defect (E). At the 33-month follow-up, contrast-enhanced MR demonstrated a nonenhancing lesion with no evidence of recurrence (F).

Collecting System Injury Prevention

Shultze et al. first demonstrated that perfusion of the collecting system with cold saline during the ablation of a central lesion prevented injury.[46] Subsequent studies have confirmed that retrograde pyeloperfusion prevents complications related to the collecting system, including hydronephrosis or ureteral strictures; however, this may result in an increased risk of treatment failure because of the heat-sink effect of pyeloperfusion.[47]

Retrograde pyeloperfusion is achieved with the cystoscopic placement of an open-ended 5-Fr ureteral catheter into the renal collecting system. After placement of the 5-Fr catheter, a Foley catheter is placed within the bladder to allow drainage (Figure 17-4). Although the first report of pyeloperfusion used normal saline, we prefer to use a nonelectrolyte-based fluid such as D5W. The perfusion pressure is then set to 80 cm H_2O and 1-L bags of D5W that have been stored at 2°C–6°C are used.

Postprocedure Care

Postprocedure care includes appropriate postanesthesia nursing care with most patients treated as outpatients. Postprocedure laboratory tests do not generally need to be ordered, unless clinically indicated. Mild pain is expected and can be managed with oral pain medications. There is no general consensus on the use of periprocedure antibiotics. Their use is largely dependent on the individual interventionalist.[48] Generally, gram-negative coverage, such as 1 g of ceftriaxone, is used if the patient has undergone pyeloperfusion, has a history of urinary tract diversion, or recurrent urinary tract infections. Fevers, severe flank pain, hypotension, and hematuria are concerning symptoms and warrant further workup.

Postablation imaging is just as important as the ablation itself and is essential for appropriate patient management because recurrence has been seen as long as 31 months postablation.[49] There has been no consensus on the frequency of postablation imaging in the literature, with initial scans ranging from 0 to 5 weeks and subsequent follow-up of 3 months, 6 months, and then yearly.[21,41,50] We perform surveillance imaging immediately postablation, then at 3 months, 6 months, and yearly. Whatever frequency scanning is chosen, evaluation should include the ablation zone, ipsilateral and contralateral kidney if present, and search for metastatic disease.

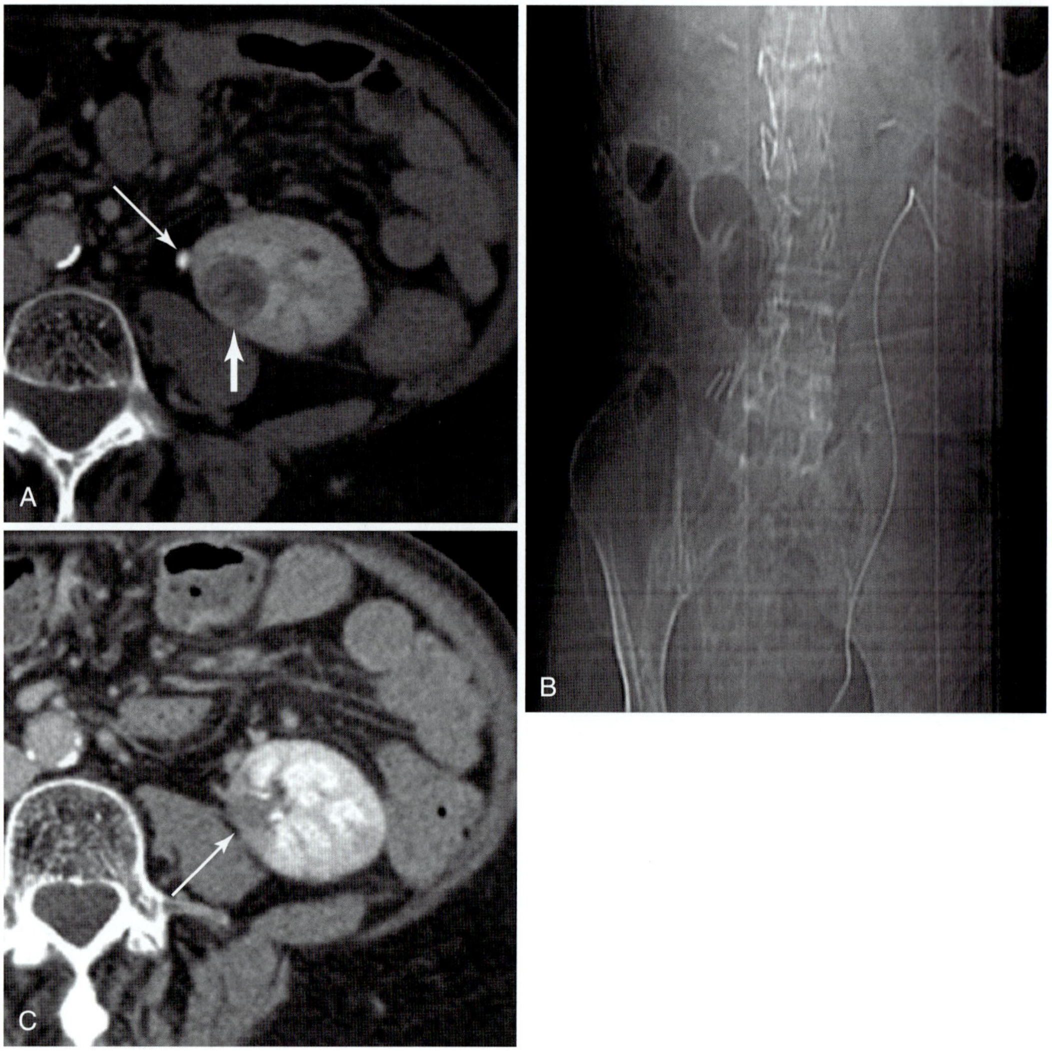

Figure 17-4 CT axial image demonstrates a left lower pole renal cell carcinoma (*thick arrow*) abutting the proximal ureter (*thin arrow*, A). Pyeloperfusion was used to protect the ureter. Scout film shows the 5-Fr angiocatheter in place (B). CT axial image demonstrated successful ablation with no enhancement (*thin arrow*) and no evidence of ureteral injury on 16-month follow-up (C).

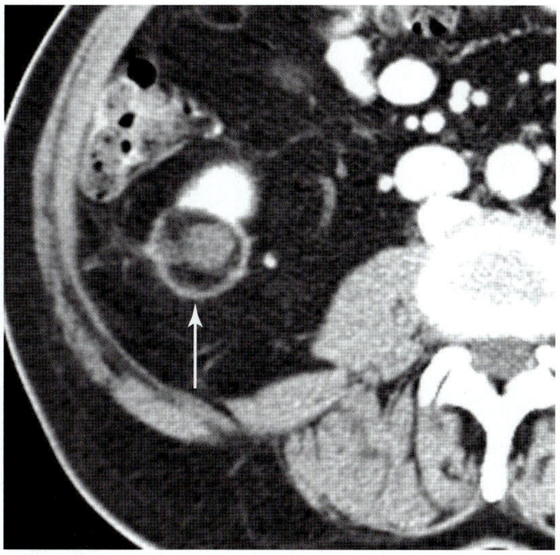

Figure 17-5 Post–radiofrequency ablation defect. Contrast-enhanced CT demonstrating "bull's eye" or "pseudo AML" ablation defect (*arrow*) with peritumoral rim of tissue at the 4-year follow-up.

The imaging findings of thermal ablation depend on the technique used. Immediate RFA ablation defects will show foci of air within the lesion, surrounding fat stranding, and no enhancement on contrast-enhanced imaging on CT. Over time, however, the foci of air and surrounding fat stranding will resolve and a "bull's eye" ablation defect with a peritumoral rim of tissue will appear, particularly in exophytic lesions (Figure 17-5). The lesion should continue to show no enhancement if successfully treated. On MR, immediate post-RFA lesions will become T2-hypointense with variable T1 signal intensity. As with CT, there should be no enhancement on postcontrast imaging. MR findings are more variable with post-RFA lesions, but the bull's-eye appearance with a central T2 hypointensity and surrounding T1/T2 heterogenous signal intensity can still be seen (Figure 17-6). Subtracted pre- and postcontrast images are vital for assessing enhancement, as the intrinsic variable T1 hyperintensity can make postcontrast imaging difficult to analyze (Figure 17-7). The size of the ablation defect may decrease over time. However, this decrease is not as pronounced as that seen with cryoablation (see Figure 17-6).[51]

Immediate cryoablation defects are seen as areas of hypodensity on CT imaging and should also show no contrast enhancement on postcontrast imaging. Subsequent imaging findings will demonstrate decreasing size of the ablation defect with continued lack of postcontrast enhancement. MR findings of immediate cryoablation defects will appear as T1 hypointensity, reflecting the ice ball. Over time, cryoablation defects will become T1-isotense and T2-hypointense. As before, there will be no enhancement on contrast-enhanced fat-suppressed T1-weighted subtraction MR images.[51]

These described imaging findings of both RFA and cryoablation treatment defects are generalizations and many lesions will have a variable appearance on follow-up, especially when treating central or mixed tumors. The keystone of imaging for recurrence is the same regardless of ablative technique, a successfully treated lesion will show no enhancement, therefore all postablation imaging must contain postcontrast images. There are two types of postablation enhancement: residual disease and recurrent disease. *Residual disease* is defined as persistent enhancement demonstrated on contrast-enhanced CT within 3 months of surveillance imaging. *Recurrent disease* is defined as previous nonenhancing lesion that now has a new focus of enhancement. Enhancement patterns of recurrence or residual disease patterns will vary depending on the type of ablation devices used. Multiple peripheral nodules can be seen with multi-tined hooked array systems, and focal areas of enhancement will be seen with straight needle systems.[42] Postablation defect growth and new foci of T2 hyperintensity within the lesion are also findings that may suggest recurrent disease.[51] The reported recurrence rate of residual or recurrent disease is approximately 4.2%, which is similar to both partial and radical nephrectomy, 3%–6%.[52,53]

Complications

Minor complications include pain, paresthesia, chyluria, transient hematuria, and subcapsular hematomas (Figure 17-8). Major complications include hemorrhage requiring blood transfusions, ureteral strictures, urinoma, abscess, and bowel injury (Figure 17-9).[21,42,50,54] Chyluria is usually asymptomatic but fairly common, occurring in approximately 41% patients undergoing percutaneous ablation. It is thought to be secondary to fistulization of lymphatics. The management of this is observation, as it will resolve.[55] There is a suggestion of a higher rate of complications with central tumors.[42,56]

Management of Complications

The large majority of complications can be managed conservatively; however, just as patient selection requires a multidisciplinary approach, so too do complications. Early consultation with the various specialists is necessary to ensure appropriate patient care.

Informed Consent

ONCOLOGIC EFFICACY

Radiofrequency ablation of renal tumors was first reported in the late 1990s with Zlotta reporting their surgical approach in 1997 and subsequently followed by McGovern who reported the first percutaneous approach in 1999.[17,57] Early studies initially reported success rates of 81%–100% in tumors 2.5 to 4 cm in size.[21,50] Subsequent longer-term studies have showed similar outcomes. McDougal et al. showed a 94% success rate in lesions followed at least 4 years with similar outcomes to surgery.[58] Levinson et al. reported an overall recurrence-free survival of 90.3%, with a mean follow-up of 5.1 years (61.6 months).[49] This study illustrated the importance of long-term follow-up in the patients as recurrence was seen at 7, 13, and 31 months postablation.[49] Zagoria et al. showed a recurrence-free survival of 88% at a mean follow-up of 5.1 years (61 months).[39] Ferakis et al. showed primary and secondary success rates of 90% and 97%, respectively, with an average follow-up of 5.1 years (61.2 months).[59]

There are limited data on the oncologic outcomes with percutaneous cryoablation, but there have been several studies that have looked at the surgical outcomes of cryoablation. Gill et al. showed a 3-year cancer-free specific survival of 98%.[60] Chalasani et al. showed a 4-year recurrence-free survival rate of 83.6% with a mean overall survival rate of 97.8%.[61] Two limited studies on percutaneous cryoablation have shown primary efficacy of 95% with 100% secondary efficacy at an

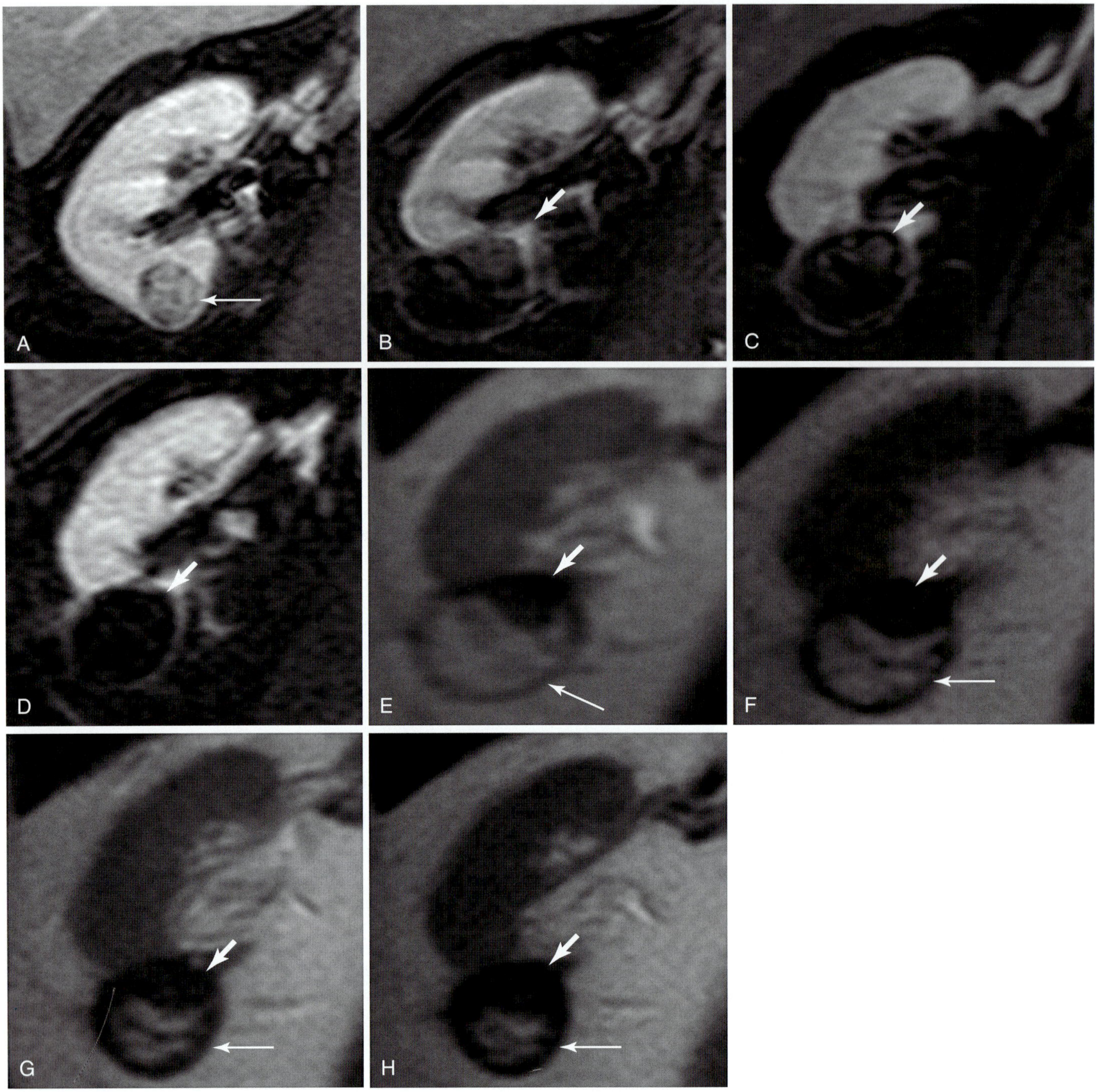

Figure 17-6 Coronal T1 postcontrast MR images demonstrate enhancing lesion in the right kidney lower pole (*thin arrow*, A). Coronal T1 contrast-enhanced MR images show ablation defect (*thick arrow*) with intrinsic T1 hyperintensity, but with no enhancement at 6 months (B), 2 years (C), and 3 years (D) of follow-up. Coronal T2 images demonstrating intrinsic T2 hypointensity of ablated defect (*thick arrow*) with surrounding rim of tissue (*thin arrow*) that over time demonstrates increase in T2 hypointensity of the lesion. Dates of scans are at 6 months (E), 2 years (F), 5 years (G), and 7 years (H) postablation.

average follow-up of 9.1 months.[62] Silverman demonstrated 92.3% complete ablation with an average follow-up of 14 months.[63] There is no difference in the oncologic outcomes when comparing laparoscopic or percutaneous approaches to cryoablation.[64] Percutaneous cryoablation has decreased complication rates and hospital stay when compared to surgical cryoablation.[64]

There has been some controversy regarding the oncologic efficacy of percutaneous ablative techniques, with one study suggesting that rates of local tumor progression were higher in ablative techniques when compared to partial nephrectomy. However, this study essentially defined local progression as primary efficacy and did not truly evaluate oncologic efficacy, as many ablations require more than one session to

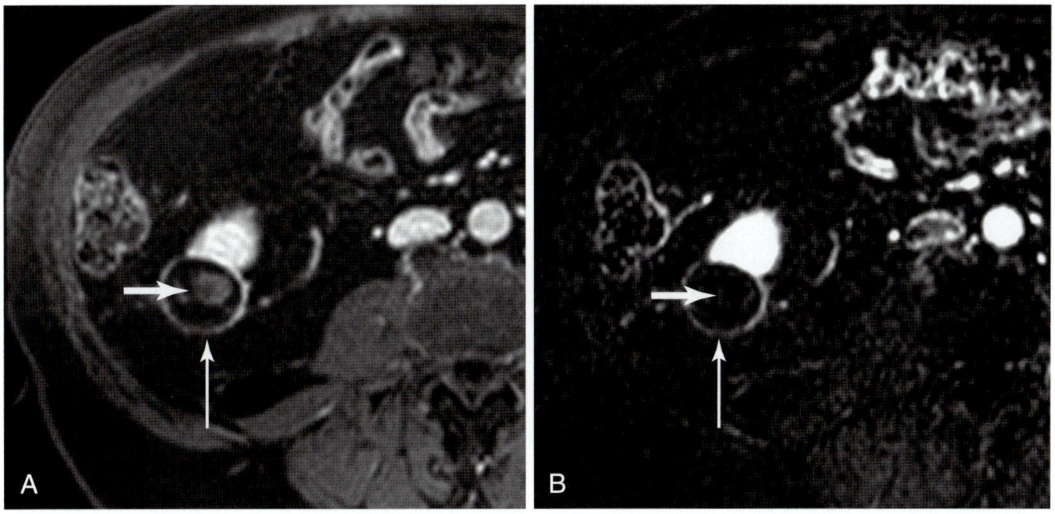

Figure 17-7 MR subtraction imaging. T1 fat-saturated precontrast MR axial images demonstrating ablation defect (*thin arrow*) with intrinsic T1 hyperintensity (*thick arrow*) (A). T1 postcontrast fat-subtracted images demonstrating no enhancement in the ablation defect (*thin arrow*) in the 4-year follow-up MRI. Notice that the intrinsic T1 hyperintensity has been subtracted from the image (*thick arrow*) (B).

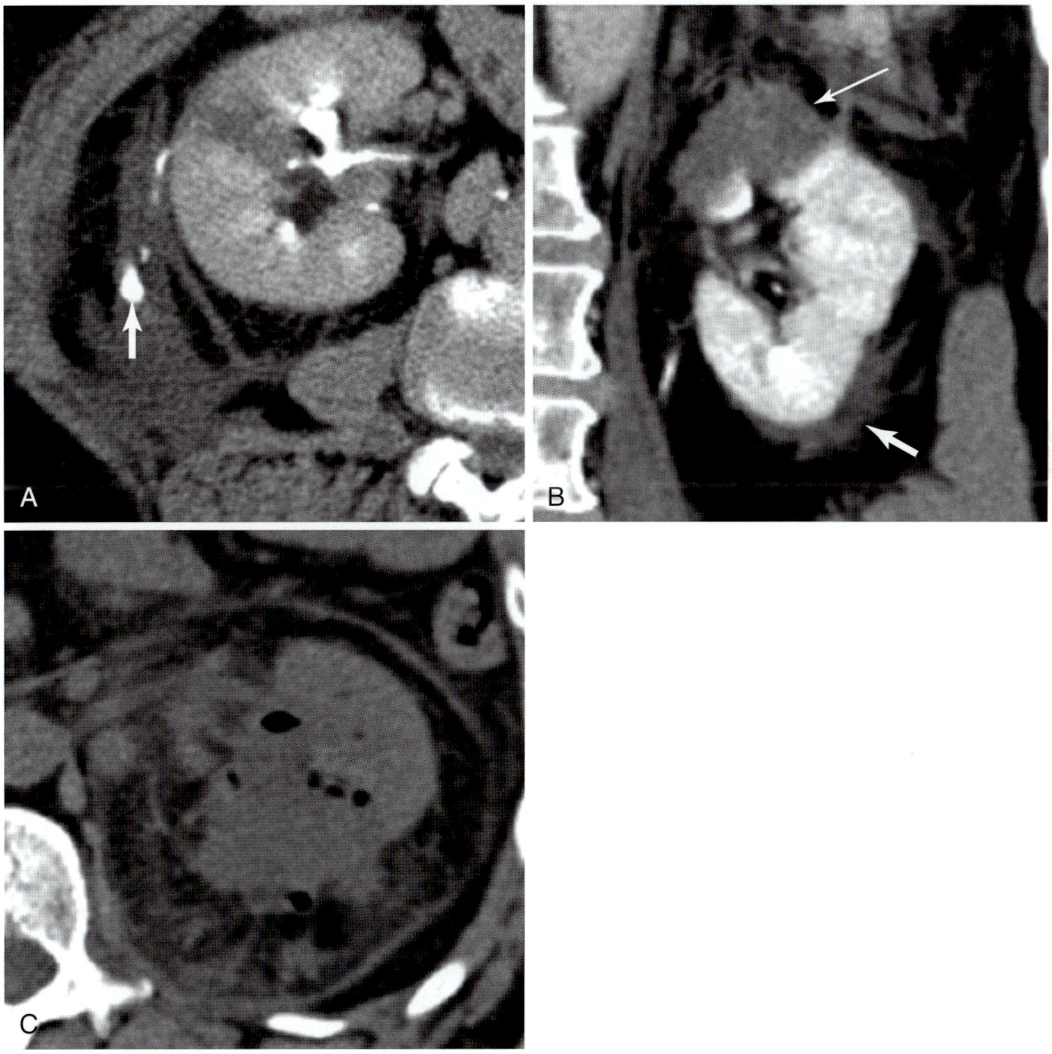

Figure 17-8 Complications associated with thermal ablation. Axial contrast-enhanced CT demonstrating urinary extravasation (*thick arrow*) immediately after thermal ablation (A). Coronal contrast-enhanced CT demonstrating ablation defect (*thin arrow*) and hematoma (*thick arrow*) (B). Both complications resolved with conservative therapy. Non-contrast-enhanced CT showing emphysematous pyelonephritis in a patient who underwent ablation of lower pole lesion, which was close to the ureter and did not undergo pyeloperfusion (C).

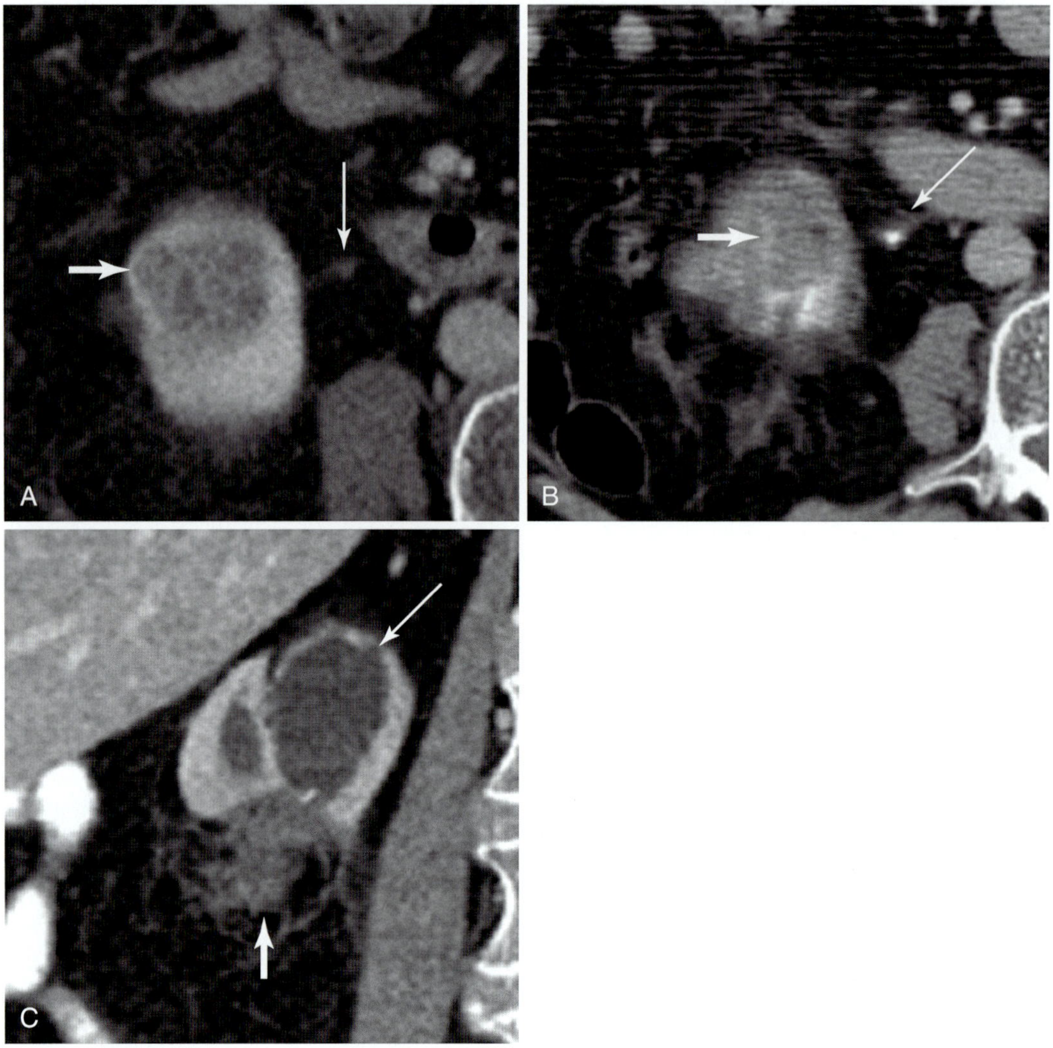

Figure 17-9 Axial contrast-enhanced CT image showing renal cell carcinoma in the lower pole of the right kidney (*thick arrow*) within 5 mm of the ureter (*thin arrow*, A). Postablation contrast-enhanced CT image shows successful ablation and periureteral standing concerning for injury. Coronal enhanced CT image shows postablation defect (*thick arrow*) with hydronephrotic kidney (*thin arrow*, C).

be successful.[65] Subsequent studies have demonstrated no statistically significant difference between lesions undergoing ablation when compared to partial nephrectomy, with both having similar 3-year recurrence-free survival.[66] When comparing oncologic efficacy with radiofrequency and cryoablation ablative techniques, there is no difference.[67]

Nephron-sparing surgery has been shown to have longer preservation of renal function, overall survival, and equivalent oncologic control as total nephrectomy.[14,15] Wehrenberg-Klee et al. showed that neither cryoablation nor radiofrequency ablation significantly affects renal function among patients with chronic kidney disease. Change in GFR went from 41.2 mL/min/1.73 m^2 to 40.9 mL/min/1.73 m^2. [68] Other studies have also shown no change in renal function.[64,69] There have been data to suggest that in patients with von Hippel-Lindau (VHL) disease, there is a decrease in renal function after multiple ablations.[70]

Controversy regarding the presence of residual tumor despite negative imaging exists, particularly with RFA. One study analyzed tumors immediately postablation and found histologic evidence of viable tumor cells within the ablation zone.[71] A second study biopsied ablation defects 6 months after RFA and found 13 patients with histologic findings concerning for RCC. Of these patients, 46.2% demonstrated no postcontrast enhancement on imaging. This surprisingly high rate of false negatives was not seen in patients who underwent cryoablation. Both these studies used hematoxylin and eosin staining for pathologic analysis, and an explanation for these findings is that the coagulative necrosis associated with RFA causes heat fixation, preserving the appearance of RCC even though these cells are nonviable and thereby making hematoxylin and eosin staining suboptimal in RFA biopsy samples.[72] A third study showed discrepancy between radiologic findings of nonenhancement and tumor presence as two of three patients with residual viable tumor did not have enhancement of CT imaging. A major limitation to this study was that these scans occurred 1 week after ablation, which underscores the need for appropriate timing of follow-up imaging.[73]

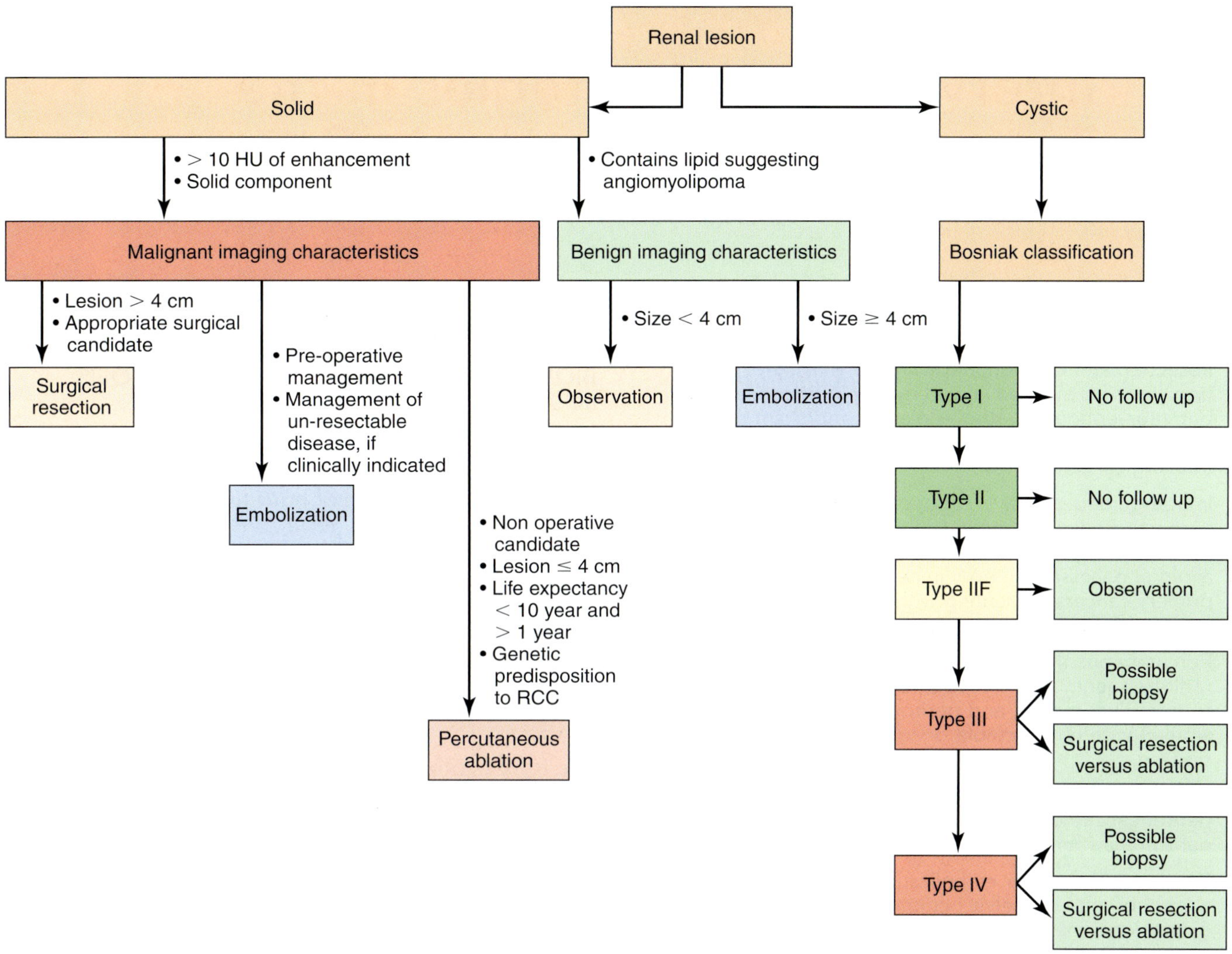

Figure 17-10 Algorithm for treatment choice.

CONSIDERATIONS FOR BENIGN DISEASE (ANGIOMYOLIPOMA)

Percutaneous management of benign disease is predominately focused on angiomyolipomas. Angiomyolipomas are benign tumors composed of blood vessels, smooth muscle, and fat cells. The presence of multiple, bilateral tumors suggests an association with tuberous sclerosis, whereas solitary, unilateral tumors suggest a sporadic form. The clinical implication of these benign tumors is bleeding, particularly in lesions greater than 4 cm in size. Nephron-sparing techniques are favored in the management of these tumors and embolization is the predominant treatment option for lesions greater than 4 cm.[74] Radiofrequency ablation has been described to treat angiomyolipomas with excellent outcomes.[75]

Conclusion

Imaging-guided techniques are quickly becoming an integral component in the treatment algorithm for patients with renal tumors. Although thermal ablative therapies have limited long-term data on their oncologic efficacy, the current literature is promising. Given this lack of evidence, it is imperative that patients are counseled on the treatment risk and benefits, including but not limited to the lack of full oncologic data seen with long-term surgical studies. Despite these limitations, the current literature suggests that in experienced hands, thermal ablation is a promising treatment option for the appropriately selected patient. A proposed treatment algorithm is presented in Figure 17-10.

Acknowledgments

The author would like to acknowledge Dr. Steven Raman for his comprehensive help in both preparing and reviewing the text and for the selection of representative images.

REFERENCES

The complete reference list is available online at www.expertconsult.com.

18

Interventional Strategies in the Treatment of Gynecologic Cancers

JORDAN ANAOKAR | STEVEN S. RAMAN

KEY POINTS

- Resection and chemotherapy are the mainstays of treatment for most advanced gynecologic cancers, but interventional strategies play an important role in the diagnosis and treatment of patients who are not surgical candidates.
- Image-guided biopsy is suggested in cases of suspected ovarian cancer with peritoneal carcinomatosis to help guide neoadjuvant chemotherapy and avoid unnecessary surgery in cases of nongynecologic primary cancers presenting with omental metastases.
- Percutaneous thermoablative techniques, including radiofrequency and cryoablation, can be safely used to treat liver, pelvic, and peritoneal metastases in women with unresectable or suboptimally resected disease.
- Image-guided placement of semipermanent indwelling peritoneal catheters is an effective alternative to serial paracentesis for patients with refractory ascites.
- Transarterial catheter embolization can be used for control of massive pelvic hemorrhage from advanced gynecologic malignancies.
- Thermoablative techniques, such as high-intensity focused ultrasound (HIFU) and radiofrequency ablation (RFA), may be employed in the treatment of nonmalignant gynecologic conditions such as cervical ectopy and abdominal wall endometriosis.

Introduction

Interventional strategies are limited in the primary treatment of gynecology cancers, but they are increasingly employed as secondary therapies for patients with nonresectable disease, and image-guided techniques are used for the biopsy and management of symptoms related to these malignancies. This chapter presents the interventional techniques used in the diagnosis, management, and treatment of gynecologic neoplasms. Ovarian cancer is highlighted in this chapter because it is the leading cause of death in women with gynecologic cancers,[1] often presenting in advanced stages and with frequent recurrence that limit surgical options. However, many of these techniques can be applied in other gynecologic cancers, though their use is not as frequent. Various interventional therapies for benign gynecologic conditions are also described, with uterine leiomyomas covered in a separate, dedicated chapter.

Interventions In Gynecologic Oncology

BIOPSY OF PERITONEAL CARCINOMATOSIS IN SUSPECTED OVARIAN CANCER

Surgical cytoreduction followed by chemotherapy is the mainstay of therapy for patients with ovarian cancer. Often patients will have debulking surgery prior to tissue diagnosis, ovarian cancer may be presumed based on elevated CA-125 and imaging findings.[2] In patients with unresectable disease at the time of presentation or in those with medical comorbidities that preclude surgery, induction or neoadjuvant chemotherapy is typically administered first.[3] Unfortunately, the diagnosis of ovarian cancer is not always clear and a tissue diagnosis is warranted prior to these treatments. Additionally, some medical therapies rely on pathologic or molecular analysis.

Advanced ovarian cancer can sometimes be indistinguishable from peritoneal and adnexal metastases from other primary tumors, and up to 20% of women undergoing surgical debulking for suspected ovarian cancer are found to have metastatic disease from a nongynecologic source.[4,5] Moreover, in women with a history of a primary cancer known to demonstrate peritoneal spread, such as breast or gastrointestinal tract malignancies, new ovarian or peritoneal lesions do not always represent spread of disease. At least two series have demonstrated a diagnosis of a different primary Müllerian cancer (ovarian or primary peritoneal) on resection.[6,7] There also can be considerable overlap with the imaging appearance of benign complex ovarian masses.[8] In these situations, a site-specific diagnosis is imperative to avoid unnecessary surgery or inappropriate chemotherapy.

Image-guided biopsy (IGB) of omental, peritoneal and pelvic masses is a safe and effective alternative to surgical biopsy via exploratory laparotomy or laparoscopy.[6,9-11] In the largest published study to date of IGB in 149 women with peritoneal carcinomatosis, a site-specific diagnosis was made in 93% of patients.[6] Smaller series in women with peritoneal carcinomatosis and suspected ovarian cancer also had favorable results, with reported accuracy rates of 92%[11] and 87%.[12]

Both ultrasound and CT-guided techniques have been described, modality selection depends largely on the patient and his or her disease burden as well as operator comfort.[6,9-13] For patients with bulky disease likely to be visualized sonographically, ultrasound may be the appropriate choice as it is typically faster, allows for real-time visualization of vasculature, and spares the patient and physician from ionizing radiation. However, isolating peritoneal or omental masses from the adjacent bowel under ultrasound guidance can be challenging for a less experienced operator. CT may be a better choice in these cases or with smaller, more inaccessible lesions. Often CT and ultrasound are used in conjunction, as the portability of ultrasound allows operators to image the target lesions using both modalities in the same room and choose the most appropriate modality at the time of the procedure (Figures 18-1 and 18-2).

All patients should undergo a diagnostic CT of the abdomen and pelvis with intravenous and oral contrast shortly prior to the procedure to identify disease burden and distinguish peritoneal disease from adjacent bowel or liver. Ultrasound-guided biopsies require no patient preparation, though one may request a full bladder for a better acoustic window. Multiple authors have described CT-guided techniques that employ oral contrast prior to the procedure to opacify and help identify bowel from adjacent disease.[6,11,12] With both techniques, the procedure can be combined with a diagnostic or therapeutic drainage of ascites.

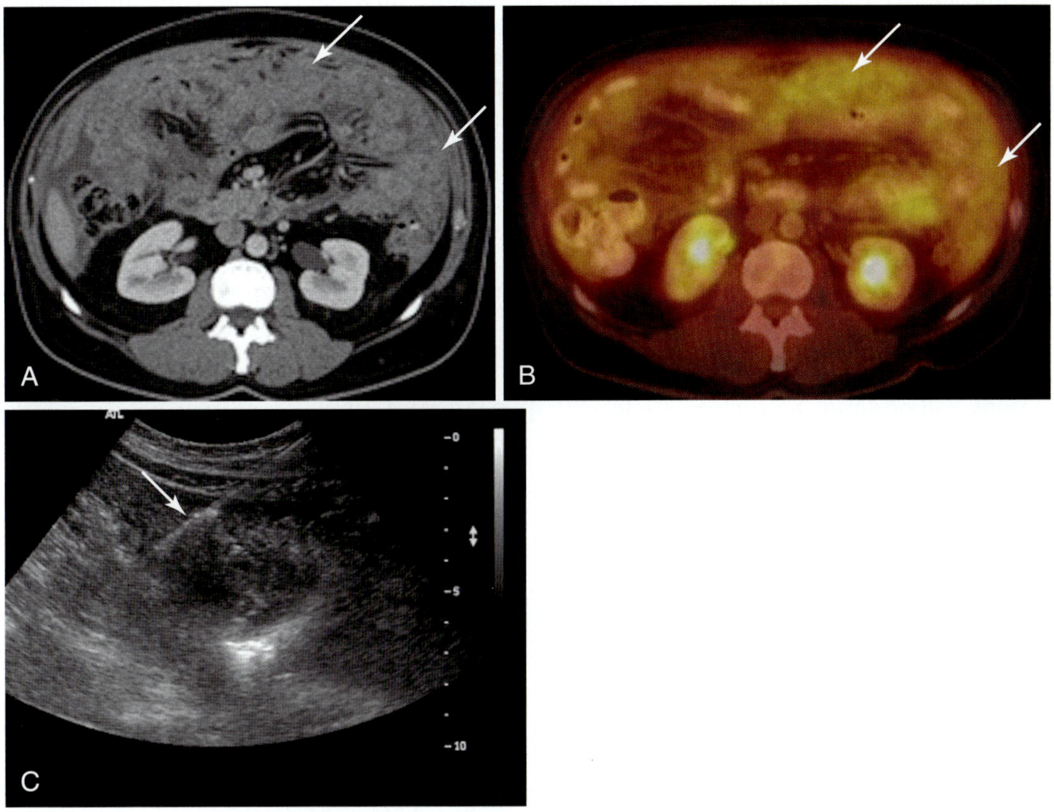

Figure 18-1 Biopsy of peritoneal carcinomatosis under ultrasound guidance. (A) Axial CECT demonstrates diffuse enhancing soft tissue peritoneal implants (*arrow*) with increased metabolic activity on FDG-PETCT (B). (C) A focal peritoneal implant was visualized and successfully biopsied under ultrasound guidance using an 18-gauge needle (*arrow*).

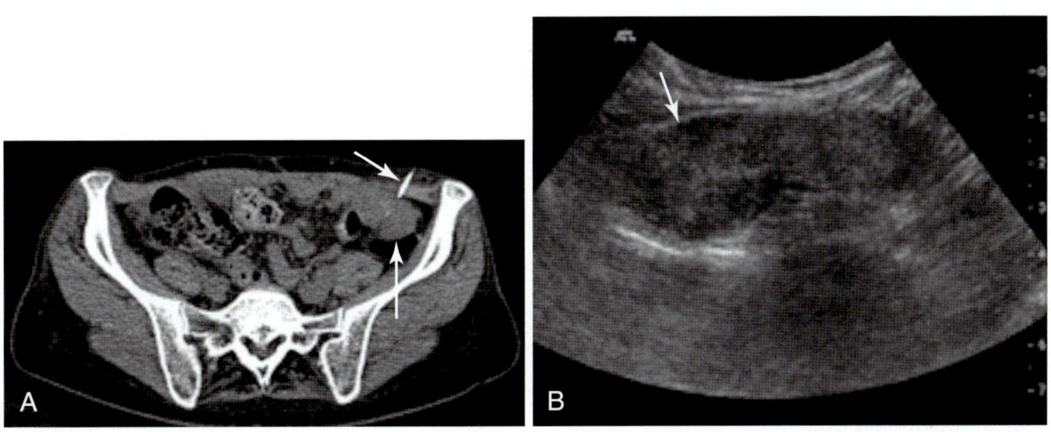

Figure 18-2 CT-guided biopsy of a peritoneal implant in a patient with a history of papillary serous adenocarcinoma of the ovary following total abdominal hysterectomy with bilateral salpingectomy and omentectomy and six cycles of adjuvant carboplatin and paclitaxel (Taxol). (A) Axial CT shows the biopsy needle (*short arrow*) at the periphery of a soft tissue peritoneal mass (*long arrow*). (B) Ultrasound was used in conjunction with CT during the procedure to confirm location of the mass. The biopsy was successful, with a histologic diagnosis consistent with metastatic disease from her ovarian primary.

Although trace fluid may improve sonographic visualization, removal of large-volume ascitic fluid prior to biopsy can help minimize the risk of hemorrhage.[12]

The safety of larger-gauge (18 gauge and below) core biopsy needles for use in peritoneal or omental disease is well documented, these are preferred to the finer gauge (20-gauge and higher) self-aspirating needles because the increased specimen size allows for assessment of the tissue architecture and further analysis with immunohistochemistry if necessary.[6,9-12] Coaxial systems, commonly available as a 17/18-gauge or 19/20-gauge introducer/biopsy needle combinations, are preferred as they allow the operator to take several specimens through a single needle track. This is also advantageous for small, difficult-to-reach lesions as the introducer needle can help anchor the target lesion, facilitating multiple passes.

Both CT- and ultrasound-guided biopsies are quick, taking roughly 15–20 minutes and can safely be performed in an outpatient setting. Other than local pain and bruising at the puncture site, there have been few reported complications, the most serious being a rectus sheath hematoma that was managed conservatively[6] and focal abdominal wall cellulitis.[9] Though there is a theoretical risk of tracking tumor into the abdominal wall, as this has been reported in a laparoscopy scar,[14] there have been no reported cases following IGB or during percutaneous interventional treatments. IGB is fast, safe, accurate and an important tool in the diagnosis and management of women with suspected ovarian cancer.

INTERVENTIONAL TECHNIQUES FOR LOCAL CONTROL OF METASTATIC DISEASE

For women with advanced-stage ovarian cancer and peritoneal, nodal, or hepatic metastases, there is a survival benefit to aggressive cytoreduction despite widespread disease. In a study of patients with Stage IV ovarian cancer, Bristow et al. reported a median survival of 50.1 months for women with optimal debulking of both their intra- and extrahepatic disease, defined as a maximal diameter of residual tumor $\leq$1 cm. However, anatomic limitations meant that optimal debulking was achieved in only 16% of patients, and in women with successful resection of their extrahepatic disease but residual tumor in the liver, the median survival fell to 27.0 months.[15] Their experience reflects a challenge for many oncologists and surgeons treating women with ovarian cancer, as many of them present with advanced disease and roughly 50% will have hepatic involvement at the time of death.[16]

Percutaneous thermoablative techniques, including radiofrequency ablation (RFA), microwave ablation, and cryotherapy, are well-established tools for treating hepatic tumors, and the techniques are described elsewhere in this book. Although more commonly used in the treatment of hepatocellular carcinoma or colorectal metastases, both have been applied in the treatment of hepatic metastases from ovarian cancer as well as nodal and peritoneal metastases from gynecologic cancers.[17,18]

Although RFA of hepatic tumors is typically reserved for patients with disease confined to the liver,[19] this is not the case for ovarian cancer, as it can be used as part of the overall strategy of cytoreduction. Unfortunately, the literature on the use of RFA in ovarian cancer is limited to a few case studies, small series, or cases in a larger series of hepatic metastatic lesions.[20-24] In the largest reported series of six patients, Gervais et al. achieved a mean local progression-free interval of 2.5 years after percutaneous RFA.[21] RFA can also be used as an adjunct to surgical resection when there is bilobar involvement or when intraoperative ultrasound demonstrates small, deep parenchymal lesions that may have been missed on preoperative CT or MR: In a three-person case series of patients undergoing resection and intraoperative RFA, Mateo et al. reported progression-free survivals of 9, 13, and 39 months.[22] The minimally invasive nature of RFA also offers the option of following patients with the test of time approach in which lesions are ablated with close imaging surveillance in an effort to minimize the number of hepatic resections that would not benefit the patient either because of rapid progression of extrahepatic disease or lack of disease elsewhere[21,25] (Figure 18-3).

Data on the application of cryoablation for gynecologic malignancies is more sparse and limited to a handful of patients in larger series. To our knowledge, the use of cryoablation for hepatic lesions from metastatic gynecologic disease has been reported in eight cases: one percutaneous[26] and seven intraoperative.[27] Unfortunately, half of these patients succumbed to their disease shortly after treatment without follow-up of their hepatic lesions. Each of the four remaining patients demonstrated recurrence of their hepatic disease within a year of treatment.[27]

Our experience includes nine women with 27 metastatic lesions from advanced ovarian or endometrial cancer treated with RFA (70%), cryoablation (26%), and microwave ablation (4%). Complete ablation was achieved with 14 lesions (52%) with an average local progression-free survival of 18 months. In the other 13 cases (44%), partial ablations were performed for debulking and palliative purposes. All patients survived the procedure without complication. Of our 8 patients with adequate follow-up, 2 (25%) remained free of disease, 1 (12.5%) developed distant metastases, and 1 (12.5%) had both local and distant progression. The other 4 women died from extensive metastatic disease at 1, 12, 14, and 21 months following their ablation sessions. Though limited, our own experience with percutaneous thermoablative techniques has also demonstrated that these techniques are safe and can be effective for local control or palliation.[18]

Transarterial chemoembolization (TACE) has been successfully employed in the treatment of hepatocellular carcinoma (HCC) as well as colorectal and neuroendocrine metastases, and the first case series of its use for ovarian metastases was recently published.[28] Sixty-five patients with no response, disease progression on, or toxicity to platinum and taxane-based chemotherapy underwent a minimum of three (mean 5.03) TACE procedures. The chemotherapeutic protocol evolved over the course of their experience, with the initial protocol of only mitomycin eventually supplemented with gemcitabine, and then later a therapeutic regimen of mitomycin, cisplatin, and gemcitabine was used. The embolization material was standardized to include a maximum of 10 mL lipiodol followed by an injection of 200–450 mg of degradable starch microspheres (200 μm) for vessel occlusion. A 14-month median survival was achieved, with survival rates of 58% at 1 year, 19% at 2 years, and 13% at 3 years. Survival times from the start of therapy showed no significant difference among the groups treated with the different chemotherapeutic regimens. From a treatment perspective, they selected perhaps the most challenging subset of ovarian cancer patients, as the presence of capsular or shallow lesions from peritoneal seeding was an exclusion criterion. Patients with deeper parenchymal lesions from hematogenous spread have poor survival compared to patients with resectable

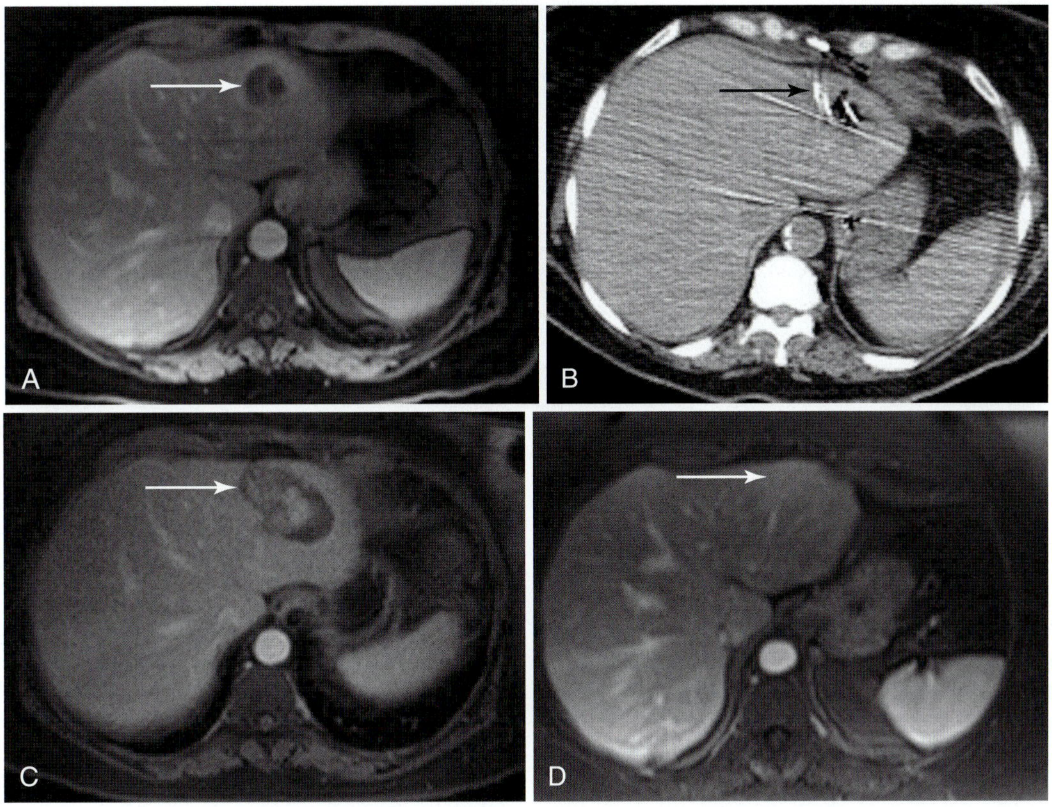

Figure 18-3 Radiofrequency ablation of an ovarian cancer metastasis to the liver. (A) T1-weighted MR with gadolinium demonstrates a cystic, peripherally enhancing mass on the peritoneal surface of the left hepatic lobe in a woman with granulosa cell ovarian cancer, treated several years prior with primary resection and chemotherapy. (B) RFA was performed for local control. The three tines of the RFA are seen within the mass on this image. Fluid from attempts to hydrodissect and increase the distance between the ablation target and abdominal wall is present in the left upper quadrant. (C) Immediate postprocedural gadolinium-enhanced MR demonstrates the zone of ablation, which nearly completely resolved on follow-up imaging (D) 4 years later. *(Image courtesy Dr. Steven Raman.)*

disease from peritoneal spread.[29] These results compare favorably to survival times of 9 and 10 months reported for other cases of nonresectable hematogenous ovarian metastases.[29] Although more data are needed regarding the use of TACE in these patients, it appears to be a reasonable strategy in the management of patients with unresectable hepatic involvement.

Finally, the safety and feasibility of high-intensity focused ultrasound (HIFU), a newer transcorporeal thermoablative technique, for treating liver tumors has been validated,[30-33] but to date, no report exists of its use in patients with hepatic metastasis from gynecologic cancers. Nevertheless, this is likely to be a promising noninvasive treatment option for these patients in the near future.

INTRAPERITONEAL CATHETERS FOR PALLIATIVE TREATMENT OF REFRACTORY MALIGNANT ASCITES

Recurrent ascites can be a significant source of distress for patients with advanced gynecologic malignancies and negatively affect the quality of their last few months of life. The large-volume ascites that develop in these patients can cause orthopnea, dyspnea, abdominal discomfort, vomiting, lower-extremity edema, and even difficulty with ambulation.[34-37] There is no standardized approach for the management of rapidly accumulating ascites beyond treatment of the primary disease. Diet modification and diuretic use are not very effective. Internal peritoneovenous or transjugular intrahepatic portosystemic shunts (TIPS) are not commonly used in the setting of cancer. Often these patients will undergo repeat paracentesis for palliative relief. However, each procedure introduces a risk of infection, peritonitis, bleeding, bowel perforation, and hypotension.[36] Moreover, ascites reaccumulates quickly, necessitating frequent trips to the hospital for drainage, sometimes multiple trips per week. Because of the pain and inconvenience of repeat procedures, many patients delay interventions for as long as possible and present with tense ascites, requiring large-volume taps, which increase the risk for hypotension and renal insufficiency related to large fluid shifts and protein loss.[35,38]

Indwelling, semipermanent intraperitoneal drains are an effective alternative to serial paracentesis, allowing patients or their caregivers to safely manage their ascites at home by removing small aliquots of liquid with vacuum bottles at regular intervals. A variety of catheters have been used for this purpose, including tunneled Tenckhoff® catheters, tunneled and untunneled Pleurex® catheters, a Cope-type loop drainage catheter, a tunneled silastic catheter with Dacron cuff, tunneled and untunneled peritoneal catheters, and tunneled peritoneal Port-A-Caths®. Tunneled catheter systems are generally preferred, as they are associated with a lower risk of peritonitis than the untunneled systems.[36]

These intraperitoneal drains can be placed under CT or ultrasound guidance (Figure 18-4). An 18-gauge needle fitted with a syringe is first used to access the peritoneal cavity. Once

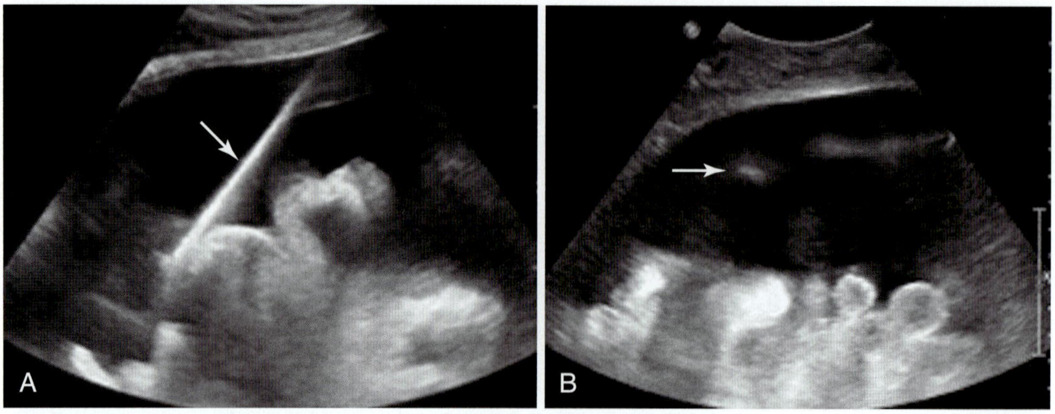

Figure 18-4 Insertion of indwelling peritoneal catheter: (A) An introducer needle (*arrow*) is seen entering the peritoneal cavity. (B) Subsequent images demonstrate the indwelling catheter within the peritoneal space (*arrow*), with a slightly smaller volume of ascitic fluid.

the cavity has been entered and ascitic fluid aspirated, a 0.035-in. guide wire is inserted through the needle and then the needle is removed. For tunneled systems, the fenestrated end of the catheter is attached to a tunneler, then passed subcutaneously from an incision approximately 5 cm away to the puncture site, pulling the catheter subcutaneously until the plastic cuff comes to rest under the skin approximately 1 cm from the second incision. Serial dilations are performed so that a 16-Fr peel-away introducer could be placed over the guide wire and into the peritoneal cavity. The catheter is then inserted through the peel-away introducer until all of the fenestrations are within the peritoneal cavity. The catheter is clamped closed, the incisions sutured, and the catheter is sutured to the skin.[34,37] Contraindications to placement include coagulopathy, active abdominal infection, and the presence of loculated ascites.[37]

The rate of complications such as bacterial peritonitis and development of loculated ascites is similar to large-volume paracentesis, [35] but the indwelling catheters allow patients to avoid multiple trips to the hospital. Additional adverse events include leakage around the catheter, mild cellulitis, hypotension, catheter-related infections and catheter occlusion, both of which can be minimized with appropriate drainage care.[36] For many patients with recurrent malignant ascites, these drains are in important palliative treatment that can help improve their quality of life in the late stages of their disease.

INTERVENTIONAL TECHNIQUES FOR PALLIATIVE TREATMENT OF PAINFUL METASTATIC DISEASE

RFA and cryoablation have been used to palliate painful metastatic disease. Cryoablation has even been used in the treatment of lesions in the lung, spleen, superficial soft tissues, and retroperitoneum from gynecologic primary cancers.[39] MR-guided high-intensity focused ultrasound (MRgFUS) is being tested for pain relief in patients suffering from bone metastases.[40-42] One case report utilized MRgFUS for pain relief in patients suffering from recurrent cervical carcinoma. A 29-year-old patient with recurrent squamous cell carcinoma of the cervix, after radical hysterectomy, chemotherapy, and radiation, had a pelvic mass unresponsive to conventional treatment, causing her intractable pain. Following two treatments by MRgFUS, the patient experienced a marked reduction in pain and an increase in Karnofsky Performance Status (KPS)—a measure of functional status—from 50 to 80%.[43]

TRANSCATHETER ARTERIAL EMBOLIZATION FOR CONTROL OF HEMORRHAGE FROM GYNECOLOGIC MALIGNANCIES

Pelvic hemorrhage is an uncommon but serious complication of advanced gynecologic malignancies. Transcatheter arterial embolization for the management of intractable bleeding from pelvic cancers was first described in the mid-1970s,[44,45] but the technique is more commonly used in the treatment of obstetric emergencies, such as postpartum hemorrhage or bleeding related to cervical ectopic pregnancies, or in the treatment of symptomatic uterine fibroids.[46] However, there are a handful of studies and scattered case reports indicating that embolization is effective at achieving partial or complete control of bleeding in this setting.[47-51]

The principles of embolization related to gynecologic malignancies are similar to those from other etiologies of pelvic hemorrhage. The extensive vascular network in the pelvis and potential for collateralization necessitates a bilateral approach.[46,47] Unlike some trauma or obstetric hemorrhages in which the site of bleeding may be readily identified on angiography, uncontrollable bleeding related to neoplasms often does not show specific foci of extravasation.[48] However, there is still a benefit to empiric embolization in these cases, and bilateral embolizations of the internal iliac arteries is recommended.[46] A more selective approach can be used when there is visualization of active extravasation. Appropriate embolic agents include Gelfoam or embolization coils when the site of bleeding is identified[52] (Figure 18-5). Particulate agents such as polyvinyl alcohol spheres have also been safely and effectively used.[50]

As with any embolization procedure, there is potential for nontarget embolization resulting in ischemia or infarction. However, these treatments are often the best option for the emergent control of life-threatening hemorrhage and outweigh these risks.

SELECTED INTERVENTIONS FOR SELECTED BENIGN GYNECOLOGIC CONDITIONS

Cervical Ectopy

Cervical ectopy, or ectropion, is a normal condition that results from extension of the endocervical columnar epithelium out over a portion of the visible ectocervix, and is associated with infection, typically chlamydial cervicitis. The subsequent

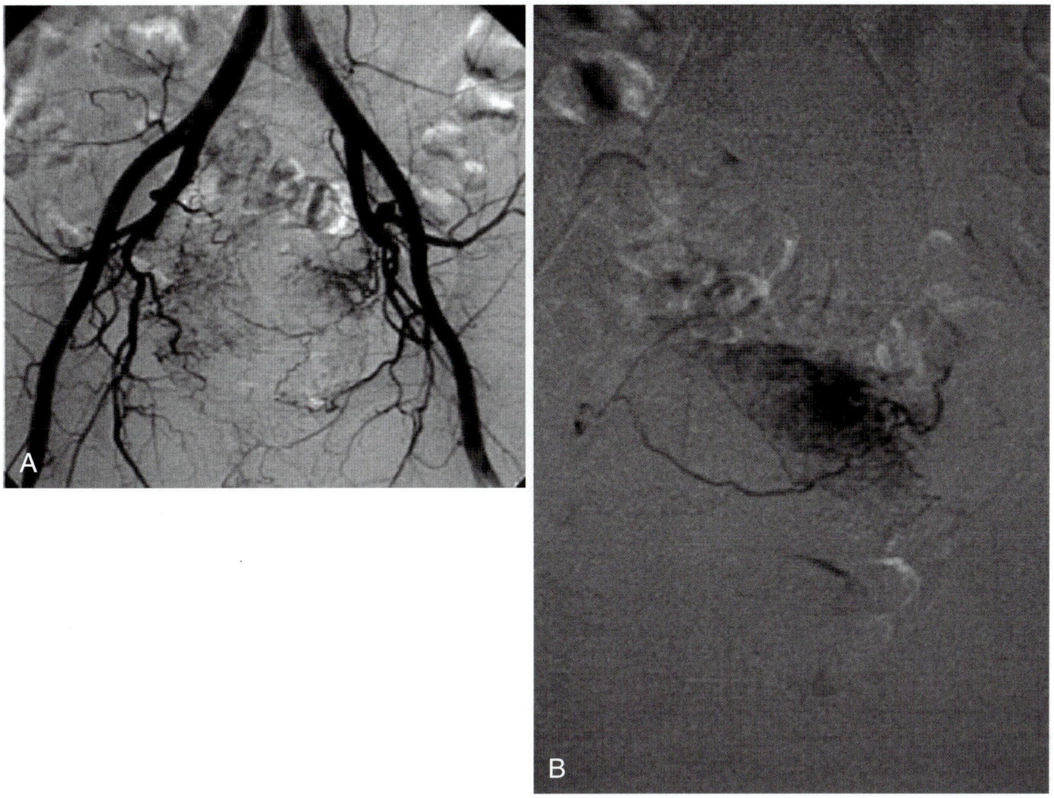

Figure 18-5 Transcatheter embolization for control of hemorrhage related to recurrent cervical cancer. 54-year-old woman with a history of cervical cancer, status-post total abdominal hysterectomy and bilateral salpingo-oophorectomy, with known tumor recurrence, presenting with intractable vaginal bleeding. (A) Pelvic arteriogram shows tumor neovascularity supplied by branches of the bilateral internal iliac arteries. (B) Selective injection of one of the feeding branches shows tumor neovascularity without evidence of contrast extravasation. Subsequent embolization was performed with Gelfoam. *(Reprinted with permission from Wu CC, Lee MH: Transcatheter arterial embolotherapy: a therapeutic alternative in obstetrics and gynecologic emergencies,* Semin Intervent Radiol *23(3):240-248, 2006.)*

inflammation and repair results in reactive changes, which are characterized by epithelial disorganization and nuclear atypia.[53,54] For chronic cervicitis refractory to medical management, surgical options, such as cryocautery, electrocoagulation, and laser therapy, are available to mitigate symptoms and to prevent neoplastic transformation. However, these are destructive procedures that induce necrosis of treated tissue, which may cause subsequent cervical scarring stenosis and, hence, secondary infertility and cervical-origin dystocia.[55] HIFU as a treatment option for cervical ectopy offers several advantages: sonication may be precisely delivered at a target depth without collateral damage to interposed, nontarget tissues in the path of the ultrasound beam.[56] Infected tissue is treated through inactivation of pathogenic microorganisms and their metabolic products, thus improving local irritation without tissue loss. Subsequently, the cervix is preserved, with function and elasticity of the cervix unaffected.[57] In one study, 200 patients with symptomatic, benign ectopy of the cervix were allocated alternately to the ultrasound and laser groups.[58] The Nd:YAG laser was used for tissue vaporization destruction, whereas the therapeutic ultrasound device (Seapostar, Chongqing Haifu[30] Technology, Co. Ltd., Chongqing, China) was applied to the other group. Anesthesia was not used and all patients tolerated the procedure. Although there were no differences in the symptomatic cure rate (97% vs. 98%) or success rate in treatment (95% vs. 96%) of the ectopic areas between the ultrasound and laser groups, respectively, the rate of side effects (including vaginal reactive discharge and colporrhagia) was found to be much lower in the ultrasound group than that in the laser group (8% vs. 45%).

Abdominal Wall Endometriosis

Abdominal wall endometriosis (AWE) is a much less common manifestation of extrapelvic endometriosis, associated with prior obstetric or gynecologic incisions during cesarean delivery, hysterectomy, and amniocentesis.[59,60] The implanted tissue responds to menstrual cycles, and patients may feel a palpable abdominal wall nodule.[61] Medical therapy, which includes hormonal suppression of ovulation with danazol or a gonadotropin-releasing hormone antagonist, can mitigate symptoms but is associated with high risk of recurrence.[62] Treatment of AWE includes hormonal treatment, curative surgical resection, and wide excision with at least a 1-cm margin to prevent local recurrence. However, with large lesions, especially those involving both muscle and fascia, patch grafting may be needed to strengthen the abdominal wall to prevent postoperative hernia.[63,64]

Early reports suggest that RFA and HIFU may provide nonsurgical therapeutic options for symptomatic AWE: There is a single case report of RFA used for treatment of recurrent AWE in a woman refusing surgical intervention. The patient experienced improvement in her pain from a 6–7 out of a possible 10 on a visual analog pain scale prior to the intervention to a 0 at 1 at 12 weeks after the procedure. Apart from

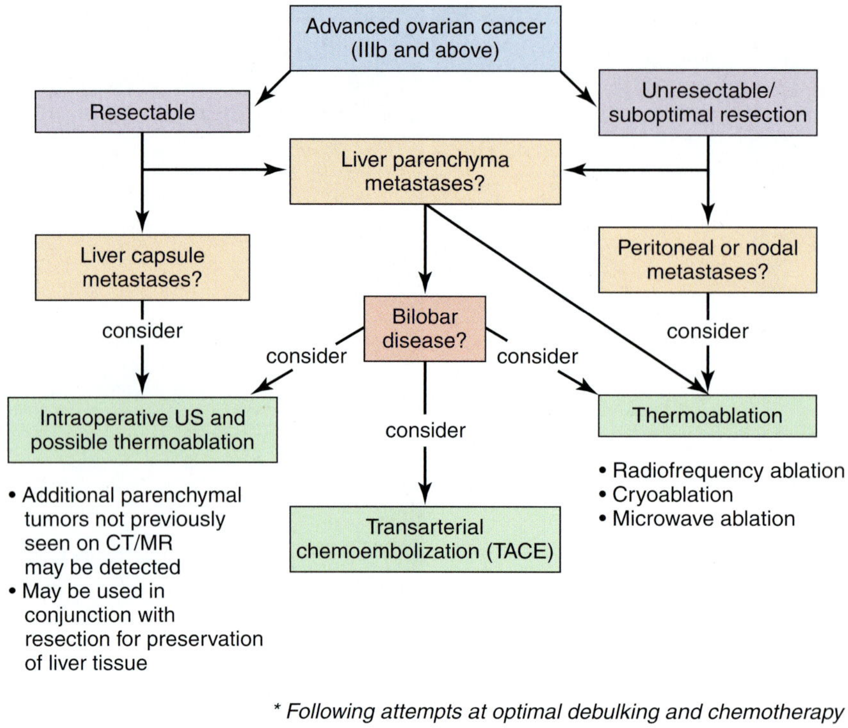

Figure 18-6 Algorithm for choosing image-guided interventional techniques.

moderate skin erythema near the puncture site, no major complications occurred.[65]

Evaluation of AWE ultrasound-guided HIFU ablation was recently published: 21 consecutive patients with AWE were treated as outpatients and the median AWE size was 2.4 cm (range 1.0–5.3 cm).[66] Treatment was considered complete when the entire nodule and its nearby 1-cm margin became hyperechoic on ultrasound. All AWEs were successfully ablated after one session of HIFU ablation. the ablation time lasted for 5–48 minutes (median 13 minutes) and no major complications occurred. The cyclic pain disappeared in all patients after a mean follow-up of 18.7 months (range 3–31 months). The treated nodules gradually shrank over time, and 16 nodules became unnoticeable on follow-up serial ultrasound examination, suggesting that under the guidance of high-frequency diagnostic ultrasound, HIFU ablation with adequate safety margins can obtain therapeutic results similar to that of surgical resection. Though promising, further randomized, controlled study is needed before ultrasound-guided HIFU ablation can be recommended as a nonsurgical treatment for AWE:

Conclusion

Image-guided interventional techniques are increasingly important in the diagnosis, treatment, and palliative care of patients with advanced gynecologic malignancies. Percutaneous and intraoperative RFA has been proven as a valuable treatment option and gives patients with otherwise unresectable disease a chance at optimal cytoreduction and improved survival. Although its application for treating hepatic metastases from gynecologic malignancies has not been published, HIFU may also be a safe and effective nonsurgical alternative. In addition to trying to reduce tumor burden, these thermoablative techniques can be also employed as palliative treatment for painful metastases. Image-guided placement of semipermanent peritoneal drains for at-home management of recurrent ascites allows patients to avoid numerous trips to the hospital for serial large-volume paracenteses. Although surgical cytoreduction and chemotherapy is the cornerstone of therapy for gynecologic malignancies, these techniques are valuable adjuncts, particularly in treating patients with advanced disease. An example of a potential algorithm for choosing these techniques is presented in Figure 18-6.

Acknowledgments

The authors would like to thank Dr. Steven Raman for his assistance with some sections of this chapter.

REFERENCES

The complete reference list is available online at www.expertconsult.com.

19

Image-Based Interventional Therapies for Benign Uterine Neoplasms

NITA NAYAK

KEY POINTS

- Uterine leiomyomata are common benign neoplasms that may cause symptoms related either to tissue bulk or bleeding for many women.
- Triage to the ideal treatment depends not only on fibroid characteristics and location within the uterus but also the patient's fertility goals, nature of presenting symptoms, and consideration of potential complications.
- In addition to watchful waiting and traditional treatment, including medication for symptomatic relief, hormonal therapy, and surgical excision, patients now have the option of minimally invasive, image-guided procedures: uterine artery embolization (UAE) and many forms of thermal ablation (radiofrequency ablation and high-intensity focused ultrasound [HIFU]).
- UAE, associated with significant fibroid volume reduction and symptom relief, as well as less major adverse events and a shorter recovery as compared with hysterectomy, is also shown to lead to the need for reintervention in almost one third of patients, negating the cost-effectiveness at 5 years posttreatment.
- HIFU, especially when guided by MR imaging, has shown to be clinically effective in reducing fibroid volume and reducing symptoms, with fewer major complications and less lifetime total costs compared to currently available treatments.
- Clinical outcomes for minimally invasive, image-guided procedures are improving with improved technical skill and greater treatment volumes, but randomized trials analyzing longer-term outcomes (>5 years) and post-procedure fertility outcomes have not been reported to date.

Introduction

Uterine leiomyomas (fibroids) are benign, hormonally driven, well-encapsulated neoplasms originating from uterine smooth muscle, affecting an estimated 20%–35% of all reproductive-age women; some studies report that a cumulative lifetime incidence of leiomyomas occurs in 70% of U.S. white and 80% of African American women.[1] Risk factors include African or African American background, family history, early menarche, nulliparity, obesity, hypertension, and polycystic ovary syndrome.[2] Although the majority of women with uterine leiomyomas are asymptomatic, approximately 20%–30% of women have related symptoms, typically presenting in the fifth decade of life and lasting into menopause, with subsequent decrease in symptoms.[1] Uterine fibroid-related symptoms are secondary to either mass effect (bulk) or excessive endometrial effect (bleeding). Bulk-related symptoms include back and pelvic pain, pelvic pressure, urinary frequency, dyspareunia, and defecation disorders. Bleeding-related symptoms include menorrhagia, metrorrhagia, menometrorrhagia, and dysmenorrhea, and the associated anemia.[3] Submucosal fibroids, or those that significantly distort the endometrial cavity, are also thought to contribute to mass-related infertility.[4] Leiomyoma-related symptoms, among the most common of all gynecologic disorders, are thought to be responsible for more than 360,000 hysterectomies in the United States annually, with an overall estimated annual cost of care exceeding $2 billion.[5]

Imaging Characteristics of Uterine Leiomyomas

Leiomyomas are readily detectable on pelvic ultrasonography, typically appearing as solid, hypoechoic masses originating from the uterine myometrium with varying degrees of echogenicity depending on fibrous, calcified, and degenerating components. There is no interruption of the endometrium (unless submucosal in location, which may cause adjacent cavity distortion), differentiating these lesions from endometrial polyps or more concerning endometrial carcinoma. Although ultrasonography most commonly identifies fibroids, MR imaging offers superior soft tissue contrast and tissue characterization of individual fibroids, multiplanar imaging, and characterization of perfusion, which helps triage patients to one or more therapeutic options, including surgical resection, uterine artery embolization (UAE), and high-intensity focused ultrasound (HIFU) ablation. It is also superior in diagnosing concomitant adenomyosis, which may contribute to UAE treatment failure.[6] Based on MR imaging and enhancement patterns, individual leiomyomas can be classified as classical, hypercellular, or degenerating. Classical fibroids appear hypointense on T2-weighted sequences and enhance on gadolinium-enhanced T1-weighted sequences (Figure 19-1, *A*). Hypercellular fibroids, which are T2 hyperintense, enhance avidly on gadolinium-enhanced T1-weighted sequences. Degenerating fibroids have variable T1 and T2 signal and do not exhibit contrast enhancement. The tissue characterization of these different subtypes of fibroids can help determine the best choice of treatment, as classical fibroids have been found to respond better to HIFU than hypercellular fibroids, while degenerating fibroids respond poorly to both HIFU and UAE.[7]

LOCATION OF UTERINE LEIOMYOMAS

Leiomyomata are also described in terms of their location in the uterus, and these subtypes can display varying responses to

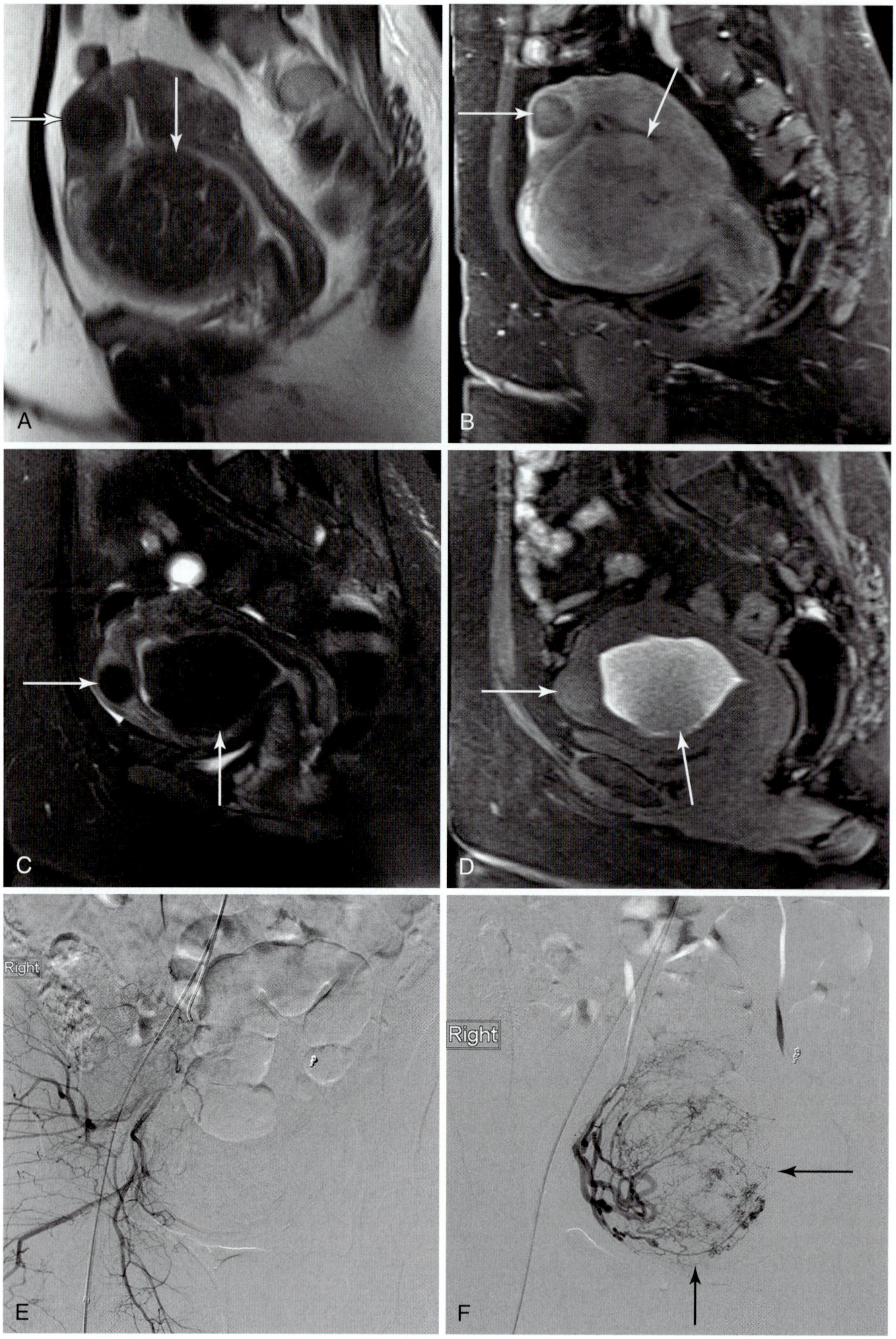

Figure 19-1 Uterine artery embolization (UAE). Sagittal MRI images of uterine fibroids (*arrows*) on T2-weighted (A) and contrast-enhanced fat-saturated gradient T1-weighted (B) images before and (C and D) after UAE. Subtracted angiographic images before (E) and after (F) embolization of the feeding artery, with resultant reduction in perfusion of the fibroid (*arrows*).

specific treatments as well. Intramural leiomyomas, completely contained within the uterine wall, are most common and mostly asymptomatic, but if large, may cause bulk symptoms. Subserosal lesions are found along the outer contour of the uterus, and when large, can also cause bulk symptoms. Fibroids abutting or extending into the endometrial cavity are termed submucosal, and even small lesions can cause uterine bleeding. This subtype can potentially become intracavitary following UAE, predisposing to fibroid expulsion and postprocedure complications, the risk for which can best be gauged by preprocedure magnetic resonance imaging (MRI), with assessment of fibroid size to endometrial interface.[6] Intracavitary leiomyomas grow into the endometrial cavity on a fibrovascular stalk and commonly result in bleeding symptoms. Those growing outside the uterus on a fibrovascular stalk are termed pedunculated and can cause mass effect on adjacent organs, and voiding or defecation symptoms.

TRADITIONAL TREATMENT OF UTERINE LEIOMYOMA

Traditional options for therapy of uterine leiomyoma-related symptoms may be divided into medical, surgical, or watchful waiting/alternative therapy. Medical treatments, like nonsteroidal anti-inflammatory drugs (NSAIDs) or contraceptive steroids, or alternative therapies, such as acupuncture or herbal therapies, may be effective in the short term or for bridging perimenopausal patients whose fibroids may still spontaneously involute,[8-10] but most symptomatic patients progress over time, requiring more durable treatment. Hormone therapy, namely gonadotrophin-releasing hormone (GnRH) agonists, are also used and act by suppressing circulating estradiol and progesterone levels via the pituitary–ovarian axis. This results in significant fibroid shrinkage, but long-term use of these compounds is not recommended because of the side effects of bone loss.[9] Surgical therapy, including laparoscopic, hysteroscopic, robotic-assisted, or open hysterectomy, is the standard of care and is considered the definitive therapy for fibroid-related bulk symptoms, bleeding, and infertility. Although these are extremely common and safe surgical procedures, there is a major complication rate (such as hemorrhage requiring transfusion, urinary tract, and bowel damage) of 8.9% for abdominal, 14% for vaginal, and 19% for laparoscopic hysterectomy (the latter including the risk of conversion to laparotomy).[11] Removal of the uterus and surrounding attachments also has been thought to increase a woman's postmenopausal risk of pelvic floor disorders (pelvic prolapse and laxity).[12,13] For women who desire the option of future fertility or who wish to retain their uterus, open or laparoscopic surgical resection of individual leiomyomas (myomectomy) is performed.[14] Although generally safe, the most frequent complications include perioperative blood loss requiring transfusion, fever, and ileus.[15] There is a postoperative recurrence of up to 51% over time, and 10%–25% of patients will require a major surgery after the first myomectomy.[16]

MINIMALLY INVASIVE TREATMENTS

Uterine Artery Embolization

UAE, also called uterine fibroid embolization (UFE), is the most widely available nonsurgical treatment option for moderate and large symptomatic uterine leiomyomas, and was first developed in the early 1970s for control of postpartum hemorrhage.[6] The procedure itself typically lasts from 50 to 75 minutes in 90% of patients.[17] With slightly differing techniques between institutions, the goal of therapy is the same: to occlude the uterine artery branches that supply only the fibroid tumors, causing cutoff of blood flow and subsequent infarction, while sparing normal myometrial vessels through extensive collateral blood supply (Figure 19-1, *B*). Utilizing local anesthesia and conscious sedation, vascular access is obtained with a wire via a unilateral femoral artery approach, which is advanced up to the aortic bifurcation; a small visceral catheter, typically 4–5 French (Fr), is placed over the wire to select the contralateral internal iliac artery. Digital angiography is then performed in the posterior–anterior projection to identify the origin of the uterine artery, which usually arises as a first or second branch of the anterior division of the internal iliac artery, and is usually dilated in the presence of a uterine fibroid tumor (Figure 19-2). Using a coaxial microcatheter, 3 Fr in size, the portion distal to the cervicovaginal branch, supplying the fibroid of interest, is then selectively catheterized. Embolic particles, most commonly trisacryl microspheres or polyvinyl alcohol (PVA) microspheres, from 350 to 700μm in size, are injected; depending on the size of the leiomyoma, anywhere from 100 to 1500 mg may be used. The contralateral uterine artery is catheterized in similar fashion and embolized, with the procedure deemed complete when no arterial flow is visualized in the perifibroid arterial plexus, with slow antegrade flow maintained in the main uterine artery (Figure 19-3).

Thermal Ablation

More recently, uterine fibroids are being treated by thermal ablation, one of the newest and least invasive treatment option for uterine fibroids, particularly in those who wish to retain the option of future fertility.[18] Thermal ablation was initially performed using a neodymium-doped yttrium aluminum garnet (Nd:YAG) laser to deliver energy to fibroids via laparoscopy or hysteroscopy, but now can be performed by electrosurgical radiofrequency ablation (RFA), in which needle electrodes deliver heat energy.[19] Exposure to temperatures exceeding 60°C instantaneously and irreversibly injures soft tissue through protein denaturation and coagulative necrosis (Figure 19-4). Unlike UAE, which results in tissue infarction with cell membrane disruption and spillage of intracellular contents, hyperthermic ablation allows for thermal fixation, which preserves cellular architecture.[20] Coagulated lesions shrink in size from water volume loss and inflammatory response reabsorption, and the consistency changes from very firm to soft and gel-like, which may also contribute to the resolution of symptoms. A similar concept is ablation by freezing the fibroid tissue, or cryomyolysis, which utilizes gas-cooled probes to deliver high-pressure argon gas, causing irreversible cell injury at a temperature of −20° C and forming elliptical "ice balls" in the affected tissue (Figure 19-5), promoting vascular thrombosis that ultimately necroses the fibroid.[21]

Varying techniques are used for needle-based thermal ablation among institutions, including needle electrode design (bipolar vs. monopolar, single tine vs. multiple tines), mode of deployment (transabdominally, transcervically, transvaginally), the modality used for real-time visualization (laparoscopy, sonography), and the hardware/software monitoring energy delivery to tissue. Typically, a 15-gauge needle electrode is inserted with the tip positioned at the center of the target myoma,

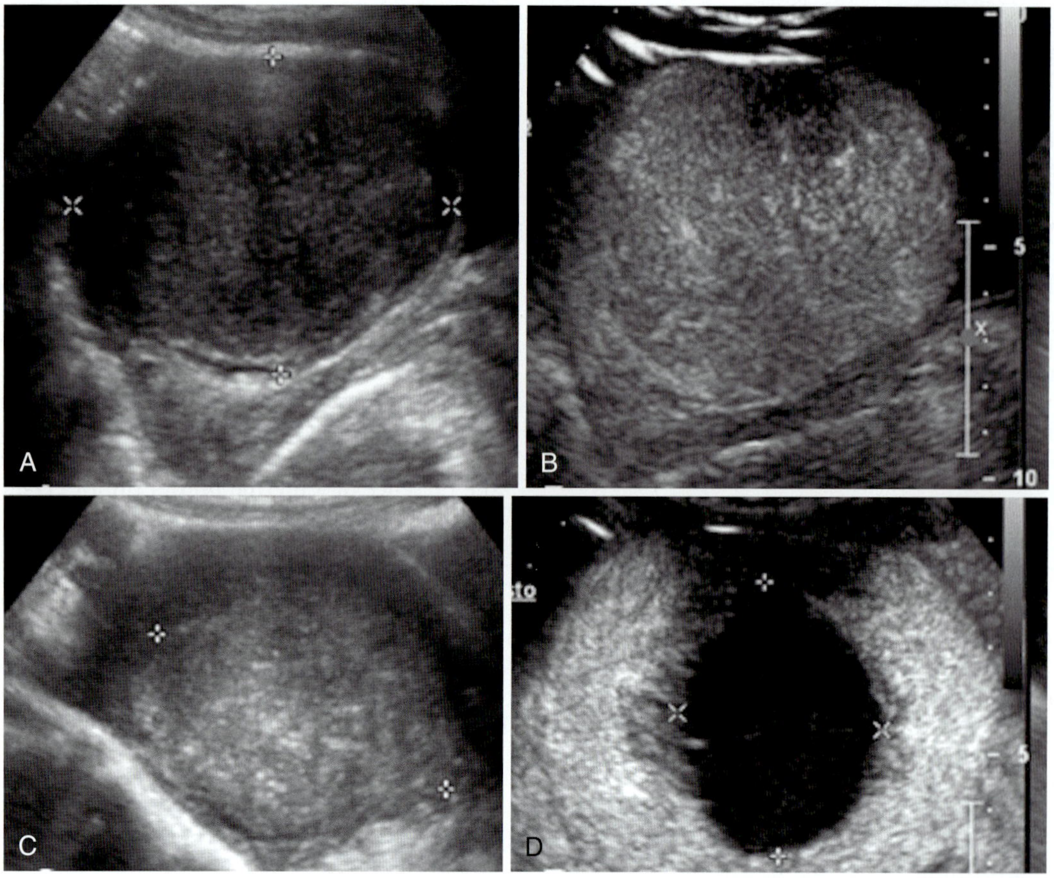

Figure 19-2 A 41-year-old woman affected by a 7-cm symptomatic uterine fibroid. (A) B-mode ultrasonograph shows a hypoechoic mass in the uterus. (B) Contrast-enhanced ultrasonography (CEUS) confirms rich vascularization inside the mass. (C) B-mode ultrasonograph 6 months after percutaneous RFA: the treated fibroid appears nonhomogeneous and reduced in size. (D) CEUS confirmed a huge area of necrosis with a peripheral rim of enhancement in a normal uterus without any residual disease. *(Images reprinted courtesy Carrafiello G, Recaldini C, Fontana F, et al: Ultrasound-guided radiofrequency thermal ablation of uterine fibroids: medium-term follow-up,* Cardiovasc Interv Radiol *33(1):113–119, 2010.)*

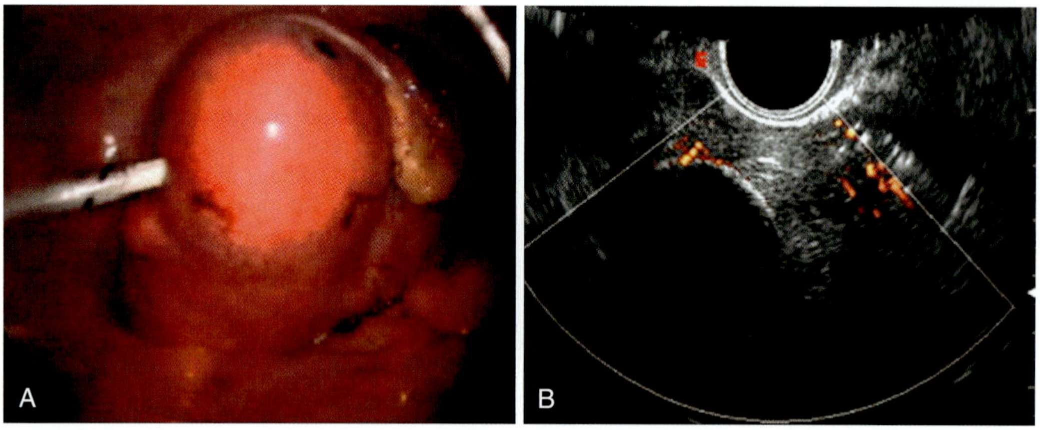

Figure 19-3 Monitoring of the extension of the iceball. (A) Laparoscopic view of the cryoprobe inserted into the fibroid during freezing. (B) Transvaginal ultrasound view during cryomyolysis. *(Images reprinted courtesy of Exacoustos, C., et al: Ultrasound-assisted laparoscopic cryomyolysis: two- and three-dimensional findings before, during and after treatment,* Ultrasound Obstet Gynecol *25: 393–400, 2005.)*

with manually deployable prongs designed to laterally bracket the target tissue in order to produce a spherical area of coagulative necrosis. The needle electrode is connected to a generator that displays the temperature of the electrode tip, as well as tissue impedance characteristics and ablation time, and allows for cauterization of the needle track on completion via modification of the power settings.[22] The desired fibroid tissue damage induced by these procedures is monitored by real-time imaging, namely, ultrasonography or MR. Although empirically more costly, MR-guided ablation has several theoretical advantages over ultrasound-guided ablation: MRI provides much higher, near-real-time, multiplanar unenhanced soft tissue contrast

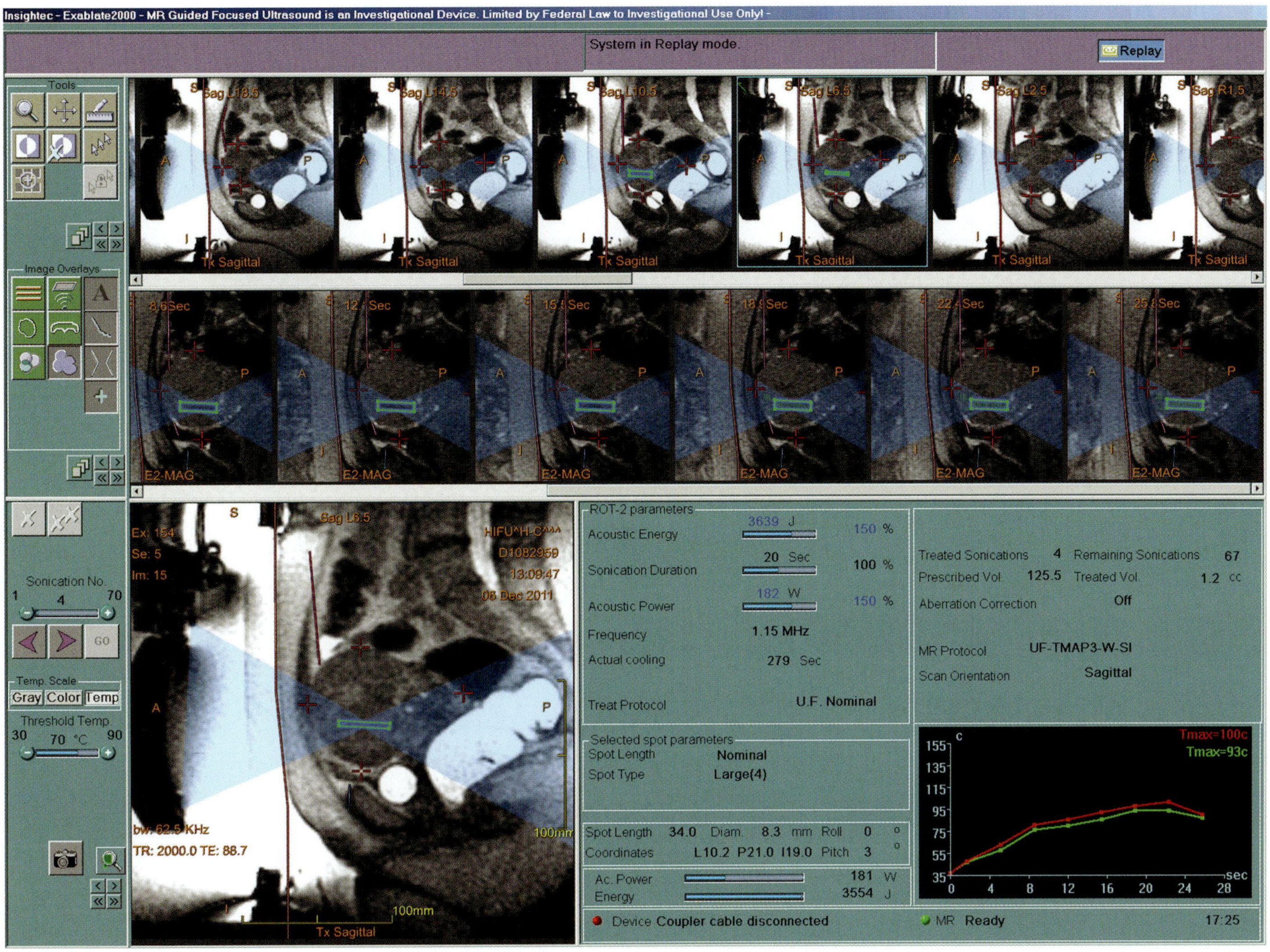

Figure 19-4 Planning and treatment image during magnetic resonance-guided focused ultrasound (MRgFUS) treatment of a fibroid. The top row of images are contiguous sagittal T2-weighted single-shot images of the fibroid, and the second row temperature-monitoring images of the ablation zone, identified as a green rectangle. The graph in the left lower corner of the images shows the near-real-time change in temperature. *(Image courtesy Dr. Steven Raman.)*

and spatial resolution and provides near-real-time, MR-based thermal mapping of the ablated tissue and surrounding nontarget soft tissues. This real-time feedback of thermal gradient enables a complete ablation of the targeted site that avoids adjacent tissues[23] and allows for the evaluation of thermal sites posttreatment.

High-Intensity Focused Ultrasound

HIFU is another mode of thermal ablation, delivering a noninvasive, targeted dose of low-frequency, high-intensity cyclic acoustic pressure to cause focal thermal toxicity and coagulation necrosis. Unlike thermal or cryoablation, HIFU obviates the need for (and potential complications of) direct access to the fibroid tissue. HIFU can treat a variety of disorders, including solid tumors, such as uterine leiomyomas and malignant tumors in liver, bone, pancreas, and prostate.[24] For the current first-generation technology, with motion correction in development, minimally mobile lesions like uterine fibroids present an ideal target. HIFU devices are available from several manufacturers, combining the therapeutic HIFU transducer with either MR guidance (ExAblate, InSightec, Hiafa, Israel; Sonalleve, Philips, Best, Netherlands) or ultrasound guidance (Seapostar, Chongqing Haifu [HIFU] Technology, Co. Ltd., Chongqing, China).[18] The Insightec Exablate 2000, known widely by its marketing name, MR guided Focused Ultrasound Surgery (MRgFUS), received approval from the United States Food and Drug Administration (FDA) in 2004 for the noninvasive treatment of uterine leiomyomas.

MRgFUS incorporates a HIFU transducer unit and is built into a table designed to fit into a gantry in a 1.5- or 3.0-Tesla magnet. InSightec's ExAblate system 2000 is compatible exclusively with General Electric Healthcare's standard Signa line of 1.5-T MR machines. Potential risks from the procedure include bowel, skin, or nerve injury and possible deep venous thrombosis (DVT). Patients are placed prone on the table with the lower abdomen and pelvis on a degassed water bath over the transducer, with a coupling gel pad placed in between. The anterior pelvic wall is shaved to the symphysis pubis to minimize the chance of air bubble entrapment by hair in the water bath. A Foley catheter is always placed to control bladder distension (bladder fill) as necessary for

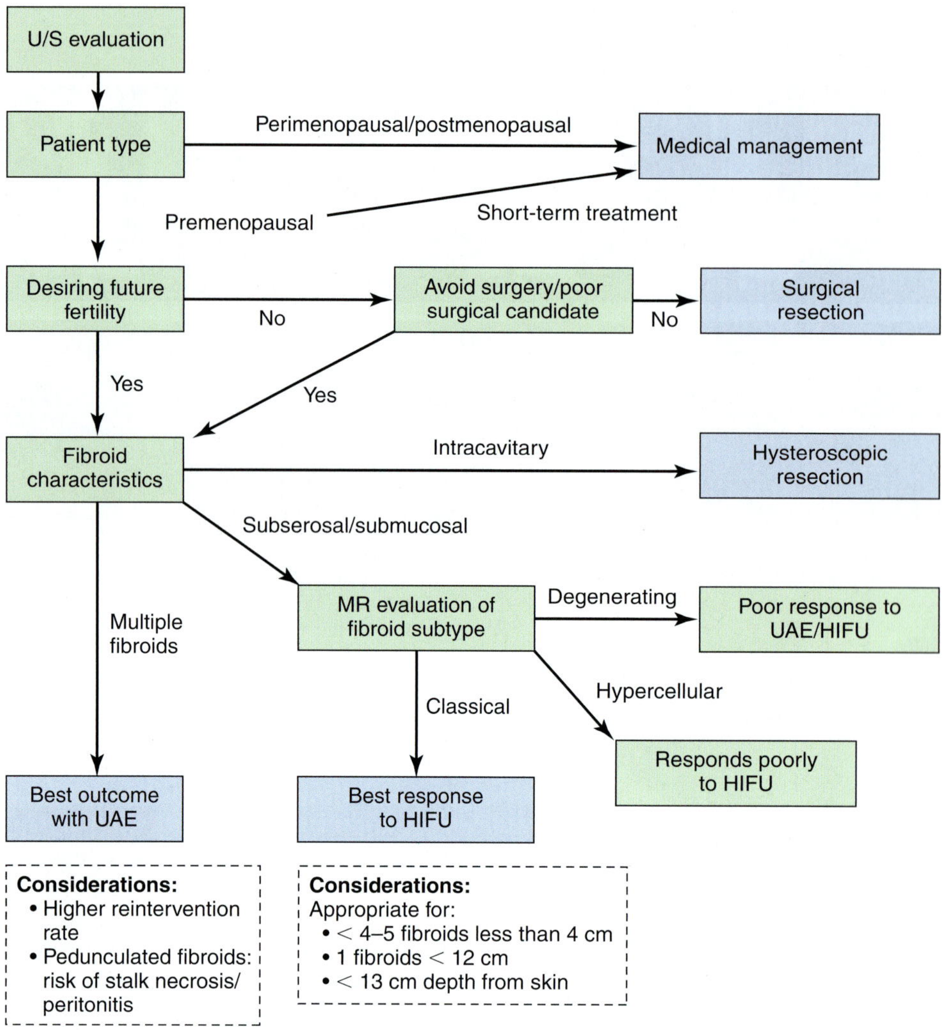

Figure 19-5 Treatment of symptomatic uterine fibroids

optimal uterus position. In selected instances, sonographic gel, water, or air may be needed to fill the rectum (rectal fill) via a small-gauge rectal tube to displace the uterus anteriorly and move the bowel out of the treatment field. Manual displacement of the bowel via suprapubic massage can also be performed for optimal positioning of the fibroid. A pre-treatment MR of the pelvis is performed with T2-weighted coronal, sagittal, and axial sequences, which serves as the template scan to map the procedure and select for individual leiomyomas. The treatment volume of the target lesions is then calculated by dedicated software from the measured circumference. Imaging can then display near-real-time temperature and phase maps using the receiver channels built into the ExAblate table. The bowel, pubic bone, lumbosacral spine, and nerves are all demarcated to prevent unintended target sonication.

On the ExAblate system, transducer power ranges from 0 to 3000 W/cm^2, with an ultrasound frequency of 1.0–1.3 MHz. Over an approximately 20-second period, energy deposition can vary between 2000 and 4000 J into the target site per each sonication. The target site is ellipsoid with dimensions of 8–40 mm parallel to the sonication beam and 1–10 mm perpendicular to the beam direction at the 17 cm focal distance from the therapeutic transducer (up to 13 cm deep to the skin within the patient's pelvis). Newer devices will allow for deeper pelvic penetration by physical movement of the transducer. Low-power test sonications are delivered to the target lesions to ensure precise aim and to correct for sonication-related distortion in the coronal and sagittal planes. High-power treatment sonications, lasting from 15 to 20 seconds, are then delivered to the selected treatment volume, followed by a cooling duration of 45–90 seconds to minimize risk of skin burns.

With the currently available system, up to approximately 120 sonications may be needed to ablate a given volume in the maximum 3-hour period. Temperature at the target sonication is noninvasively derived by phase changes on MR imaging every 3–4 seconds, creating an MR thermal map and allowing for adjustments to the therapeutic energy and sonication time. Postprocedure dynamic contrast-enhanced MRI can then assess nonperfused tissue. Patients are monitored for 1–3 hours posttreatment for recovery from conscious sedation and then discharged home. Normal activities may be resumed almost immediately, typically the following day, with a small subset needing a more prolonged recovery.

Other Gynecological Applications Of HIFU

Adenomyosis is the ectopic location of endometrial and fibrous stroma in the myometrium, and is a common, often misdiagnosed, gynecologic disorder, with symptoms mimicking those of uterine fibroids (menometrorrhagia, menstrual cramps, dyspareunia, and dysmenorrhea). Medical therapies can provide symptomatic relief, but they are short-lived; currently, the definitive therapy for uterine adenomyosis is hysterectomy, with minor surgical procedures, including endomyometrial ablation, laparoscopic myometrial electrocoagulation, and adenomyoma excision, used with varying degrees of success.[25] The use of HIFU for treatment of adenomyosis, though not approved by the U.S. FDA, has shown potential as an effective modality in China; multiple studies have reported reductions in mean uterine volumes up to 25% after 12 months posttreatment, with significant symptomatic improvement and without serious adverse effects.[26]

Cervical ectopy, or ectropion, is a normal condition that results from extension of the endocervical columnar epithelium out over a portion of the visible ectocervix, and is associated with infection, typically chlamydial cervicitis; the subsequent inflammation and repair results in reactive changes, which are characterized by epithelial disorganization and nuclear atypia.[27,28] For chronic cervicitis refractory to medical management, current surgical options, such as cryocautery, electrocoagulation, and laser therapy, are available to mitigate symptoms and to prevent neoplastic transformation, but are destructive procedures that induce necrosis of treated tissue and subsequent cervical scarring, stenosis, and, hence, secondary infertility and cervical-origin dystocia.[29] HIFU as a treatment option for cervical ectopy offers several advantages, primarily that sonication may be precisely delivered at a target depth without collateral damage to interposed, nontarget tissues in the path of the ultrasound beam.[30] Infected tissue is treated through inactivation of pathogenic microorganisms and their metabolic products, thus improving local irritation without tissue loss. Subsequently, the cervix is preserved, with function and elasticity of the cervix not affected.[31] One study found no differences in the symptomatic cure rate (97% vs. 98%) or success rate in treatment (95% vs. 96%) of the ectopic areas between the ultrasonography- and laser-treated groups, respectively, but the rate of side effects (including vaginal reactive discharge and colporrhagia) was much lower in the ultrasonography group (8% vs. 45%, respectively).[32]

Treatment-specific Patient Selection Criteria And Evaluation

Once individual symptoms are causally related to uterine fibroids, all options (medical, interventional radiology, surgical, and alternative) should be presented. Most women who desire an image-based interventional therapy are evaluated jointly by a radiologist and a gynecologist, and patient selection is relatively straightforward; potential patients are excluded if they have contraindications for MR imaging (e.g., non-MRI compatible implanted metallic devices), uterine pathology other than leiomyoma, active pelvic infection, a pelvic mass outside the uterus, concurrent pregnancy, obesity exceeding table capacity, or intolerance to a prolonged stationary position (restless leg syndrome, etc.).

Ideal UAE candidates include women with symptomatic fibroids who desire uterine preservation and/or the avoidance of surgical intervention. Most patients with multiple, submucosal fibroids are good candidates for embolization, though large baseline fibroid volume has been associated with poorer outcomes and treatment failure.[33] Preprocedure evaluation should include a comprehensive history and physical examination, a recent gynecologic examination and Pap smear, an endometrial biopsy for patients with dysfunctional uterine bleeding, and imaging documenting the presence of uterine fibroids. Exclusion criteria include pregnancy; patients with severe renal insufficiency not receiving dialysis; history of pelvic irradiation; ovarian, endometrial, uterine, or cervical carcinoma; pelvic inflammatory disease or other pelvic infection and endometritis.[17] Pedunculated submucosal or subserosal fibroids on a narrow stalk should be identified prior to UAE, as embolization of these fibroids can lead to stalk necrosis and detachment of the fibroid from the uterus, causing either transcervical expulsion of necrotic fibroid tissue or peritonitis, persistent pain, and/or infection. An acceptable criterion to most interventional radiologists is stalk diameter greater than one third to one half the diameter of the fibroid, best assessed by preprocedure MRI.[6]

Initially, HIFU was contraindicated by the FDA for premenopausal women with symptomatic fibroids desiring future fertility; however, in 2009 the FDA modified this to a relative contraindication after more published data suggested treated women were able to successfully conceive and carry pregnancies to term.[34] At the 2008 international symposium, limitations to patient selection for MRgFUS were assessed on a 10-point Likert-type scale in a survey of 13 providers (5 gynecologists [39%] and 8 radiologists [61%]): 1, which indicated no impediment to therapy, to 10, which represented an absolute contraindication to therapy.[35] Factors that were not considered impediments (score <3) included concomitant mild adenomyosis, primary complaint being heavy bleeding, bulk pain, pelvic pain; possible impediments (score 3–5) included a desire for future fertility and pedunculated subserosal fibroid; significant impediments (score >5) included abdominal scarring, concomitant severe adenomyosis, gadolinium nonenhancement, high T2 signal intensity, pedunculated submucosal fibroid, size >10 cm and postmenopausal status. Other relative contraindications include inability to comprehend instructions or communicate sensations during treatment (safe treatment involves timely feedback of sensations such as leg, buttock, skin, or back pain to the operator). Other factors for exclusion are those common to many procedures, such as unstable cardiac status or cerebrovascular disease, hemolytic anemia, anticoagulation therapy, or underlying bleeding disorder.[36] Patients with nondisplaceable bowel that cannot be shifted out of the sonication beam path with provocative measures, or with cutaneous scars in the beam path (which may absorb ultrasound energy, causing cutaneous pain or burns), including those that could not be seen on the MR images, may be excluded. Other pathology or technical factors that would preclude the beam from entering the fibroid, including clips/metal in the beam path, history of liposuction, primary adenomyosis, too many fibroids (three or more >5 cm), nonenhancing (degenerated) leiomyomas, intracavitary lesions amenable to hysteroscopic resection, pedunculated leiomyomas, T2 hyperintense leiomyomas, and lesions suspicious for cancer (cervical or endometrial carcinoma or sarcoma), also factor in patient selection.[37]

Certain groups of patients are at risk for failing screening; a recent study analyzing screen failures prior to MRgFUS for uterine fibroids showed that African American women were more likely to fail screening because they presented with a significantly larger number of fibroids compared to non-African American women, and they possessed significantly more technical problems risking interference with safe delivery of treatment.[38] With current technology, larger volumes or numbers of lesions or deep lesions may not be fully treated in the 3-hour treatment window, though these limitations may ease as technology improves. The clinically eligible patient will undergo a prone screening MR study, which includes multiplanar T2- and T1-weighted sequences and dynamic gradient-echo 2D or 3D T1 sequences after power injection of an extracellular gadolinium chelate (0.1 mmol/kg). A radiologist trained to determine patient suitability then analyzes images; as size and fibroid number directly influence the success of both MRgFUS and UAE, leiomyomas should be described in terms of size, location, and T1 and T2 enhancement characteristics. Patients are deemed technically appropriate for first-generation MRgFUS if their leiomyomas are of proper size (<12 cm), number (four to five <4 cm or one <12 cm), signal quality (T2 hypointense, enhancing), and depth from skin (<13 cm).[39] Location of lesions within the uterus also independently influences the outcome, to a lesser extent. Intramural lesions are preferred, and subserosal lesions may also be acceptable as long as at least 30% of the circumference of the leiomyoma is within the uterine wall. If less than 30% of the circumference is contained, the lesion is considered "pedunculated" and is best treated with surgical myomectomy because of the theoretical risk of posttreatment torsion and detachment into the pelvis. Similarly, intracavitary leiomyomas are amenable to hysteroscopic resection.[40]

Patients with a total fibroid volume of more than 500 cm^3 may be pretreated with a gonadotropin-releasing hormone (GnRH) agonist, for example, leuprorelin (Lupron), for 3 months, reducing fibroid volume by 30%–60% and enabling treatment of a greater percentage of the overall leiomyoma.[41] Based on experience from myomectomy, where preoperative administration of GNRH agonists are used to temporarily decrease bulk, bleeding-related symptoms, and leiomyoma size, one study reported that GnRH-treated patients required half the energy (Joules) for a given nonperfused volume (NPV), confirming enhanced MRgFUS therapy after pretreatment.[42]

Clinical Outcomes of Minimally Invasive Interventions

UAE has consistently demonstrated safety and efficacy with minimal morbidity, without the need for general anesthesia and allowing for same-day hospital discharge. Reported ranges in mean uterine volume reduction are 38%–61%, and of fibroid size reduction, 58%–66%.[6,43] Common postprocedure side effects (Table 19-1) include pelvic pain, natural fibroid expulsion, and postembolization syndrome associated with high fever, leukocytosis, and general malaise lasting from a few hours to a few days, but major complications are rare: uterine necrosis and infection requiring emergent hysterectomy, ovarian failure, and vaginal dryness related to nontarget embolization or overembolization, and rarely, death, attributed to sepsis and possible acute pulmonary embolism described in two case reports.[45] However, several multicenter trials show consistently lower major complication rates, as well as shorter hospital stays, related to UAE, as compared with surgical management; in the HOPEFUL (2007) and REST (2007) trials, UAE patients experienced a 4.5%–19% adverse event (including major complications) rate compared with 14.8%–25% in surgical patients, most occurring within the first year.[45,46] The FIBROID Registry reported short- and mid-term outcomes based on the Uterine Fibroid Symptoms and Quality of Life (UFSQOL) Questionnaire, administered to patients at baseline, 6 months, 12 months, and then annually for 2 additional years after the procedure, with higher scores indicating worse symptom severity.[47] The mean score of fibroid patients was 59.83, compared to the mean score of 22.5 in a normal population, suggesting that the patients enrolled in the FIBROID Registry were highly symptomatic as a result of their fibroids. At 6 months, the mean symptom score was 19.87, and 19.23 at 12 months; these significant improvements suggest that UAE was highly effective at relieving symptoms. The major limitation of UAE is the need for further intervention; studies demonstrated that 14% of patients required further intervention (repeat UAE, myomectomy, or hysterectomy) within 2 years posttherapy, with up to 23%–32% undergoing additional therapy after 5–7 years.[45,46] Technical failure was attributed to the size and position of the fibroid and the technical difficulties during embolization.[45] Treatment failure may also occur with concurrent adenomyosis,

TABLE 19-1 Common Post Procedure Side Effects

Severity of complication	Type of complication	Hysterectomy (%)	UAE (%)
Severe	Death	0	0
	Pulmonary embolus	0.4–1.3	0
	Organ failure	0.2	0
Major	Permanent amenorrhea (<40 years)	0	0.2
	Blood transfusion	2.4–7.4	0.6
	Structural damage	0.5–3.5	0.8
	Sepsis	0.4–4	1.5–6
	Thrombosis	0.4	0
Minor	Minor infection/ Postembolization syndrome	10.9–13.5	5.9–25
	Hematoma	1.3	0.6–2.9
	Adverse drug reaction	0.7	1.2
	Permanent amenorrhea (>40 years)	0.2	1.4
	Urinary retention	2.2	1.4
	Fibroid expulsion	0	3–6.3

Data from Dutton S, et al: UK Multicentre retrospective cohort study comparing hysterectomy and uterine artery embolization for the treatment of symptomatic uterine fibroids (HOPEFUL study): main results on medium term safety and efficacy, *Br J Obstet Gynaecol* 114:1340–1351, 2007; Spilsbury, K., et al: Morbidity outcomes of 78,577 hysterectomies for benign reasons over 23 years, *Br J Obstet Gynaecol* 115(12):1473–83, 2008; Manyonda, I, et al: Uterine artery embolization versus myomectomy: impact on quality of life—results of the FUME (Fibroids of the Uterus: Myomectomy versus Embolization) Trial. *Cardiovasc Interv Radiol*. 2011; and Edwards R D, et al. Uterine artery embolization versus surgery for symptomatic uterine fibroids. The REST investigators, *N Engl J Med*. 356:360–370, 2007.

sometimes not detected by preprocedure ultrasound, as well as from inadequate embolization secondary to uterine artery spasm or aberrant arterial supply through the ovarian arteries.

Reintervention rates, which may be more clinically meaningful than fibroid volume reduction, have been reported to be less than 10% from 3 to 36 months for RFA.[22] Ren et al.[49] evaluated the therapeutic efficacy of ultrasound-guided HIFU in the treatment of uterine fibroids by using imaging and histopathologic examination, enrolling 119 consecutive patients and treating 187 uterine fibroids. Sixty-two fibroids received an ultrasound-guided needle puncture biopsy 1 week before and after HIFU treatment to both confirm the diagnosis and assess the early therapeutic efficacy, respectively. Hematoxylin–eosin staining and electron microscopy (EM) were performed to characterize more subtle, phenotypic changes in order to determine treatment success, and immediate therapeutic effects were assessed at follow-up using Doppler ultrasound and computed tomography or MRI. All patients were followed for 6–12 months to observe long-term therapeutic effects. No severe complications after HIFU ablation were demonstrated, and 51 (82.3%) of 62 biopsy specimens revealed obvious signs of necrosis under light microscopy. More subtle changes suggesting nonviability could be found by EM in the cellular structure in 60 specimens (96.8%). Follow-up imaging showed absent or reduced blood supply in the lesions after HIFU ablation, and the median reductions in tumor size as a percentage of initial tumor volume at 1, 3, 6, and 12 months after HIFU treatment were 21.2%, 29.6%, 44.8%, and 48.7%, respectively. Subsequent clinical outcomes demonstrated 9.7% of patients requiring secondary procedures (4 hysterectomies and 10 microwave ablation) for therapy failure or fibroid recurrence.[50] HIFU was effective in treating symptoms, with 85.5% of women reporting substantial relief from prior symptoms 12 months after treatment and a high proportion of completely asymptomatic post-treatment patients (59.3%), without major complications.

Several phase 1 studies have established the basic safety and feasibility of MRgFUS for treatment of symptomatic uterine leiomyomas, without demonstration of major complications.[51] Although ultrasound-guided HIFU is less expensive and theoretically more accessible compared to MRgFUS, there are substantial disadvantages, including the inability to monitor temperature, distinguish intervening bowel loops from inferior soft tissue, and poor bone resolution. In reported studies, there is no indication of its efficacy for hypercellular fibroids, because these lesions cannot be sonographically characterized. One of the earliest studies was a multicentered study of 109 patients who received an intentionally limited thermal dose, with post-treatment contrast-enhanced images showing actual nonperfused volumes greater than the intended volume.[52] Even with the small treated volume, the mean reduction in the UFS-QOL Questionnaire symptom severity score was 27.3 points on clinical follow-up, with 79.3% of patients achieving a greater than 10-point reduction in the UFS-QOL, occurring mostly within the first 3 months, with a follow-up study[53] at the 6-month period reporting a significant reduction in all subscales of the UFS-QOL. Of note, 5% of women had skin burns, confined to the areas of the abdominal wall where hair removal was incomplete, and a single subject had skin ulceration.

After the U.S. FDA approved MRgFUS in April 2004, early restrictions on treatment were reduced, resulting in significant increases in treatment volume and time, from 120 to 180 minutes. Sonications, previously allowed only near the leiomyoma's center, were also allowed toward the edge of leiomyomas, both near the endometrium and the serosal surface. Additionally, retreatment within 14 days was permitted. In a prospective study of 160 patients comparing outcomes in the restrictive ($n = 96$) and relaxed treatment ($n = 64$) cohorts, the NPV increased from 59.4 cm^3 (16.6% of fibroid volume) to 131.6 cm^3 (25.8% of fibroid volume), respectively.[54] The UFS-QOL score also showed a 10-point decrease in a larger percentage of patients (91% vs. 72%) at the 1-year follow-up, without differences in the rates of adverse effects between the two groups, demonstrating a correlation between NPV and the change in the UFS-QOL symptom severity score from baseline. A more recent study, using a protocol with greater treatment volumes (50% of total fibroid volume compared with 33%) and greater treatment duration (180 minutes compared with 120 minutes), reported a mean fibroid volume shrinkage of 31%, with persistent symptom improvement for 1–1.5 years correlated with an NPV between 50% and 80%, and 2.5–5 years correlated with an NPV exceeding 80%.[55] A separate study of 40 patients with longer-term follow-up (3 years) found continued decreased symptom severity scores, comparable to results of prior UAE studies, with about 69% of patients not requiring additional treatments.[56]

Having a younger age at treatment and a single fibroid were associated with the need for additional treatment.[57] Other variables such as weight, smoking status, parity, age at fibroid diagnosis, presenting symptoms, baseline symptom severity score, total fibroid volume, concomitant diagnosis of adenomyosis or endometriosis, prior use of oral contraceptives, or medical history were not found to be associated with the treatment outcome.[57] As previously described, fibroids with larger treated volumes are less likely to require additional treatment. Since the FDA approval of the ExAblate device in 2004 and the increased permitted treated volumes (NPV ratios larger than 50%), published data suggest a corresponding decreased need for additional treatment as the NPV ratio is increased; newer series from outside the U.S. with mean NPV ratios of 50% have shown additional treatment in only 12%–17% of women at $\leq$12 months.[58,60] In addition to a high NPV, dynamic contrast-enhanced MRI (DCE-MRI) imaging has also been shown to predict immediate, therapeutic response of MRgFUS for symptomatic fibroids.[59] The wash-in constant K^{trans} of baseline DCE-MR, acoustic power, and ultrasound frequency were found to be independent predictors for immediate therapeutic response of volumetric MRgFUS ablation. A high K^{trans} value is deemed to be a significant predictor of poor treatment results. The authors concluded that in such cases, the choice of higher acoustic power and/or higher ultrasound frequency would enhance the ablation efficacy. As discussed previously, hyperintense leiomyomas (high T2 signal) respond relatively poorly to ablation, and have a higher reintervention rate: one study reported that fibroids with signal intensity comparable to skeletal muscle but lower than that of myometrium had a mean reduction of volume 40%; even after 12 months and an ~15-point reduction in their symptom severity score, with poorer reduction values, high reintervention rates, and low response rates seen in fibroids with higher signal intensity.[61]

Postprocedure Fertility and Pregnancy Outcomes

Desired future fertility remains a relative contraindication to UAE, given the potential complications of uterine necrosis and ovarian failure. Although this procedure allows for preservation of fertility, caution should be exercised with regard to counseling women desiring pregnancy in the future. However, current literature has documented numerous successful pregnancies and successful live births after UAE, including both normal vaginal deliveries and cesarean deliveries.[44] Additionally, unlike surgery, UAE exposes the patient to pelvic radiation, and though unlikely to result in acute or long-term radiation injury, it remains important to minimize radiation dose to the pelvis, and specifically the ovaries, during the procedure.[43]

Rabinovici et al. reported 54 pregnancies in 51 women after MRgFUS, with a mean time to conception of eight months.[62] Live births occurred in 41% of pregnancies, with a 28% spontaneous abortion rate, an 11% rate of elective pregnancy termination, and 20% ongoing pregnancies beyond 20 gestational weeks, demonstrating a high rate of successfully delivered and ongoing pregnancies. Another case report[63] described a patient with fibroids that distorted the uterine cavity; 18 months after treatment by MRgFUS, the patient uneventfully carried a uterine pregnancy to term with an uncomplicated vaginal delivery. The authors suggest that MRgFUS may have a role in facilitating fertility in patients with fibroids, as the pregnancy occurred after a change in the configuration of the endometrial cavity as a result of MRgFUS. Despite these anecdotal reports, there is no formal study evaluating the effect of MRgFUS in either facilitating conception or minimizing gestational complications in women with uterine leiomyomas.

Relative Cost of Treatment

Cost analysis at 1 year posttreatment showed embolization to be more cost-effective than surgery, even including repeat hospitalization and imaging follow-up.[45] However, after this point, UAE was associated with more imaging studies and a longer mean hospital stay during the 1-year follow-up period, when compared with surgery. The initial cost benefit of UAE over surgery at 12 months is substantially reduced because of subsequent interventions, with treatments being cost neutral at 5 years.[45] In a study comparing lifetime total costs (including lost productivity) per patient for all currently available therapies, costs were found to be the lowest for the pharmacotherapy strategy ($9,200), but among procedure-based therapies, hysterectomy has the least upfront cost ($19,800), followed by MRgFUS ($27,300), UAE ($28,900), and myomectomy ($35,100).[64] The quality-adjusted life-year (QALY) is often used to measure disease burden, including both the quality and the quantity of life lived; treatment with UAE was associated with the most QALYs (17.39), followed by MRgFUS (17.36), myomectomy (17.31), hysterectomy (17.18), and pharmacotherapy (16.70). The cost-effectiveness ratios, or costs-per-QALY gained, were $21,800 for hysterectomy (relative to pharmacotherapy), $41,400 for MRgFUS (relative to hysterectomy), and $54,200 for UAE (relative to MRgFUS), suggesting that MRgFUS is in the range of currently accepted criteria for cost-effectiveness, along with hysterectomy and UAE. Compared directly to hysterectomy, MRgFUS was shown to lead to clinical improvement with fewer significant clinical complications and adverse events at the 6-month follow-up.[65] Another study performed in the National Health Service (NHS) Trusts in England and Wales demonstrated similar results, with the total direct medical costs of 1,000 women treated with MRgFUS at age 39 and followed until menopause or age 56 estimated at £3,101,644 ($4,817,157), compared with £3,396,913 ($5,275,740) for 1,000 women treated with currently available procedures,[66] resulting in a cost saving of £295,269 ($458,582) and an increase in QALYs by 10.658 compared with current practice.

Summary

Leiomyoma-related bulk and bleeding symptoms are among the most commonly treated gynecologic disorders in women. A multidisciplinary approach is necessary to optimize individual treatment, and pretreatment imaging is essential for triage. There are several options for noninvasive, image-guided therapies for symptomatic, classical uterine leiomyomas aside from the traditional, more invasive treatments, with particular usefulness in symptomatic women desiring future fertility. Predictably, clinical outcomes are improving with technical refinement and greater treatment volumes, but randomized trials and long-term outcomes (>5 years) have not been reported to date. An example of an algorithm for fibroid treatment is presented in Figure 19-5.

Acknowledgments

The author would like to thank Dr. Cheryl Hoffman for her assistance in preparing the section on uterine artery embolization and selection of representative images, and Drs. Steven Raman and Nelly Tan for their help and expertise in the section on magnetic resonance-guided focused ultrasound treatment and for providing a representative image.

REFERENCES

The complete reference list is available online at www.expertconsult.com.

20 Prostate Cancer Intervention

DANIEL MARGOLIS

KEY POINTS

- Prostate interventions can be used to both diagnose and treat prostate cancer.
- Although none have been shown to affect outcomes, and the data regarding side effects is heterogeneous, most show low rates of incontinence and impotence.
- Patient and treatment modality selection is a complex consideration, with diagnostic imaging providing an important component.
- Some treatments are not widely available or approved for use in all countries.
- In focal therapy, follow-up is paramount, as the entire prostate (and, in some cases, low-volume and low-grade disease) is not treated.

Introduction

Prostate cancer is the most common noncutaneous cancer and the second leading cause of cancer death in American men. Approximately one out of every six men in the United States will be diagnosed with prostate cancer in his lifetime, but only one in six of them will die of it.[1] More than 2 million men diagnosed with prostate cancer were living in 2010, and the medical costs associated with prostate cancer for 2010 are estimated at $12 billion. This relatively low death rate sets prostate cancer apart from many other cancers. Complicating this phenomenon is increasing interest in "active surveillance" of prostate cancer, the idea that small-volume, low-grade disease can be safely observed with intervention reserved for the identification of progression of disease.[2,3]

The goal of treatment is to both discriminate cancer that should be treated from that for which treatment can be safely deferred, and then to minimize the adverse effects of treatment while still achieving cure. This is complicated by the fact that the nerves involved in potency and continence lie alongside the prostate. A *New England Journal of Medicine* article reporting on 1201 men from multiple sites found incontinence rates of up to 20% for surgery and erectile dysfunction in up to 60% for radiation therapy at 2 years.[4] Yet, the majority of prostate cancer is organ-confined at the time of diagnosis with current detection algorithms. This has driven interest in minimally invasive treatments for prostate cancer.

One persistent controversy in prostate cancer treatment is the concept of the "index tumor." Prostate cancer can be a multifocal process, but there is growing interest in finding the largest, most aggressive of these tumors and treating it, while monitoring the rest for progression.[5]

Detection and Characterization of Prostate Cancer

The current paradigm for prostate cancer detection is screening with serum prostate-specific antigen (PSA) sampling and digital rectal examination (DRE). The PSA serum test is not approved for screening, but only for therapy monitoring, in the United States, and its use in this regard is controversial. Literature both supports and refutes a reduction in mortality from screening, with a concomitant increase in costs.[6,7] An additional wrinkle is that not all prostate cancer secretes PSA, which can also be elevated in benign conditions such as prostatic hyperplasia (BPH) and prostatitis. Additionally, the United States Preventive Service Task Force has issued a draft whereby it assigned PSA screening a grade D recommendation, meaning that it recommends *against* the use of PSA for screening men.[8]

There are multiple ways of evaluating PSA: Commonly, a measurement of 4.0 ng/mL or higher is considered suspicious, with 4.0–10.0 a "gray zone" of overlap with levels seen in BPH and prostatitis.[9] The percent free PSA is higher in benign conditions, but there is a large degree of overlap between ratios seen in cancer and benign conditions. PSA density compares the value against the size of the prostate, with lower densities seen in BPH, but again a large degree of overlap. The best indicator of suspicion is PSA velocity or doubling time, which reflects the rate of change over time, but even this is controversial and, of course, it requires at least two time points.[10]

Regardless of the utility of prostate cancer screening, if either the PSA test or DRE is abnormal, most physicians will refer the patient for biopsy. The biopsies are normally done systematically rather than targeted, and the number of cores varies between 6 (one per sextant) and over 20 in saturation biopsy procedures, but most physicians perform 10–12 cores, or 2 per sextant. Transrectal ultrasound (TRUS) is used to localize the prostate, but not commonly suspicious regions within it.[11] The false-negative rate for standard 12-core systematic prostate biopsies varies in the literature but conservatively measures about 20%.[10] The biopsies are reported in terms of the percentage and length positive and the Gleason score, which consists of the dominant and subdominant pattern ranging from 1 to 5. Therefore, a result of "30% (1.5 mm) Gleason 3+4=7" means that of the prostate tissue in the sample, 30%, or 1.5 mm, was predominantly Gleason pattern 3 with some pattern 4.

Current Conventional Treatment

Currently, the standards of care for prostate cancer include medical therapy, surgery, and radiation therapy. Surgical extirpation of the prostate has shown the highest long-term success for organ-confined prostate cancer. Traditionally, this was performed as an open surgery, but laparoscopic and robot-assisted surgery have overtaken this approach recently.[12] Although the markedly improved visual resolution and fine control over the surgical field afforded by robot-assisted surgery purports to afford improved outcomes, both in cancer control and side effects, this has not been proved.

Radiation therapy can be performed for organ-confined and locoregional disease, including after surgery. External-beam radiotherapy (EBRT) is often supplanted or augmented with image-guided, intensity-modulated techniques sometimes called "stereotactic body radiotherapy (SBRT)," with different trade names (e.g., Leksell Gamma Knife from Elekta AB, Cyberknife from Accuray, or Novalis Tx from Varian) used in marketing. Radioactive seed placement in brachytherapy affords some of the lowest rates of associated morbidity, but is usually reserved for localized low-grade disease.[4] High dose rate (HDR) brachytherapy involves placement of plastic catheters transperineally into the prostate, through which a robot places highly radioactive seeds for a limited amount of time in order to give specified radiation doses to tissue based on three-dimensional image-based planning software. HDR brachytherapy patients usually require only a 23-hour clinic stay, but this is not yet widely available.

Medical therapy can encompass hormonal modulation by lutein hormone releasing hormone agonists (e.g., leuprolide) or antiandrogenic compounds (e.g., bicalutamide) as well as chemotherapy. Surgical orchiectomy can also be considered for hormone modulation.

For patients with small-volume, low-grade disease, active surveillance rather than definitive management (surgery, radiation therapy, or other focal therapy) is sometimes considered, but even here the criteria vary by institution and some patients will exit surveillance because of anxiety.[13]

Image-guided Diagnosis

The first area of prostate cancer management where radiology can play a role is in improved diagnosis. This is primarily achieved by both noninvasive imaging and image-guided biopsy.

Although ultrasonography is an excellent modality to identify the location of the prostate, and can often resolve structures within it, it has shown relatively poor ability to discriminate benign from suspicious areas.[14] Magnetic resonance imaging (MRI) has steadily improved over the past couple of decades in its ability to characterize the prostate, not only localizing suspicious areas, but also suggesting the aggressiveness of these areas.[15,16] Initially used for surgical planning, high-resolution T2-weighted images are acquired with the use of an endorectal coil, supported with information from magnetic resonance spectroscopic imaging (MRSI) used to identify an alteration of the normal choline–citrate ratio to suggest malignant transformation of tissue. The application of diffusion-weighted imaging (DWI) and its concomitant apparent diffusion coefficient (ADC) map, and dynamic contrast-enhanced (DCE) perfusion imaging, has nearly obviated the endorectal coil for all but the most demanding protocols, as modern scanners with high-performance gradients sacrifice only the very fine detail of the prostate capsule necessary for a highly detailed differentiation of stage T2 (organ confined) disease from T3 (extraprostatic extension). MRSI, although the most specific component of multiparametric MRI, is also sometimes omitted.[17,18]

A dedicated limited protocol which incorporates thin-section, small-field-of-view turbo spin-echo T2-weighted imaging of the prostate in 2 or 3 planes along with DWI incorporating b-values from at least 100 s/mm^2 to at least 800 s/mm^2 and DCE perfusion imaging can accurately identify suspicious areas in less than ½ hour of scanner time. Criteria for prostate cancer on MRI are listed in Table 20-1.[19] Generally, each component is ranked on a 1–5 scale, with the sum (or average) giving the relative level of suspicion (see Table 20-1). Some centers will use purely quantitative ADC and pharmacokinetic perfusion values (e.g., k^{trans}), whereas others will use the qualitative appearance of the DWI and ADC map and curve types; the important consideration is that the reporting be standardized.

The oncologic interventionalist can then decide if any potential targets are worth sampling and has the option of multiple methods of doing so. Image fusion with transperineal CT-guided biopsy is an option but one not documented in the literature except after anorectal resection. Direct MRI-guided biopsy and MRI-ultrasound fusion biopsy are two well-documented choices.

Direct MRI-guided biopsy has been in development for more than a decade.[20] The setup commonly involves the patient prone with an external phased array and a dedicated biopsy guidance apparatus for a transrectal approach. Standard T2-weighted images are acquired with the biopsy guide attached to the table. Dedicated planning software is then used for biopsy guidance with fine adjustments of the biopsy guide. The biopsy device is then passed through the guide, with optional imaging of the device in place (Figure 20-1). A core is acquired, and the position can then be adjusted to acquire an adjacent core as needed.[21,22] There is currently one FDA-approved device in the United States (DynaTRIM, Invivo Inc., Gainesville, FL), with at least two others in development, one of which incorporates a dedicated endorectal coil.

MRI-ultrasound fusion imaging is another consideration. Previously, this was done with "mental" image fusion. In other words, a planning MRI is acquired, and the same area is identified during TRUS based on the location of the target. One or more 18-gauge cores are then acquired. This is relatively straightforward to incorporate into standard systematic sextant biopsies. However, although this technique has been shown to significantly increase yield after a negative biopsy up to 55%, its reliability is uncertain.[23] Prostate tissue characteristics can be quite different from MRI to ultrasound, complicating the coregistration.

New software and hardware combinations purport to fuse MRI and ultrasound data, either with image coregistration (Urostation, Koelis, La Tronche, France) or with mechanical localization (Artemis, Eigen, Grass Valley, CA).[24-26] For this method, the targets and prostate are outlined on dedicated software, with semiautomatic registration of the prostate. The data are then transferred to the ultrasound interface. The prostate is scanned using a sweep of the ultrasound probe and its registration on the ultrasound data set is registered to the MRI data. The ultrasound interface then displays a three-dimensional representation of the prostate and targets with the direction of the probe and biopsy throw superimposed. The ultrasound probe is manipulated until the planned biopsy throw would intersect the target, and the biopsy device is then deployed (Figure 20-2). These methods also allow for concomitant sextant biopsies. Some experts have found that, with experience, the image fusion becomes less important as they become

TABLE 20-1 Standardized Criteria for Prostate MRI Reporting

Score	T2 (Peripheral)	T2 (Central)	DWI/ADC	Perfusion	Spectroscopy
1	Uniform high signal intensity (SI)	Heterogeneous TZ adenoma with well-defined margins: "organized chaos"	No reduction in ADC compared with normal glandular tissue. No increase in SI on any high b-value image (≥b800)	Type 1 enhancement curve	Citrate peak height exceeds choline peak height >2 times
2	Linear, wedge-shaped, or geographic areas of lower SI, usually not well demarcated	Areas of more homogeneous low SI, however well marginated, originating from the TZ/BPH	Diffuse, hyper SI on ≥b800 image with low ADC; no focal features; however, linear, triangular, or geographic features are allowed	Type 2 enhancement curve	Citrate peak height exceeds choline peak height >1, <2 times
3	Intermediate appearances not in categories 1/2 or 4/5	Intermediate appearances not in categories 1/2 or 4/5	Intermediate appearances not in categories 1/2 or 4/5	Type 3 enhancement curve	Choline peak height equals citrate peak height
4	Discrete, homogeneous low signal focus/mass confined to the prostate	Areas of more homogeneous low SI, ill-defined: "erased charcoal sign"	Focal area(s) of reduced ADC but isointense SI on high b-value images (≥b800)	For focal enhancing lesion with curve type 2–3	Choline peak height exceeds citrate peak height >1, <2 times
5	Discrete, homogeneous low signal intensity focus with extracapsular extension/ invasive behavior or mass effect on the capsule (bulging), or broad (>1.5 cm) contact with the surface	Same as 4, but involving the anterior fibromuscular stroma or the anterior horn of the PZ, usually lenticular or water-drop shaped.	Focal area/mass of hyper SI on the high b-value images (≥b800) with reduced ADC	For asymmetric lesion or lesion at an unusual place with curve type 2–3	Choline peak height exceeds citrate peak height >2 times

Scores are ranked from 1 to 5 for T2-weighted imaging (with different criteria for the central and peripheral zones), diffusion-weighted imaging (DWI, using the high b-value and ADC map images), dynamic contrast perfusion images (based on focality/asymmetry and curve type: 1 = progressive, 2 = plateau, and 3 = washout) and, when acquired, spectroscopic imaging.

From Barentsz JO, Richenberg J, Clements R, et al: ESUR prostate MR guidelines 2012, *Eur Radiol* 22(4):746-757, 2012.

attuned to how targets on MRI will appear on ultrasound and can identify them even in the absence of direct image fusion; this is even true of some urologists who are invested in imaging technology and work closely with their radiologists, such that these biopsies may be performed with a conventional TRUS setup after review of MR images.

In both cases, because a transrectal approach will be undertaken, patients undergo a cleansing enema prior to arrival, and adequacy of the preparation is performed by DRE. Antibiotic prophylaxis, often a fluoroquinolone such as ciprofloxacin combined with a third-generation cephalosporin such as ceftriaxone, is taken before and also after the procedure. Analgesia is achieved with local anesthetic, such as 1% lidocaine administered just lateral to the prostate bilaterally, or (less effectively) with lidocaine jelly. Conscious sedation can also be employed. Commonly, at least two cores per target are acquired. Care should be taken to avoid the midline urethra. Complications are rare and include pain, bleeding, and prostatitis. Although a urethral fistula is possible, it is extremely uncommon.

Focal Therapies for in Situ Prostate Cancer

In order to minimize the morbidity associated with prostate surgery and radiation therapy in organ-confined disease, the concept of focal therapy has been developed as a middle ground between active surveillance and conventional definitive therapy.[27] There are a number of choices of focal therapy modality, and a number of potential approaches. The choice of both is based in part on the extent of disease, in part on the expertise of the physician, and in part on the desires of the patient. The treatment can be as radical as ablation of nearly the entire prostate, sparing only one neurovascular bundle, or so focal as to only encompass the dominant prostate tumor excluding any subdominant tumors (Figure 20-3).[28] Focal treatment modalities include cryotherapy, high-intensity focused ultrasound (HIFU), photodynamic therapy (PDT), laser (photothermal) ablation, and, potentially, high dose rate brachytherapy, to name but a few. This section will cover HIFU, cryotherapy, and laser ablation. PDT is primarily a whole-gland treatment scheme, whereby a vascular-targeted photosensitizer is given intravenously and light is delivered using optical fibers placed using a brachytherapy grid, while the patient is otherwise kept in total darkness (Figure 20-4).[29] This procedure is relatively uncommon given the exquisite skin sensitivity to light resulting from the photosensitizer. High dose rate brachytherapy is primarily a whole-gland treatment regimen as well, but can be delivered focally. However, the treatment strategy and subsequent brachytherapy catheter placement is most commonly performed by the radiation oncologist.

A consensus of experts recommends that potential focal therapy patients should have unilateral low- to intermediate-risk disease with clinical stage ≤cT2a, and that the choice of treatment type and extent will depend on the tumor volume and location and overall prostate size.[30] Until recently, focal therapy usually involved treatment of the entire prostate, but an important consideration given imaging guidance is whether to only treat the "index" tumor, or the dominant suspicious area. How accurately it can be targeted, and the confidence in imaging and biochemical markers (such as PSA) to continue to survey the prostate for the need for additional treatment, will guide how "focused" the treatment is planned. This same

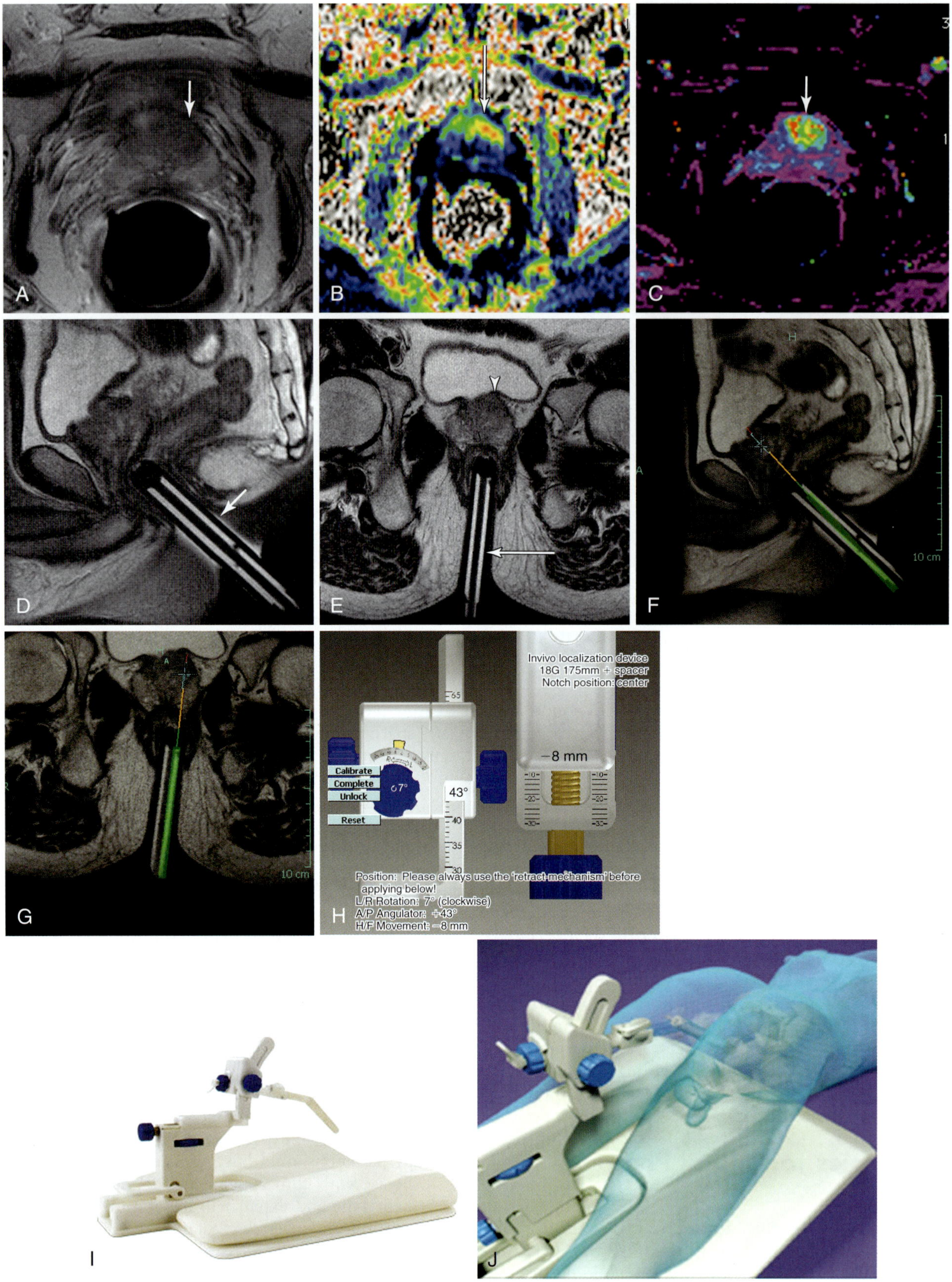

Figure 20-1 MR-guided biopsy. Diagnostic axial T2-weighted turbo spin-echo (A) and ADC color map (B) and K_{ep} perfusion color map (C) images reveal an anterior base lesion with ill-defined T2-hypointensity and corresponding restricted diffusion and washout (*arrow*). Planning sagittal (D) and oblique axial (E) T2-weighted turbo spin-echo images show the lesion (*arrowhead*) and biopsy guide in place (*arrow*). Planning software sagittal (F) and oblique axial (G) images show the biopsy guide in place with the target (plus-sign) and recommended adjustments to the biopsy guide (H). Examples of the external biopsy guide alone (I) and with phantom patient overlay (J). *(From Invivo.)*

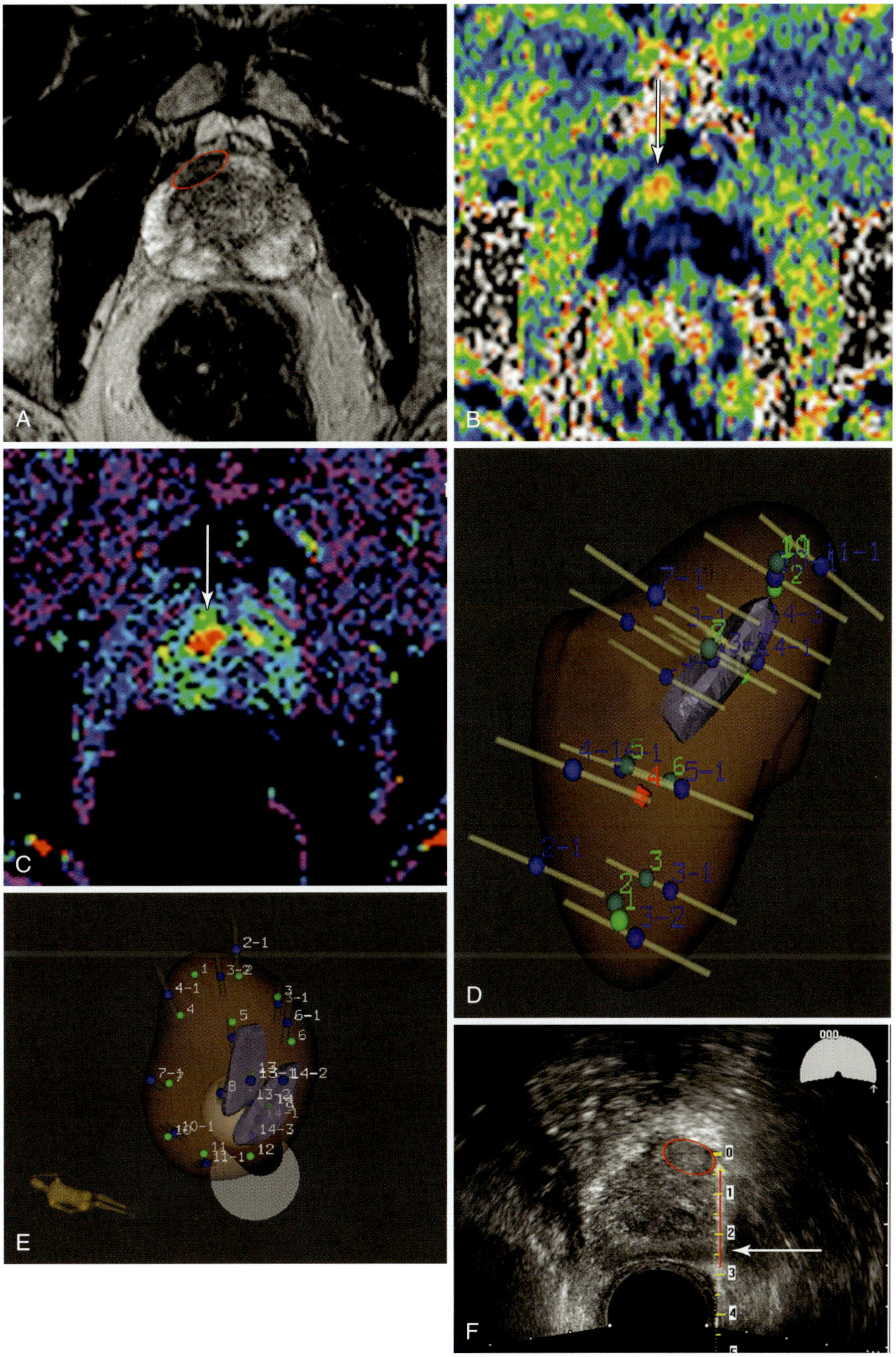

Figure 20-2 MR-ultrasound fusion targeted biopsy. Diagnostic axial T2-weighted (A), ADC color map (B), and K^{trans} perfusion color map (C) images show an area of restricted diffusion and increased perfusion (*arrows*) outlined on the T2-weighted image. Three-dimensional lateral (D) and frontal (E) planning software diagrams show the prostate (*transparent brown*), target (*violet*), systematic core targets (*green dots*) and targets (*blue dots*) with biopsy throw (*beige lines*) superimposed. Intraprocedural ultrasound image (F) shows the biopsy guide (*arrow*) and target (*red outline*).

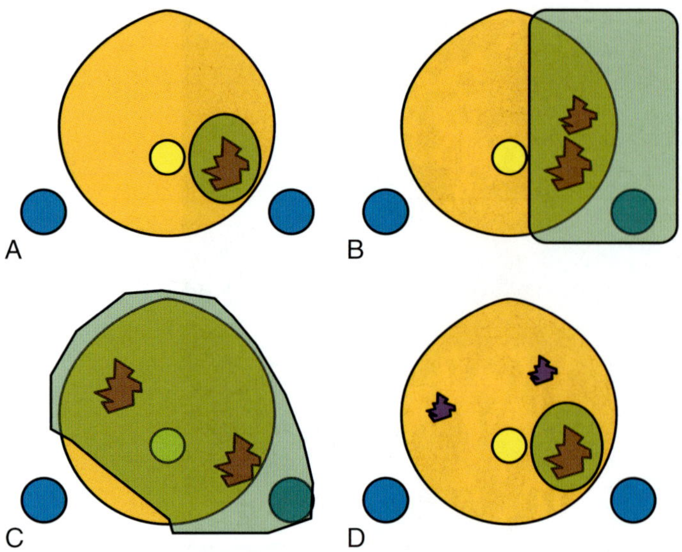

Figure 20-3 Examples of focal therapy types (axial cross-section). True focal therapy (A) treats (*green circle*) only the aggressive tumor (*red area*) and spares the neurovascular bundle (NVB, *blue circle*) as well as the urethra (*yellow circle*) and remainder of the prostate (*orange*). Hemiablation (B) treats the entire half of the prostate where the lesion or lesions lie, including the ipsilateral NVB, but sparing the contralateral NBV and urethra. Subtotal ablation (C) is more commonly used in this case, with only a small portion of the prostate and the NVB spared. It should be noted that true focal therapy could be considered even in the presence of multifocal disease (D) *if* those other foci are small volume and low grade (*purple areas*).

consensus, however, specifically recommends template biopsies to confirm localization of disease, with MRI considered "an investigative tool" that would "require validation in prospective clinical trials" although this is not the practice of all the signers to the article in question.

HIGH-INTENSITY FOCUSED ULTRASOUND

HIFU has the advantage that it is, potentially, completely noninvasive. There are two ways to guide the therapy, in combination with diagnostic ultrasound or using MRI guidance. The technique for the latter is more formally described in the chapter on uterine fibroid treatment, and, because it requires a sonographic window that would be obscured by the pubic symphysis, its pursuit for prostate cancer treatment has as yet been limited.

Therapeutic ultrasound is performed at lower frequency, usually 0.8–3.5 MHz, compared with diagnostic ultrasound, although modern ultrasound-guided HIFU units allow for imaging and therapy with a single transducer. During therapy, sound waves are focused to deposit the maximal power in a cylindrical volume of tissue, with the size usually on the order of a grain of rice (1–3 mm in diameter and 8–15 mm in length). Tissue ablation is accomplished by two processes. The deposition of thermal energy causes heating and resultant coagulative necrosis. Alternating cycles of compression and rarefaction from pressure alteration results in inertial cavitation as microbubbles of gas are drawn out of cells, which ultimately also results in coagulative necrosis. High-intensity devices deliver greater than 5 W of power per square centimeter.[27,31]

Treatment units allow for planning of multiple adjacent ablation zones in order to accomplish larger volumes of treatment. Treatment planning is therefore accomplished using dedicated treatment planning software on the HIFU machine, and the treatment time varies based on the amount of tissue to be treated (Figure 20-5). Treatment of the entire gland may take up to 2 hours or more.

There are two HIFU systems commercially available. It should be noted that neither are approved by the United States Food and Drug Administration (FDA) for treatment of prostate cancer, but rather for uterine fibroids, although this modality is in clinical trials for prostate cancer ablation in the United States. The two available models are the Ablatherm® HIFU from EDAP-TMS (Lyon, France) and Sonablate® 500 from Focus Surgery (Indianapolis, IN). Both are approved in Europe for prostate treatment, and the former is approved in Canada, Russia, Australia, and South Korea and the latter in Japan.

Considerations in the choice of technology include safety monitoring of the rectum (available in both devices), focal length, and power density variation (available on the Sonablate 500) and power deposition either by preprocedure planning software (with Ablatherm) or by monitoring grayscale changes taken to signify steam generated by successful coagulation (on Sonablate 500).

Potential complications of HIFU, especially whole-gland treatments, include urethral stricturing, and for that reason, treatment is often combined with transurethral resection of the prostate (TURP). Rates of biochemical failure are difficult to determine, as the technique varies from series to series, but has been reported from as low as 0% (for PSA <1 ng/mL) to as high as 44% (PSA <0.1 ng/mL) in various series. Rates of incontinence also vary from as low as 0.5%–15% Stamey Grade I, and rates of erectile function are poorly characterized, if at all, in most series. More serious adverse effects include fistula formation reported in up to 2% of early series, although this is very rarely seen with modern equipment.[32,33] Also, given the relative novelty of this treatment and indolent nature of low-grade prostate cancer, mortality outcomes are not yet known. It is likely for this reason that its approval is lagging in the United States.

CRYOTHERAPY

The tumoricidal effect of cryotherapy (or cryoablation) is likely primarily due to the formation of ice crystals, which burst cells through expansion. There is also the potential ischemic necrosis from vascular injury, dehydration, thrombosis from endothelial damage, and associated platelet activation, and possibly cryoactivation of an immune response to the tumor. The factors that determine efficacy include the nadir temperature, duration of freezing, rate of temperature normalization, and number of freeze–thaw cycles. Like any thermally ablative technique, heat sinks such as vessels may limit efficacy. In general, 3 minutes at −40°C is sufficient for tumoricidal effect.[27,34] However, many sites now rely on two freeze–thaw cycles for each probe position, with 8–11 minutes per freeze.

Modern cryotherapy devices use ultrasound guidance with a relatively small (17-gauge) treatment probe that allows for freezing with argon and thawing with helium gas. The technique is similar to that originally proposed.[35] Normally, two to four probes are used per focus, with an additional probe placed contralaterally adjacent to the urethra or external sphincter but used for warming (Figure 20-6). Urethral warming has been

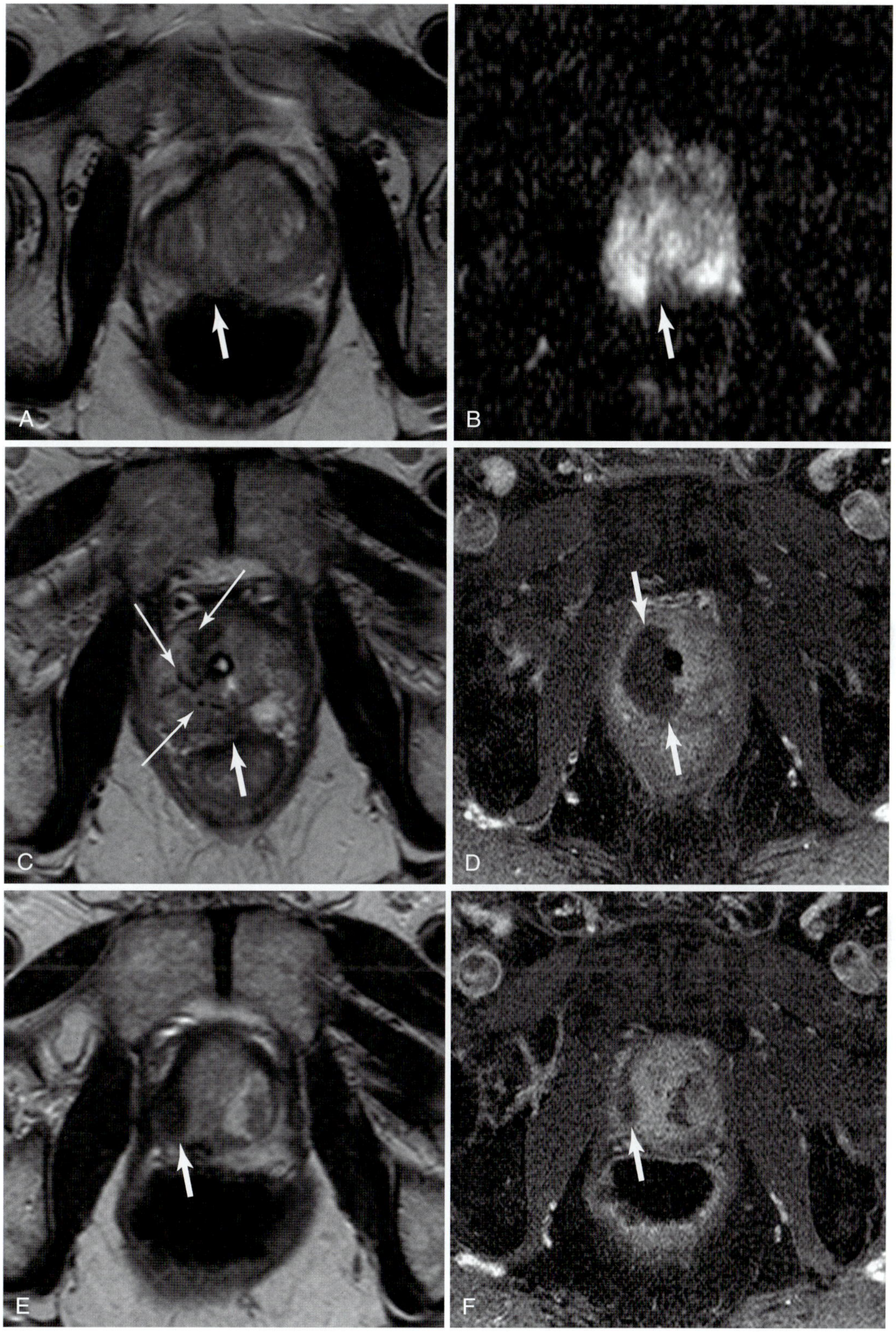

Figure 20-4 Photodynamic therapy (PDT) example of hemiablation. Axial T2-weighted imaging (A) and ADC map (B) show a low signal focus in the medial posterior right peripheral gland. Intraprocedural T2-weighted imaging (C) shows the lesion (*thick arrow*) with fibers for light conduction (*thin arrows*) still in place in the right gland. Postcontrast gradient T1-weighted image (D) shows a zone of absent perfusion including the suspicious area (*arrows*). Follow-up images at 3 months show the right side is now much smaller, and low signal on T2-weighted imaging (E) with decreased perfusion on postcontrast gradient T1-weighted images (F).

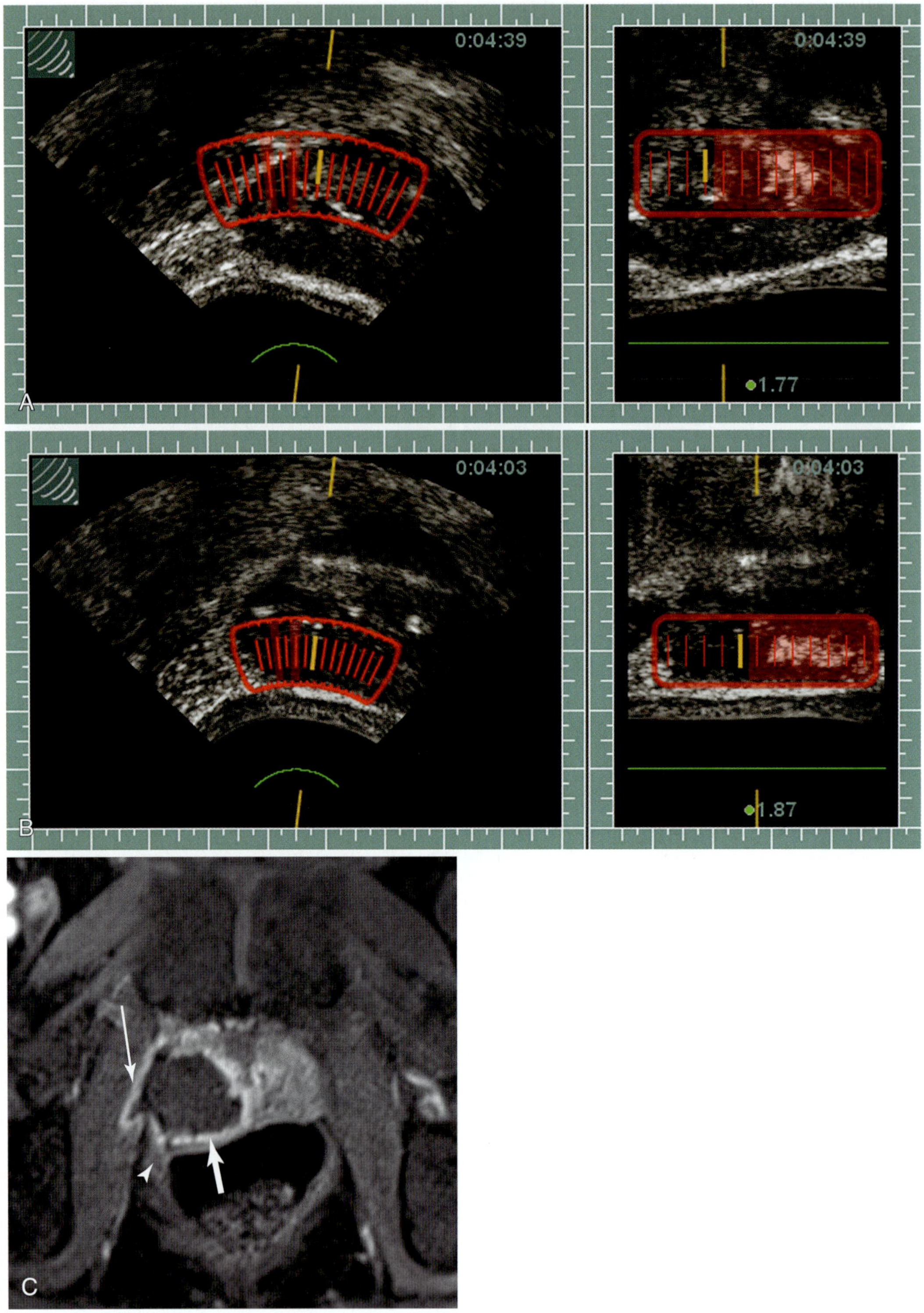

Figure 20-5 High-intensity focused ultrasound. Intraprocedural ultrasound images show planning of ablation in the anterior (A) and posterior (B) right prostate. Follow-up axial postcontrast gradient T1-weighted image (C) shows ablation of the right prostate (*thick arrow*) and likely some tissue peripheral to the anterolateral prostate (*thin arrow*) but not at the expected location of the neurovascular bundle (*arrowhead*). *(Images courtesy of Hashim Ahmed, University College London.)*

added to the original technique to reduce the likelihood of urethral sloughing. In addition, planning software, using three-dimensional ultrasound data combined with a traditional brachytherapy transperineal template for probe placement has made whole-gland treatment or hemiablation more straightforward. However, the prospect of true focal therapy of just the index lesion using real-time TRUS guidance remains a possibility, with the relative drawback that the ice ball limits resolution of tissue beyond it on ultrasound. Whether to use the transrectal approach, which may be crowded for multiple probe placements, or the transperineal brachytherapy-grid approach, varies based on user preference.

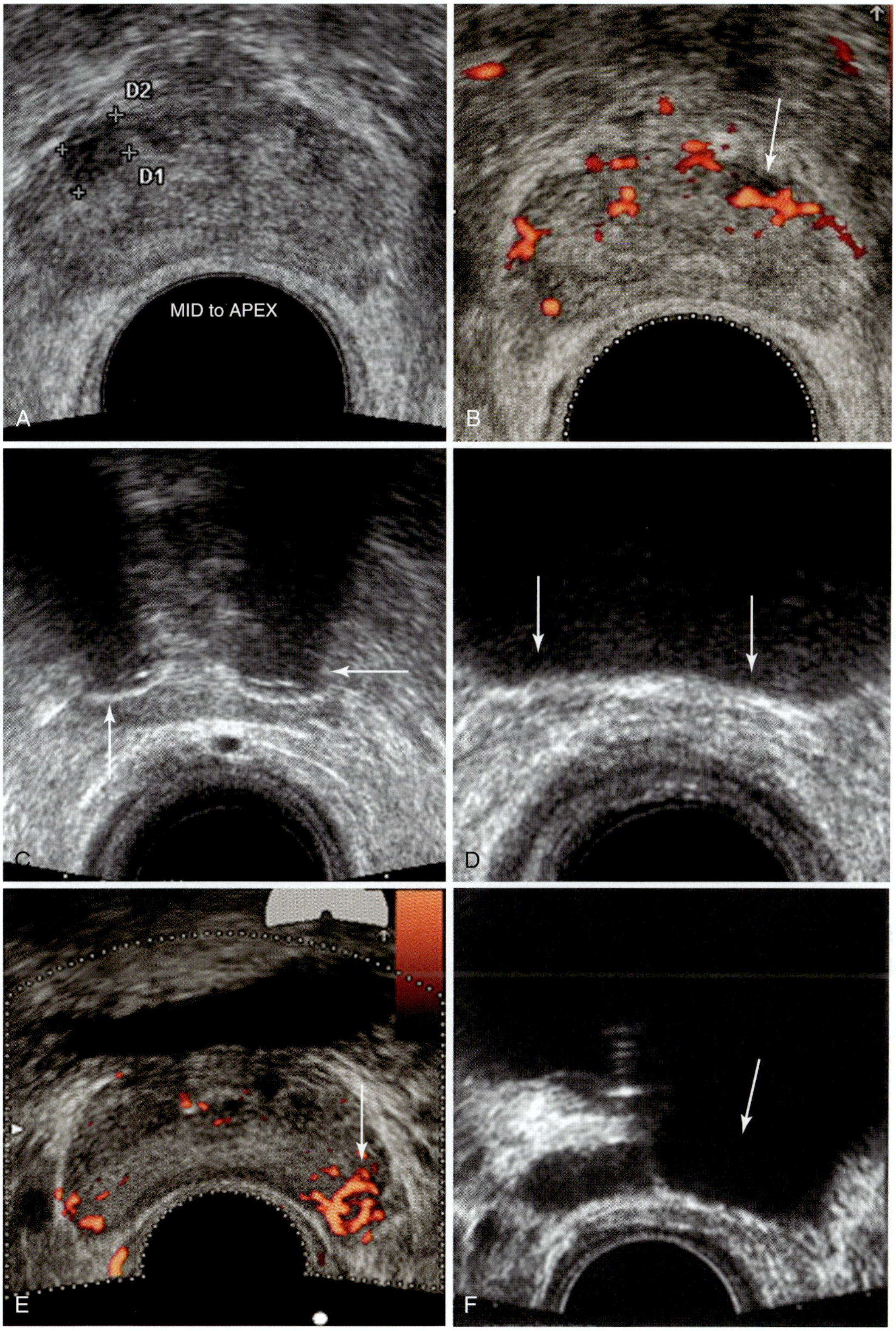

Figure 20-6 Cryoablation. Axial ultrasound images delineating a hypoechoic nodule in the right anterior apical midgland (A) and a hypoechoic nodule with increased power Doppler signal (B, *arrow*). This patient was referred for total prostate ablation. An initial image (C) shows the hypoechoic and reflective ice balls forming (*arrows*) around the cryoprobes with posterior acoustic shadowing, progressing to involvement of the entire prostate (D), which is now hypoechoic with shadowing. Two treatments of 11 and 8 minutes were applied for this result. A second patient with a single nodule in the posterior left peripheral gland that has increased power Doppler signal (E, *arrow*) underwent successful focal cryoablation (F, *arrow*). *(Images courtesy of Duke Bahn, Prostate Institute of America.)*

Another limitation of cryotherapy is the relatively limited data to support it for truly focal therapy. There are a number of series with more than 100 patients for whole-gland treatment with follow-up for as long as 12 years. However, not all of these reported continence or erectile function, although the former ranged from 0.4% to 16.7%, with the highest values largely seen in older generations of hardware. Also, biochemical failure, though not all reported using the same criteria, ranged from a low of 10% to a high of 65% (again, with older equipment) but many series report 20% or greater failure even in low D'amico criteria risk groups.[36-38] More modern series of truly focal prostate cryotherapy, however, have shown better results, with low complication rates.[39]

PHOTOTHERMAL LASER ABLATION

This section will focus on the use of laser energy to treat prostate malignancy. Laser treatment of benign prostatic hyperplasia is discussed in a later section of this chapter; although, like any therapy, laser treatment specifically for prostatic hyperplasia could alter the appearance of the prostate on imaging, the technique is significantly different from the focal cancer treatment approach. Focal photothermal laser ablation (PTLA) therapy is alternately known as laser-induced interstitial thermotherapy (LITT) or focal laser ablation (FLA). The use of laser for tissue ablation of cancer has a specific advantage to the interventional radiologist: MRI compatibility. This allows for not only image-guided targeting but, potentially, intraprocedural temperature monitoring (as in MR-guided HIFU).[40] Contrast-enhanced ultrasound (CEUS) could also be used to monitor tissue perfusion, as microbubbles do not enter treated tissue because of shutdown of perfusion.

The prostate is also ideally suited for PTLA because the ablation size is limited by its optical absorption, and it is relatively nonvascular, which prevents heat sink effects. There is also evidence to suggest that laser energy penetrates tumor cells to a greater degree than benign tissue with resultant larger coagulation zones in tumors. The choice of wavelength is largely determined by the device used, with the Nd:YAG laser using a wavelength of 1064 nm, but newer, cheaper, and smaller units tend to use lower wavelengths, approximately 800–980 nm. The high water content of tissue allows for extensive absorption of energy in the infrared range and therefore efficient energy transfer and heating.[41]

Similar to other forms of thermal therapy, tissues are heated to produce the desired effects. Although coagulative necrosis will occur at temperatures above 60°C, irreversible cell death is achievable at lower temperatures exceeding 42°C with a longer duration of treatment. Vaporization of cellular protoplasm and subsequent desiccation and shrinking of tissue occurs in excess of 100°C. Repeat treatment will cause a rapid rise in temperature, with charring (carbonization) above 300°C, which markedly impedes transmission of photothermal energy. Therefore, water-cooled fibers have been designed to prevent temperature spikes close to the diffusing tip of the fiber, with ablative zones of up to 8 cm possible using up to 50-W lasers (as opposed to the 5-W lasers more common without cooling). Fibers are generally made of quartz with diameters between 250 and 1000 μm and have cylindrical or flat diffusing tips up to 40 mm long.

There are multiple systems in use for interstitial laser therapy that can be adapted for use in the prostate. The Visualase Inc. Thermal Therapy System and its components and the MRI analysis software and workstation have all been cleared through the FDA 510(K) premarket notification mechanism specifically for MRI-guided tissue treatment, as they have been found to be substantially equivalent to other approved devices. It is specifically approved to necrotize or coagulate soft tissue through interstitial irradiation or thermal therapy under magnetic resonance imaging (MRI) guidance for wavelengths 800 nm through 1064 nm. Much of the literature supporting MRI-guided preclinical and human trials of laser ablation of prostate tissue has used this system.

For MRI-guided therapy, the procedure is similar to MRI-guided biopsy or brachytherapy treatment. Patients are normally placed in the prone lithotomy position. The fibers can either be placed transrectally using the biopsy system, or via a MRI-compatible brachytherapy planning template for a transperineal approach, with appropriate patient preparation identical to MRI-guided prostate biopsy or brachytherapy placement respectively. Specialized or brachytherapy planning software can be used for the brachytherapy-style approach. A 14-gauge MRI-compatible catheter and trocar is advanced into the target, with the trocar replaced by the interstitial fiber once in place (Figure 20-7). MRI thermometry software can then be used to monitor the efficacy of treatment and place safety temperature limits around the urethra and rectum to prevent their injury. For truly focal therapy, using the cooled laser fiber, only a single treatment may be needed per lesion.

For ultrasound-guided therapy, a system whereby TRUS is combined with a brachytherapy grid, with the patient in dorsal lithotomy position but otherwise the same patient preparation works similar to MRI-guided treatment. The main difference is that treatment efficacy is monitored with CEUS rather than MRI.

Very few series have been published regarding human trials of PTLA, with scant evidence of side effects and long-term follow-up. However, in one small series (up to 12 patients), no significant incontinence or impotence has been observed. However, in this ultrasound-guided cohort, only 50% were disease-free by biopsy; PSA results were not explicitly reported in this series.[40,42,43]

Importance of Image Guidance

The original papers on cryotherapy and HIFU of the prostate describe whole-gland treatment, and until recently, this was how "focal" therapy was considered. The use of imaging to guide treatment of the index lesion holds the promise of decreased morbidity with similar biochemical control rates, and ensures that the target lesion is identified and treated. However, this advantage is predicated upon the ability to identify and adequately treat localized disease.

The choice of focal treatment imaging modality will largely depend on the technology available and the type of therapy desired.[44,45] Ultrasound is widely available and relatively inexpensive. However, grayscale ultrasound does not discriminate malignant from benign lesions in the prostate. Although color Doppler ultrasound (CDUS) improves the detection rates of prostate cancer in some series, its ability to do so has been shown to be unreliable in others.[45] However, CEUS has been shown to significantly improve detection rates on TRUS-guided biopsy, but no studies compare it to MRI.[46] Additionally, microbubble contrast is not without risk, and has received a "black box" warning in the United States,

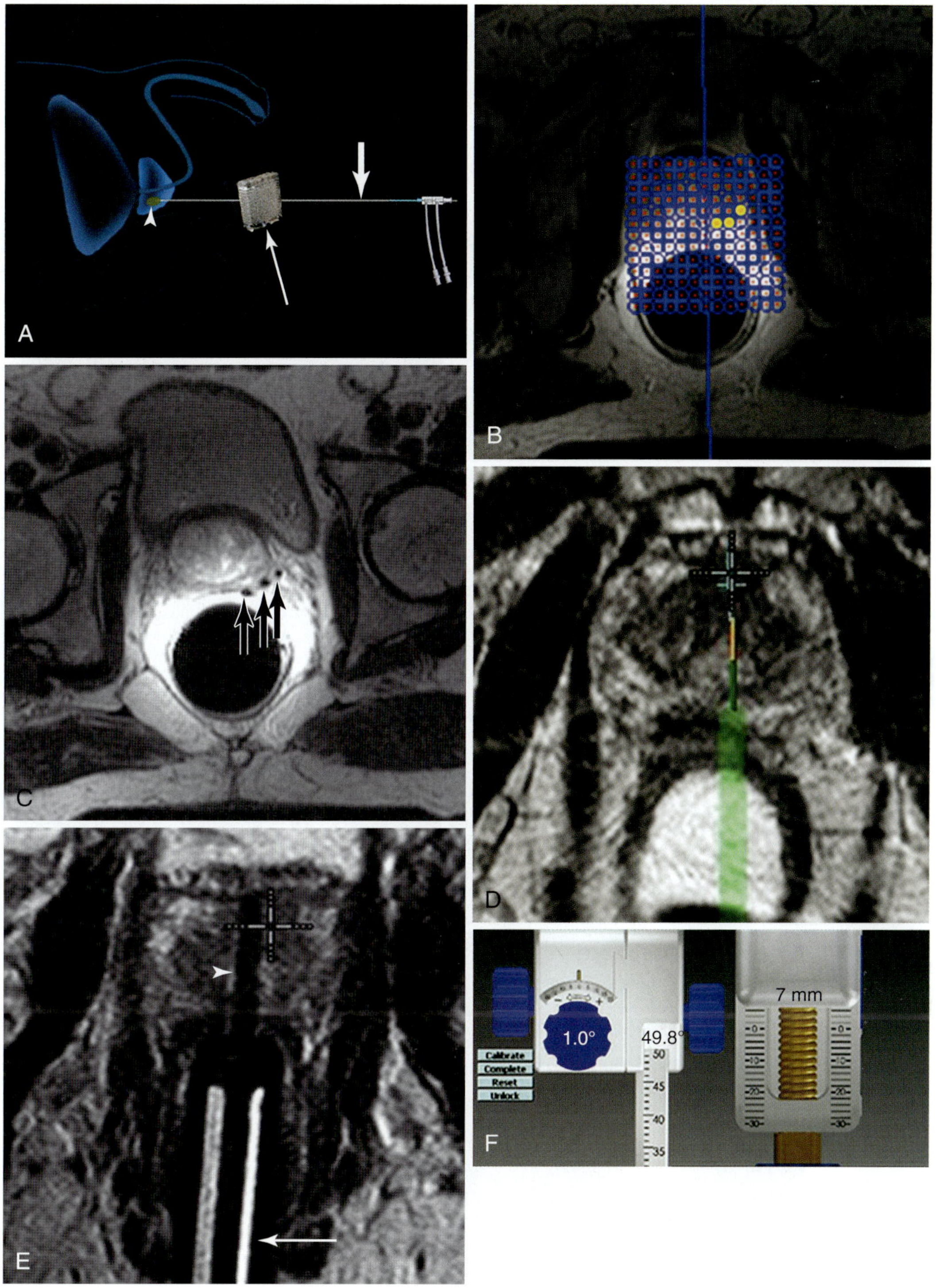

Figure 20-7 Photothermal Laser Ablation (PTLA). Diagram (A) showing the laser catheter (*thick arrow*), perineal template (*thin arrow*), and intraprostatic target (*arrowhead*). Planning T2-weighted axial images showing template overlay (B) and catheters in place (C, *arrows*). Example of transrectal treatment planning using biopsy planning software (DynaTRIM, Invivo Inc.) with trajectory (*green line*) overlaid on oblique axial T2-weighted image (D) showing target (*plus sign*). Procedural axial oblique T2-weighted image (E) showing guide (*arrow*) and fiber (*arrowhead*) adjacent to target. Planning diagram (F) is identical to that used to adjust the guide for biopsy. In a separate patient, using the transperineal approach, oblique coronal T2-weighted images showing the fiber (*arrowhead*) and Foley catheter (*arrow*) with thermal *Continued*

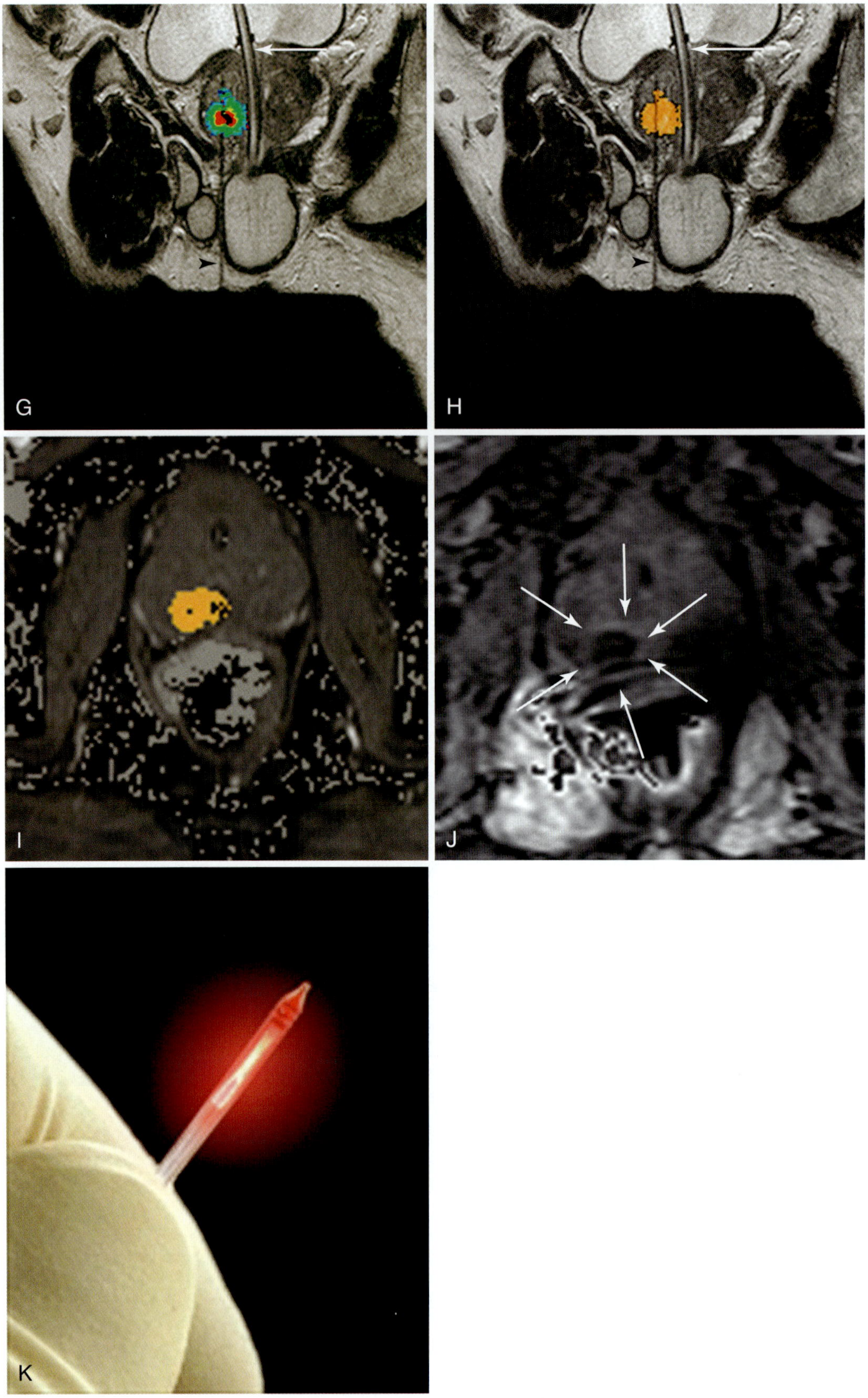

Figure 20-1, cont'd (G) and Arrhenius-based thermal injury (H) maps overlaid. Correlation of thermal injury map (I) and postcontrast gradient T1-weighted images (J) in a different patient showing excellent agreement. Example of fiber active tip (K). *(Images courtesy Visualase, Inc.)*

where it is not approved for use other than in echocardiography. Ultrasound elastography has traditionally used physical pressure to deform tissue and thus determine its "stiffness," but newer techniques use high-frequency ultrasonic shear waves to quantify tissue elastic properties.[47] It holds great promise, but has not been proven.

MRI provides a high degree of specificity for in situ tumor identification. However, there are many drawbacks to performing procedures using direct MRI guidance. Time on the magnet is expensive. Many materials and devices are not MRI-compatible. The gantry of most systems makes performing interventions with the patient inside the bore difficult, if not impossible, such that the patient may have to be slid in and out multiple times during treatment set-up. The advantage of real-time three-dimensional temperature monitoring and direct visualization of the target may trump these disadvantages.

A third option is image fusion. MRI-localized targets can be treated using ultrasound or CT with image fusion software, such as the Eigen, Inc. Artemis device or Philips Traxtal. This allows for the ease of use of ultrasound or CT and the specificity of MRI.[24-26]

The degree to which the prostate is treated largely depends on the size, number, and location of the "index" (largest and most aggressive) lesion and any other lesions felt significant. The concept of only treating "significant" lesions is gaining popularity as these patients would be expected to undergo continued surveillance with PSA and, potentially, imaging. How the index lesion is defined varies based on the series reviewed, but it is generally the largest lesion, measured on T2-weighted imaging, with the most abnormal functional (diffusion, dynamic contrast enhancement perfusion, and/or spectroscopic) characteristics.[44,48-50]

Another consideration is the accuracy of targeting. As described in the respective sections, the degree of biochemical failure for each treatment modality is not insignificant. Even MRI-guided therapy risks undertreatment, as low-grade disease may not be conspicuous on MRI.

For hemiablation of the prostate, ultrasound is likely the most cost-effective choice. The prostate is well delineated, as is the urethra, and this is often the modality of choice for cryotherapy, photodynamic therapy and, understandably, HIFU. Hemiablation is usually reserved for patients with either a single, large unilateral index lesion or multiple ipsilateral significant tumors. Focal therapy of a small lesion could be accomplished with either direct MRI-guided treatment or MRI image fusion with TRUS. Although there is some variability of targeting, literature supports accuracy to within 3 mm for most conventional software.[24-26]

Determinants of Success (or Failure)

The concept of the "trifecta" of prostate cancer treatment is absence from incontinence, erectile dysfunction, and detectable disease (either by PSA or repeat biopsy). The first two should be advantages of focal therapy that does not injure the neurovascular bundles, but the last consideration is more elusive. The criteria used to define abnormal PSA, either >0.2 ng/mL for surgery or two successive rises above the nadir for the American Society for Therapeutic Radiology and Oncology (ASTRO) "Phoenix" criteria, and the number of cores taken can all affect detection of recurrent disease.[52,53] PSA surveillance can be even more difficult if there is a background of (untreated) BPH. It can also be difficult to interpret systematic sextant biopsies in a patient who has undergone hemiablation with atrophy of the treated prostate.

Biochemical (PSA) outcomes are complicated by the residual normal tissue and BPH. In radiation therapy, the entire prostate is treated, but the treatment is gradual, so that long-term trends in PSA are evaluated. With surgery, no significant prostate tissue remains, so an absolute nadir of near-undetectable is used (PSA is produced in other tissues, such as breast tissue, to a minimal degree). Using PSA kinetics or density is a consideration, but this has not been validated. PSA density, first described by Stamey, correlates PSA serum values with the size (and therefore mass) of the prostate, with benign tissue producing on average 0.30 and cancer 3.5 ng/mL per gram prostate, and should therefore be adjusted for any overall change in prostate size.[54] PSA kinetics, such as doubling time or velocity, have also been shown to be more predictive than overall PSA in detecting significant disease. How these would change after prostate focal therapy is unknown, but they should normalize in the absence of residual disease with 1 ng/mL/year as the normal maximum for velocity and 2 years the minimum for doubling time. PSA nadir could conceivably be calculated based on the percentage tissue treated, but the accuracy of such a calculation would be difficult to estimate, and residual treated tissue would have an unknown contribution to serum PSA.[55] For any of these estimates of PSA, there is the difficulty that the major contributor, the index lesion, should cease to produce it, with a disproportionate but incalculable drop in PSA.

As these patients would continue to undergo surveillance, and their PSA would not be expected to completely extinguish, they would be expected to be referred for repeat biopsies. Because the therapy would have been targeted, it makes sense that the biopsies would be, too, in order to sample the treated tissue, in addition to systematic sextant biopsies. Another consideration is that residual low-grade (Gleason pattern 3) disease would not be unexpected and should not be considered treatment failure, as it is often not evident on imaging. How to interpret this finding, and what should be considered significant (e.g., only Gleason pattern 4 on at least 25% of two systematic cores) is not established or validated.[56] The number of biopsies, including template saturation biopsies, is also up for consideration.

Yet another consideration is the use of imaging alone. Many patients are beginning to inquire if they can substitute MRI for biopsy (especially nonendorectal coil MRI, which is likely appropriate in the surveillance population). However, treatment effects can render the prostate quite distorted with abnormal parameters on functional imaging. MRI has been shown accurate for detection of recurrent disease in irradiated prostates.[57] Whether this would hold true for thermal therapies is as yet unknown. As in most ablative therapies, the appearance of enhancing tissue in the ablation zone is considered suspicious, either on CEUS or MRI, but how to interpret the distorted remainder of the prostate, and whether functional abnormalities could be seen in the peri-ablation zone is unknown. It is likely that imagers, who could perform targeted biopsy of suspicious tissue, would have a low threshold to do so.

An example of an algorithm for management of prostate cancer from the standpoint of the interventional oncologist is presented in Figure 20-8.

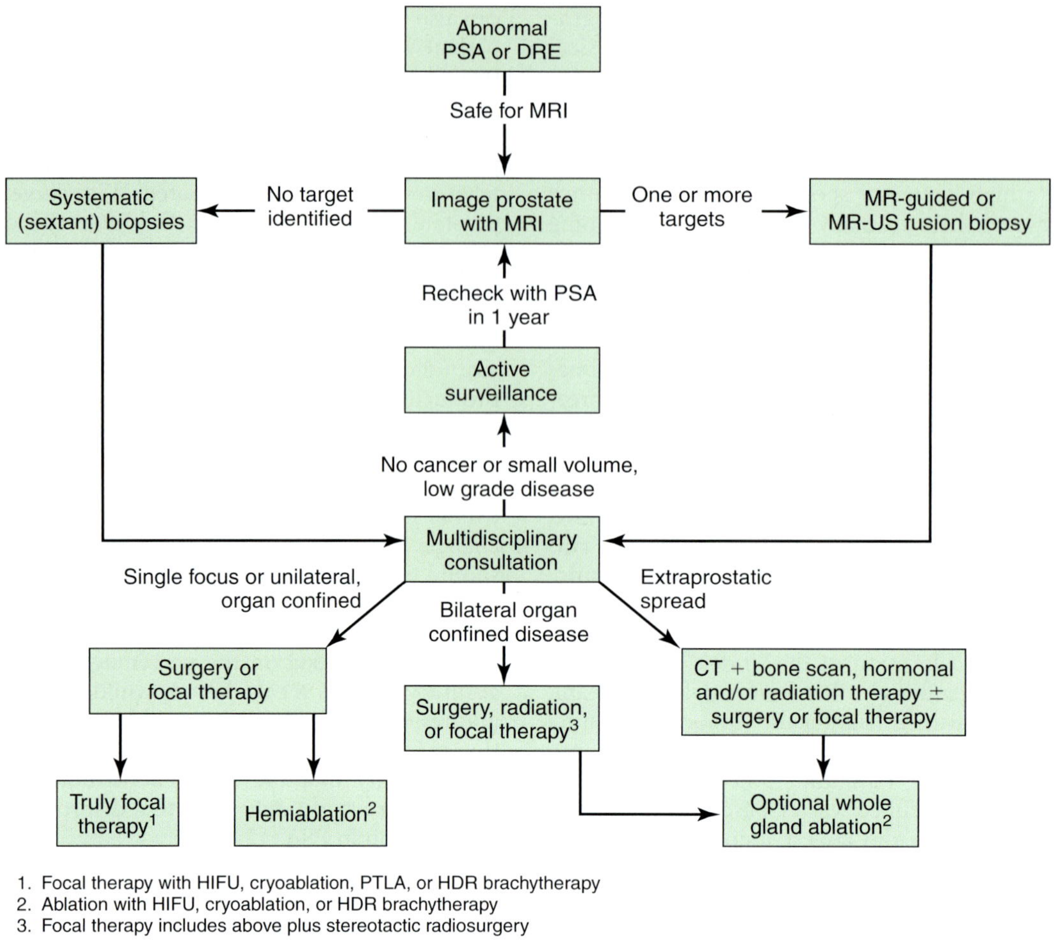

Figure 20-8 Algorithm for Prostate Cancer Management.

Interventions for Biochemical Failure (Recurrence)

Image-guided interventions can be an important part of the management of men who fail primary definitive treatment of prostate cancer. These are primarily men who have undergone radical prostatectomy or radiation therapy for prostate cancer with a decrease in serum PSA level and a subsequent rise. There are more than 100 definitions for biochemical failure in the literature, but two definitions have become widely accepted. For patients who have undergone radical prostatectomy, the American Urological Association Prostate Guidelines for Localized Prostate Cancer Update Panel recommends defining biochemical recurrence as an initial serum prostate-specific antigen level of ≥0.2 ng/mL, with a second confirmatory level of prostate specific antigen of >0.2 ng/mL who then experience a rise in PSA.[52] For patients who underwent external beam radiation therapy (EBRT), the ASTRO "Phoenix" criteria define biochemical failure as two successive rises above the nadir, with the time point designated "at call" rather than backdated.[53] This would apply to EBRT patients regardless of hormonal therapy, but would be used only for brachytherapy patients who had not also received hormone modulation. As is evident from a review of the literature that purports to support the use of focal therapy for prostate cancer, adoption of a standard definition is important not only for validation of clinical trials but as a benchmark against which to base patient management.

In the case of biochemical failure, there are a number of options for salvage treatment of in situ prostate cancer. These include surgery for patients who previously underwent EBRT, brachytherapy, cryoablation, and HIFU, with some literature to support other forms of focal therapy such as PTLA and PDT.[58] Identifying the ideal candidate for salvage focal therapy is less well established. However, a general consensus would be one with serum PSA <10 ng/mL, Gleason score of <8, and clinical stage T2 or less before EBRT. In addition, PSA kinetics, such as doubling time, at the time of biochemical failure may be predictive of the outcome of salvage focal therapy as it may correlate with the likelihood that disease remains locally confined, with disease-free survival at 5 years of 57% and 23% for salvage cryotherapy patients with a serum PSA less than or 10 ng/mL or more, respectively.[59] Although metastatic disease is often occult on standard imaging (CT and skeletal scintigraphy) with PSA levels less than 1 ng/mL, these modalities should also be considered to exclude metastatic disease, although its presence does not entirely preclude the possibility of focal therapy, as described below.

The first consideration for patients with biochemical failure is documentation of recurrent in situ or prostatic bed disease. Here, image-guided biopsy can play an important role, although the distortion in the anatomy and effects of therapy can render interpretation much more complicated compared with the untreated prostate. The standard of care for biochemical failure of EBRT is to repeat systematic sextant biopsies, although the utility is questionable; a positive biopsy within 2 years of EBRT is not indicative of eventual failure and some patients with positive biopsies will eventually "convert" to negative.[60] Also, these biopsies should be reviewed by a pathologist familiar with the appearance of successfully treated prostate cancer after radiation therapy to avoid the possibility of confusing radiation changes with high-grade disease.

With respect to approach, direct MR-guided, MR-image fusion, and MR-informed TRUS have all shown efficacy over systematic biopsies.[57,61] Treatment effects often result in overall lower signal on T2-weighted imaging and a uniform decrease in apparent diffusion coefficient, such that asymmetry and perfusion imaging play an increasingly important role in identifying a target. Magnetic resonance spectroscopic imaging (MRSI), which can also be difficult to interpret because of depletion of citrate after radiation therapy, has nonetheless been shown useful in identifying recurrent disease.[62] This also holds true for recurrent disease in the surgical bed, where residual tissue that displays increased perfusion, restricted diffusion, or elevated choline on MRSI may indicate recurrent disease, especially at the vesicourethral anastomosis.[63,64]

Salvage cryotherapy is probably the most widely used focal therapy for biochemical failure. In fact, its initial use was in biochemical failure and only after it appeared effective was it considered for primary focal therapy.[65] At 7-year follow-up, biochemical disease-free survival rates were in excess of 70% for good- to intermediate-risk patients and nearly 50% for high-risk patients.[66] Treatment planning is otherwise identical to primary therapy with the same consideration of subtotal ablation, hemiablation, and truly focal therapy depending on biopsy and imaging results. One potential advantage to cryotherapy is its ability to activate an immune response to the treated tumor, which may help in systemic control, although this is purely conjectural at this point. As mentioned in the section on primary cryotherapy, rates of complication have markedly diminished with modern techniques, including urethral warming. Rates of complication for salvage cryotherapy are difficult to quantify because of the underlying risk of side effects from the primary therapy.

HIFU can also be considered for salvage treatment, although there exists much less experience with it, and reported literature is heterogeneous in terms of definition of treatment failure and side effects.[58,67] However, in the largest series of 167 patients, progression-free survival (PSA <2+nadir) at 3 years was 53%, 42%, and 25% for low-, medium, and high-risk groups, respectively.[32] The most recent report of salvage HIFU in 84 men with a median follow-up of 20 months found 38% of men with some symptoms of incontinence, a significant decrease in the mean international index of erectile function score, four fistulae from either the first or second HIFU procedure, and the need for intervention for bladder outlet obstruction in 20%.[61] Two-year progression-free survival was 43% (including PSA-nonresponders) or 48% (excluding PSA-nonresponders), using a definition of ASTRO-Phoenix criteria (PSA >nadir+2 ng/mL) and/or a positive biopsy and/or start of hormone therapy.

A single reported case of PTLA for recurrent prostate cancer after prostatectomy shows promise.[68] This patient experienced neither impotence nor incontinence and the appearance of successful ablation on procedural MRI. The patient's PSA level decreased from 2.0 to 0.42 ng/mL at 2 months after therapy.

Interventions for Prostatic Hyperplasia

Although similar in principle to PTLA for prostate cancer, treatment of BPH by PTLA differs in a few important aspects. It is primarily performed by urologists, does not use imaging guidance, and is achieved with an intraurethral catheter.[69] There are many variations on this technique including the direction of delivery, depth of penetration, and wavelength used. The first report of laser therapy used a neodymium:yttrium-aluminum-garnet (Nd:YAG) laser in 1992, followed in 1996 by holmium laser enucleation of the prostate (HoLEP), which has produced superior relief of bladder outlet obstruction as compared to transurethral resection of the prostate and has proved equally as effective as open prostatectomy for the management of large prostates (>100 g), with lower morbidity.[70] In addition to HoLEP, several newer but less well studied laser techniques currently are available. These include photoselective laser vaporization utilizing the potassium-titanyl-phosphate (KTP or "green light") laser, thulium laser enucleation, and high-power diode laser vaporization.[69] These therapies differ in terms of depth of penetration, which is greater with HoLEP and thus its use for enucleation. These are largely accomplished cystoscopically. However, PTLA can also be used for the same effect with MRI or ultrasound guidance.

PROSTATIC ARTERY EMBOLIZATION

Neither bland embolization therapy nor chemotherapy/radiotherapy-augmented embolization have been used for prostate cancer therapy. However, prostate arterial embolization (PAE) is gaining in popularity as a minimally invasive treatment for BPH. A recent study in 15 patients with a mean follow-up of 7.9 months found technical success in 14 of the 15 patients (93.3%).[71] International Prostate Symptom Score decreased a mean of 6.5 points ($P = 0.005$), quality of life improved 1.14 points ($P = 0.065$), International Index of Erectile Function increased 1.7 points ($P = 0.063$), and peak urinary flow increased 3.85 mL/second ($P = 0.015$). A PSA reduction of 2.27 ng/mL did not appear significant ($P = 0.072$) but a decrease in mean prostate volume did, quantified as 26.5 mL ($P = 0.0001$) by ultrasound and 28.9 mL ($P = 0.008$) by magnetic resonance imaging. There was one major complication, bladder wall ischemia, and four clinical failures (28.6%).

These patients stopped all prostatic medication 1 week before embolization with no medication to treat BPH after successful PAE. Patients started an acid-suppressing drug (omeprazole 20 mg once daily), and an antiinflammatory agent (naproxen 1000 mg twice daily) for 2 days before the procedure and continued to receive them for 10 days after PAE. The day of PAE, patients received omeprazole 20 mg and naproxen 1000 mg in the morning before PAE. Naproxen 1000 mg was also given 8 hours after PAE. During embolization, ketorolac 30 mg and metamizole 2 g were given intravenously for analgesia and sedation. Embolization was performed under local anesthesia by unilateral approach, usually the right femoral artery. Initially, pelvic angiography was performed to evaluate the iliac and prostatic arteries. Then, a 5-Fr Cobra-shaped catheter (Cordis, Warren, NJ) was introduced in the right femoral artery to catheterize the left hypogastric artery and reach its anterior division.

The inferior vesical artery and finally the prostatic vessels were selectively catheterized with a 3-Fr coaxial microcatheter (Progreat; Terumo, Tokyo, Japan). Another angiographic study was performed to confirm the position of the catheter in the ostium of the prostatic artery before embolization. For embolization, nonspherical 200-μm PVA particles (Cook, Bloomington, IN) were used. The end point chosen for embolization was slow flow or near-stasis in the prostatic vessels with interruption of the arterial flow and prostatic gland opacification. When embolization of the left prostatic arteries was finished, a Waltman curve was formed on the Cobra catheter and the right prostatic arteries were embolized in the same way.

Future Directions

The field of prostate focal therapy is young and rife for development. One of the major limitations is heterogeneity in the literature regarding efficacy and morbidity. Another is nonuniformity of available or approved technologies, resulting in marked regional variation in practice patterns. However, image guidance for prostate therapy is a hot topic, with many sites of development.

HIFU is currently delivered with a transrectal approach, with more than a decade of development. However, different approaches have been suggested. The transabdominal approach used for fibroid treatment, discussed in a separate chapter, is not as easily applied to the prostate because of a suboptimal sonic window.[72] However, improvements in geometry may allow the real-time temperature monitoring and functional identification of suspicious areas to be applied to this modality. Additionally, transurethral deployment of a HIFU transducer has been investigated in a preclinical model, also with direct MR thermal mapping.[73]

PDT is generally used for hemiablation or subtotal ablation, whereas PTLA is more commonly used for a focal approach. The combination of these two technologies with laser-activated gold nanoparticles may augment the tumoricidal properties of laser therapy, improving efficacy while reducing the risk of adverse effects.[74]

Irreversible electroporation is a compelling technology, with microsecond pulses of direct current applied directly to tissue with resultant cell membrane damage. It appears to spare blood vessels and connective tissue. Promising preclinical results have not yet been shown in human trials, and this technology is not yet approved by the FDA for prostate treatment. However, the NanoKnife ® from AngioDynamics, Inc, Latham, NY, is approved for the ablation of soft tissue, similar to the approval for PTLA in the United States.[75]

MRI-compatible robots are being tested for both biopsy guidance and therapy. They decrease scanner time as patients do not need to be drawn out of the bore of the magnet for repositioning, and allow the potential of real-time imaging of manipulations.[22]

As interest grows in minimally invasive approaches to prostate cancer care, growth in the field of focal therapy is imminent. Current treatment modalities have shown promise, and the lay media is rife with tales of "medical tourists" who travel abroad for treatments not yet approved in their homeland. As these technologies become proven, one hopes this practice will be unnecessary.

Acknowledgments

The author would like to acknowledge the help of Steven Raman, Leonard Marks, and Shyam Natarajan in image acquisition, Jelle Barentsz and Jurgen Fütterer for guidance regarding prostate MRI and MR-guided biopsies, Hashim Ahmed for assistance with and images of HIFU, Duke Bahn for images of cryoablation, and Anil Shetty, John Feller, Stuart May, Scott Eggener, Aytekin Oto, Stephen B. Solomon, Jonathan A Coleman, and Al Barqawi for images of photothermal laser ablation.

REFERENCES

The complete reference list is available online at www.expertconsult.com.

PART 4

Head and Neck Oncology

WHITNEY POPE

21

Imaging of Head and Neck Cancer

ALI R. SEPAHDARI | WHITNEY POPE

Introduction

Head and neck cancers are a complex, heterogeneous group of diseases with a variety of treatment options. Surgery, chemotherapy, and radiation all have a role. Outcomes data are often ambiguous, and the same tumor may be treated differently at different institutions, depending on the local expertise and experience. Cross-sectional imaging plays a central role in assessing the extent of disease, and in planning treatment strategies.

Anatomy

A detailed understanding of cross-sectional anatomy in the head and neck is critical in interpreting pretherapy imaging studies. Figure 21-1 details the anatomy of the paranasal sinuses, nasal cavity, and anterior skull base. Figure 21-2 details the anatomy of the upper aerodigestive tract.

Imaging Strategy

Computed tomography (CT), magnetic resonance (MR), and ^{18}F-fluorodeoxyglucose positron emission tomography (FDG-PET) are complementary imaging modalities, each with unique advantages. CT is widely available, making it a workhorse modality. The very rapid acquisition time of a CT study with modern scanners, on the order of seconds, makes CT an especially useful modality for patients who are unable to lie still for the approximately 45 minutes required for an MR examination. CT also depicts bony anatomy and cortical bone erosion better than any other modality.

MR provides superior soft tissue contrast, and distinguishes between tumor, edema, and muscle with greatest accuracy. MR has the highest sensitivity for bone marrow infiltration and perineural tumor spread,[1] and is superior for assessing the extent of disease in the oral cavity, where artifact from dental amalgam often obscures the soft tissues. In the sinonasal region, MR readily distinguishes among tumor, edema, and retained secretions, where CT is often unable to do so. In the larynx, MR is more sensitive for laryngeal cartilage invasion,[2] and probably equally specific, depending on the criteria that are applied.

FDG-PET, when combined with CT, is the best exam for nodal staging, and is the most effective way to detect disease recurrence in the posttreatment neck.[3] Limitations include false positives due to physiologic uptake, inflammation, and infection. False negatives include small tumors, tumors that are obscured by areas of normal physiologic uptake, and malignant tumors that are not FDG avid.[3]

Assessing Local Extent of Disease

Local extent of disease is in many cases the most important factor that determines the initial treatment plan. Radiologic imaging and clinical examination are complementary in assessing the local extent of disease. Superficial mucosal tumor is better seen by direct inspection or endoscopy than by cross-sectional imaging. It may be impossible to pass an endoscope beyond a bulky mass to see the full extent of a mucosal mass. Although fixation to deep tissues on clinical examination can provide some information on the deep extent of disease, this finding is confirmed and often better detected with cross-sectional imaging. Invasion of bone, intracranial extension of disease, and perineural spread of tumor are findings that are typically discovered by cross-sectional imaging.

Nodal Staging

For any head and neck tumor, the size and extent of the primary tumor must be determined, and the regional lymph nodes must also be assessed. Determination of lymph node involvement may be based on morphologic features or on size criteria. Lymph node size is determined in the axial plane, which typically bisects the long axis of the lymph node, as most cervical lymph nodes have a craniocaudal orientation. One may measure either the longest dimension in the axial plane, or the shortest dimension in the axial plane. For either measurement, 10 mm is considered the upper limit of normal. The exception to this is the highest level IIA lymph node, that is, the jugulodigastric node. A normal jugulodigastric lymph node may measure up to 11 mm in the shortest dimension in the axial plane, or up to 15 mm in the longest dimension in the axial plane. Regardless of size, a lymph node is abnormal if it demonstrates necrosis or extracapsular tumor extension (Figure 21-3).

Lymph nodes are grouped by region. Superficial lymph nodes, such as facial chain, periparotid, intraparotid, preauricular, and occipital lymph nodes, are described by location. Retropharyngeal lymph nodes, which lie medial to the internal carotid arteries near the skull base, are grouped into medial retropharyngeal lymph nodes (uncommonly seen) and the more common lateral retropharyngeal lymph nodes (nodes of Rouviere). Cervical chain lymph nodes are grouped into seven levels, determined by anatomic landmarks (see Figure 21-2).[4] If a lymph node overlaps two regions, it is assigned to the level that contains the majority of its bulk. Level I lymph nodes are anterior to the posterior edge of the submandibular gland. These may be further subcategorized into Level IA (medial to the anterior belly of the digastric muscle) and Level IB (lateral to the anterior belly of the digastric muscle). Level II lymph nodes are found posterior to the posterior edge of the submandibular gland, lateral to the internal carotid artery, anterior to the posterior edge of the sternocleidomastoid muscle, and superior the inferior edge of the hyoid bone. These may be divided into Level IIA (anterior to the internal jugular vein or touching the internal jugular vein), and Level IIB (posterior to the internal jugular vein). Level III lymph nodes are bordered superiorly by the inferior edge of the hyoid bone, medially by the medial edge of the common carotid artery, inferiorly by

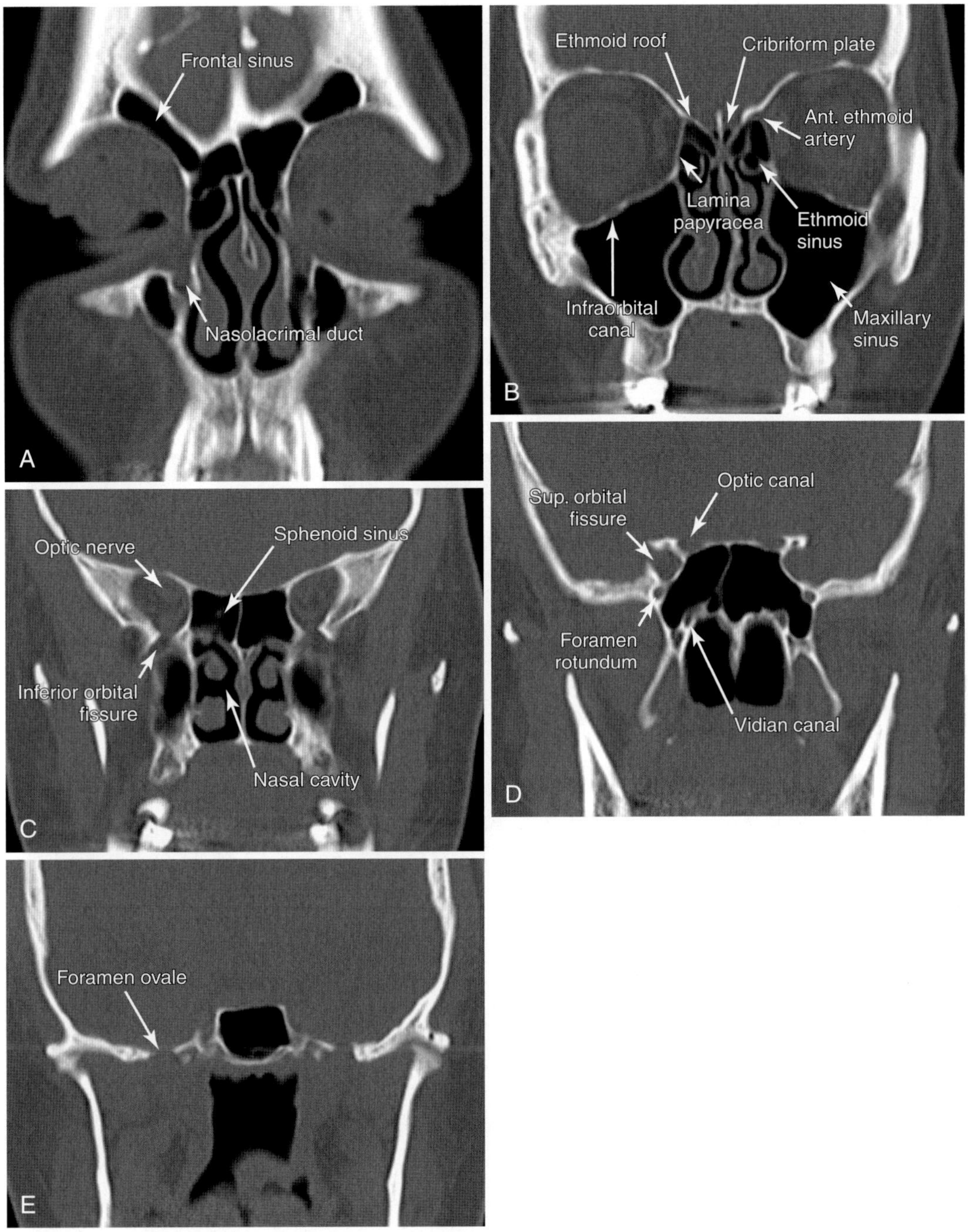

Figure 21-1 Normal anatomy: sinuses, nasal cavity and skull base—coronal CT

the inferior edge of the cricoid cartilage, and posteriorly by the posterior edge of the sternocleidomastoid muscle. Level IV lymph nodes are bordered superiorly by the inferior edge of the cricoid cartilage, medially by the medial edge of the common carotid artery, posterolaterally by a line drawn through the lateral edge of the sternocleidomastoid and the lateral edge of the anterior scalene, and inferiorly by the clavicle. If the clavicle is visible in the axial plane, then a lymph node is said to be in the supraclavicular station. Because of varying anatomy between individuals, the level IV station may be quite small or even nonexistent. Level VA lymph nodes are located posterior to the posterior edge of the sternocleidomastoid muscle, from the skull base to the inferior edge of the cricoid. Level VB lymph nodes are located posterolateral to a line drawn from the lateral edge of the sternocleidomastoids to the lateral edge of the anterior scalene muscles, below the inferior edge of the cricoid, and above the clavicle. Level VI lymph nodes are below the inferior edge of the hyoid bone, medial to the common carotid arteries, and superior to the manubrium of the sternum. Level VII lymph nodes are in the superior mediastinum, medial to the common carotid arteries, below the top of the manubrium of the sternum, and above the brachiocephalic vein.

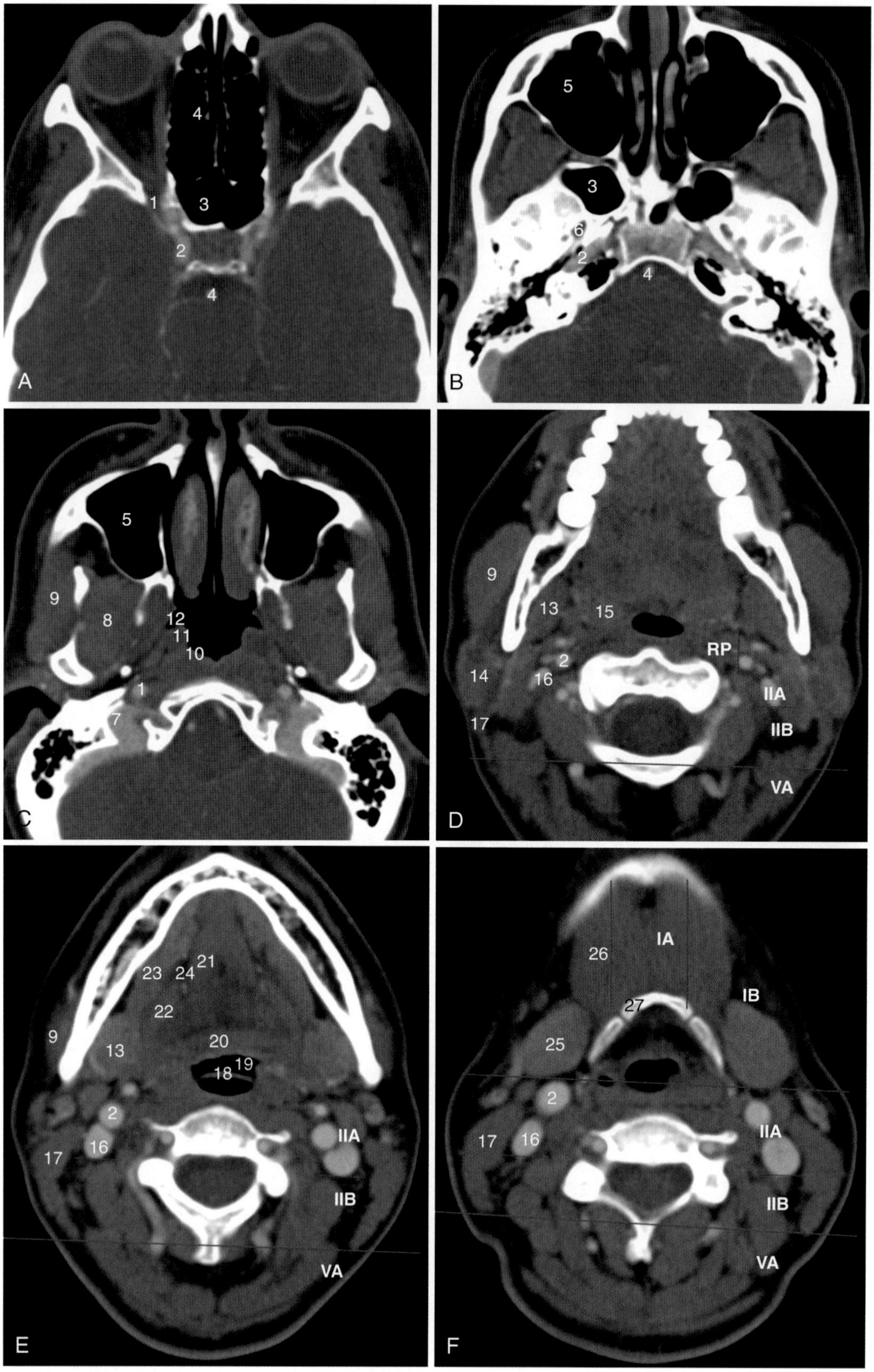

Figure 21-2 Normal anatomy: nasopharynx, oral cavity, oropharynx, hypopharynx—axial CT

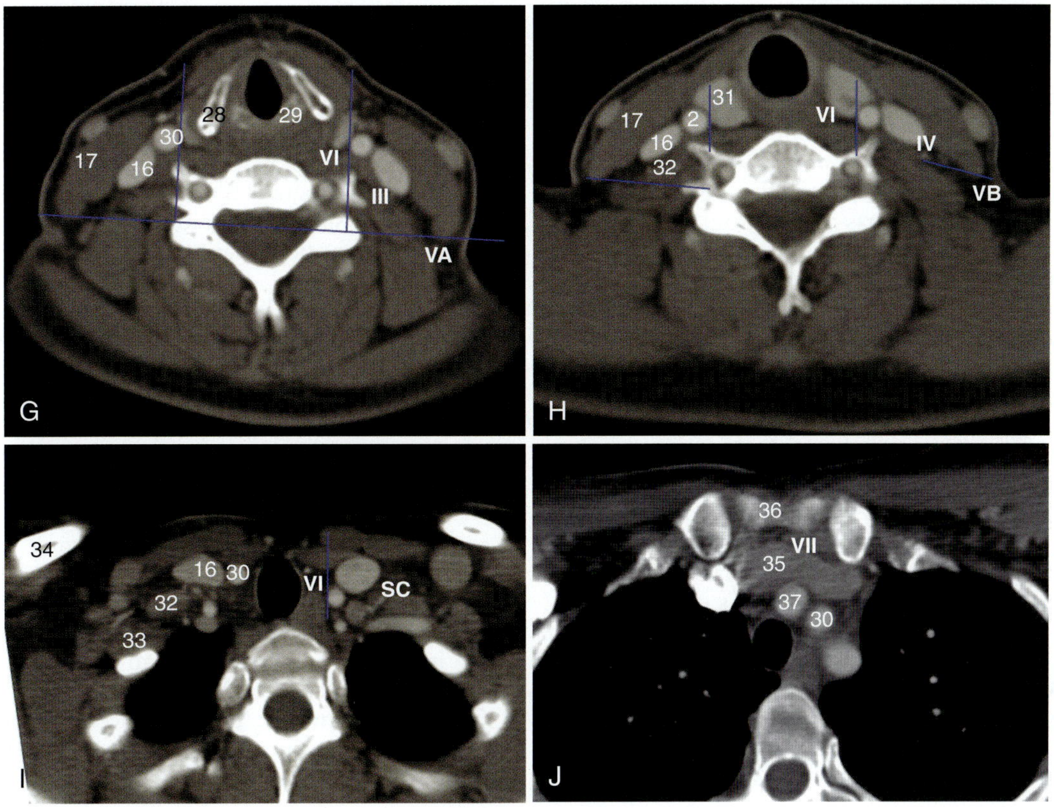

Figure 21-2, cont'd

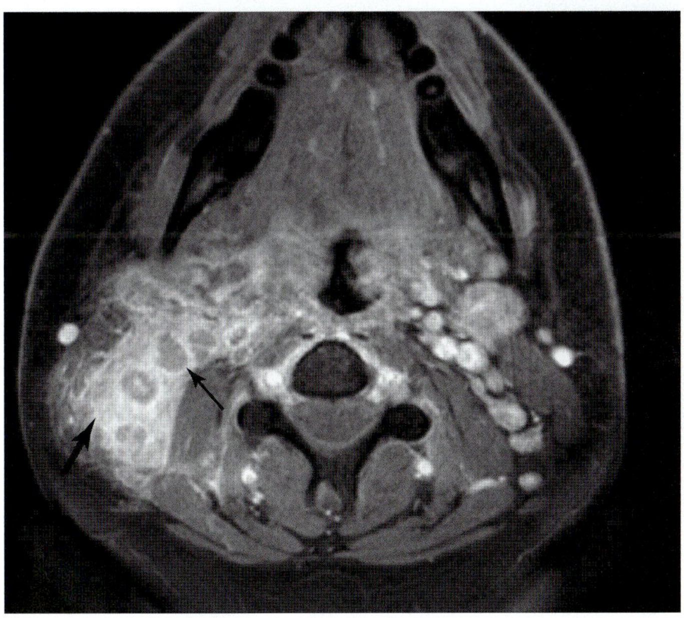

Figure 21-3 Lymph node necrosis and extracapsular tumor extension

Perineural Spread

Perineural spread is a specific pattern of local disease extension that warrants separate discussion, because of the complexity of the involved anatomy. The cranial nerves and their branches may be conduits for spread of disease. Although a variety of benign lesions such as nerve sheath tumors, meningioma, infection, and granulomatous disease may spread along nerves, this pattern of disease is most commonly seen with malignancy. Care should be taken to distinguish between perineural *invasion* and perineural *spread*. Perineural invasion is not detectable by imaging; it is a feature of the primary tumor that is seen on histopathology, and is associated with worse prognosis. Perineural spread refers to the phenomenon of tumor using the nerve as a pathway to spread away from the primary site. Perineural spread can happen early in the disease course, can be a pattern of recurrence, and can be responsible for the only presenting symptoms. It is the responsibility of the radiologist to detect perineural spread so that an appropriate treatment plan can be selected. Adenoid cystic carcinoma and squamous cell carcinoma are the tumors that are most commonly associated with perineural spread. Perineural spread may also be seen with other minor salivary gland tumors, lymphoma, melanoma (particularly the desmoplastic subtype),[5] and sarcomas. Pain, paresthesia, and motor denervation (when V3 and/or facial nerve are involved) are the most common complaints, though up to 40% of patients may be asymptomatic or have nonspecific complaints.[6,7] Furthermore, presence of symptoms is not specific for perineural spread.

PATHWAYS OF SPREAD

V1: Perineural spread along V1 typically relates to cutaneous malignancy.[6] The supraorbital and supratrochlear nerves, branches of the frontal nerve, are most commonly involved.[8] Tumor can then spread back along the main V1 trunk to the superior orbital fissure, cavernous sinus, and Meckel's cave.

V2 (Figure 21-4): The main trunk of V2, the maxillary nerve, runs through foramen rotundum, through the cavernous sinus, and continues to Meckel's cave. Tumor may reach the maxillary nerve through several pathways. Minor salivary gland tumors arising from the palatal mucosa may extend through the greater and lesser palatine foramina, to the pterygopalatine fossa, and then to the maxillary nerve. Cutaneous carcinomas arising from the cheek or temporal region may extend along the zygomaticofacial and zygomaticotemporal nerves and then to the pterygopalatine fossa. Tumors of the maxillary sinus may extend along the anterior and posterior superior alveolar nerves to reach V2, and tumors of the face or maxillary sinus may spread along the infraorbital nerve.

Vidian nerve (see Figure 21-4): Tumor that reaches the pterygopalatine fossa, through the pathways described above, may extend along the Vidian nerve and progress intracranially. Tumor may then extend further along the greater superficial petrosal nerve (GSPN) to the geniculate ganglion and to other branches of the facial nerve. Tumor that has reached Meckel's cave may also extend down to GSPN and then anteriorly along Vidian nerve.

V3 (see Figure 21-4, Figure 21-5): Tumor arising in the masticator space or prestyloid parapharyngeal space may extend along V3, through foramen ovale and to Meckel's cave. Tumor that reaches Meckel's cave by spreading along V2 may spread antegrade along V3. Parotid gland tumors that involve the facial nerve may also spread to V3 via the auriculotemporal nerve. The auriculotemporal nerve passes immediately posterior to the mandibular condyle and splits around the middle meningeal artery before passing through the otic ganglion and connecting with V3. Tumor that spreads retrograde along V2 to reach Meckel's cave may also then spread antegrade along V3. When tumor involves V3, denervation change may be seen in the muscles of mastication.

Facial nerve (see Figure 21-5): Primary salivary gland tumors and malignancies that involve the parotid gland secondarily may extend along the facial nerve, through the stylomastoid foramen, and along the facial nerve as it courses through the temporal bone. Tumor involving the Vidian nerve may also extend along the GSPN to the geniculate ganglion and main facial nerve, and tumor involving Meckel's cave may extend inferiorly to involve the adjacent GSPN.[6] Tumor involving V3 may extend to the facial nerve along the auriculotemporal nerve. The chorda tympani, a branch of the facial nerve, is also connected to the lingual nerve branch of V3, though this is not generally considered an important pathway of perineural spread of tumor.

Hypoglossal nerve: Tongue cancers can spread retrograde along the course of the hypoglossal nerve, and secondarily involve cranial nerves IX, X, and XI.

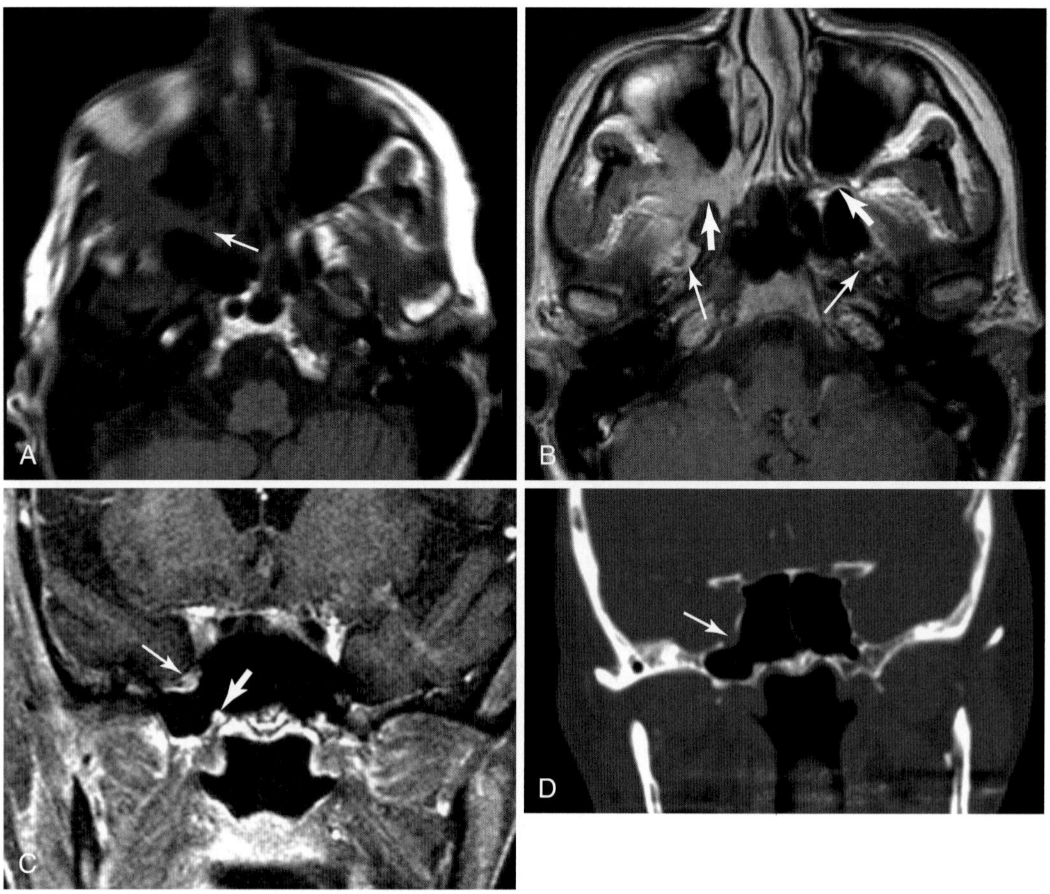

Figure 21-4 Perineural tumor—V2, vidian, V3

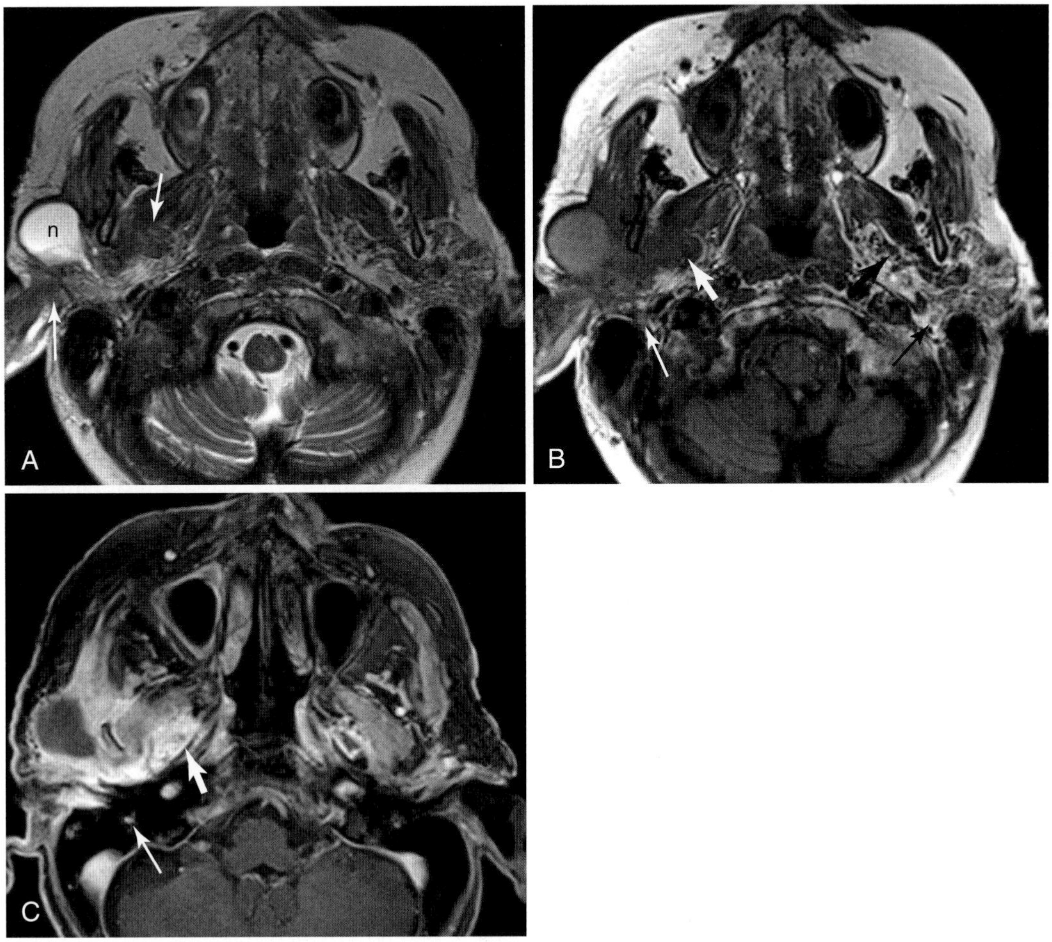

Figure 21-5 Parotid squamous cell carcinoma, perineural spread and intracranial

IMAGING OF PERINEURAL SPREAD

MRI is the preferred modality for detecting perineural spread. According to most reports, CT is 80%–90% sensitive and specific for perineural spread.[1,9] MRI is considered much more sensitive than CT, with >95% sensitivity, and equal or greater specificity.[1] According to an early report, MRI does not detect the full extent of perineural spread with high sensitivity,[10] though current performance is probably much better with modern equipment.

Direct signs of perineural spread on MRI include obliteration of the fat around the involved nerve, enhancement of the nerve, or thickening of the nerve. Any single one of these features should be considered evidence of disease,[1] with one important caveat: the mastoid, tympanic, and geniculate segments of the facial nerve frequently enhance in normal subjects, because of enhancement of perineural and epineural venous plexus.[11,12] Thus, to be considered involved by disease, the facial nerve should show abnormal thickening *and* enhancement, a marked asymmetry in enhancement, or denervation change in affected muscles. Obliteration of fat at the stylomastoid foramen is also helpful in confirming extension along the facial nerve from a parotid tumor (see Figure 21-5). CT is sometimes able to demonstrate perineural spread by showing enlargement of the involved foramen, or obliteration of fat surrounding the involved nerves. A standard MR imaging protocol tailored for detection of perineural spread should include axial and coronal T1-weighted images, axial and coronal T2-weighted images (including at least one plane with fat suppression), and axial and coronal contrast-enhanced T1-weighted images with fat suppression.

Indirect signs of perineural spread include denervation change in the target muscles of motor nerves. There are several stages of denervation change. Initially, muscle volume is slightly increased, T2 is prolonged, and the affected muscle enhances diffusely. There may be subtle loss of the normal T1-bright fat interspersed among the muscle fibers. Next, the muscle volume normalizes, and some fatty infiltration is seen, evidenced by intrinsic T1 hyperintensity. Enhancement persists, and is best detected on fat-suppressed postcontrast images. In the next stage of denervation, T2 hyperintensity and enhancement resolve, and fatty replacement continues. In the final stage of denervation, the muscle volume is reduced and there is diffuse fatty infiltration of the muscle. In general, these stages are seen in muscles innervated by the trigeminal and hypoglossal nerves. Small muscles innervated by other nerves (such as the facial nerve) typically progress directly to fatty atrophy without clearly defined intermediate stages by current imaging techniques. It is important to be aware of these changes so as not to confuse denervation edema with direct tumor extension or an inflammatory process.[14] In addition, reflex sympathetic dystrophy can involve the muscles of mastication following skull fracture or craniotomy.[15] Localized edema and inflammation can also be associated with contusion, laceration, or temporomandibular joint inflammation.[15] Identifying denervation change also sometimes improves confidence in detecting perineural spread.

Sinonasal Tumors

Neoplasms affecting the sinonasal cavity are rare, constituting only 0.2% to 0.8% of all malignancies, and approximately 3% of malignancies in the head and neck.[16] Symptoms are often present for up to 6 months before the diagnosis is made.[17] Wood dust,[18] chemical, and metal occupational exposures[17] are known risk factors. Sinonasal tumors are often difficult to recognize clinically, often presenting with nonspecific complaints such as congestion, which are attributable to inflammatory disease, which frequently coexists. Even when CT imaging is performed prior to endoscopic sinus surgery, tumors can be mistaken for inflammatory disease, and the diagnosis only comes as a surprise during surgery. Proptosis, epiphora, and cranial neuropathies are rare, and indicative of advanced disease. The maxillary sinus is the most common site of malignancy (approximately 55%), followed by the nasal cavity (35%), frontal sinus (9%), and finally the ethmoid and sphenoid sinuses (<1% each).[17] Nasal cavity tumors are evenly divided between benign and malignant lesions, with inverted papilloma the most common benign lesion and squamous cell carcinoma (Figure 21-6) and minor salivary gland tumors as the most common malignancies. Paranasal sinus tumors are much more likely to be malignant. Other sinonasal malignancies include lymphoma, melanoma, olfactory neuroblastoma (Figure 21-7), neuroendocrine carcinoma, and sinonasal undifferentiated carcinoma. Unless there is evidence of frankly invasive tumor with bone destruction, it is difficult to tell benign from malignant tumors by imaging features.

The role of imaging in sinonasal tumors is to determine the local extent of disease so that the appropriate treatment modality can be selected. Important landmarks include the medial orbital wall (lamina papyracea) and the orbital floor (see Figures 21-6 and 21-7). Violation of either of these structures makes a complete resection extremely difficult and potentially disfiguring. The integrity of the cribriform plate and ethmoid roof should also be assessed. Intracranial extension does not preclude a complete resection, but does typically demand an open approach with a bifrontal craniotomy. Proximity of tumor to the optic nerve is important in radiation planning. Sphenoid sinus tumors may involve the carotid canals, cavernous sinus, and sella turcica, precluding safe complete resection.

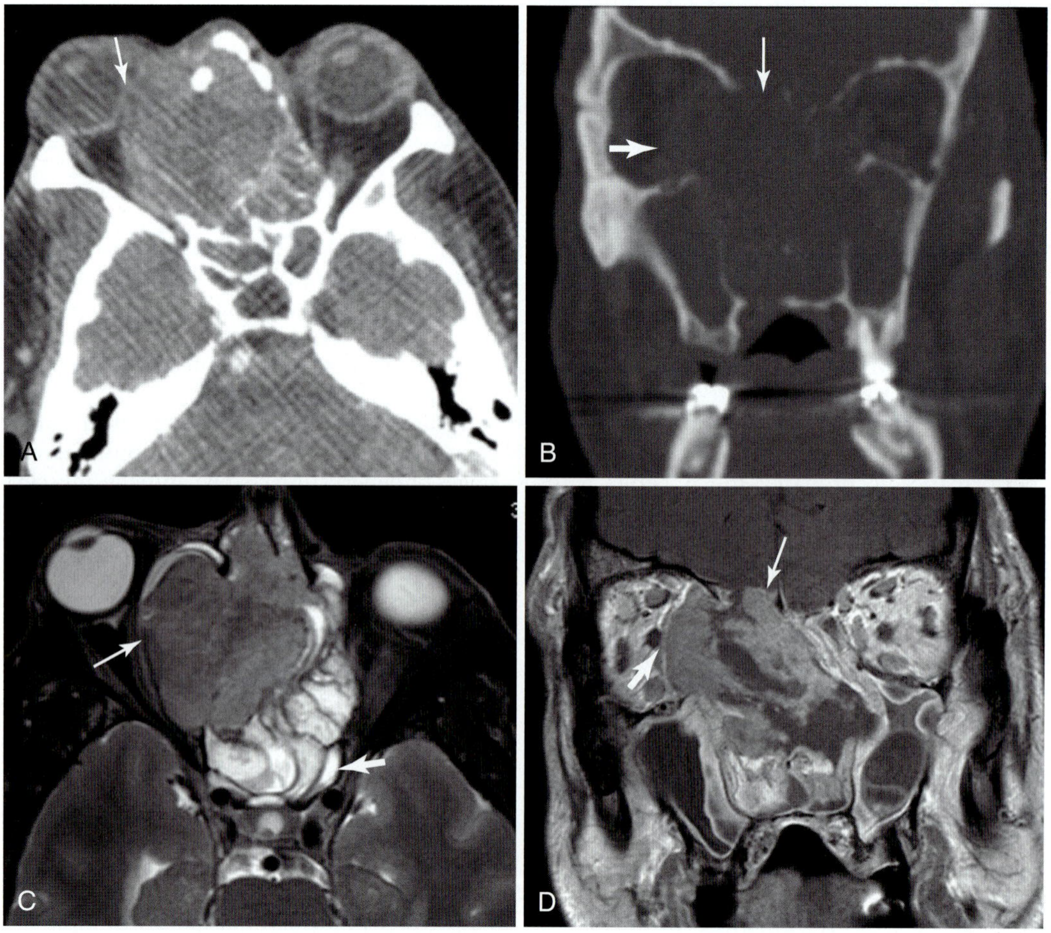

Figure 21-6 Sinonasal squamous cell carcinoma invading orbit

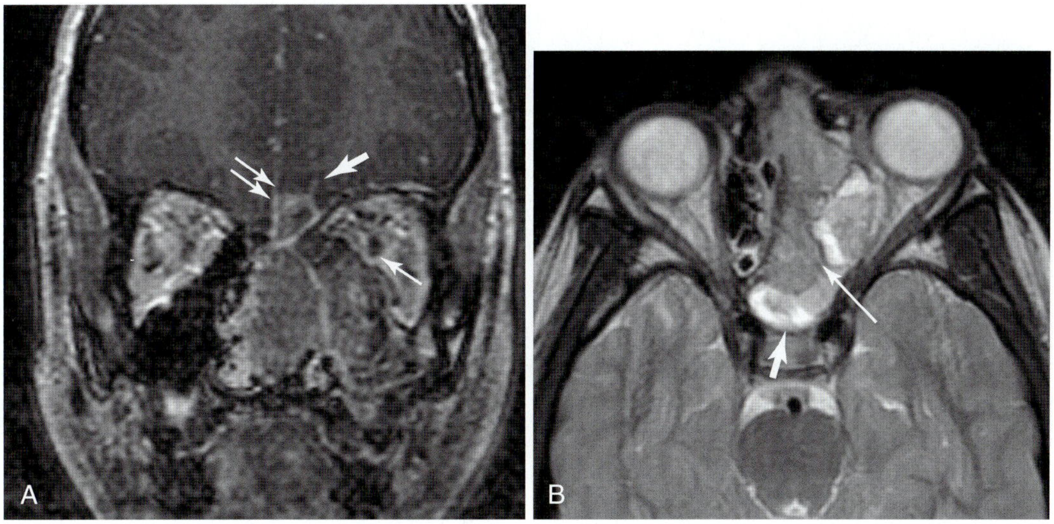

Figure 21-7 EsthesioNB

Oral Cavity Tumors

Oral cavity tumors may arise from the lip, the gingival mucosa, buccal mucosa, floor of mouth, or oral tongue (anterior two thirds of the tongue, anterior to the circumvallate papillae). Squamous cell carcinoma is by far the most commonly encountered histology, representing more than 90% of malignancies in this region.[19] Men are affected twice as often as women, and peak incidence is between the sixth and eighth decades. Smoking and alcohol are the major epidemiologic risk factors.[19] There is a recently discovered association of posterior oral cavity and oropharyngeal tumors with human papilloma virus.[20] Despite being associated with higher T stage and great burden of nodal disease at presentation, human papillomavirus (HPV)–positive squamous cell carcinoma (SCCA) typically responds very well to radiotherapy. Cystic lymphadenopathy is strongly associated with HPV-positive SCCA. Other lesions such as minor salivary gland tumors or lymphoma may be encountered. Regional lymph node drainage is primarily to levels I, II, and III. Lip tumors are rarely imaged, unless disease is so extensive that the full extent cannot be determined by clinical examination. When a lesion of the buccal mucosa and gingival mucosa is encountered, attention should be directed toward the adjacent bone for evidence of invasion (Figures 21-8, 21-9, 21-10), and toward adjacent deep spaces of the neck. Involvement of the retromolar trigone is important for surgical

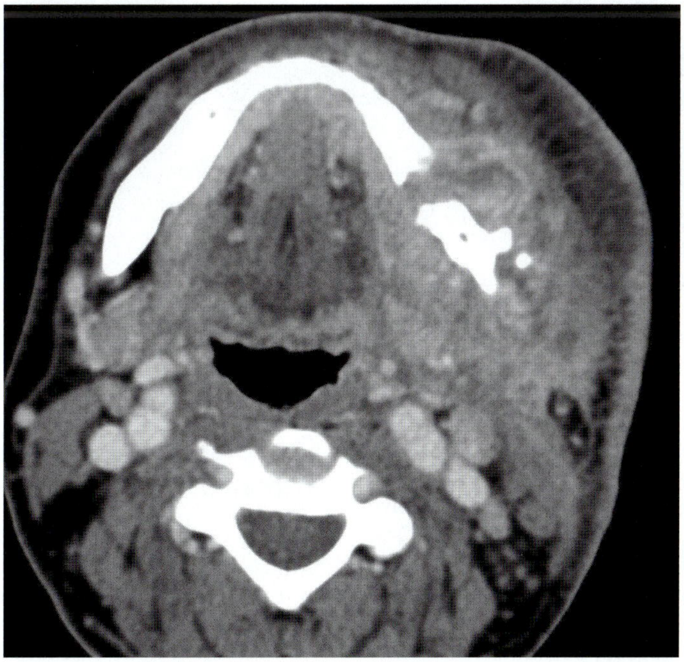

Figure 21-8 Buccal gingival squamous cell carcinoma invading mandible

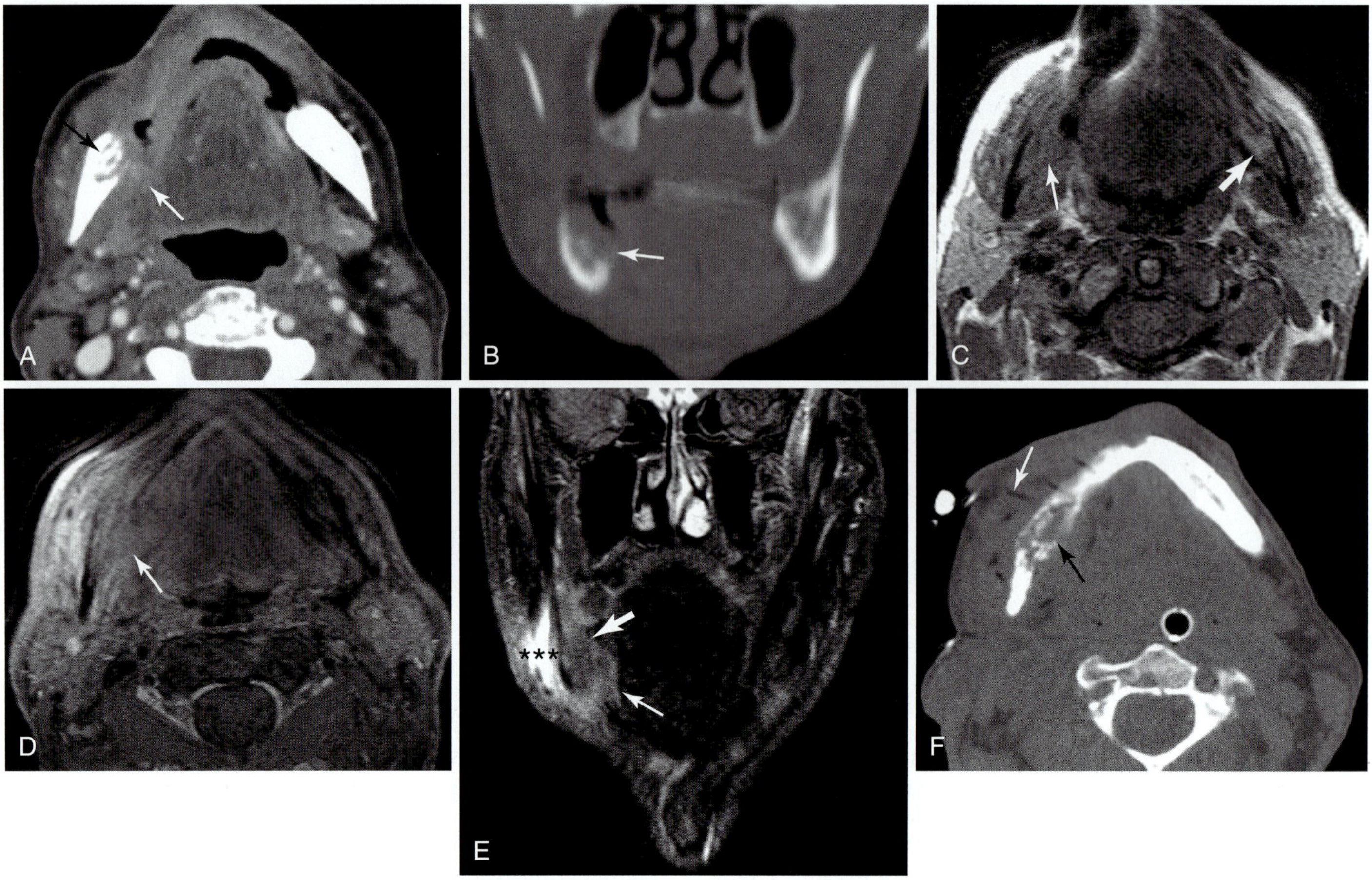

Figure 21-9 Buccal gingival squamous cell carcinoma invading mandible 2

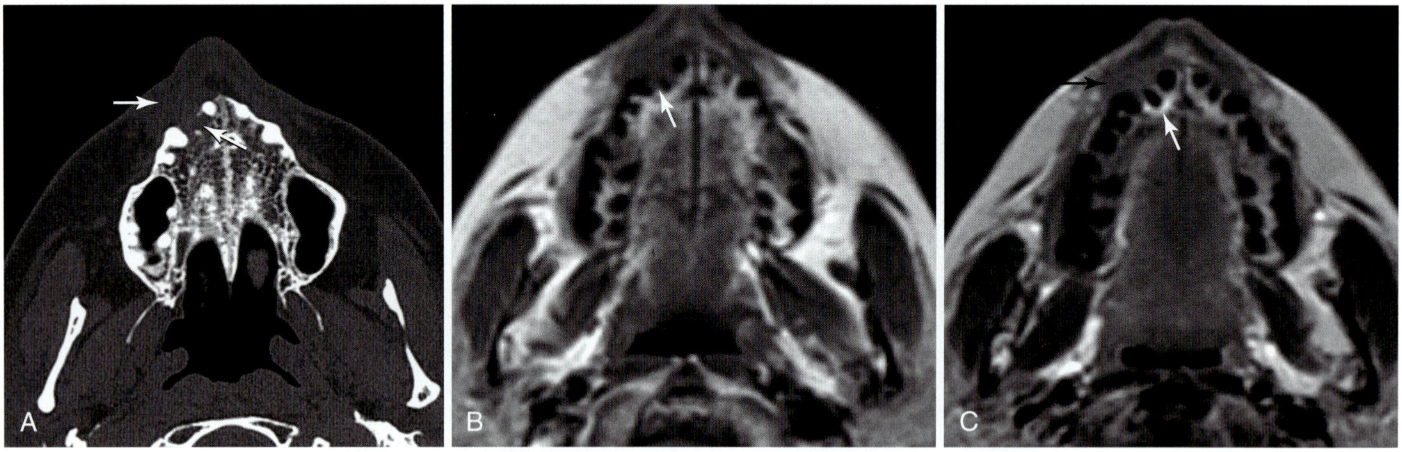

Figure 21-10 Buccal gingival lymphoma

planning (Figure 21-11) Lesions of the oral tongue and floor of the mouth may invade the extrinsic tongue muscles, involve the neurovascular bundle in the sublingual space, and involve the submandibular (Wharton) duct (Figure 21-12). Oral tongue tumors that cross the midline typically cannot be resected with an organ-sparing procedure. In addition to assessing the deep extent of disease, cross-sectional imaging can help assess the extent of mucosal spread, particularly as some anatomic sites may be difficult to visualize by endoscopy.

Oropharyngeal and Hypopharyngeal Tumors

Tumors of the tongue base, vallecula, palatine tonsil, and pharyngeal wall constitute tumors of the oropharynx. As with the oral cavity, squamous cell carcinoma is by far the most commonly encountered histology. Tumors of the oropharynx, particularly the tongue base and tonsil, may be difficult to detect by clinical examination. In this regard, cross-sectional imaging is

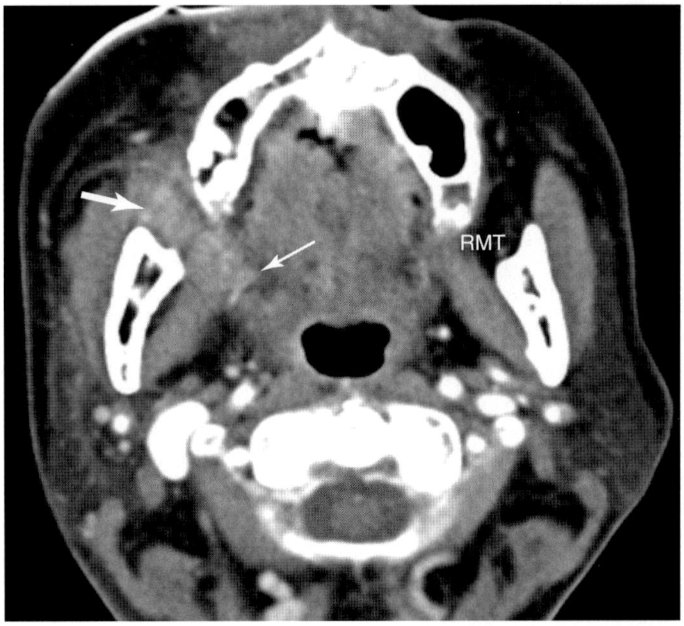

Figure 21-11 Retromolar trigone cancer

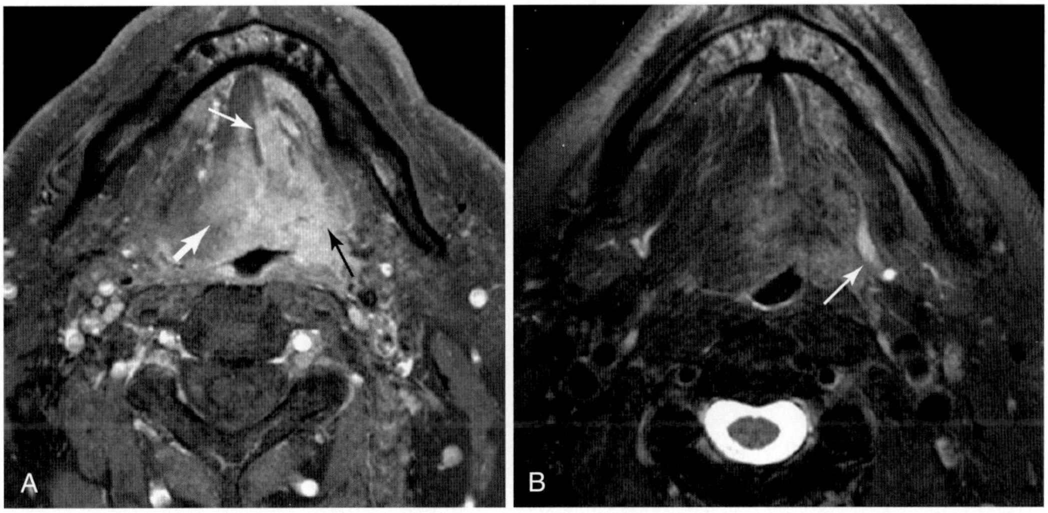

Figure 21-12 Oral tongue adenoid cystic carcinoma—crossing midline and involving NVB

helpful in establishing the diagnosis and guiding biopsy. Tumors that are very exophytic are easier to treat with surgical excision (Figure 21-13), whereas highly endophytic, infiltrative tumors can be very difficult to resect (Figure 21-14). Base of tongue tumors may infiltrate the neurovascular bundle and cross the midline, precluding an organ-sparing surgery. Tonsil and posterior oropharyngeal wall tumors may invade the retropharyngeal and parapharyngeal space (see Figure 21-14), though they typically spare the prevertebral space because of the dense barrier of the prevertebral fascia. Imaging helps detect the degree of deep soft tissue infiltration and extent of mucosal disease. Lymph node drainage is to levels II, III, and retropharyngeal stations.

NASOPHARYNGEAL TUMORS

Nasopharyngeal carcinoma is the most common malignancy of the nasopharynx, arising from the mucosa (Figure 21-15). It is rare in the United States and Europe, occurring in 1 per 100,000, but is 30 times more common in Taiwan, Hong Kong, and southern China.[21] The World Health Organization classifies nasopharyngeal carcinoma in three types. Type 1 is squamous cell carcinoma. Type 2a is keratinizing undifferentiated carcinoma. Type 2b is nonkeratinizing undifferentiated carcinoma. The Type 2b nonkeratinizing undifferentiated form is most common, and is most strongly associated with Epstein-Barr virus infection. A unilateral neck mass is the most common presenting sign (36%–80%), followed by bloody nasal discharge (18%), unilateral hearing loss (12%), and unilateral nasal obstruction (5%).[21] Other tumors may involve the nasopharynx, including lymphoma arising from or involving the pharyngeal tonsils.

Key imaging findings in the initial workup of nasopharyngeal carcinoma include invasion of the parapharyngeal space, invasion of the masticator space, invasion of the skull base,

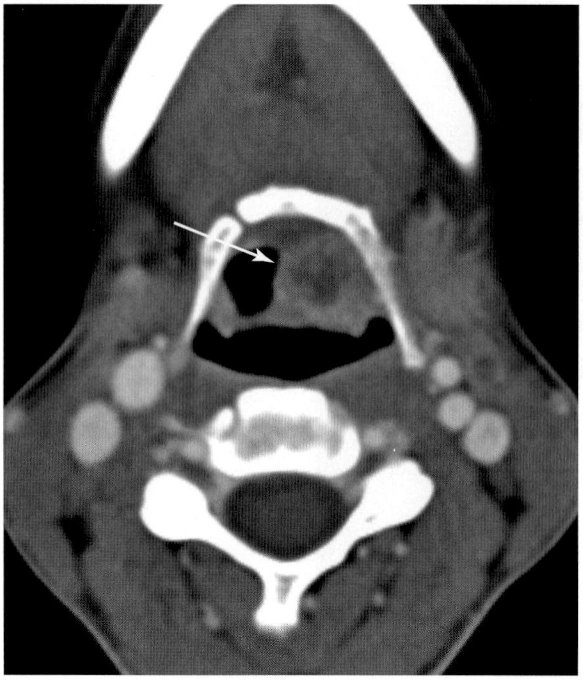

Figure 21-13 Exophytic vallecula cancer

frank intracranial extension, perineural spread, and nodal involvement. MRI is vastly superior to CT in assessing the extent of local disease, and probably equivalent in detecting nodal disease, depending on the quality of the MRI unit used and the patient's ability to cooperate with the study. Regional lymph node drainage pattern is to the retropharyngeal lymph nodes, and to levels II and V (see Figure 21-3). Lymphadenopathy is frequently bulky and confluent at presentation, and may be the presenting complaint.

LARYNGEAL TUMORS

Laryngeal tumors, typically squamous cell carcinoma, are divided into supraglottic, glottic, and subglottic sites. The bottom edge of the laryngeal ventricle is the dividing line between the supraglottic larynx and the glottic larynx. The subglottic larynx begins 1 cm below the bottom edge of the laryngeal ventricle. It is often difficult to see a primary mucosal tumor with cross-sectional imaging. The role of imaging is to assess infiltration of the paraglottic fat, the preepiglottic fat, involvement of the laryngeal cartilages, the anterior commissure, and the subglottic region (Figure 21-16). CT is equivalent or superior to MR in many cases, and has the advantages of lower cost, greater availability, higher spatial resolution, and shorter examination time. However, MR is typically superior for detecting cartilage invasion.[2]

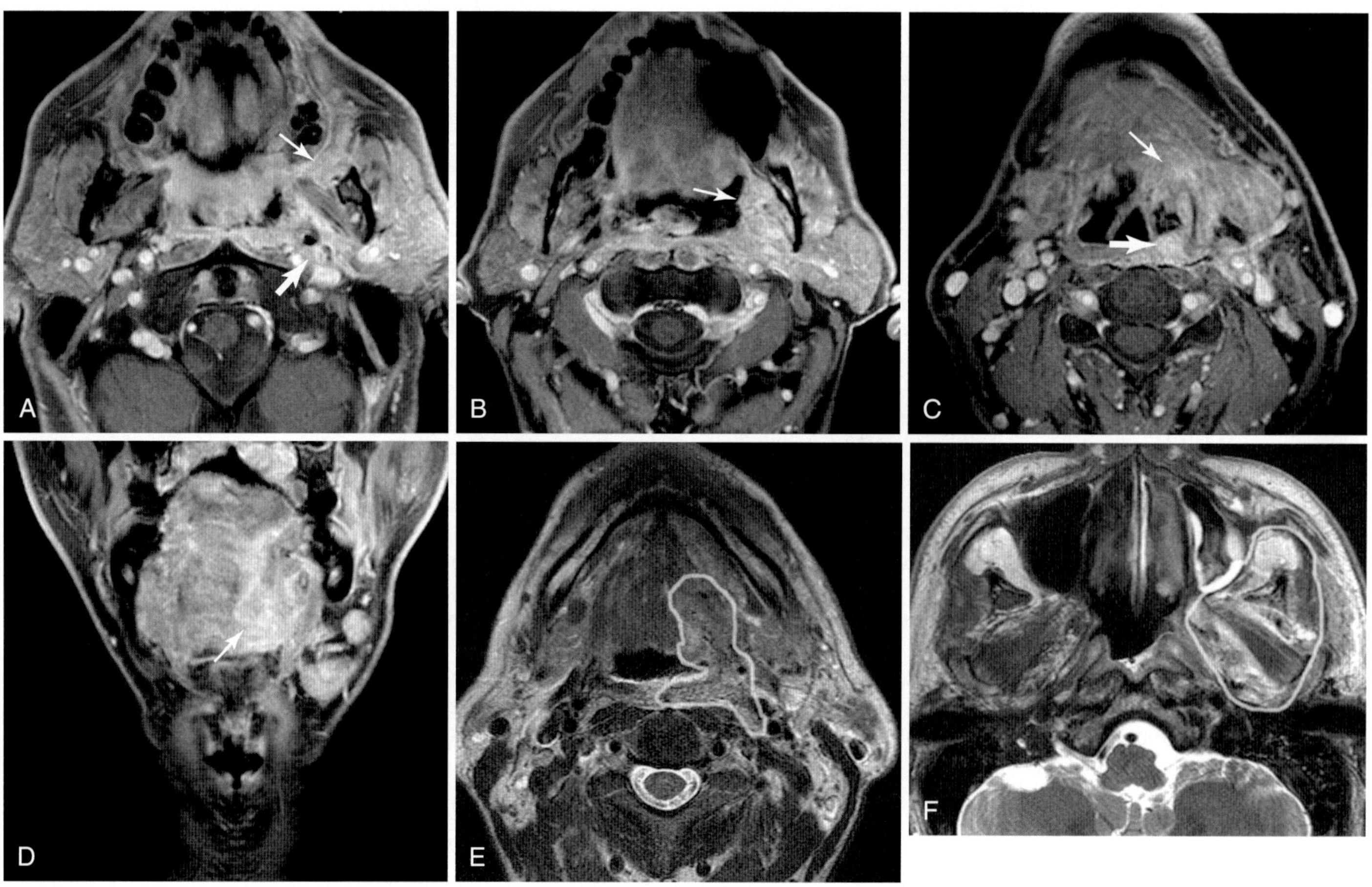

Figure 21-14 Oral cavity and oropharyngeal squamous cell carcinoma involving retromolar trigone

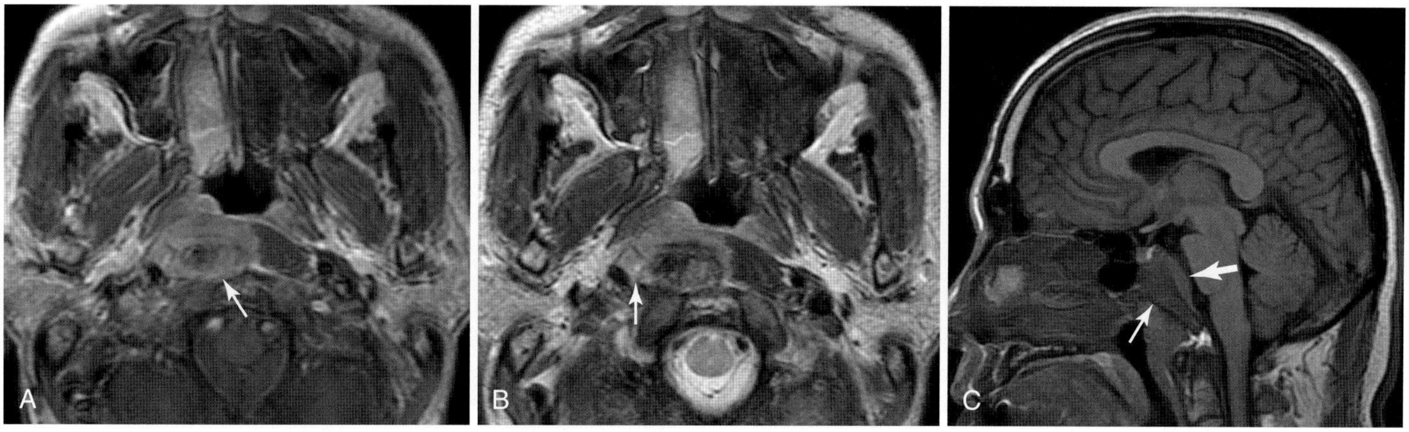

Figure 21-15 Nasopharyngeal carcinoma

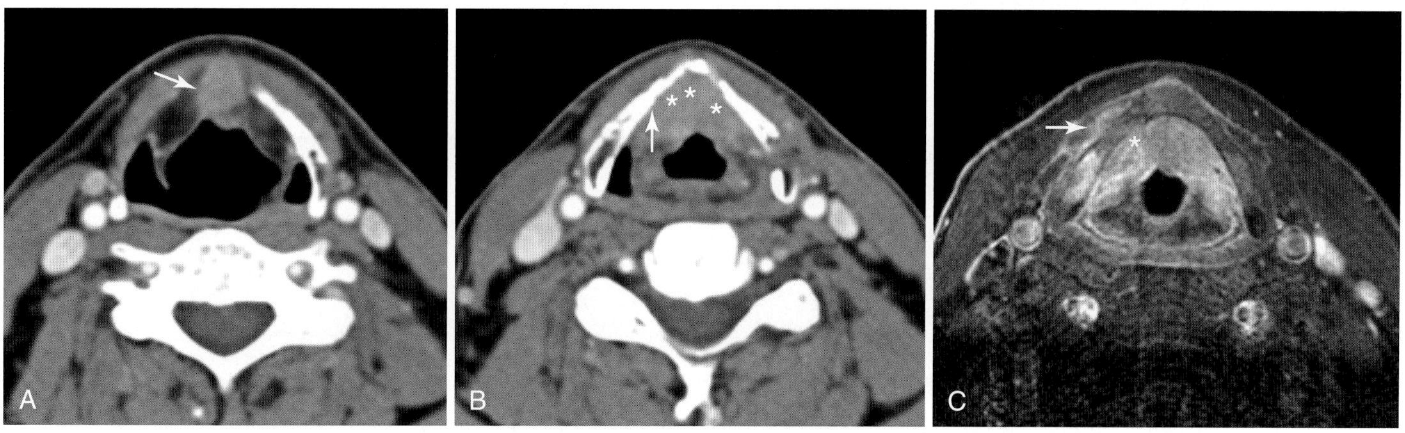

Figure 21-16 Laryngeal cancer with cartilage involvement

Supraglottic laryngeal tumors may spread to level II and III regional lymph nodes. The glottic larynx, in contradistinction, is very sparsely supplied by lymphatic network. Thus, lymphadenopathy is extremely rare for glottic laryngeal tumors, unless they have already spread to the supraglottic region or widely invaded adjacent soft tissues.

THYROID TUMORS

Imaging is frequently unable to distinguish between benign and malignant thyroid masses. Gross extension beyond the thyroid capsule is specific for malignancy, but is insensitive. Lymphadenopathy also suggests malignancy. In general, fine-needle aspiration should be performed for any thyroid nodule greater than 1.5 cm in diameter, or any lesion greater than 1 cm in diameter that demonstrates microcalcifications on ultrasound.[22] Cross-sectional imaging is most useful in assessing the extent of nodal disease at presentation, and in detecting pulmonary metastases. Diagnostic radioiodine scanning (ideally with I-123) is complementary in assessing for distant disease. Thyroid cancers are a heterogeneous group of diseases with varying behaviors. Papillary thyroid cancers (Figure 21-17) tend to follow a long clinical course, even after they have involved regional lymph nodes. Medullary (Figure 21-18) and anaplastic thyroid cancers, on the other hand, typically behave very aggressively. Serum thyroglobulin is an effective biochemical marker for surveillance. Ultrasound, CT, and MRI are all useful for detecting recurrent disease in the neck. Radioiodine scanning and FDG-PET are complementary in detecting distant recurrence.[23,24] The role of imaging is typically to define the extent of recurrent disease that is detected by serum analysis, to plan an appropriate treatment strategy.

SALIVARY GLAND TUMORS

Salivary gland tumors are divided into major salivary gland and minor salivary gland tumors. The major salivary glands comprise the parotid, submandibular, and sublingual glands. The minor salivary glands are distributed throughout the mucosa of the upper aerodigestive tract, particularly the mouth and palate. Approximately 60%–80% of salivary gland tumors occur in the parotid gland. In general, the probability of malignancy of a salivary gland mass is inversely proportional to the size of the gland. Only 20%–30% of parotid tumors are malignant. Approximately 50% of submandibular tumors are malignant, and approximately 75% of minor salivary gland tumors are malignant.[25] There is significant overlap in the appearance of benign and malignant salivary gland tumors. Although benign

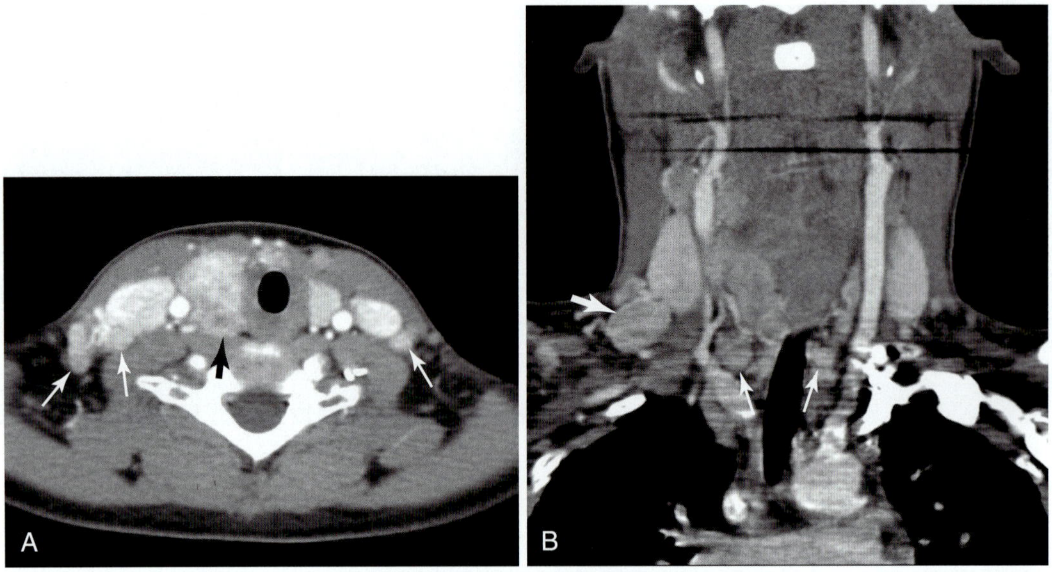

Figure 21-17 Papillary thyroid cancer

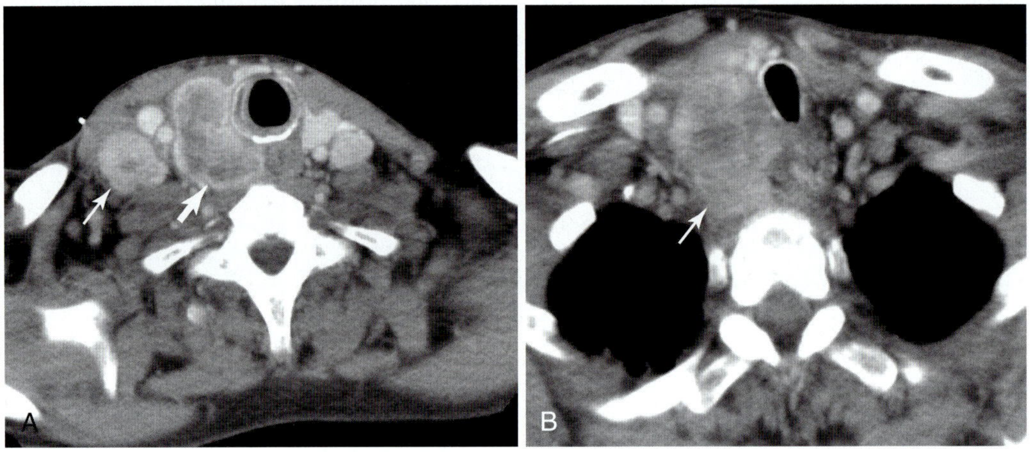

Figure 21-18 Medullary thyroid cancer

tumors are typically well defined, they can show surrounding inflammatory reaction. Malignant tumors occasionally show a very invasive growth pattern, crossing fascial planes, spreading along nerves, and destroying bone (see Figure 21-5). However, many malignant salivary gland tumors are reasonably well circumscribed and overlap in appearance with benign tumors. In general, low T2 signal and ill-defined margins are features that suggest malignancy, whereas bright T2 signal and well-defined margins are more typical of benign lesions.[26] The purpose of imaging is to confirm that a mass is of salivary gland origin, to assess the relationship of a mass to the facial nerve (in the case of parotid masses), and to assess the extent of disease, including features such as perineural tumor spread (see Figure 21-5).[27]

Summary

The regional anatomy of the head and neck is complex, containing many critical structures that may affect resectability and ability to tolerate radiation therapy. CT and MRI are the primary modalities for assessing tumors of the head and neck, and provide complementary information. High-quality imaging is essential in assessing the extent of local disease and presence of nodal metastases at presentation, and in detecting tumor recurrence after treatment.

REFERENCES

The complete reference list is available online at www.expertconsult.com.

22

Transcatheter Chemotherapy for Malignancies in the Brain, Head, and Neck

BRUNO DAMASCELLI | VLADIMIRA TICHÀ | GIANLUIGI PATELLI

Introduction

Intraarterial chemotherapy has long been investigated as a potentially superior treatment modality for tumors of the cervicocephalic, thoracic and abdominopelvic regions, and the limbs. Tumors of the brain, head, and neck have attracted the most attention for several reasons. For brain tumors, particularly high-grade gliomas, the therapeutic benefits from systemic therapy are minimal, even for drugs with recognized activity and a demonstrated dose–response relationship. Theoretically, local infusion should achieve a higher drug concentration in the tumor. This would provide a potentially important palliative option for brain metastases, which are rapidly debilitating and fatal. By the time these tumors are radiologically detectable, there is impairment of the blood–brain barrier, which until then had protected the cancer cells from the action of chemotherapeutic agents administered systemically. Direct intraarterial administration should assist in overcoming drug resistance by ensuring higher concentrations of the drug at the site needed most.

For tumors of the oral cavity, hypopharynx, and larynx, other considerations arise. The early onset of local pain, interference with feeding and speech, and general deterioration call for a treatment that produces the rapid response necessary for the physical and psychological recovery of these patients, who often have advanced disease at presentation. The ability to provide a therapy that could avoid devastating operations would have a major impact on quality of life, particularly because these operations do not improve the prognosis.

Recent percutaneous catheterization techniques, deriving from neuroradiologic practice, have reopened the possibilities for intraarterial therapy. New criteria for preliminary diagnosis and response assessment, and new drug formulations, have revolutionized pharmacokinetic criteria, so higher concentrations can be achieved not only in the area of the tumor but with a significant difference between the tumor and surrounding tissue.

Background of Intraarterial Chemotherapy for Tumors of the Head, Neck, and Brain

HIGHER LOCAL CONCENTRATIONS

Certain characteristics must be taken into consideration when choosing drugs for locoregional treatment by direct intraarterial infusion.[1-3] Drugs with a particular pharmacokinetic profile, with rapid systemic clearance, are considered to offer an advantage over intravenous administration. Single-drug or combinations of drugs such as carmustine, cisplatin, carboplatin, etoposide, methotrexate, gemcitabine, irinotecan, anthracyclines, and taxanes as macrocomplexes have long been identified as having potential for intraarterial use. Some drugs cross the blood–brain barrier intact but do not reach concentrations that can destroy micrometastases.[4-6]

The potential pharmacokinetic superiority of intraarterial chemotherapy is manifested at the first pass through the tumor circulation. The positive consequences of the first pass are more evident for some drugs than others, namely, those that have a high extraction fraction by the tumor coupled with rapid systemic clearance through metabolism or excretion.

THE BLOOD–BRAIN BARRIER

Primary or metastatic brain tumors merit a chapter apart because the blood–brain barrier, if intact, does not allow drugs to pass into the brain tissue at high enough concentrations to prevent the infiltration of microscopic metastases.[7,8] Intraarterial chemotherapy, when applicable, should not be considered a stand-alone option but should be combined with external radiotherapy to control microscopic disease. When the blood–brain barrier is not intact, the radiopotentiating or radiosensitizing properties of some chemotherapy drugs are potentially predictive of greater efficacy.

CHEMOSENSITIVITY

Chemosensitivity must be considered, when discussing higher or lower drug concentrations and longer or shorter exposure of primary or metastatic tumors, whether in the brain or head and neck.[9,10] Chemosensitivity is generally classified as high, intermediate or low. Chemotherapy has proved effective even with systemic administration in patients with brain metastases from spindle-cell carcinomas, breast cancer, and germ cell tumors. Intraarterial infusion tends to enhance the therapeutic response even if the site—generally not just one—classifies the treatment as palliative with the aim of improving the patient's quality of life.

NEW CHEMOTHERAPY FORMULATIONS

As for some extraencephalic tumors, a new formulation of liposome-encapsulated anthracyclines has achieved higher intratumoral drug concentrations. Anthracyclines are active in glioblastoma in vitro, with a close dose–response relationship.[11] Recent studies with systemically administered liposomal doxorubicin for recurrent high-grade gliomas appear to provide in vivo confirmation of greater antitumoral efficacy.[12] This takes into consideration a developing area of chemotherapy that is based on the enhanced permeability and retention effect due to the characteristics of the tumor's capillary and lymphatic network.[13,14]

All tumors have an imperfect vascular and lymphatic architecture. Tumor neovascularity demonstrates profound alterations in the structure of the vessel walls and in the anatomic artery–capillary–vein sequence, with arteriovenous shunts and vascular lakes. These findings are clearly visible in histology slides and can be evident in vascular radiology diagnostic examinations and in high spatial and temporal resolution multislice contrast CT studies. Depending on the tumor size and histologic type, the permeability of the vascular wall allows the passage of substances in the form of macrocomplexes of considerable size, even of the order of 150–200 nm. The longer retention of the macrocomplexes in the tumor interstitium is partly due to inefficient lymphatic drainage by the tumor lymphatic network, which is also abnormal.

The majority of cytostatic drugs are phase-specific and those that have a shorter contact time do not normally have as good a chance of interfering with a significant number of tumor cells synchronized in a favorable phase for a lethal encounter. Pharmaceutical engineering has intentionally in some cases—and unintentionally in others—created a sort of camouflage for some cytostatic molecules. They can thus reach a higher intratumoral concentration, and their intracellular penetration is better too, with many more cells killed.

Liposome-encapsulated drugs provide an example of low pharmacologic signaling.[15] An example of potentially more effective disguise is incorporation of the taxane paclitaxel into albumin microparticles. Two specific formulations have been used in intraarterial chemotherapy for tumors of the head and neck and of the brain: liposomal doxorubicin (Caelyx, Janssen-Cilag SpA, Belgium), Myocet (Chepalon, PA), and paclitaxel in albumin microparticles[16] (Abraxane, Celegen Corporation, NJ). Anthracyclines are among the most active agents in a variety of tumors and experimentally they appear active on primary brain tumors. Liposome-encapsulated doxorubicin and conventional doxorubicin have different pharmacokinetic and therapeutic behavior.[17] Liposomes are vesicles that closely resemble cell membranes; they can have a monolamellar or multilamellar structure, and range from 20 nm to 1 μm in diameter. Once administered into the circulation, liposomes tend to persist longer in the vessels as they travel through normal tissue. The loss of structural integrity of the liposome in the plasma is only a question of time and these corpuscles are sequestered fairly fast by the macrophage system, so when used systemically the time of drug release is not optimal; intraarterial administration helps avoid this issue.

To avoid rapid recognition by the reticuloendothelial system and subsequent destruction, monolamellar liposomes coated with chains of polyethylene glycol (peg), a hydrophilic polymer, have been designed. These "stealth" liposomes remain in the circulation longer with a greater chance of penetrating the tumor sites while respecting healthy tissue. A special formulation of nonpegylated liposomes with a size of 150 nm is available on the market.[18-20] These are loaded with doxorubicin shortly before administration. In view of its size, the macrocomplex should accumulate more in the tumor interstitium because of slower drainage. These liposomes should also release doxorubicin more readily because of lower membrane resistance.

Taxanes are a class of antitumoral drugs that has had the same clinical impact as anthracyclines and cisplatin as regards its results but seemed to be completely excluded from the possibility of intraarterial administration because the original formulations contained alcohol and a surfactant agent, Cremophor, which are both irritants for the endothelium and can induce frequent, severe allergic reactions.[21] In the late 1990s, at the Special Radiological Procedures section of the Radiology Unit of the National Cancer Institute in Milan, Damascelli and colleagues began to use the paclitaxel-albumin macrocomplex ABI-007,[22] developed to allow easier and less toxic parenteral administration of the taxane, selectively by the intraarterial route in various malignancies.[16] Attention focused on squamous cell carcinoma of the head and neck, a historical target of intraarterial chemotherapy.[23] The vehicle used—albumin—seemed to increase the permeability, further raising the drug concentration inside the tumor.[24] Cancer cells develop the molecular transport mechanism of albumin to the maximum, as it is their main energy source, with receptors in the tumor vessel endothelium responsible for this transport. The receptors form caveolae or sacs in which the drug is enveloped and then emptied into the tumor interstitium where free paclitaxel penetrates the tumor cells and causes cell death by interfering with the microtubule system. If antitumoral efficacy depends on the effective dose in the tumor, it follows that regardless of the mechanisms of final transport, the greater local availability ensured by intraarterial administration is a considerable strength of this modality, when practicable.

Intraarterial Chemotherapy Technology and Technique for Brain and Head and Neck Tumors

Two main techniques have been developed for transcatheter intraarterial chemotherapy: one with surgical placement and the other with percutaneous placement.[25-27] Surgical catheter placement is used only for tumors fed by branches of the external carotid artery. The technique entails preparation of the superficial temporal artery anteriorly to the tragus of the ear, arterial cut-down, and insertion of a small-diameter catheter (2-F). The position of the catheter tip can be adjusted by injecting a vital dye (Patent Blue Violet) and checking which cutaneous or mucous region is stained. If the tongue is stained, the catheter tip will be just below the lingual artery; if the palate is stained, it will be just below the internal maxillary artery. Because of the size of the catheter, contrast medium can give rise to inadequate images, even with digital angiography.

Percutaneous catheterization of the neck vessels, generally through the femoral artery, is much more flexible, offering the possibility of treating both sides in a single session and selecting the appropriate region with ready reproducibility and acceptable invasiveness. The procedure is done in serial sessions, normally at 3-week intervals, under local anesthesia and with a minimal hospital stay. The utmost care is recommended for percutaneous access, choosing the smallest-diameter catheters, alternating the side of access and using simple manual compression or dedicated devices for hemostasis.

Damascelli and colleagues have developed a disposable coaxial infusion circuit that facilitates the maneuvers of prolonged catheterization.[28] To reduce the risk of thromboembolism, the guide catheter is perfused with heparinized saline throughout the diagnostic stage and the infusion of cytostatic drugs. Superselective catheterization, generally reserved for branches of the external carotid artery, is done with microcatheters and microguides served by an independent flushing line. The drug can be infused using a pump capable of overcoming the resistance offered by the microcatheter and by arterial pressure (Figure 22-1). The drug dose, dilution, and infusion time are chosen on the basis of the characteristics of the molecule used, the actual position of the catheter, and the expected toxicity.

TOXICITY

Intraarterial chemotherapy for brain and head and neck tumors began on an absolutely empirical basis with drugs and doses based on systemic treatment. There are no clinical trials defining the maximum tolerated dose and dose-limiting toxicity for intraarterial chemotherapy but only reports of general toxicity or local adverse events reflecting the site of administration. In some cases, optical ischemic neuropathy and also hearing loss have been reported, the latter related to cisplatin treatment. Supraophthalmic infusion seems to involve a greater risk of acute neurologic toxicity such as epileptic fits, confusion, headache, and focal deficits. The drugs implicated are carmustine, cisplatin, and other nitrosoureas.[3] Damascelli et al. conducted a limited study, treating recurrent high-grade glioblastoma and brain metastases from lung cancer with two drugs: liposomal doxorubicin (Myocet) and paclitaxel/albumin (Abraxane). No ophthalmic or neurologic toxicity was observed with infraophthalmic infusion of either drug into the internal carotid artery. The dose of liposomal doxorubicin was 40 mg/m^2 and three out of five patients received respectively five, seven, and eight doses, at 4-week intervals. Abraxane was used up to 250 mg/m^2, again

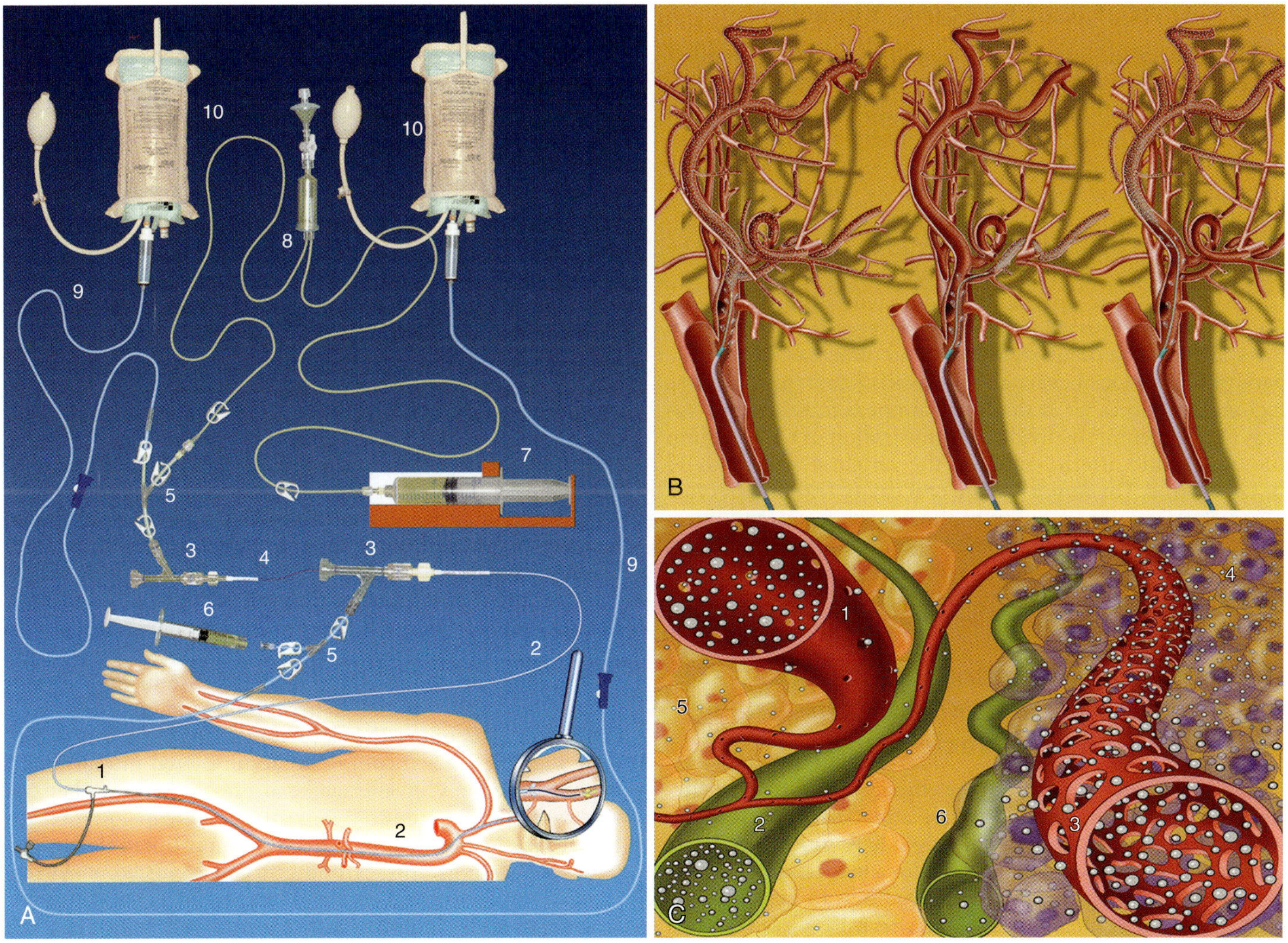

Figure 22-1 (A) Infusion circuit for intraarterial chemotherapy of head and neck tumors: 1, vascular introducer; 2, guide catheter; 3, Y connectors; 4, coaxial infusion catheter; 5, three-way connectors with clamps; 6, high-pressure injection syringe; 7, power pump for drug infusion; 8, air bubble trapping and removal system; 9, flushing lines with flow regulator; and 10, saline solution in pressurized bags. (B) Coaxial catheterization of the external carotid branches and injection of a chemotherapeutic agent in macrocomplexes. Flushing is maintained with a heparinized saline solution between the guide catheters and the microcatheters. (C) Increased permeability and retention of macromolecules by the tumor tissue. More macromolecules pass into the tumor tissue because of the pathologic permeability of the capillaries and more are retained in the tumor interstitium because of limited drainage by the abnormal lymphatics. 1, Capillary with intact endothelium; 2, normal lymphatic drainage; 3, break in the endothelium of tumor capillaries; 4, tumor tissue; 5, normal tissue; and 6, abnormal tumor lymphatics.

in a small series of patients, with no central neurologic toxicity or bone marrow depression.

More information is available on intraarterial chemotherapy of tumors of the head and neck. The toxicities were primarily peripheral neurotoxicity, bone marrow depression, and nephrotoxicity.[29] The authors conducted phase 1 and 2 studies with Abraxane,[16,23,28] in which the dose-limiting toxicity was peripheral paralysis of the facial nerve. This adverse reaction was more frequent at doses above 150 mg/m^2 and with infusion into the external carotid artery (6 cases out of 60), whereas in superselective infusion into the lingual artery no peripheral neurotoxicity was recorded. For the dose of 150 mg/m^2 used in subsequent cycles at 3-week intervals, bone marrow depression and gastrointestinal disturbances were rare, whereas general fatigue, albeit short-lasting, was frequently reported and alopecia occurred in all patients.

Complications Related to Catheterization of the Cerebral Vessels and Cervicofacial Feeding Vessels

The complications related to catheterization of the vertebral arteries and of the common carotid artery, hence of the internal and external carotids, do not differ in frequency and severity from those encountered in common diagnostic and interventional angiographies done by neuroradiologists and are mainly mechanical. Intimal dissection, thrombosis, and distant embolism are not influenced by drug administration but by the quality of the materials used, by the operator's experience, and by the strategies adopted in the procedure.

Surprisingly, the external carotid system has proved more fragile than the internal carotid district because of the structures it feeds, particularly nerves and mucosae. Reversible paralysis of the facial nerve and mucositis[28] are typical adverse regional reactions.[30,31] If the brain tumor is multifocal or supra- and subtentorial, divided administration of the dose into the two carotid arteries and into the vertebral artery should be considered. For tumors of the oral cavity and oropharynx, superselective catheterization of the lingual, facial, and internal maxillary artery is one tentative way of avoiding exposure of the cranial nerves to the drug. Bilateral catheterization is necessary for head and neck tumors that cross the midline.

Current Indications for Intraarterial Chemotherapy of Tumors of the Brain and the Head and Neck

Phase 3 studies have compared the efficacy of intraarterial chemotherapy with nitrosoureas and cisplatin—drugs whose toxicity profiles are far from negligible—and have shown a negative impact on the quality of life in return for a modest survival benefit. Results are awaited from recent studies with intraarterially administered liposomal doxorubicin, which has already shown significant survival benefits with acceptable general toxicity, mainly bone marrow depression, when given systemically.

Intraarterial chemotherapy of primary central nervous system lymphomas and brain metastases has given more encouraging results, particularly on metastases. The agents used, methotrexate and carboplatin (recently also combined), showed a certain efficacy, with acceptable neurologic and systemic toxicity. Decidedly more encouraging are the results on control of squamous cell carcinomas of the head and neck, mainly tumors of the oral cavity, oropharynx, and hypopharynx. As we noted earlier, these malignancies often trigger a personal and family emergency because they cause such rapid deterioration in the quality of life and have a poor prognosis. Intraarterial chemotherapy appears to offer the best features for so-called induction chemotherapy and historically, with the introduction of cisplatin into clinical use, the response rate has been better than with combined systemic treatment.[29] High-dose cisplatin must be accompanied by intensive pharmacologic treatment to prevent renal toxicity.

Systemic treatment with taxanes has proved effective. Initially used to treat recurrences, these molecules have now been combined with cisplatin and 5-fluorouracil in induction chemotherapy regimens.[32,33] A formulation of the taxane paclitaxel bound in albumin nanoparticles has been registered in the United States and Europe for the treatment of metastatic breast cancer that has not responded to chemotherapy even with paclitaxel in the conventional formulation. Damascelli and colleagues used this product, initially designated as ABI-007 and now known as Abraxane, for intraarterial infusion in patients with advanced squamous cell carcinoma of the head and neck.[16] In the phase 1 and the recently published phase 2 study,[28] the primary endpoints were reached, confirming the feasibility of intraarterial chemotherapy using the new agent, with high rates of partial and complete responses, 25% and 50%, in 60 consecutive cases. The most frequent nonhematologic toxicities were neurologic, essentially paralysis of the facial nerve, gastrointestinal, flulike syndrome, and alopecia. High-grade hematologic toxicity was seen only in four patients. Procedure-related complications were minimal, and catheterization was highly reproducible by a dedicated group of radiologists experienced in percutaneous arterial catheterization.

Discussion

Intraarterial chemotherapy for primary or metastatic brain tumors and for tumors of the head and neck is coming under renewed scrutiny because of a number of small studies that have shown better survival of these patients, and improvement in quality of life.

High-grade glioblastomas recurring after surgery or radiotherapy with or without temozolomide chemotherapy—to cite the regimen currently adopted as standard of care—cause significant neurobehavioral changes because of rapid tumor growth with intracranial hypertension and neurochemical disturbances. Pending the development of genetic and biologic therapies, macrocomplexes administered intraarterially appear to be the only alternative at present because they can achieve high intratumoral concentrations with low toxicity. Liposomal doxorubicin has already demonstrated this in systemic applications. Intracarotid infusion avoids bone marrow exposure, reducing an important aspect of general toxicity. In a small series studied by Damascelli and colleagues, not yet published, intraarterial infusion was not associated with any neurotoxicity (Figure 22-2). Response assessment in glioblastomas is mainly clinical and functional. Neurobehavioral improvement or lack of deterioration and the possibility of reducing steroid therapy are important.

For the treatment of brain metastases (Figure 22-3) there is another macrocomplex that is readily manageable in intraarterial

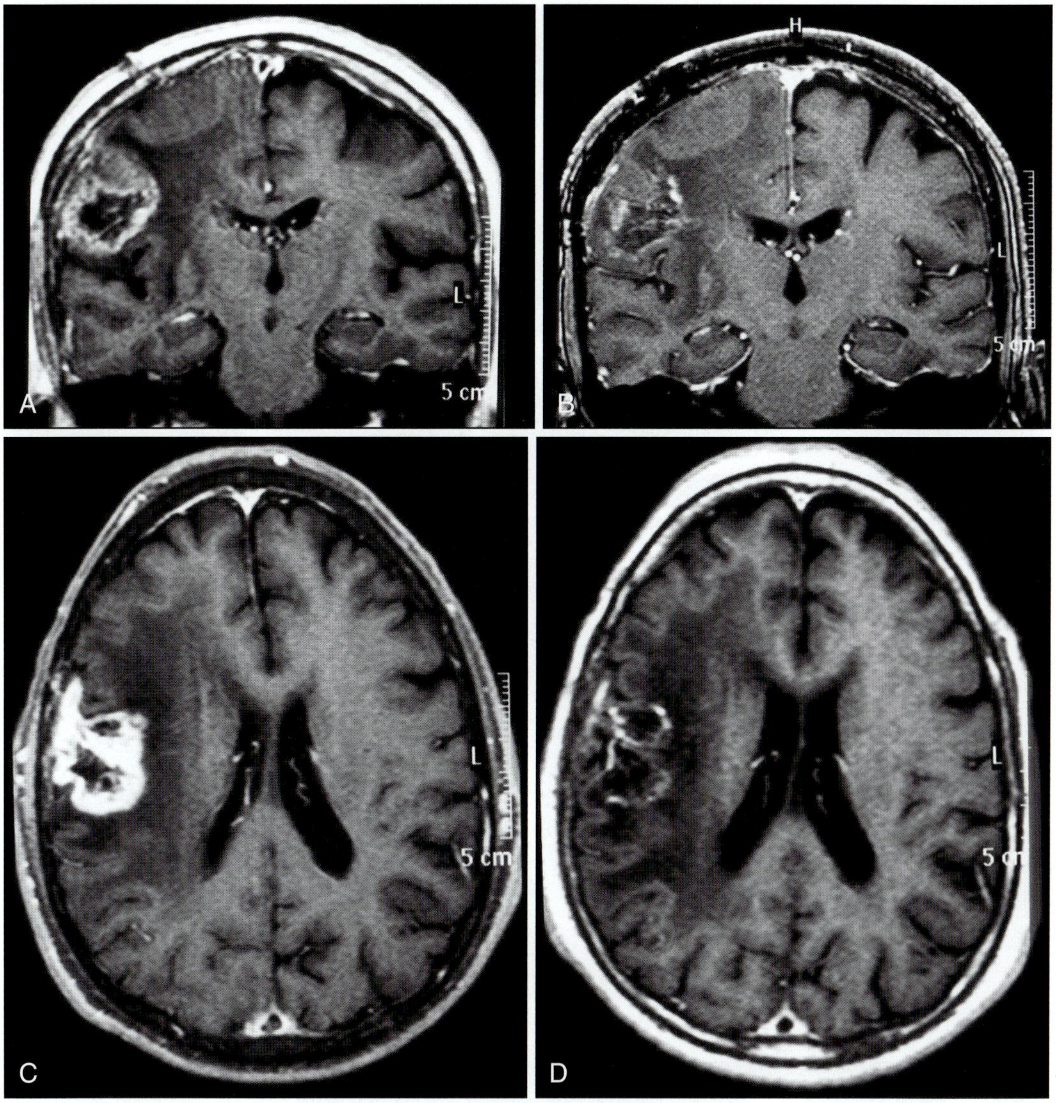

Figure 22-2 Right parietal glioblastoma recurring after surgery, radiotherapy, and chemotherapy with temozolomide. (A and C) Pretreatment magnetic resonance scans. (B and D) Radiological response after eight cycles of intraarterial infusion of liposomal doxorubicin (Myocet) into the right internal carotid artery.

administration: paclitaxel bound in albumin nanoparticles, which are similar in size to the larger liposomes. The size of the macrocomplex allows for trapping in the tumor interstitium with consequent greater drug release at the appropriate site.

This fortuitous combination of a cytostatic drug with human albumin particles opens up a new frontier for different types of cancer and so far has been explored in systemic treatment of metastatic breast cancer and squamous cell carcinoma of the head and neck (Figure 22-4). The latter study was developed originally by the authors. Intraarterial injection of Abraxane combines exploitation of the increased permeability and retention shown toward macromolecules by the tumor capillary network with an active transport mechanism, known as transcytosis, exerted on albumin by the endothelial cells. Glycoprotein 60, a receptor found on the surface of endothelial cells, triggers the formation of vesicles known as caveolae, which convey the albumin/paclitaxel complex into the tumor interstitium at four times the speed of the conventional paclitaxel formulation with the surfactant Cremophor. The increase in albumin uptake is partly due to the tumor's production of secreted protein, acidic and rich in cysteine (SPARC), which is expressed by a certain number of tumors, particularly those of the head and neck.[34] SPARC is overexpressed in squamous cell carcinomas and is an unfavorable prognostic factor. Although only one study on a small number of patients is available, it showed that among patients with head and neck cancer treated intraarterially with Abraxane, the response rate was higher in SPARC-positive than SPARC-negative cases. Identification of SPARC-positive patients would permit further refinement of the therapeutic potential of albumin-bound paclitaxel, particularly for intraarterial administration, which would prolong the local tumoricidal effect with less systemic toxicity. The local toxicity is still under investigation but it appeared to be controlled with dose adjustment (Figures 22-5 and 22-6).

Because the macrocomplexes considered here have radiosensitizing properties,[35-37] the possibility of combining intraarterial infusion with radiotherapy should also be considered.

REFERENCES

The complete reference list is available online at www.expertconsult.com.

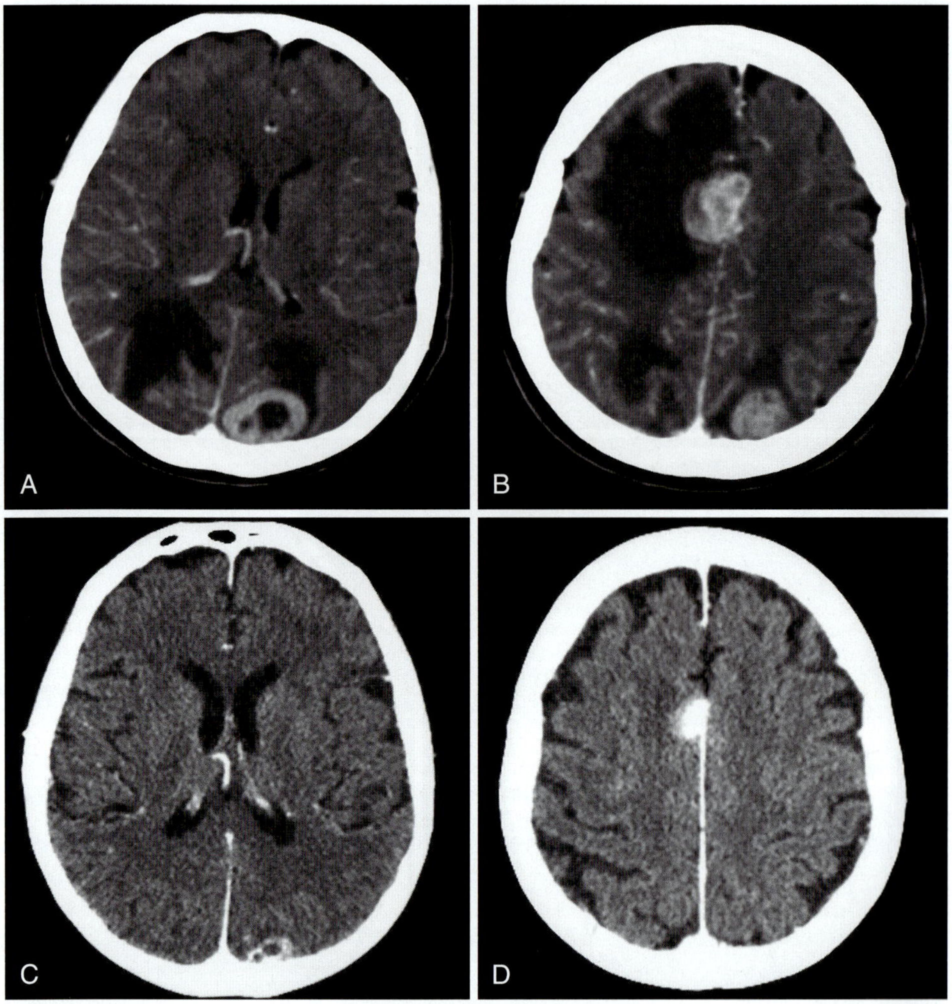

Figure 22-3 Brain metastasis from squamous cell carcinoma of the lung with progression after radiotherapy. (A and B) Brain sections before intraarterial infusion of paclitaxel-albumin (Abraxane) into the internal carotid arteries. (C and D) Result after three treatment cycles.

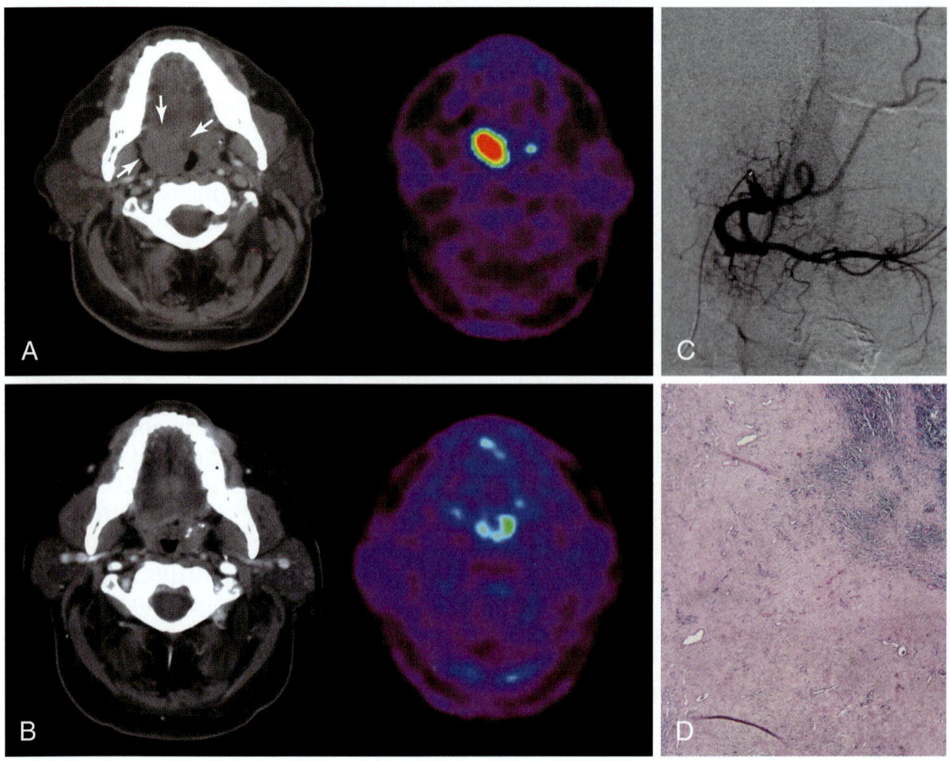

Figure 22-4 Squamous cell carcinoma of right tonsil. (A) Computed tomographic and positron-emission tomographic scans with morphologic demonstration of the tumor and its metabolic activity. (B) Complete radiologic response after three cycles of intraarterial chemotherapy with paclitaxel-albumin (Abraxane). (C) Selective angiography. (D) Complete pathologic response.

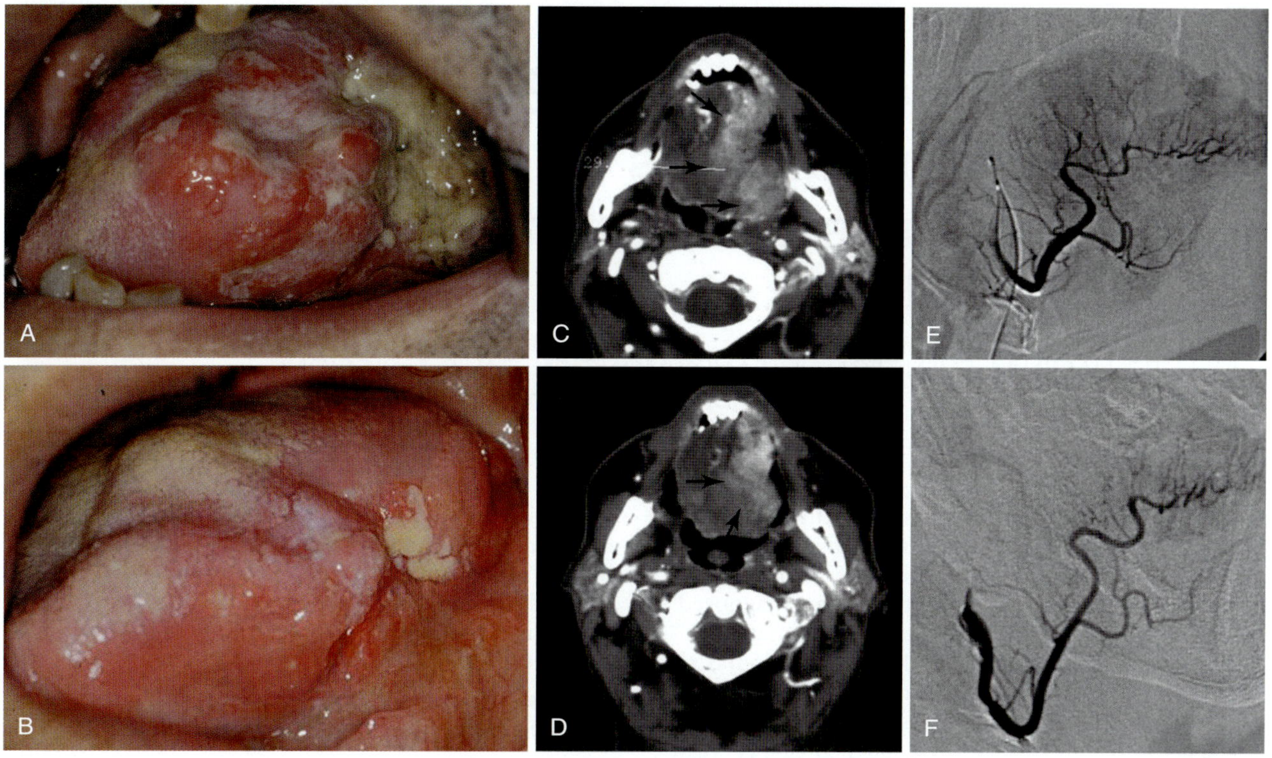

Figure 22-5 Advanced squamous cell carcinoma of the left half of the tongue. (A) Photograph on presentation. (B) Response after intraarterial chemotherapy with paclitaxel-albumin (Abraxane). (C) Computed tomographic (CT) scan before treatment. (D) CT scan after three cycles of treatment: reduction in tumor size and pathologic contrast agent uptake. (E) Left lingual angiography before treatment. (F) Left lingual angiography after three treatment cycles: note reduction in tumor circulation

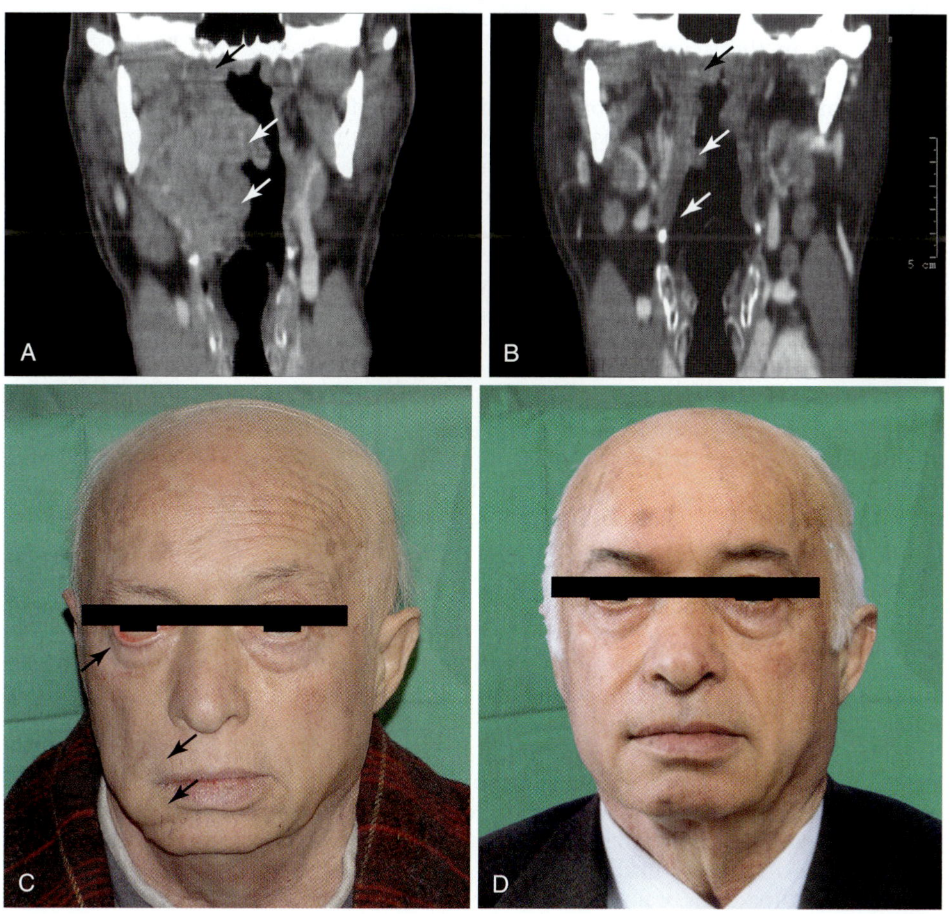

Figure 22-6 Advanced squamous cell carcinoma of the oropharynx. (A) CT scan at presentation. (B) Radiologic response after three cycles of intraarterial infusion of paclitaxel-albumin (Abraxane) into the external carotid artery. (C) Right facial nerve paralysis with lagophthalmos secondary to paclitaxel neurotoxicity. (D) Resolution of paralysis after 6 months.

23

Head: Intracranial - Gliomas, and Meningiomas and Extracranial - Orbits, Internal Auditory Canals, and Skull Base

BENJAMIN M. ELLINGSON | SANDY MONG | DAVID E. PICCIONI | SARAH N. KHAN | ALI R. SEPAHDARI | WHITNEY POPE

Primary central nervous system tumors constitute a relatively rare, but significant, fatal health problem in the United States and the rest of the world. Every year in the United States approximately 44,000 new primary brain tumors are diagnosed,[1] or 14 in every 100,000 citizens.[2-6] Of these, approximately 60% are malignant and 45% are gliomas.[1] Malignant gliomas are the second leading cause of cancer mortality in people under the age of 35, the fourth leading cause in those under the age of 54, and kill approximately 13,000 people per year.[1] Epidemiologic evidence suggests children younger than age 14 years and patients older than age 70 years have a higher incidence of primary brain tumors compared with other age groups[7] Median age at diagnosis for primary brain tumors is between 54 and 58 years old[2-6] Metastatic brain tumors arising from other primary cancer types are substantially more common, affecting more than 150,000 patients each year in the United States.[8-10]

Glioblastoma is a particular type of infiltrative malignant glioma with a very poor patient prognosis and few effective treatment options. Despite advances in surgical procedures, radiation, and chemotherapy, median survival is only around 14 months for glioblastoma patients when treated with radiotherapy and concurrent temozolomide, followed by adjuvant temozolomide ("Stupp protocol").[11] Tumor cell invasion into normal parenchyma, otherwise undetected by standard neuroimaging techniques, along with resistance to treatments remains the primary reason for poor prognosis in glioblastoma. Low-grade gliomas have a substantially longer median survival, ranging from 6 to 10 years when including both astrocytomas and oligodendrogliomas.[1] Except for medulloblastoma and embryonal tumors,[12] younger patients generally have a better survival rate than older patients, and patients with any type of glioma who survive more than 2 years from diagnosis have more than a 75% chance of surviving more than 5 years.[3]

Primary Brain Tumor Classification

Central nervous system tumors are currently classified based on histologic features and the particular tumor cells of origin. Examination of histologic features includes assessing the general degree of tumor cellularity (i.e., cell density), architecture of the tumor, organization of cellular arrangements (e.g., rosette formations, whirling patterns, angiogenesis), cytologic features of the tumor cells themselves (e.g., identification of cellular processes, cytoplasm characteristics), and cytologic atypia suggestive of malignancy. The use of specialized histochemical or immunohistochemical stains, including glial fibrillary acidic protein (GFAP), further help differentiate the particular type of brain tumor. Table 23-1 summarizes the main classifications of primary intracranial central nervous system tumors.

Neuroimaging In Brain Tumors

Modern neuroimaging techniques and biomarkers in brain tumors are intimately tied to clinical understanding of in vivo human brain tumor behavior. Almost all brain tumor treatment decisions are based on neuroimaging findings and interpretations (Figure 23-1).

Gliomas

The World Health Organization (WHO) classifies primary nervous system tumors into grades I to IV in order of increasing malignancy and worse prognosis.[62] According to the WHO classification, gliomas can be divided into either diffuse or localized subtypes, for which diffuse gliomas can be further subdivided into astrocytomas, oligodendrogliomas, and mixed oligoastrocytomas, depending on the particular histologic features of the tumor. Glioblastoma, or grade IV astrocytoma, can be subdivided into primary and secondary glioblastoma. Secondary glioblastomas arise from malignant transformation of grade II/III gliomas, as opposed to primary glioblastomas, which arise de novo. Ependymomas and choroid plexus tumors, which are also considered of glial origin, constitute most of the remaining proportion of primary brain tumors in adults.

ASTROCYTOMA

Astrocytomas (WHO grade II) are diffusely infiltrative gliomas composed of neoplastic astrocytes. Astrocytomas typically have ill-defined boundaries, low cellularity, and few nuclear atypia.[62,63] Lacking malignant features such as endothelial microvascular proliferation, high mitotic activity and proliferation rate, and microscopic necrosis, astrocytomas are typically of low aggressivity compared to higher-grade tumors. Postcontrast T1-weighted MR images of low-grade astrocytomas typically lack contrast enhancement, as contrast uptake is indicative of blood–brain barrier compromise commonly caused by microvascular

TABLE 23-1 Classification of Primary Intracranial Central Nervous System Tumors

I. GLIAL CELL TUMORS (GLIOMAS)
- a. Low-grade gliomas (WHO I and II)
  - i. Pilocytic astrocytoma (WHO I)
  - ii. Maxopapillary ependymoma (WHO I)
  - iii. Subependymal giant cell astrocytoma (WHO I)
  - iv. Subependymoma (WHO I)
  - v. Ependymoma (WHO II)
  - vi. Astrocytoma (WHO II)
  - vii. Oligodendroglioma (WHO II)
  - viii. Mixed oligoastrocytoma (WHO II)
- b. Anaplastic gliomas (WHO III)
  - i. Anaplastic astrocytoma (WHO III)
  - ii. Anaplastic oligodendroglioma (WHO III)
  - iii. Anaplastix mixed oligodendroglioma (WHO III)
- c. Glioblastoma (WHO IV)
- d. Special subtypes
  - i. Pleomorphic xanthoastrocytoma
  - ii. Desmoplastic infantile astrocytoma
  - iii. Gliofibroma
  - iv. Choroid plexus papilloma
  - v. Choroid plexus carcinoma

II. NEURONAL AND MIXED NEURONAL-GLIAL TUMORS
- a. Neuronal tumors
  - i. Gangliocytoma
  - ii. Neurocytoma
- b. Mixed neuronal-glial tumors
  - i. Ganglioglioma and anaplastic ganglioglioma
  - ii. Desmoplastic infantile ganglioglioma
  - iii. Dysembryoplastic neuroepithelial tumors

III. MEDULLOBLASTOMA
- a. Medulloblastoma
- b. Nodular medulloblastoma
- c. Medullomyoblastoma
- d. Melanotic medulloblastoma

IV. MENINGEAL TUMORS
- a. Meningioma
- b. Atypical meningioma
- c. Anaplastic meningioma
- d. Meningioma variants (meningiothelial, fibrous, transitional, psammomatous, angiomatous, microcystic, secretory, metaplastic, etc.)

proliferation, characteristic of malignant transformation. Diffusion MR estimates of apparent diffusion coefficient (ADC), a measure of water mobility inversely proportional to cell density and proportional to extracellular space,[13-18] is often low in distinct regions thought to contain viable tumor, while elevated in regions of infiltration and/or edema.

Anaplastic Astrocytoma

Anaplastic astrocytomas (WHO grade III) are malignant astrocytomas with many of the histologic features of grade II astrocytomas, but lacking the endothelial microvascular proliferation and necrosis found in glioblastoma (WHO grade IV) tumors. Anaplastic astrocytomas are typically more highly cellular compared to low-grade astrocytomas and exhibit mitotic activity (Ki-67), typically of 12%–14%.[64,65] Increased cytoplasmic pleomorphism and elevated cellularity in anaplastic astrocytomas manifest as lower mean ADC values compared with low-grade astrocytomas,[66] whereas slightly higher cerebral blood volume is also observed in high- compared to low-grade astrocytomas.[31] Anaplastic astrocytomas typically demonstrate a higher degree of infiltrative features on standard and advanced magnetic resonance imaging (MRI) compared to low-grade astrocytomas, including blurring of the gray–white matter interface, and have higher rates of enhancement (Figure 23-2).

OLIGODENDROGLIOMA

Oligodendrogliomas (WHO grade II) comprise 2.1% of all primary brain and CNS tumors and 6.6% of all primary brain and CNS gliomas.[67] Oligodendrogliomas occur approximately three times more often in white compared with black patients,[67] and occur most often in the fourth and fifth decades of life. Almost two-thirds of patients with oligodendrogliomas present with seizures.[68] Oligodendrogliomas are often gelatinous masses that tend to blur the white–gray matter interface on anatomic MRI. Oligodendrogliomas also often exhibit cystic degeneration and necrosis on MRI (Figure 23-3). Calcifications within oligodendrogliomas are often detectable as hypointensities on gradient recall echo (GRE) or susceptibility-weighted MRI sequences, while presenting as hyperdensity on computed tomography (CT). Similar observations on MRI are also common because of hemorrhages within oligodendrogliomas. Histologically, oligodendroglioma tumor cells have indistinct cytoplasm and round nuclei, giving them a "fried egg" appearance, and are often distributed along regions of neovascularization with distinctive vascular patterns or "chicken wire" patterns.[63] These geometrically distinct vascular patterns manifest as elevated blood volume on perfusion imaging compared with the same-grade astrocytomas, and the tightly packed oligodendroglioma tumor cells often result in a lower ADC compared with astrocytomas. Grade II oligodendrogliomas do not present with histopathologic features of anaplasia or malignant transformation; therefore, these tumors may have low a mitotic index (Ki-67) between 2% and 5%.[69]

Anaplastic Oligodendroglioma

Anaplastic oligodendrogliomas (WHO grade III) often occur as a result of anaplastic transformation of oligodendroglioma WHO grade II tumors, but can also occur de novo. Although they maintain many of the histologic features of low-grade oligodendrogliomas, anaplastic oligodendrogliomas have additional malignant features including increased mitotic activity, endothelial cell proliferation, microscopic necrosis, increased nuclear and cytoplasm pleomorphism, and tumor cell infiltration. Anaplastic oligodendrogliomas have both better clinical and prognostic outcomes compared to anaplastic astrocytomas, primarily because of the increased chemosensitivity in oligodendrogliomas.[70,71]

MIXED AND ANAPLASTIC OLIGOASTROCYTOMA

Mixed oligoastrocytomas (WHO grade II) and anaplastic oligoastrocytomas (WHO grade III) are primary brain tumors consisting of both neoplastic oligodendroglial and astrocytes. Although no definitive histologic criteria exist for diagnosis of oligoastrocytomas, identification of neoplastic cells from both populations appears to be necessary, either diffusely distributed or focally isolated. As with oligodendrogliomas, mixed oligoastrocytomas or anaplastic oligoastrocytomas have a more favorable prognosis compared with pure astrocytomas of the same grade or with glioblastoma.[72] The extent of the oligodendroglial component of these tumors correlates with improved overall survival.

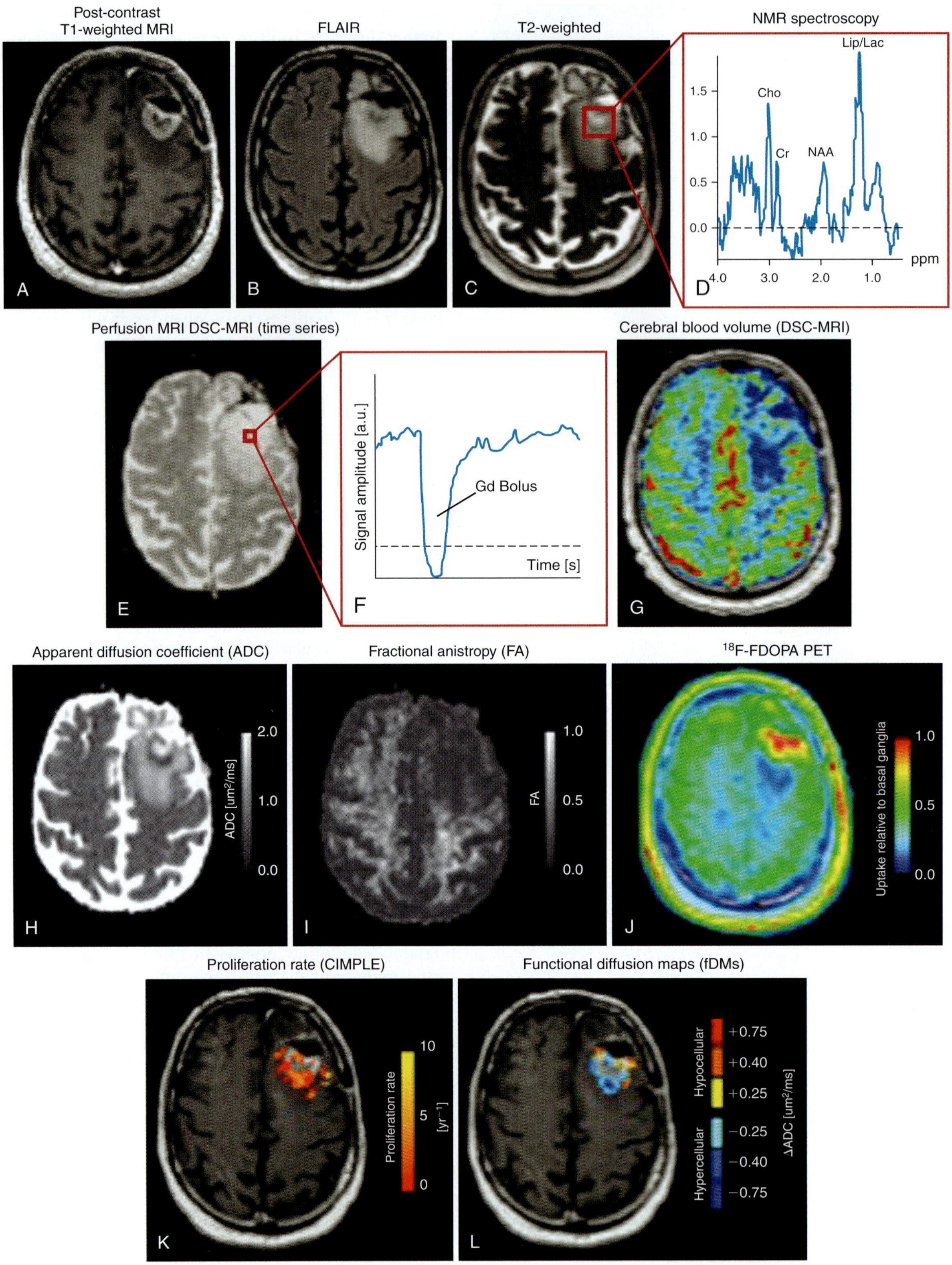

Figure 23-1 Common and advanced neuroimaging techniques used for diagnosis, surgical planning, and clinical monitoring of brain tumors. (A) Postcontrast T1-weighted MRI images showing contrast enhancement in the left frontal lobe. (B) Fluid-attenuated inversion recovery (FLAIR) images showing mixture of edema and tumor infiltration in hyperintense regions. (C) T2-weighted MRI images. (D) Single-voxel NMR spectroscopy showing elevated lipids and lactate (Lip/Lac), indicative of necrosis, along with elevated choline (Cho) and creatine (Cr) and reduced *N*-acetyl aspartate (NAA), a neuronal marker. (E) Raw dynamic susceptibility contrast (DSC)-MRI time series. (F) DSC-MRI time series for a single voxel showing transient signal loss during bolus passage of a gadolinium-chelated (Gd) contrast agent. (G) Relative cerebral blood volume (rCBV) calculated from DSC-MRI time series. (H) Apparent diffusion coefficient (ADC) showing reduced ADC in hypercellular tumor regions. (I) Fractional anisotropy (FA) images derived from diffusion tensor images (DTI) showing reduced FA in tumor regions indicative of white matter compromise. (J) ^{18}F-FDOPA PET showing elevated uptake relative to the basal ganglia in contrast-enhancing regions. (K) Proliferation rate estimates from CIMPLE maps created using serial diffusion MRI data. (L) Functional diffusion maps (fDMs) showing decreased ADC in regions believed to contain hypercellular tumor.

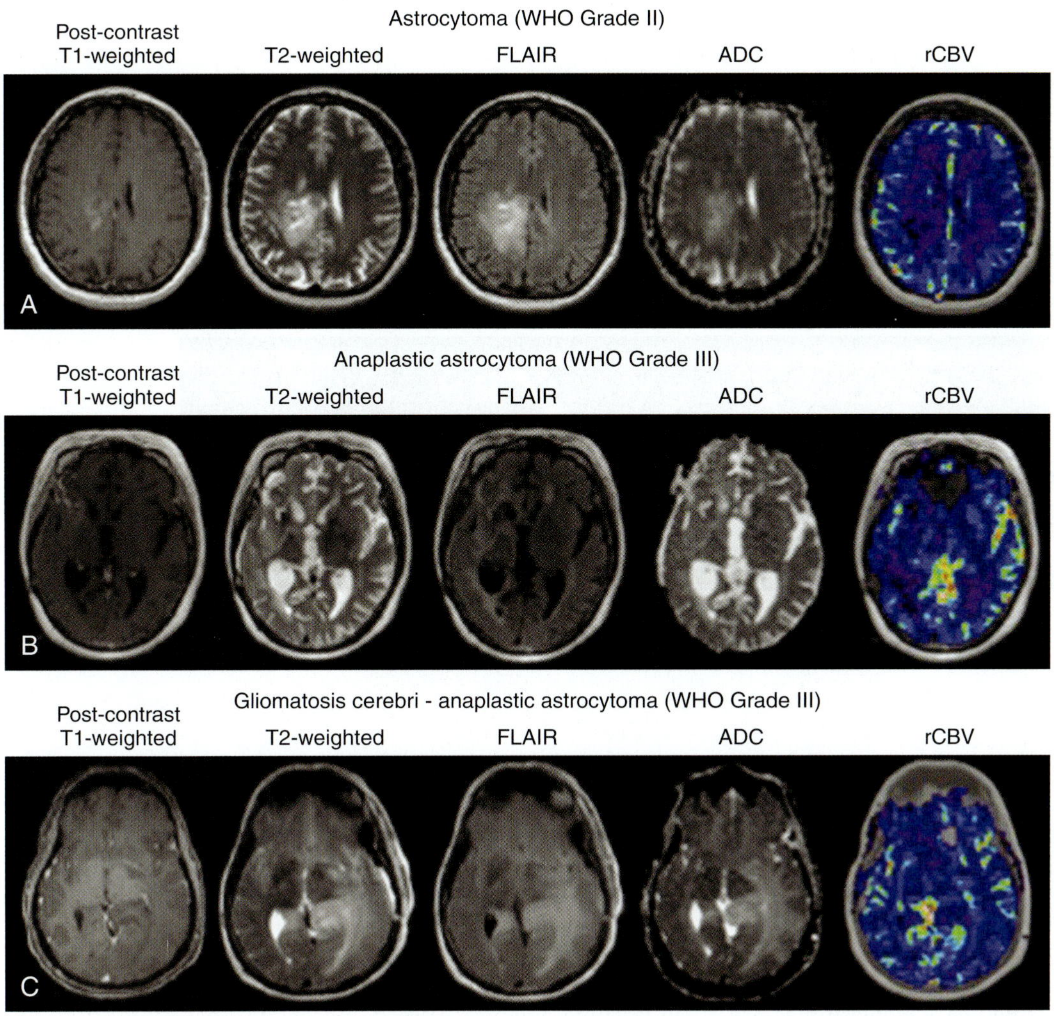

Figure 23-2 Neuroimaging of WHO grade II astrocytoma and grade III anaplastic astrocytoma. (A) 52-year-old woman with WHO grade II astrocytoma. Images were acquired after stereotactic radiation therapy. (B) 65-year-old woman with recurrent WHO grade III anaplastic astrocytoma. Images are shown after subtotal resection, radiotherapy and temozolomide, and four cycles of adjuvant temozolomide. (C) 48-year-old man with WHO grade III anaplastic astrocytoma and features of gliomatosis cerebri. Images were acquired prior to surgery.

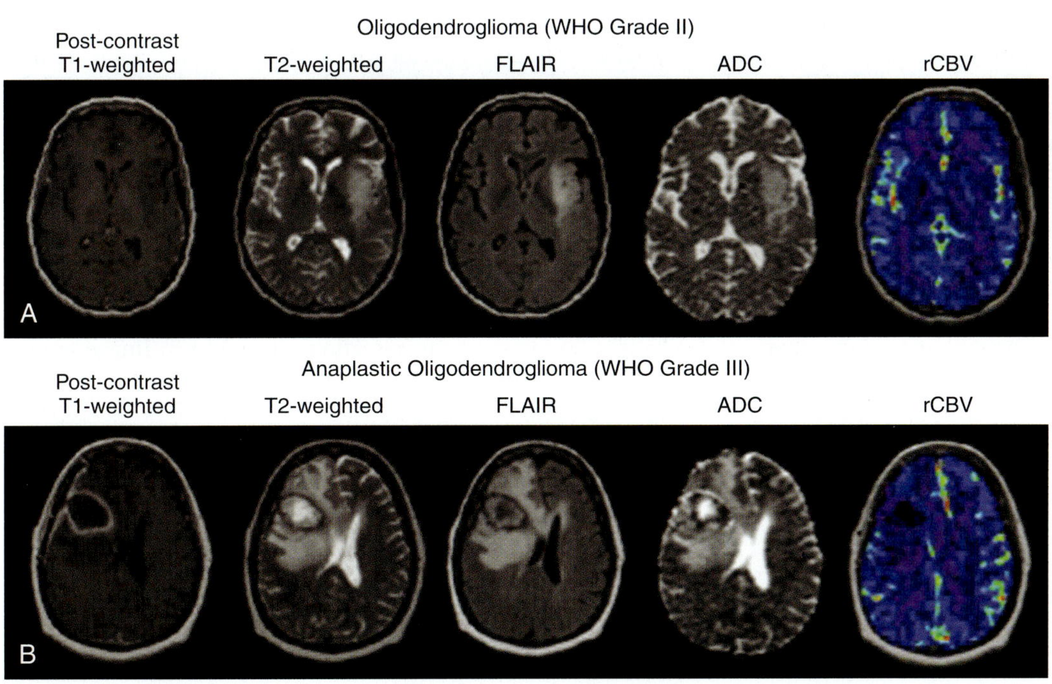

Figure 23-3 Neuroimaging of grade II oligodendroglioma and grade III anaplastic oligodendroglioma. (A) 49-year-old woman with a recurrent low-grade (WHO grade II) oligodendroglioma. Images were acquired after stereotactic biopsy, treatment with PCV followed by high-dose tamoxifen, and ending with failure on temozolomide. (B) 56-year-old woman with a recurrent anaplastic (WHO grade III) oligodendroglioma. Images were acquired during tumor progression after surgical resection, concurrent radiotherapy and temozolomide, followed by three cycles of adjuvant temozolomide.

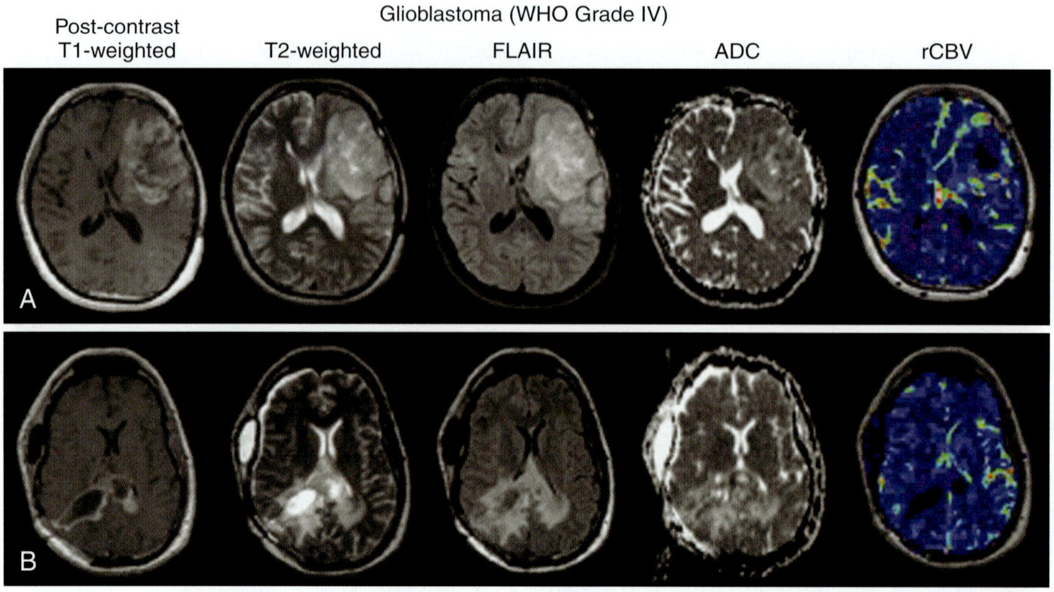

Figure 23-4 Neuroimaging of glioblastoma (WHO grade IV). (A) 27-year-old man with a recurrent left frontal glioblastoma. Images were obtained after resection and failure of radiotherapy and temozolomide. (B) 36-year-old man with recurrent glioblastoma crossing the corpus callosum. Note the central necrotic region in both patients surrounded by a highly vascular, contrast-enhancing rim and peritumoral edema.

GLIOBLASTOMA

Glioblastoma, previously referred to as *glioblastoma multiforme (GBM)*, are the most malignant and most common primary brain tumors, constituting nearly 54% of all primary gliomas.[67] Glioblastomas occur most frequently in older patients, and patterns in glioblastoma location suggest that the most frequent region of tumor occurrence moves from anterior to posterior with increasing age. Glioblastomas are highly infiltrative, proliferative, and aggressive brain tumors with a very poor patient prognosis. Despite advances in surgical resection, radiotherapy, and chemotherapy, median survival for patients with glioblastoma is around 14.6 months (radiotherapy and temozolomide) and 12.1 months for radiotherapy alone.[11] Microscopically, glioblastomas exhibit many of the malignant features of anaplastic gliomas, with the addition of endothelial microvascular proliferation and pseudopalisading necrosis. Anatomic MRI exhibits contrast enhancement on postcontrast T1-weighted images in the majority of cases,[73-75] and this contrast enhancement often occurs in a "ring-shape" enhancement with an area of central T1 hypointensity indicative of macroscopic necrosis. Perfusion imaging demonstrates elevated blood volume and blood flow in regions of contrast enhancement, corresponding to regions with elevated angiogenesis. T2-weighted or fluid-attenuated inversion recovery (FLAIR) images often show extensive tumor infiltration, along with "fingers of edema" presented as hyperintense regions on T2-weighted images respecting the gray–white matter interface at the cortical ribbon. T2-isointense or T2-hypointense regions within T2-hyperintense regions may signify dense bulk tumor regions in glioblastoma (Figure 23-4).

Surgical Planning and Guidance

Imaging plays a large role in current surgical planning and intraoperative guidance for the treatment of gliomas. A number of imaging techniques are useful in surgical management of patients with gliomas. fMRI, MRI with diffusion tensor imaging (DTI), intraoperative monitoring, and image-guided needle biopsies are all useful in planning and execution. The overall goal of imaging is to assist the surgeon in obtaining a maximal resection *while preventing neurologic complications.* Extent of resection has been shown to correlate with overall survival.[76]

Preoperative fMRI is used to localize critical areas involved in learning, memory, speech, motor, and sensory function.[77,78] fMRI testing maps areas of basic functions with regard to the tumor location. Mass effect from tumor or edema can distort the normal architecture of the brain, making localization by traditional landmarks difficult. fMRI facilitates surgical planning by localizing areas of eloquent cortex prior to surgery.

MRI with DTI provides information about major white-matter tracks associated with eloquent cortex (Figure 23-5). It can determine if tumor is displacing critical white-matter tracks, enabling the surgeon to resect the tumor without causing significant neurologic deficits.[79] Whereas fMRI helps the surgeon avoid critical areas of the cerebral cortex, MRI with DTI identifies the major white matter pathways and connections, assisting the surgeon with resection in the white matter and avoiding major fiber tracts. Interoperative MRI can account for brain shift that occurs during surgery, either from changes in pressure or resection of tumor.[80] Image-guided needle biopsy provides real-time feedback on the location of the biopsy needle, increasing the accuracy of a blind needle biopsy to a few millimeters. These techniques minimize the potential for neurologic complications from surgery while helping the surgeon safely resect as much tumor as possible.

Treatment

GRADE II GLIOMAS

Treatment of grade II astrocytomas, oligoastrocytomas, and oligodendrogliomas are similar and are largely customized to the

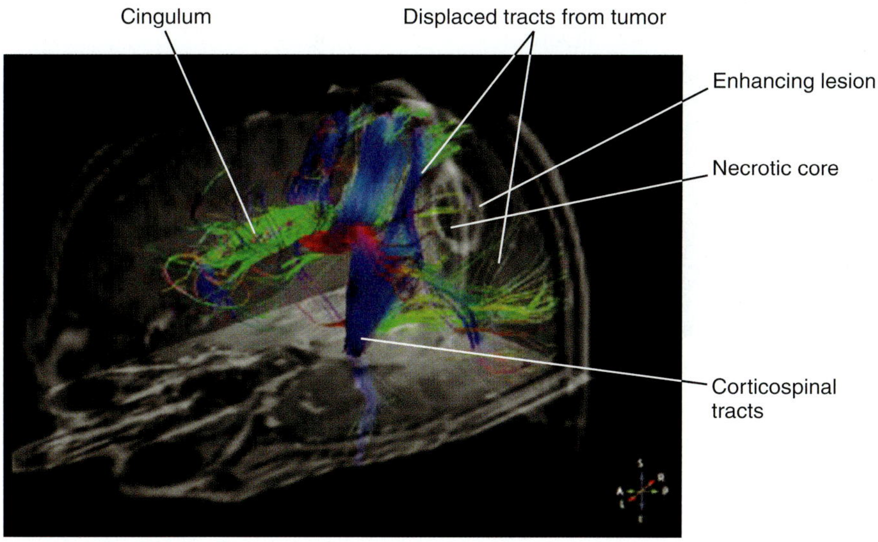

Figure 23-5 DTI tractography used for preoperative planning of brain tumor resection. (*Blue*: S = superior, I = inferior; *Red*: L = left, R = right; *Green*: A = anterior, P = posterior).

clinical situation and tumor location. Although guidelines exist for treatment, there is no level 1 evidence to define a standard treatment course. If maximal resection is not feasible, subtotal resection or biopsy should be considered for debulking and tissue diagnosis. Radiation has shown a clear benefit in grade II gliomas. However, there is some debate about when to start radiation therapy. When upfront radiation was compared to radiation at tumor progression, there was no difference in overall median survival (7.4 vs 7.2 years),[81] but there was an increase in progression-free survival in the upfront setting and better control of symptoms such as seizures. The decision to treat is left to the clinician and often depends on the remaining tumor bulk, extent of resection, and involvement in or near eloquent cortex. Temozolomide chemotherapy alone, though less effective than radiation, is sometimes used up front in patients wishing to delay radiation in order to postpone long-term cognitive side effects of radiation therapy. Patients with low-grade gliomas are followed with serial MRI imaging, initially every 3–6 months for the first 5 years, and then at least yearly thereafter.[82]

GRADE III GLIOMAS

Treatment of anaplastic astrocytomas and anaplastic oligodendrogliomas is also similar. Again, much of the clinical management is dictated by expert consensus, and data from phase III studies is largely lacking. The initial treatment for grade III gliomas is gross total resection as assessed by routine MRI. When gross total resection is not possible, subtotal resection and biopsy are used for tissue diagnosis.

Following resection, treatment is most often 6 weeks of radiation therapy followed by chemotherapy.[83,84] Radiation therapy is fractionated into 30–33 treatments over 6 weeks. Chemotherapy is usually temozolomide, 5 days of treatment followed by 23 days off, for one 28-day cycle. Temozolomide was initially approved by the FDA for recurrent anaplastic astrocytomas. The PCV regimen of procarbazine, lomustine (CCNU), and vincristine have also been used.[85] This regimen has been largely replaced by temozolomide alone, given the improved tolerability of temozolomide in comparison to PCV.[86]

Patients are followed with serial MRI imaging, starting with the first postsurgical scan 2–6 weeks following radiation therapy, prior to the start of adjuvant chemotherapy (Figure 23-6). Patients are monitored by MRI for response or progression every 2–4 months for 2–3 years, then less frequently afterwards. If recurrence is local, a second surgery can be considered, with or without the addition of carmustine (BCNU) wafers to the surgical cavity, followed by a change in the chemotherapy

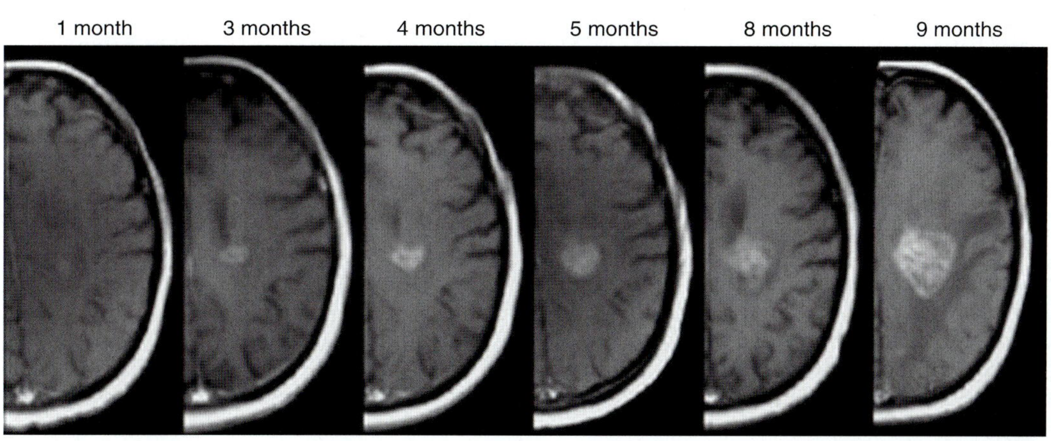

Figure 23-6 Glioblastoma growth (progression) evaluated with post-contrast T1-weighted images from the start of adjuvant temozolomide therapy.

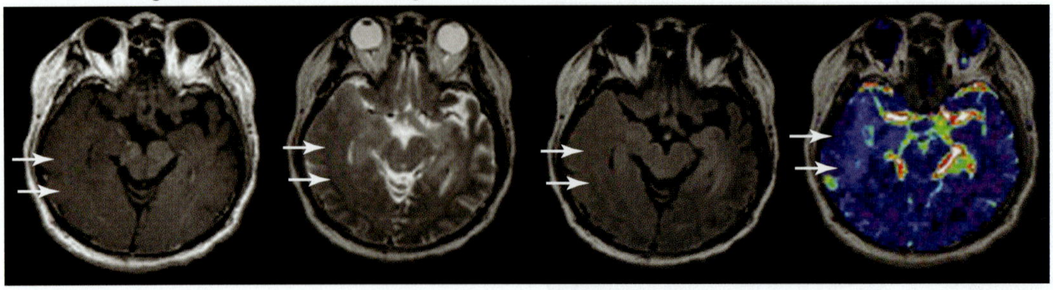

Figure 23-7 Tumor progression after failure of bevacizumab can sometimes occur as nonenhancing, infiltrating tumor growth. For this example, arrows show regions in the right temporal lobe with mass effect, subtle T2 hyperintensity, and elevated rCBV.

regimen.[87] Reirradiation is also considered, especially if recurrent disease is outside the original field of radiation, but this is controversial.

GLIOBLASTOMA (WHO GRADE IV)

The standard of care treatment for glioblastoma and gliosarcoma has become the Stupp regimen.[11] This consists of maximal resection if possible, followed by 6 weeks of daily chemotherapy with temozolomide plus radiation therapy, which is fractionated into 30–33 treatments over that initial 6-week period. Postsurgical imaging is recommended within 72 hours in order to assess the extent of resection and possible ischemia before postsurgical blood products cause significant T1 shortening (hyperintensity on precontrast T1-weighted images), as this can often mask residual contrast enhancement on postcontrast T1-weighted images. A second postoperative imaging session is usually acquired 2–6 weeks after 6 weeks of concurrent radiation and temozolomide in order to assess the response to the initial treatment regimen, prior to initiating adjuvant cycles of temozolomide. The goal of this imaging regimen is to first assess the initial extent of resection. Near gross-total resection is associated with a good prognosis. Next, imaging is obtained a few weeks after initial radiation and chemotherapy to establish a baseline tumor burden once postsurgical and initial postradiation changes have stabilized. This baseline is used to assess for tumor progression (Figure 23-7). Adjuvant temozolomide is typically given 5 consecutive days every 28-day cycle as described above. Bevacizumab is a monoclonal antibody to vascular endothelial growth factor, which is FDA approved for recurrent glioblastoma, and is used alone or with other chemotherapy agents, such as irinotecan.[88,89] Patients are encouraged to participate in clinical trials at disease recurrence. Participation in clinical trials at the time of initial diagnosis is becoming more common as well.

Meningiomas

EPIDEMIOLOGY AND PRESENTATION

Meningiomas are the most common extraaxial intracranial tumors and constitute 6.6% of all intracranial tumors.[90] These benign tumors originate from nonneuroepithelial progenitor cells, the arachnoid cap cells of the leptomeninges that are imbedded in arachnoid villi of the skull vault and base. Though most common in the parasagittal area, meningiomas may arise anywhere in the skull, including the falx, cavernous sinus, tuberculum sellae, lamina cribrosa, foramen magnum, and torcular zone.[129] The WHO classification system, revised in 2007, grades meningiomas as benign (I), atypical (II), and anaplastic (malignant) (III) on the basis on both histologic features and invasion of adjacent structures including brain, bone, sinus, and nerve.[130]

Most often affecting middle-aged females, meningiomas progress asymptomatically until gradual enlargement leads to mass effect, compression of adjacent structures, and intracranial hypertension. Presenting symptoms depend on the location of tumor, and focal findings may be directly related to the size and location of tumor and presence of associated hydrocephalus. Common symptoms may include pain around the location of tumor, cranial nerve deficits, seizures, dizziness, behavioral disturbances, visual impairment, and eye proptosis. Parasagittal meningiomas of the frontal lobe may lead to Jacksonian seizures of the lower limbs or headache.[129] Meningiomas of the anterior falx may present with headache and gradual personality changes with apathy and dementia.[129] Suprasellar meningiomas may be heralded by hormonal disturbances[131,132]; clinoidal meningiomas may lead to visual impairment, cranial nerve palsies, and exophthalmos,[132] while peritorcular meningiomas may present with neurologic symptoms due to compression of the occipital lobe, such as headache, occipitally localized pain, papilledema and homonymous field deficits, ataxia, dysmetria, hypotonia, and nystagmus.[133]

One of the most frequently found genetic defects of meningiomas are truncating mutations in the neurofibromatosis 2 gene (merlin) on chromosome 22q.[134] Other somatic genetic defects have been characterized as well in meningiomas of both the sporadic and neurofibromatosis type 2 (NF2)-associated types.[135] Meningiomas also elaborate a variety of soluble proteins such as the angiogenesis-promoting vascular endothelial growth factor (VEGF), which may contribute to the vascularized nature of these tumors and their prominent surrounding edema, and which may be used to predict recurrence.[136,137] Additionally, meningiomas contain estrogen and progesterone receptors, which may be connected to its increased incidence in women, its tendency to enlarge during pregnancy, and an association with breast cancer.[138]

IMAGING CHARACTERISTICS

MR is the preferred diagnostic modality for meningiomas,[139] whereas CT may be helpful in the setting of patient contraindications to MR, and its ability to demonstrate adjacent bony reaction or infiltration and intratumoral calcifications. On CT, meningiomas are well-circumscribed, unilobular, extraaxial masses with smooth borders and broad-based dural attachments. On CT, they are most commonly isodense to cortex, and enhance homogenously and strongly after contrast administration.[13] Meningiomas may exhibit a characteristic mottling in association with dural surfaces related to their hypervascularity.[129] Bony reaction including adjacent hyperosteosis can appear in up to 18%–50% of cases as well.[129,139] These tumors may also contain punctate microscopic calcifications in up to a quarter of cases and may be calcified in up to 20% of cases.[95]

Meanwhile, MR can provide the necessary detail for meningioma diagnosis and for subsequent treatment planning and prognosis (Figure 23-8). The majority of tumors are hypointense to isointense relative to normal brain tissue on T1-weighted images due to hypercellularity and low water content.[95] In contrast, they may appear isointense to hyperintense on T2-weighted images.[95] The classic "dural tail sign," the intense enhancement of the thickened dural attachment, is attributed to either reactive hyperemia, or tumor infiltration, or both, and has a reported sensitivity of 58% and specificity of 94%.[140] Additional classic features include white matter buckling (an inward bowing of the gray and white matter junction), the presence of a "pseudo-capsule" that represents the vascular flow void at the dural base of the tumor, and the presence of a CSF attenuation cleft between the cortex and meningioma that dermarcates the tumor.[139]

Imaging features that may affect the feasibility of surgical resection include enhancing tumor invasion into adjacent dura, invasion into dural venous sinuses, and degree of associated peritumoral edema,[141] among other factors. In particular, peritumoral edema may be increased around malignant meningiomas, and thus correlated with increased risk of recurrence.[139] The correlation of preoperative T2-weighted signal intensity patterns with postoperative histologic subtypes has been attempted, with conflicting results.[17,18] If reproducible, such radiographic–pathologic insights can be used to assist interventionalists in the selection of open resection versus minimally invasive intervention and radiotherapy.

Embolization involves introduction of a microcatheter into the ECA and into the feeding dural vessels with angiography to confirm that it supplies the meningioma, followed by injection of polyvinyl alcohol (PVA) particles until stasis is achieved, followed by placement of pushable platinum coils more proximally in the feeding artery to achieve complete arterial occlusion.[139] Both during and after embolization, advanced MR perfusion with intraarterial injections may be performed.[145] The postembolization intraarterial MR perfusion studies can be used to evaluate for changes in tumor vascularity, and determine the volume of treated versus untreated tumor.

TREATMENT OF MENINGIOMAS

Close follow-up with serial imaging is possible in patients with small, asymptomatic slowly progressing meningiomas, but requires particular vigilance in younger patients who are more likely to experience more rapid tumor growth.

Meanwhile, surgical resection is preferred for meningiomas causing symptoms and can achieve a complete cure in up to 80% of cases, if the tumor is superficial and bony invasion is not present.[149] In patients who undergo gross total resection (GTR) who later experience recurrence, 12% of these cases recur within 5 years of GTR and 19% recur at 20 years.[150,151] Preoperative embolization may facilitate subsequent removal of highly vascularized tumor from adjacent tissue, and is associated with exceedingly low rates of ischemic and hemorrhagic complications[152] (Figures 23-9 and 23-10). The Simpson Criteria, a scale to evaluate completeness of resection, has been used to predict likelihood of recurrence or tumor regrowth after resection: grade I (complete removal with resection of underlying bone and associated dura) is associated with an ~9% 10-year

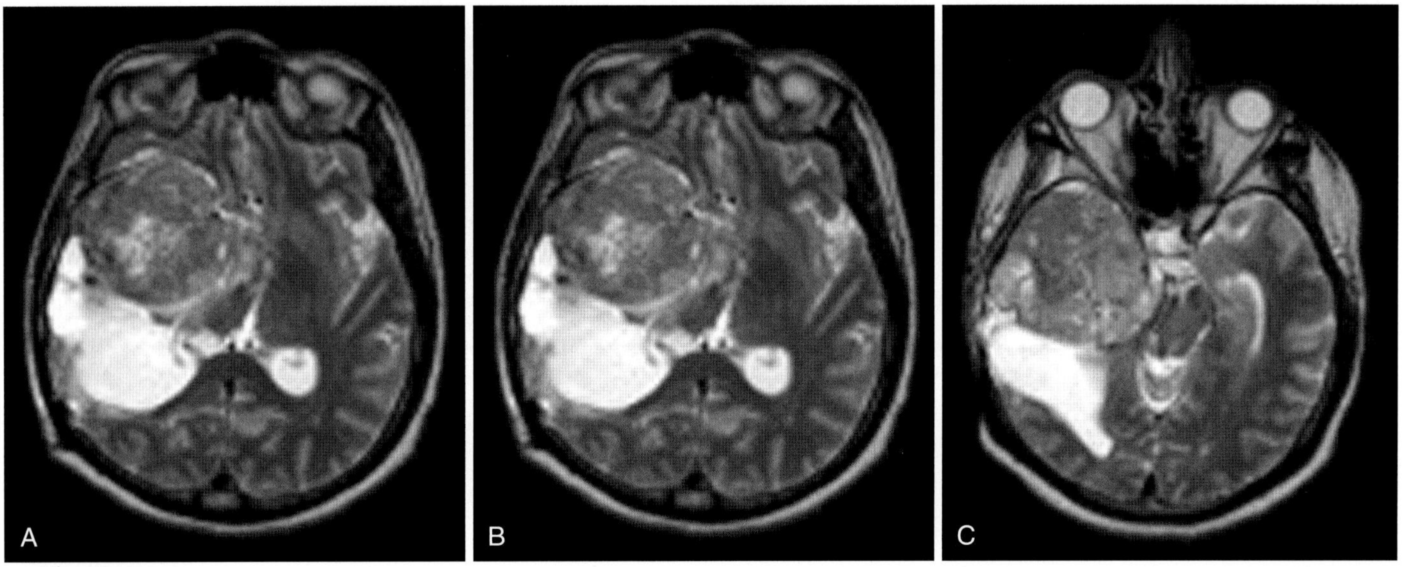

Figure 23-8 (A–C) 30-year-old man with history of recurrent right sphenoid wing meningioma, presents with facial numbness. Axial TSE T2 images demonstrating heterogeneously enhancing extraaxial mass centered in the right middle cranial fossa, likely dural based. The tumor causes mass effect on right and frontal temporal lobes, right insula, basal ganglia, and midbrain. T2 hyperintensity within the white matter is representative of vasogenic edema.

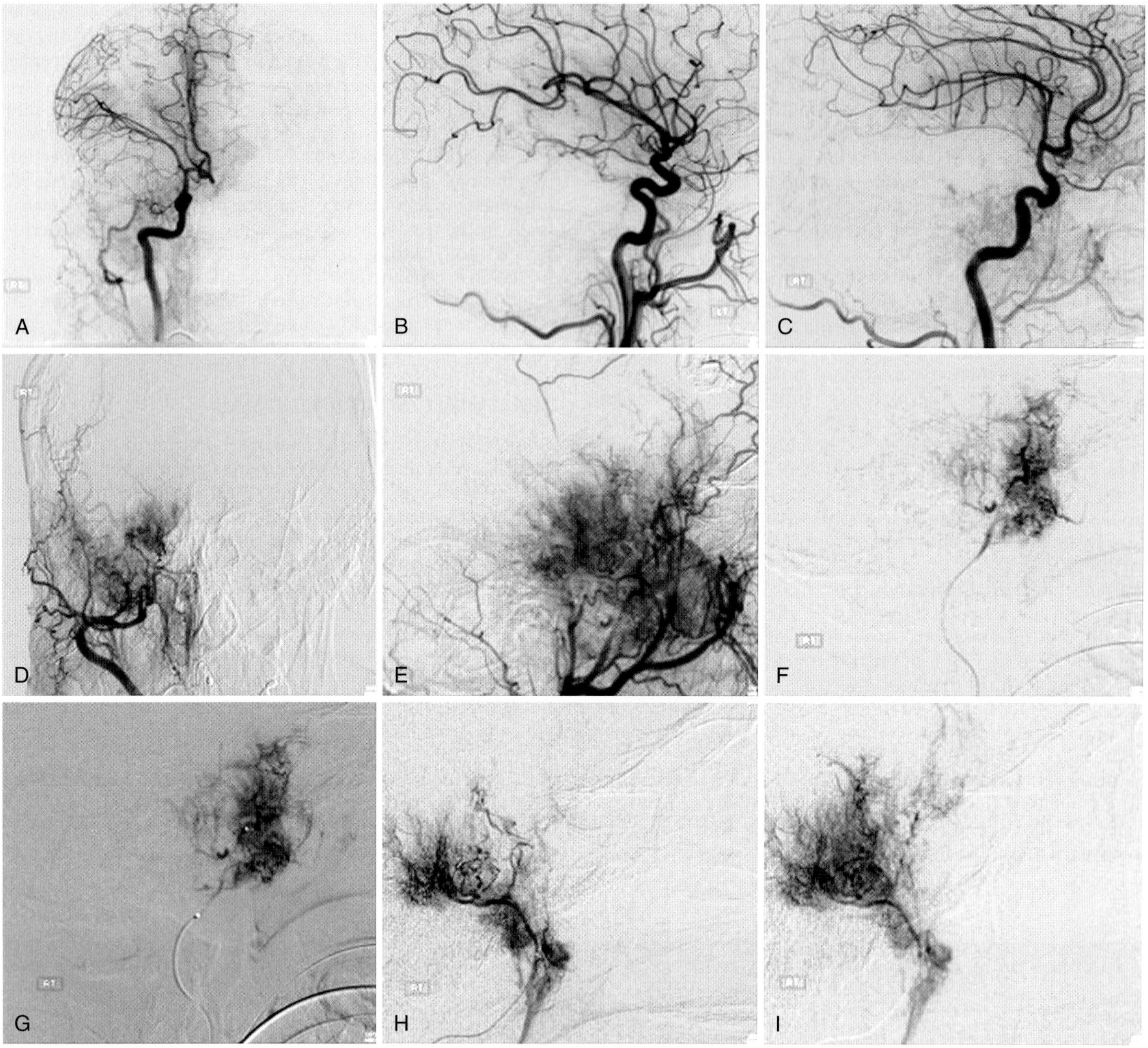

Figure 23-9 Thirty-year-old man with recurrent right sphenoid wing meningioma, postresection. Preembolization (images A–G) demonstrate tumor blush. Embolization performed of right middle meningeal artery, right accessory meningeal artery, and right middle deep temporal artery with PVA particles (150–250 μm) and coils. Postembolization (images H–M), 80%–90% of the vascular supply to the tumor has diminished. (A) Preembolization: selective angiography of right internal carotid artery injection, anteroposterior (AP) projection. (B) Preembolization: selective angiography of left common carotid artery, lateral projection. (C) Preembolization: selective angiography of right internal carotid artery, lateral projection. (D) Preembolization: selective angiography of right external carotid artery, AP projection. (E) Preembolization: selective angiography of right external carotid artery, lateral projection; dense neovascularization is present. (F) Preembolization: superselective angiography of right accessory meningeal artery, lateral projection; tumor blush is present. (G) Preembolization: superselective angiography of right accessory meningeal artery, lateral projection. (H) Postembolization: superselective angiography of right middle deep temporal artery, lateral projection. (I) Postembolization: superselective angiography of right middle deep temporal artery, lateral projection.

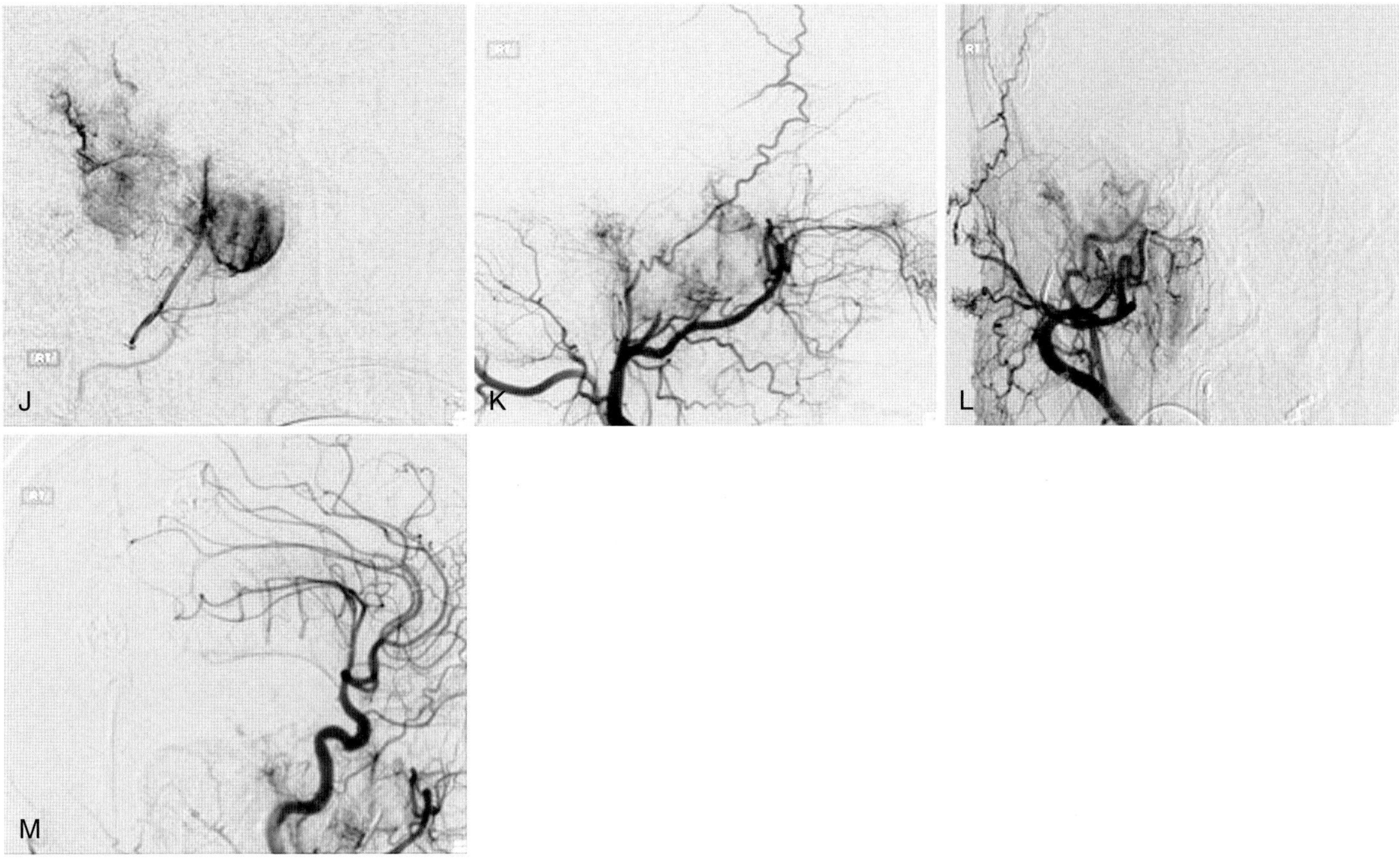

Figure 23-9, cont'd (J) Postembolization: superselective angiography of right middle deep temporal artery, lateral projection. (K) Postembolization: selective angiography of right external carotid artery, lateral projection; reduced tumor blush is present. (L) Postembolization: selective angiography of right external carotid artery injection, AP projection; reduced tumor blush, with coils in place. (M) Postembolization: selective angiography of right common carotid artery, lateral projection.

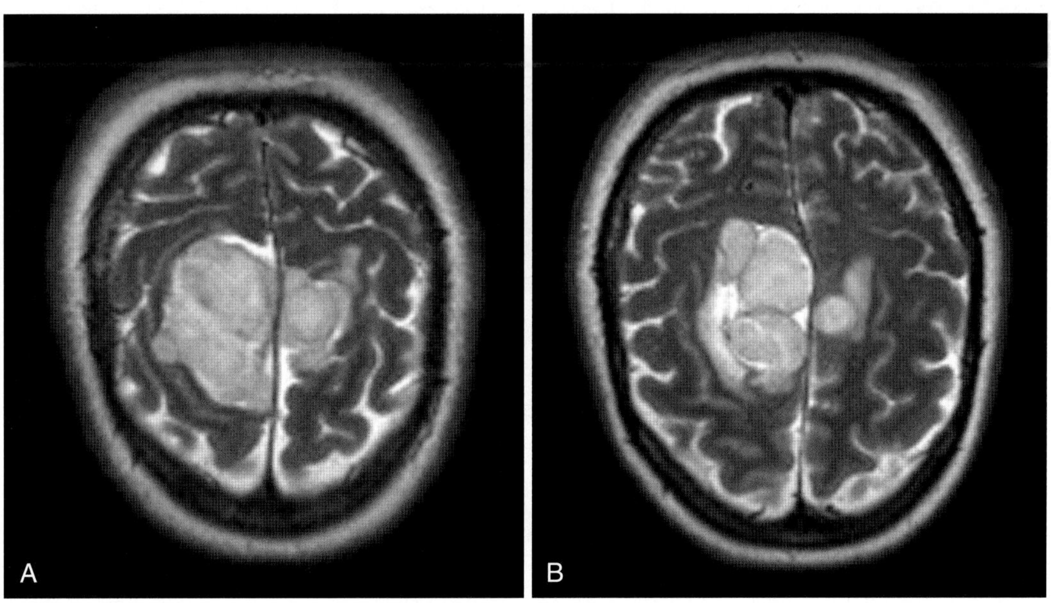

Figure 23-10 (A, B) 51-year-old woman with new-onset seizures. Axial TSE T2-weighted images demonstrate large lobulated tumor originating from the falx, extending bilaterally without significant ventricular shift. Findings are consistent with meningioma. 51-year-old woman with large bilateral falcine dural based meningioma, invading the superior sagittal sinus. Embolization was performed with 2:1 glue mixture of *n*-BCA and Ethiodol, injected into right and left middle meningeal arteries.

Continued

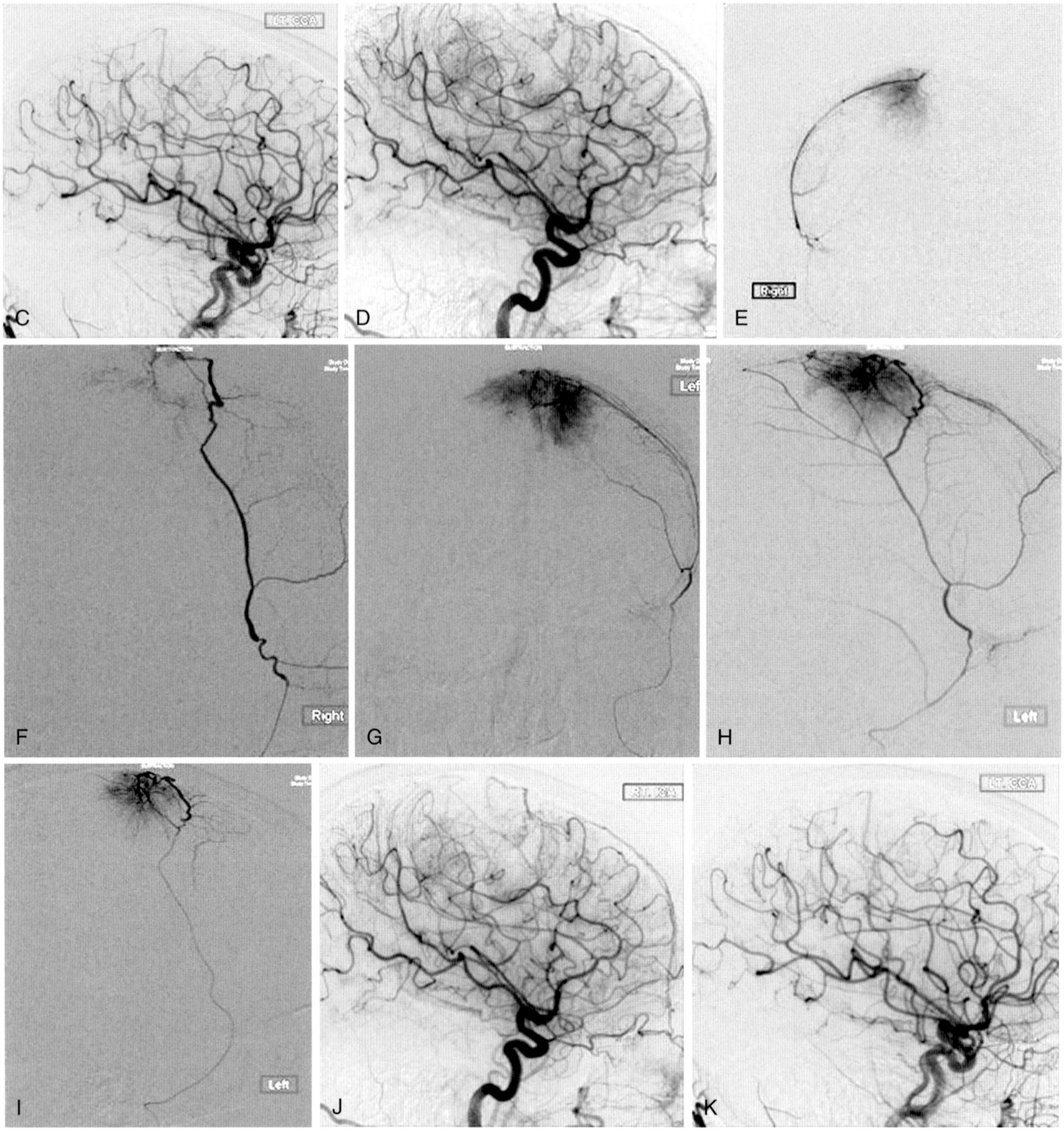

Figure 23-10, cont'd Images (C) and (D) display preembolization vascular anatomy. Images (E)–(I) demonstrate superselective microcatheter angiography with tumor blush. Images (J) and (K) are postembolization, demonstrating reduced tumor vascularity. (C) Preembolization: selective angiography of left common carotid artery, lateral view. (D) Preembolization: selective angiography of right internal carotid artery, lateral view. (E) Embolization: superselective angiography of right middle meningeal artery, anteroposterior (AP) view. (F) Embolization: superselective angiography of right middle meningeal artery, lateral view. (G) Embolization: superselective angiography of left middle meningeal artery, AP view. (H) Embolization: superselective angiography of left middle meningeal artery, lateral view. (I) Embolization: superselective angiography of left middle meningeal artery, lateral view. (J) Postembolization: selective angiography of right internal carotid artery, lateral view. No significant residual tumor blush. (K) Postembolization: selective angiography of left common carotid artery, lateral view. No significant residual tumor blush.

recurrence; grade II (complete removal with coagulation of dural attachments) is associated with ~19% 10-year recurrence; grade III (complete removal without dural resection or coagulation) is associated with ~29% 10-year recurrence; and grade IV (subtotal resection) is associated with ~40% 10-year recurrence rate.[129]

The addition of postoperative irradiation to surgery, particularly for grade II and higher tumors, can improve progression-free survival, achieving 5-year recurrence rates comparable to those of complete surgical resection, and improving local control in around 80%–90% cases.[129] Recurrence-free survival for patients undergoing such multimodal therapy results can be as high as 97% at 5 years and 96% at 10 years.[153] Stereotactic radiation such as gamma knife radiosurgery (GKS) may be offered as primary treatment for atypical, malignant, or recurrent meningioma, and may be particularly well suited in certain patients with tumors that are well-circumscribed and smaller than 3 cm and/or inaccessible for surgery (such as cavernous sinus meningiomas and petroclival meningiomas). A recent summary of radiosurgical outcomes for meningiomas noted a tumor control rate of >90% in nearly all case series, and a complication rate of <5% with doses <15 Gy.[129]

Systemic treatment with chemotherapy or hormonal therapies such as Mifepristone and chemotherapies for unresectable meningiomas has achieved varying degrees of success. For example, Mifepristone did not confer a dramatic survival advantage to the patients treated for meningioma palliation, and also caused significant rates of endometrial hyperplasia and may induce hypothyroidism.[154] Similarly, in vitro and in vivo efficacy for hydroxyurea and combination therapies such as Adriamycin and dacarbazine varies, alongside significant side effects.[155-157] Bevacizumab treatment has been attempted given the observation of VEGF expression in these tumors, and led to the reduction in the size of an anaplastic meningioma.[158]

Because the majority of meningiomas are benign WHO grade I with a 5-year recurrence rate of 7%–22% after gross total resection[129] and a median time to recurrence of 7.5 years,[159] surveillance MR may be conducted 3 months after resection or radiotherapy, followed by imaging every 6 months for the next 2 years, and then annually in stable patients. In the small fraction of cases with atypical meningioma with 5-year recurrence reported in the range of 29%–40%[129] and a median time to recurrence reported as 2.4 years,[159] control MRIs should be scheduled as frequently as every 3 months during the first year, and may later be modeled on the same routine as for benign meningiomas once radiographic stability is verified. For anaplastic meningiomas with a reported 5-year recurrence of up to 78%[159] and a median time to recurrence around 3.5 years,[159] follow-up may be as frequent as every 3–6 months for the first year, and subsequently spaced out as appropriate pending clinical stability.

INTERVENTIONAL MANAGEMENT OF MENINGIOMA

The embolization of meningiomas is well established to obliterate tumor blood supply prior to surgical resection. This has been shown to reduced postoperative bleeding, shorten resection time, and reduce postoperative complications.[160] The embolization of meningiomas at the skull base is particularly important as management of bleeding in this area during surgery is a challenge.[161] Intraarterial MR perfusion can be used to identify the specific arterial branch supplying a tumor, as there would be unwanted effects from embolization of a vessel that supplies both tumor and normal tissue.

Dynamic susceptibility contrast MR perfusion imaging with intraarterial contrast administration was found to be more useful than conventional angiography in five patients undergoing preoperative embolization.[145] Results showed significant differences in the portion of the tumor fed by a specific artery based on conventional angiographic findings and MR perfusion findings. Additionally, only very low gadolinium contrast doses were necessary because of intraarterial delivery (1/10th of original strength). MR perfusion assessed tissue fed by selected arteries and clearly demonstrated treated and untreated portions of the tumor after embolization. In some cases, MR depicted residual postembolization enhancement that could not be appreciated by conventional angiography.

In a report of 17 years' experience in 63 patients of success with preoperative embolization of intracranial meningiomas, total or subtotal devascularization was achieved in 60% of patients and partial devascularization was achieved in the remaining 40%.[162] Reasons for partial devascularization were described as (1) if the other feeding arteries would easily be accessible surgically, (2) the feeding arteries were inaccessible for a microcatheter approach, (3) the risk of unsafe embolization or reflux of embolization material was high. Complications over the 17 years included 1 death and 2 permanent disabilities, but these were between 1982 and 1989 using techniques that are no longer up to the current standard.

Certain risks accompany the embolization of meningiomas. Patients with meningioma whose tumor-feeding arteries run posteromedially toward the petrous apex or cavernous have been identified as increased risk of cranial nerve palsy after embolization with cellulose porous beads.[163] Embolization of meningiomas supplied by the ophthalmic artery are high risk because of the complication of interrupted retinal artery blood flow leading to retinal ischemia and visual compromise. In a report using ethylvinyl alcohol polymer (Onyx) over particles or spheres for more controlled embolization, all cases had preservation of ophthalmic artery retinal branches.[164] No hemorrhages or thromboembolic complications occurred. One patient with a lesser sphenoid wing lesion experienced oculomotor nerve palsy after embolization. This was secondary to bleeding, and it resolved with surgery.

Minimally Invasive Treatments

The standard therapies for brain tumors are surgical resection, radiation therapy, and chemotherapy. Whole brain radiation therapy in metastatic brain tumors has been reported to increase survival by only 4–6 months, hence the drive for new treatment options and active enrollment of patients in clinical trails.[165] Thermal ablation techniques can provide an alternative noninvasive approach. Embolization is performed preoperatively to reduce blood loss and improve surgical outcomes, or as palliation in nonsurgical candidates. Endovascular treatment approaches to glioma and retinoblastoma are areas of continuing investigation, but do not yet have an accepted clinical role as in the management of meningiomas.

RADIOFREQUENCY ABLATION

Radiofrequency ablation uses thermal energy to destroy cells, allowing scope for its use in the management of brain tumors. The mechanism of cell death is postulated to be the denaturation of the protein membrane cytoskeleton, destruction of DNA replication, the altered passage of ions (calcium/potassium), and water out of the cell resulting in coagulative necrosis.[166] The technique uses a high-frequency alternating electric current through an electrode to provide thermal energy to surrounding local tissue. Thermal energy is generated from the frictional movement of electrons in the alternating electric current. The temperature generated around the electrode tip is proportional to the square of the RF current, which in turn decreases as the square of the distance from the electrode.[167] Temperatures between 42°C and 50°C are required for cell death[166]; however, now target temperatures of up to 100°C are used to accelerate the formation of necrotic tumor debris.[168] Imaging is used to localize the tumor and monitor the ablation process. The signal intensity of an ablated lesion is similar to the appearance of intracranial hemorrhage.[169] The minimally invasive nature of this technique, short treatment time, and ability to treat unresectable and recurrent tumors are advantages. Limitations are as follows: ablation of tumors next to blood vessels is a challenge as flowing blood carries heat away and the maximum area that can be ablated at a time is restricted in size with the current equipment. Factors for limited radiofrequency lesion size include current intensity, tip temperature, duration of radio frequency application, size of electrode, and tissue properties.[170,171]

MR-guided stereotactic radiofrequency ablation has been successful in a sample of 12 patients with primary and metastatic brain tumors (adenocarcinoma, melanoma, osteosarcoma, oligodendroglioma, and glioblastoma multiforme).[172] The lesions were heated to 80°C for 10 minutes until tumor destruction. MR imaging was used for planning, during the procedure, and for follow-up at 10 months, when all tumors were found to be smaller in size.

Radiofrequency ablation has also been useful with recurrent head and neck squamous cell carcinoma, in 4 patients who were not suitable for repeat surgery or radiation.[173] Substantial reduction in tumor size and tumor-associated pain was reported, with minimal perioperative morbidity and no mortality.

In a recent study, 21 patients with recurrent and unresectable head and neck cancers who failed other therapies were offered radiofrequency ablation.[168] The end point of the study was defined as progressive disease (at least 20% increase in the maximum diameter of the target lesion) or nonprogressive disease (less than 20% increase in the maximum diameter of the target lesion). Results showed 62% of the patients who received pre- and post-procedural CT scans were found to have nonprogressive disease. An increase in quality-of-life scores in 8 of 11 patients was found. Two major life-threatening adverse events were noted from the procedure: a carotid artery hemorrhage after 18 days resulting in death and stroke in 2 patients. Other less serious adverse events included increase in size of preexisting orocutaneous fistula, cellulitis, central venous catheter infection, and pneumonia.

LASER ABLATION

Laser-induced interstitial therapy is another minimally invasive technique that destroys tissue by thermal destruction. Image guidance can assist with catheter placement and procedure monitoring. Fiber-optic catheters carry the laser energy directly to the target tissue. Laser therapy offers speed and precision over other thermal ablation techniques.

Laser coagulation therapy has been used in two patients with recurrent glioblastomas. Areas of the tumor that received treatment showed volume reduction after therapy, whereas the areas that were not treated showed growth progression. A survival benefit of four times that of the natural history of the disease was suggested in the patients who received partial irradiation.[174] In another study, 16 patients with recurrent glioblastoma multiforme treated with laser-induced interstitial thermotherapy were found to have a median survival time of 11.2 months after laser therapy, compared to a natural history of <5 months, or with first-line chemotherapy (temozolomide) of 5.4–7.1 months.[175] The following complications were reported: neutropenia ($n = 3$), thrombocytopenia ($n = 1$), high transaminases ($n = 1$).

Similarly, four patients with cerebral metastatic lesions who failed prior treatments underwent laser therapy under local anesthesia. All patients tolerated the procedure well, and follow-up MR scans showed an initial increase in lesion volume at 7 days followed by a gradual decrease in volume over 90 days. No tumor recurrences were noted.[176] In another recent pilot study of seven patients with a total of 15 intracranial resistant metastatic tumors treated with real-time MR-guided laser-induced thermal therapy, apparent lesion volume initially increased by 2 weeks to maximum then decreased over 30 months.[177] The following complications were noted: blood suffusion without mass effect ($n = 1$), probe misplacement on bone-free posterior fossa ($n = 1$), transient increase in cerebellar syndrome resolving after 3 weeks ($n = 1$), transient aphasia resolving after 2 weeks ($n = 1$).

CRYOABLATION

Cryoablation or cryotherapy is another minimally invasive ablation technique that destroys tissue by coagulation necrosis. The process of freezing and thawing, along with reperfusion injury, leads to vasodilation and capillary leakage[178,179] and cell death. The lethal freezing temperature has been suggested as between –20°C and –30°C for most tissues.[180]

Cryoablation has distinct advantages over other thermal ablation techniques in the treatment of brain tumors. First, specific temperature sensitive pulse sequences are not necessary to monitor the volume of ablation with MR, as the region appeared almost signal free on T1- and T2-weighted images.[181] This effect is due to a change in the echogenicity, density, and relaxation time as the liquid in the tissue freezes.[182-186] Second, there is clear definition of the necrotic area in the brain.[187] Third, the cryoablation lesion size remains steady over the few days after therapy; this is not the case with thermal ablation techniques.[188] Intracranial hypertension and cerebral edema could ensue if a lesion continues to enlarge posttherapy. Finally, no evidence of scarring is known from the use of cryoablation in other medical fields.

Monitoring of cryoablation lesions allows for precision and safer technique. With the use of ultrasound, an ice front is visible around the transducer; however, acoustic shadowing limits the visibility of the region.[189] MR imaging has been used for monitoring of cryotherapy lesions in brain tissue, and has been suggested as technically feasible in selected patients. Li et al.

demonstrated cryotherapy planning and intraprocedural monitoring in six patients with cystic metastatic brain tumors, using a 0.23-T open MRI system.[181] Continuous multiplanar field echo T1-weighted images were obtained to plan the passage of the cryotherapy probe to avoid critical brain structures. Completely balanced steady-state (tru-FISP) imaging at 1-mm intervals in two perpendicular planes was conducted throughout the procedure to monitor the size of the cryotherapy lesion. Postprocedurally, T1-weighted fast-spin echo images were obtained to visualize the immediate therapeutic effect. All procedures were successful; MRI scans done at 3 and 7 days showed features of coagulation necrosis. At the 6-week MR follow-up, the lesions had decreased in size. However, one death occurred from secondary causes within 12 days of the procedure, raising concern for its safety. Two other patients suffered hyperthermia, headache, and nausea likely related to intracranial hypertension.

HIGH-INTENSITY FOCUSED ULTRASOUND

The use of high-frequency ultrasound to heat and destroy tissue has been in development since the 1950s. Primary cell death with ultrasound is also thought to be due to coagulation necrosis at temperatures above 60°C, which is linearly proportional to acoustic field intensity.[190] A secondary mechanism is tissue destruction by cavitation, by which the expansion and contraction of microbubbles in the ultrasound field cause destruction. Previously, the variable intensity of damage and unpredictable lesion shape with cavitation limited its therapeutic potential, but now there is evidence to suggest that the use of microbubbles may reduce the power required for the ablation.[191]

A few hurdles exist to ablation of the brain by this method. First, the ultrasound beam is defocused by the skull bone. Second, high acoustic power is required to overcome attenuation losses, which results in local overheating. It is often difficult to quantify the exact focal temperature rise in tissue due to inhomogeneous tissue structures, creating the need for procedural monitoring with other modalities (e.g., MRI). Focused ultrasound has other potential roles in tumor therapy: the occlusion of blood vessels, activation of antitumor agents, enhancement of transgene expression, induction of cell apoptosis, and opening of the blood–brain barrier.[192,193]

MR-GUIDED FOCUSED ULTRASOUND SURGERY

MR-guided focused ultrasound surgery is a novel technique, which allows for direct targeting of intracranial lesions. The application of an ultrasound beam deep into tissues causes local heating by absorption of the acoustic wave, without damage to surrounding tissue. This is done with image guidance for exquisite targeting and temperature imaging.[194] MR can also be used for temperature mapping of the target lesion, and to detect the critical temperature rise at which tumor destruction occurs.[195] The interaction between the cranium and ultrasound propagation poses a challenge of local overheating; therefore, this technique has been successful only in patients with craniotomy.[196]

This technique was not successful when applied transcranially in three glioblastoma patients, even with a hemispherical transducer operating at a lower frequency.[197] Focusing of the ultrasound beam through the cranium was successful and acoustic power of 650–800 W was applied. However, the maximum temperature rise in each patient, respectively, was 42°C, 51°C, and 48°C; thus, critical thermal coagulation temperatures were not reached. Higher power could not be applied because of technical limitations of the transducer and because one patient experienced sonication-related pain at even 650 W.

In patients who underwent craniotomy 7–10 days prior to the procedure, thermocoagulation of enhancing tumor masses was successful, with changes immediately visible by contrast-enhanced T1-, T2-, and diffusion-weighted MR scans in the treated region.[196] Maximum temperature elevations of 60°C–90°C could be reached, and thermal MRI maps showed the coagulated regions clearly. However, an unfortunate complication of new hemiparesis arose in one patient, likely from a secondary focus in the midbrain from reflection of the ultrasound beam. Disadvantages are the inability to monitor the temperature of the surrounding tissue in more than three planes, and the invasive nature of this procedure.

General Principles Of Embolization

Preoperative embolization reduces blood loss during surgery, and can be palliative therapy in nonsurgical candidates.[198] Candidates for preoperative embolization are surgically treatable patients with a hypervascular head and neck or CNS tumor who will benefit from embolization for any of the following reasons: (1) to control inaccessible arterial feeders, (2) to decrease surgical morbidity by reducing blood loss, (3) to shorten the operative time, (4) to increase the chances of complete surgical resection, (5) to decrease the risk of damage to adjacent tissue, (6) to relieve intractable pain, (7) to decrease expected tumor recurrence, and (8) to allow better visualization of the surgical field and decrease overall complications.[199] Angiography can provide intricate details of vessel anatomy and relationships to neighboring blood vessels that is critical for procedure planning. Imaging (e.g., MR) has a role in diagnosis, planning, monitoring the extent of devascularization during and after the procedure, and long-term follow-up tumor appearance.[145] Intraarterial chemotherapy allows higher doses of localized chemotoxic agents to be administered without associated systemic side effects. Endovascular approaches can allow disruption of the blood–brain barrier to infuse therapeutic agents and a future potential for the delivery of antibodies, nanoparticles, and gene vectors.

Embolization can be achieved with particles, liquids, and coils. Particles include polyvinyl alcohol, microspheres, and gel foam. Polyvinyl alcohol is easy to use and suitable for microvessels. Smaller particles cause capillary necrosis in the tumor bed, and larger particles embolize arterioles. Good forward flow in the vessel is necessary to carry embolic material to the tumor bed, or reflux of particles can occur into unwanted regions. Microspheres can be trisacryl gelatin or hydrogel. These are nonabsorbable, spherical embolic particles more suited for distal penetration.[200] Gel foam is water insoluble, porous, pliable, and lasts only 4–6 weeks. This material occludes vessels by promoting thrombus formation and is appropriate for hypervascular tumors.

N-Butylcyanoacrylate (NBCA) and ethylvinyl alcohol polymer (Onyx) are liquid embolic agents. NBCA is a liquid material that forms polymers in ionic and alkaline environments such as contact with blood. This agent embolizes proximal vessels rather than the tumor bed itself. Onyx, another liquid agent mixed with dimethylsulfoxide, also polymerizes on contact with blood but characteristically from the outer surface inwards. This advantage allows for longer injections in complex tortuous vessels.

Coils offer precision and control in deployment, making them ideal for larger vessels. Coils also occlude proximal vessels rather than the tumor bed itself, and are also the least likely to embolize distal venous structures. Coils may be coated with thrombogenic chemicals to act as a focus for coagulation and occlusion.

In certain situations, embolization of brain tumors can be a high-risk procedure: if external carotid artery–to–internal carotid artery anastomoses or if intratumoral shunting is present[201]; if the tumor shares blood supply with normal tissue; if the likelihood of reflux of embolic agents is high; or if vessels (e.g., pial vessels) are weak and fragile.[202,203] Pial vessels are associated with a high risk of arterial perforation and intracranial hemorrhage.[204]

Complications such as postoperative hyperthermia and localized pain are common. Manipulation of the external carotid artery can result in bradycardia from a trigeminocardia reflex,[205] which is reversible with administration of atropine. More serious complications are of neurologic sequelae from traveling emboli, and intratumoral hemorrhage. Embolizations involving the ophthalmic artery and external carotid artery have been associated with blindness and skin necrosis (via the cutaneous branches), respectively.[162,206] Transient cranial nerve palsies from interruption of the vascular supply (vasa vasorum) have also been found.[203]

Chemosurgery: Retinoblastoma

Systemic chemotherapy and radiotherapy are successful treatments of retinoblastoma, but the risks of systemic toxicity and secondary malignancies still exist. In addition, systemic chemotherapy alone may not eradicate tumors and further procedures such as thermal ablation or enucleation may be necessary. Superselective ophthalmic artery chemotherapy infusions appear promising, as chemotherapy is injected directly into the ophthalmic artery. Abramson et al.[207] have successfully injected melphalan into the ophthalmic artery in a procedure known as "chemosurgery." Other therapies have been administered by the same technique such as methotrexate and digoxin. The required dose of chemotherapy to be administered is patient specific and is based on eye size, vascular anatomy, wedge flow, clinical response and prior exposure to chemotherapy, and allergies and side effects from other treatments.[208]

This procedure is conducted under general anesthesia. Access is gained via the femoral artery and a microcatheter is passed over a guidewire to the ophthalmic artery via the internal carotid artery under fluoroscopic guidance, and superselective angiography is performed. Once the microcatheter is at the ostium of the ophthalmic artery, a small amount of chemotherapy drug mixed with normal saline is manually injected in pulses. After the drug is delivered, the catheter is removed.

In 2008, a phase I/II study of direct ophthalmic artery chemotherapy infusion for retinoblastoma was published.[207] Ten children with retinoblastoma (Reese–Ellsworth group V) received treatment with melphalan infusion (and carboplatin was administered in two patients) for 30 minutes via the ophthalmic artery. Four patients had received some form of prior therapy and all 10 patients were scheduled for enucleation. The patients were followed for a mean period of 8.8 months, with ophthalmic examinations, retinal photography, and electroretinograms to monitor local toxicity. Physical examinations and complete blood count examinations monitored for systemic toxicity. Nine of 10 patients were successfully catheterized; 27 total infusions were given to the 9 patients. Every case resulted in tumor regression after chemotherapy treatment. Several complications were noted: transient lid edema ($n = 3$), transient conjunctival hyperemia ($n = 3$), radiation-like retinopathy ($n = 1$), and retinal ischemia ($n = 1$). Three patients proceeded to enucleation secondary to unsuccessful cannulation ($n = 1$) and suspected continued tumor activity ($n = 2$). One patient developed neutropenia but no fevers/strokes/deaths were noted.

In 2010, a prospective trial of high concentration ophthalmic artery chemotherapy infusion as first-line treatment was published.[209] Twenty-three patients (Reese–Ellsworth group V) were treated with various combinations of drugs: melphalan ($n = 12$), melphalan and topotecan ($n = 7$), melphalan and topotecan and carboplatin ($n = 3$), and melphalan and carboplatin ($n = 1$). Twenty-eight eyes were treated over 6 months, one patient eventually had enucleation due to progressive disease. Local complications found were transient lid edema, forehead hyperemia, and loss of nasal lashes. Neutropenia was noted in six patients over 10 cycles.

This research group also studied the effect of ophthalmic artery chemotherapy infusion into both eyes simultaneously in four patients with bilateral retinoblastomas (Reese–Ellsworth group V).[210] The catheter was advanced into the ophthalmic artery of one eye, retracted back to the aorta, and then passed to the internal carotid and ophthalmic artery on the other side. The patients also received treatment with laser hyperthermia or cryotherapy. Two patients received melphalan and two patients received melphalan plus topotecan. All tumors showed reduction in size at 3-week assessment. One patient developed grade 3 neutropenia with three infusions of melphalan.

General Principles of Intraarterial Chemotherapy

Intraarterial delivery techniques increase the efficacy of chemotherapy.[211] Dose concentrations of up to five times higher with hydrosoluble drugs and up to 50 times higher with lipid-soluble drugs can be achieved by intraarterial over systemic chemotherapy[212,213] Intraarterial chemotherapy is associated with risks of increased neurotoxicity. This may arise from "streaming," in which the drug remains an aggregate and deposits heterogeneously in the target vascular therapy, or because of untailored drug doses previously intended for use in the whole body as the distribution compartment.[214]

The blood–brain barrier restricts the movement of ions with molecular weight greater than 180 Da. This poses a challenge to the passage of chemotherapeutic drugs, and strategies to overcome its barrier are often considered. In the Sherbrooke experience,[215] a published report from a phase II trial, patients with gliomas, primitive neuroectodermal tumors, primary CNS lymphomas, and metastatic disease to the brain were studied with intraarterial chemotherapy infusion after blood–brain barrier disruption with mannitol. The overall mean survival time from start of treatment was 9.1 months for glioblastoma multiforme, 13.9 months for anaplastic oligodendrogliomas, unreached for primary CNS lymphomas and 9.9 months for metastases and time to disease progression was 4.1, 9.2, 12.3, and 3.3 months, respectively. The mean survival time from diagnosis for glioblastoma multiforme was 32.2 months. Complications from this study include thrombocytopenia, neutropenia, preprocedural seizures in 5% of patients, postinfusion orbital myositis, and carotid thrombosis.

GLIOMAS: INTRAARTERIAL CHEMOTHERAPY WITH BEVACIZUMAB

Bevacizumab (Avastin), a monoclonal antibody that binds to VEGF and prolongs survival in recurrent malignant glioma.[216] However, its systemic effects of bowel perforation, pulmonary embolism, poor wound healing, and limited delivery through the blood–brain barrier limit its use of bevacizumab. Superselective intraarterial delivery of bevacizumab has overcome these barriers, with reported improvement in the appearance of gadolinium enhancement after 3 weeks of intraarterial therapy.

The response of intraarterial bevacizumab after disruption of the blood–brain barrier with mannitol has been studied, in patients naïve to prior chemotherapy and those with prior exposure to intravenous bevacizumab.[217] Patients who were naïve had a 34.7% reduction in area of tumor enhancement compared to 15.2% in patients with prior exposure. Naïve patients had a 46.9% reduction in volume of tumor enhancement, compared to 8.3% in those with prior exposure. Patients who were naïve had a 32.14% reduction in MR perfusion compared to 25.5% reduction in patients with prior exposure. Patients who were naïve had a signal decrease in T2-weighted/FLAIR signal compared to no signal change in patients who had a prior exposure. Overall toxicity from intraarterial bevacizumab was said to be similar to that of intravenous bevacizumab. No cases of intratumoral hemorrhage were found; however, there were several reports of morbidity. During the treatment, two patients experienced seizures; however, they were known to have seizure disorders. One patient developed an acneiform rash. Another patient with history of pulmonary embolus 5 months prior developed respiratory distress requiring intubation, and a different patient with a history of lower extremity thrombus returned with pulmonary embolus after 1 day of treatment. A stroke did occur in a patient after balloon insufflation caused rupture to a distal anterior cerebral vessel. This was immediately treated with coils and embolic glue, an immediate CT scan showed subarachnoid hemorrhage with intraventricular hemorrhage and ventriculomegaly, for which an external ventricular drain was placed. No deaths were reported from this study.

In a study by Medajewicz et al.,[218] patients who received intraarterial cisplatin and etoposide prior to radiation therapy rather than in those who received simultaneous chemotherapy and radiation therapy. A significant tumor response and survival benefit was noted in the patients who received intraarterial chemotherapy prior to radiation therapy than in those who received simultaneous treatment.

Pitfalls in Assessing Response

PSEUDOPROGRESSION

Pseudoprogression is defined as an increase in edema or contrast enhancement of a lesion, following treatment with radiation with or without chemotherapy, which does not represent active disease.[219] Serial MRI suggests pseudoprogression if the edema and contrast enhancement wax and wane without other changes in treatment. Pseudoprogression poses a significant problem for clinicians.[220] Changing treatment in response to pseudoprogression may deny a patient continued treatment with an effective therapy. By understanding factors that can lead to pseudoprogression, clinicians can more easily identify pseudoprogression and manage patients more effectively.

Pseudoprogression represents local inflammatory changes and changes in blood–brain barrier permeability, leading to increased enhancement and edema. It is associated with the addition of concurrent chemotherapy to radiation, as noted above in the Stupp regimen in glioblastoma. It is associated with favorable prognostic molecular markers, such as MGMT methylation and thus is actually prognostic for a good response to treatment.[221] Pseudoprogression usually occurs in the first few months following treatment with radiation and chemotherapy, and improves with time. Most cases do not develop additional neurologic symptoms. Clinical management is to continue treatment through the duration of pseudoprogression. Corticosteroids and bevacizumab are helpful in treating symptomatic lesions until the underlying edema improves.

This is in contrast to postradiation necrosis, which usually occurs later, sometimes more than a year after radiation treatment. Postradiation necrosis is associated with higher doses of radiation, hypofractionated radiotherapy, reirradiation, and stereotactic radiotherapy. Postradiation necrosis causes similar changes on MRI and may lead to edema and mass effect, and possible additional surgery.[222]

PSEUDORESPONSE

Pseudoresponse is a rapid and fairly extensive decrease in contrast enhancement in malignant gliomas following the initiation of bevacizumab therapy.[220] Bevacizumab is a VEGF antibody. It targets angiogenesis and stabilizes the blood–brain barrier. This leads to a rapid improvement in tumoral contrast enhancement on standard MRI. This rapid improvement can be seen on imaging after a single intravenous dose of bevacizumab. The administration of bevacizumab can also decrease edema and mass effect, decrease corticosteroid need, and improve clinical function and overall quality of life. However, the benefits do not translate into a significant improvement in overall survival. The radiographic response is considered a pseudoresponse because there may be a decrease in the extent of contrast enhancement (which is typically used as a surrogate for tumor size), while the underlying tumor burden remains unchanged. Although bevacizumab causes a rapid decline in the contrast-enhancing tumor, this is often accompanied by a gradual increase in non-contrast-enhancing tumor, as seen on the T2-weighted images.[223] This creates particular difficulty for the clinician in assessing response to therapy.

QUANTIFICATION OF TREATMENT RESPONSE

The quantification of treatment response is often performed using anatomic MRI or CT, although there is increased interest in more advanced imaging as surrogates for treatment response. Most commonly, the Macdonald criteria[224] are used to assess initial response (and failure) of cytotoxic treatment regimens. The Macdonald criteria[224] describe four states of tumor response: complete response (CR), partial response (PR), stable disease (SD), or progressive disease (PD).

These classifications are delineated based on the relative percentage change in bidirectional tumor measurements before and during treatment. Bidirectional measurements are defined as the product of two measurements consisting of a primary measurement along the largest extent of contrast-enhancing tumor in any orthogonal plane (sagittal, axial, or coronal) and a secondary perpendicular measurement to this primary measurement. These scan changes on MRI or CT must also take into consideration any change in corticosteroid dose, which may change the size and features of the lesion, as well as any neurologic changes that may signify disease progression even without concurrent changes on MRI or CT. Table 23-2 briefly summarizes the Macdonald response criteria.

The advent of antiangiogenic drugs, including bevacizumab, as therapeutic agents typically results in dramatic decreases in both contrast enhancement on postcontrast T1-weighted images as well as reduction in peritumoral edema.[225-229] This reduction in enhancement and edema, which could be considered a partial to complete response in some cases according to the Macdonald criteria, is due to reduction in blood–brain barrier permeability and is not thought to be a direct result of tumor destruction. As such, new criteria were established to encompass these new changes observed on MRI termed the *Response Assessment in Neuro-Oncology*, or *RANO, Criteria*.[230] The major modification proposed by the RANO guidelines is the evaluation of changes in FLAIR signal intensity as evidence of nonenhancing, infiltrative tumor growth. Of course, many new challenges have arisen in the operational use of the RANO criteria. For example, a change in FLAIR signal intensity may indicate changes in peritumoral edema without apparent changes in nonenhancing tumor. Further, the ability to measure subtle changes in nonenhancing tumor is challenging, along with combining information from enhancing and nonenhancing tumor.

TABLE 23-2 Macdonald Response Criteria[224]

Response Assessment	MR Features	Other Criteria
CR, Complete response	Disappearance of enhancing tumor (>1 month from last scan)	Neurologically stable or improved. Off Steroids.
PR, Partial response	≥50% decrease in bidirectional product	Neurologically stable/ improved. Steroids stable/reduced.
PD, Progressing disease	≥25% increase in bidirectional product	Neurologically worse. Steroids stable/ increased.
SD, Stable disease	All other situations	

From Macdonald DR, Cascino TL, Schold SC Jr, Cairncross JG: Response criteria for phase II studies of supratentorial malignant glioma, *J Clin Oncol* 8(7):1277–1280, 1990.

Although practical implementation of RANO is an ongoing discussion,[231] the RANO criteria appear to be an important advance in the clinical assessment of brain tumor response because it acknowledges the importance of nonenhancing tumor as it relates to patient outcome.

Acknowledgments

The authors would like to thank Dr. Stephanie Lee Jia Chih for her assistance with some sections of this chapter.

REFERENCES

The complete reference list is available online at www.expertconsult.com.

PART

5

Thoracic Oncology

STEPHEN T. KEE

24 Primary Lung Carcinoma

SCOTT GENSHAFT | FEREIDOUN ABTIN

KEY POINTS

- Thermal ablation is a proven method for treatment of early-stage non–small cell lung carcinoma for patients who are medically inoperable.
- Basic approaches to lung biopsy and ablation are similar.
- The risks of lung intervention include pneumothorax, hemorrhage, and air embolism.

Introduction

Lung cancer is the leading cause of cancer-related death in the United States for both men and women. Using data acquired through the North American Association of Central Cancer Registries (NAACCR), in 2012, an estimated 226,160 Americans will be diagnosed with lung cancer, and 160,340 people will die of the disease.[1] The 5-year survival rate of all lung cancers is 15.7%, based on data acquired from 1995 to 2001.[2] Primary lung cancer is classified as either non–small cell lung cancer (NSCLC) or small cell lung cancer (SCLC). Non–small cell lung cancer accounts for 87% of cases.

Smoking is implicated in up to 90% cases of primary lung cancer.[3] Other causes include environmental exposures (i.e., air pollution), occupational exposures (i.e., asbestos), pulmonary fibrosis, and exposure to ionizing radiation (i.e., radon). It is generally believed that genetic factors play a role in determining a patient's risk for ultimately developing cancer. This is supported by evidence that cancer may cluster in individual families.[4,5] Lung cancer is up to four times more common in Asian Americans in comparison to White Americans.[6] Epidermal growth factor (EGFR) mutations are common in the lung cancers of East Asians, particularly in those without a smoking history.[7]

Percutaneous thermal ablation of primary lung neoplasms, in the form of radiofrequency ablation (RFA), microwave ablation (MWA), and percutaneous cryoablation therapy (PCT), has emerged as viable alternative to surgical resection for patients with early stage disease who have medical comorbidities that put them at an increased operative risk. Interventional radiologists play a vital role in the multidisciplinary team through detection, tissue diagnosis, treatment, and posttherapeutic follow-up. This chapter will provide a basic overview of lung cancer staging, treatment options, thoracic interventional techniques, and imaging follow-up.

Staging

Lung cancers are divided into non–small cell and small cell cancer based on histology and immunohistochemistry. Both cancers are staged according to the 7th edition of the International Association for the Study of Lung Cancer (IASLC).[8,9] There are considerable differences in the treatment of these two subtypes of bronchogenic carcinoma. Treatment within each category is largely based on stage of disease. Table 24-1 provides a schematic for lung cancer staging. This chapter will primarily focus on treatment options for NSCLC.

Stage I and II tumors are considered early stage, and potentially curably through surgical resection. The 5-year survival rates for stage I and II NSCLC are 60%–80% and 40%–50%, respectively. In stage III disease, 5-year survival is 14% (IIIa) and 5% (IIIb). Stage IV lung cancer has a dismal prognosis, with 5-year survival of approximately 1%.[10]

Treatment Options

All interventional radiologists must have a working knowledge of the treatment options available to patients with NSCLC in order to be a productive member of the multidisciplinary lung cancer team. The traditional treatment for early-stage lung cancer has been resection, whereas chemotherapy and radiation have been primarily used for advanced-stage disease. Thermal ablation has proven useful in the treatment of patients with early-stage lung cancer, with a medical contraindication to resection, or in a growing population of patients who refuse resection. It is common for patients referred for thermal ablation to have previously undergone one or more of these treatments. In patients who cannot tolerate resection, ablation allows a less invasive tumor treatment, with objectives including size reduction and potential cure.[11]

SURGERY

Surgical resection is potentially curative and is the primary therapy for patients with stage I, II, and some IIIa NSCLC, who can tolerate a pneumonectomy or lobectomy. The standard practice for treatment of early-stage lung cancer has been lobectomy and lymph node dissection. This treatment has been shown to provide long-term disease-free survival.

Debate exists as to the extent of resection that is necessary for the treatment of stage Ia disease, with some now favoring a sublobar resection to preserve lung capacity. Multiple single-center studies have suggested no survival benefit for lobectomy in comparison to segmentectomy or wedge resection.[12,13] These findings are in contradistinction to the results of the Lung Cancer Study Group, which demonstrated a threefold increased incidence of local disease recurrence and 50% increased mortality for patients treated with sublobar resection in comparison to patients treated with lobectomy for stage Ia disease.[14-16] Brachytherapy has been shown to decrease the rate of locally recurrent disease after sublobar resection.[14]

Unfortunately, only one-third of patients with stage I or II NSCLC tumors are eligible for resection on the basis of pulmonary function tests. In patients who cannot tolerate resection thermal ablation, it has a role to achieve localized control and cure of disease.

TABLE 24-1 Staging of Lung Cancer

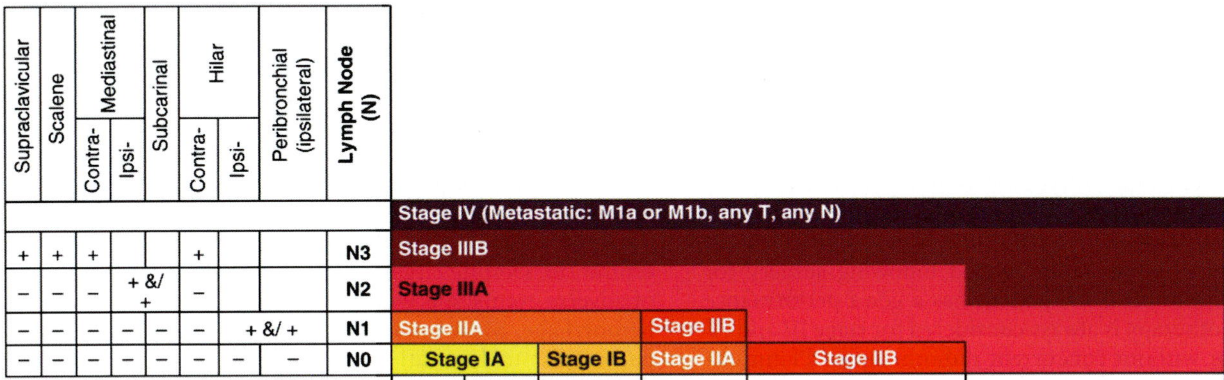

	T1a	T1b	T2a	T2b	T3	T4	Primary Tumor (T)
	≤2cm	>2cm but ≤3cm	>3cm but ≤5cm	>5cm but ≤7cm	>7cm	Any	a. Size
	No invasion proximal to lobar bronchus		Main bronchus (≥2cm distal to the carina)		Main bronchus (<2cm distal to the carina)	–	b. Endo-bronchial location
	Surrounded by lung or visceral pleura		Visceral pleura		Chest wall/diaphragm/ mediastinal pleura/ parietal pericardium	Mediastinum/trachea/heart/ great vessels/esophagus/ vertebral body/carina	c. Local Invasion
			Atelectasis/obstructive pneumonitis that extends to the hilar region but does not involve the entire lung		Atelectasis/obstructive pneumonitis of entire lung; separate tumor nodule(s) in ipsilateral primary tumor lobe	Separate tumor nodule(s) within the ipsilateral lung but different lobe as the primary mass	d. Other

Metastatic (M):

M1a:
Local intrathoracic spread:
- Malignant pleural/pericardial effusion
- Separate tumor nodule(s) in the contralateral lung

M1b:
Disseminated (extrathoracic) disease:
Liver, bone, brain, adrenal gland, etc.

UyBico S J et al. Radiographics 2010;30:1163-1181

From UyBico SJ, Wu CC, Suh RD, Le NH, Brown K, Krishnam MS: Lung cancer staging essentials: the new TNM staging system and potential imaging pitfalls, *Radiographics* 30:1163–1181, 2010.

Stage IIIa disease is treated with a combination of chemotherapy, radiotherapy, and surgery, whereas stage IIIb and stage IV cancers are treated with chemotherapy or radiotherapy without resection.

RADIATION

Although conventional radiotherapy has traditionally been associated with poor local control of disease and a high rate of radiation-associated toxicity,[17,18] the advent of stereotactic body radiation therapy (SBRT) has increased the role of radiation oncology in the treatment of NSCLC. Stage I and II lung cancers are now viewed by many in the radiation oncology community as curable disease. Timmerman et al. studied patients with medically inoperable stage I and II lung cancers treated with SBRT and demonstrated 87% locoregional control of disease and disease-free survival of 48.3% at 3 years.[19] Adjuvant radiation, in contradistinction, is not indicated for surgically resected stage I or II lung cancers.

SBRT and conventional radiotherapy are routinely used to treat stage III and IV lung carcinomas, both to achieve local control and to prevent complications of the cancer, such as superior vena cava syndrome. The delivery of SBRT is effective and well tolerated by patients. Some limitations do exist, particularly when treating central tumors. Radiation toxicity, including pleural effusion, pulmonary hemorrhage, radiation pneumonitis, and pulmonary fibrosis, increases with escalating dose and, in many cases, limits the extent of treatment.

A role for combined external beam radiation or brachytherapy with thermal ablation may exist.[20-22] These studies have used postablation radiotherapy to enhance the margin of the ablation and have shown better local control of disease when combined-modality treatment is utilized. It is also possible that a radiation-first approach to combined therapy may result in a larger subsequent ablation size through radiation-induced damage to vasculature in and around the target mass, thereby relieving a degree of heat sink (the reduction in effective ablation that results from local vasculature removing heat). This approach is the subject of active study.

CHEMOTHERAPY

The past several years have yielded important advances in the chemotherapeutic management of NSCLC. The discovery that lung cancer patients with mutations in the EGFR gene have a treatment response to certain tyrosine kinase inhibitors has signaled the dawn of targeted chemotherapy for lung cancer. The role for chemotherapy in early-stage lung cancers is a topic of debate, whereas it remains the primary treatment for patients with advanced disease.

Mutations in the tyrosine kinase–binding domain of the EGFR gene have been found in a disproportionate number of nonsmoking, east-Asian women presenting with primary lung adenocarcinoma. These changes include base-pair deletions at exon 19 and mutations at exon 21. Patients with these mutations have responded well to tyrosine kinase inhibitors, including gefitinib and erlotinib.[7,23,24] The Spanish Lung Cancer Study Group selected patients diagnosed with adenocarcinoma $EGFR^{mut}$ and treated them with erlotinib as a first- or second-line agent. These patients had a mean survival of 24 months, in comparison to a historical mean survival of 8 months.[25]

Adjuvant chemotherapy is not indicated following resection of stage I NSCLC. It is recommended following surgery for stage II disease, provided the patient has a good performance status.[26] Chemotherapy is always considered for stage III and IV disease, with or without concurrent radiotherapy.[27] Platinum-based agents have traditionally been the mainstay of treatment.

Image-guided Interventions

Interventional radiologists have an established role in providing tissue diagnosis of lung carcinoma via percutaneous biopsy, as well as treatment of localized disease with thermal ablation. This section will provide an overview of percutaneous tissue biopsy and technical approaches to lung interventions.

PREPROCEDURE ASSESSMENT

A standard preprocedure assessment of the patient is performed, including history, physical examination, and coagulation status. A high percentage of patients undergoing lung intervention are smokers and, therefore, have comorbidities of cardiac and pulmonary disease, factors that may limit tolerance of sedation and some positions on the procedure table. All attempts should be made to optimize these factors prior to elective intervention.

Goals for factors effecting hemostasis include platelets $>70{,}000$, INR <1.5, and a partial thromboplastin time (PTT) of $<1.5\%$ control value.[28] Patients on warfarin sodium (Coumadin) who are at high risk of complications of thrombosis can be bridged with subcutaneous heparin or enoxaparin. Aspirin and clopidogrel bisulfate (Plavix) should be discontinued for 7 days prior to the procedure.

Standard labs are drawn in the preprocedure area, including complete blood count (CBC), chemistry, and coagulation factors. Some interventionalists prefer the use of a blood patch following biopsy, and 10 mL of blood is obtained in a syringe for use at the completion of the procedure to reduce the incidence of pneumothorax.

BIOPSY

The first step toward treating thoracic malignancy is to establish a pathologic diagnosis through tissue biopsy. Technical aspects of placing probes for percutaneous thermal ablation mirror that for biopsy, and therefore, it is advisable to establish good biopsy technique prior to embarking upon thermal ablation.

Despite the wide availability of fluoroscopy and CT for obtaining an image-guided biopsy, lung tissue continues to be obtained largely through surgical techniques. Based on data extrapolated from the National Lung Screening Trial (NLST), up to 50% of initial diagnostic biopsies remain surgical, despite its invasive nature and added risk of general anesthesia.[29]

Image guidance provides a less-invasive method for obtaining tissue and can typically be performed with conscious sedation. Traditionally, fluoroscopy has been used to guide a fine-needle aspiration of the target lesion. With the wide availability of CT, the majority of image-guided lung biopsies are now obtained under CT guidance. CT provides superior resolution of both the target lesion and intervening tissue, which maximizes appropriate sampling and minimizes risks, such as traversing major blood vessels and airways.

Core-needle biopsy has emerged as the preferred method of obtaining lung tissue.[30] Yao et al. established that the safety profile of lung core needle biopsy is on par with fine-needle aspiration. Despite larger needle size, there is no increased risk of adverse events, specifically with regard to pneumothorax and hemorrhage. Most importantly, core needle biopsy allows the pathologist to look at a histologically intact piece of tissue, which improves diagnostic capability and decreases the chance of both a false-negative biopsy and a repeat biopsy.[32-38]

Core-Needle Biopsy Technique

At the authors institution, after detailed informed consent is obtained, the patient is brought to the CT procedure suite and placed on the table in the anticipated position for the procedure. The patient is attached to a vital signs monitor, placed on oxygen via nasal cannula, and administered conscious sedation. A combination of low-dose narcotic (opiate) and hypnotic (benzodiazepine) is preferred. Morphine sulfate has the added benefit of suppressing the cough reflex, which is particularly helpful during lung interventions.

A focused initial CT scan is performed to identify a site of percutaneous access. The site of access is then marked with a radiopaque marker and a repeat scan is performed to ensure that the marked site is appropriate. The skin is prepped, and a sterile field is created with surgical towels.

The importance of appropriate local anesthesia cannot be emphasized enough. Although conscious sedation is typically employed, lung biopsy and ablation can on occasion be performed with only local anesthesia if the patient has a significant sedation risk. As is typical of most access sites, there are two locations with pain nerve fibers that deserve special attention—in this case, the skin and parietal pleura. These sites require adequate anesthesia prior to advancing a needle into the lung parenchyma to ensure patient comfort, cooperation, and absence of movement during the course of the procedure.

Lidocaine 1% or bupivacaine 0.25% is administered to the skin and subcutaneous soft tissues with a 25-guage hypodermic needle. Care is taken not to advance the needle into the lung tissue. A small skin nick is made with a scalpel. Under CT guidance, typically an 18 or 19-guage coaxial needle is then advanced into the extrapleural space, inside the internal thoracic fascia and at the edge of the parietal pleura. The patient will frequently complain of pain when this space is entered, because of irritation of the pleura. Following confirmation of position with CT, approximately 10 mL of local anesthetic is infused into the space, which should demonstrate a visible convex wheel with mass effect on the pleura during subsequent imaging (Figure 24-1, *A*). If the patient coughs or complains of a sour taste in the mouth during the administration of pleural anesthesia, this indicates infiltration of the lung parenchyma.

Preparation for entering the lung is completed by a repeat CT, which is used to ensure that the trajectory of the needle is on target. Once the needle is placed into the lung, very little

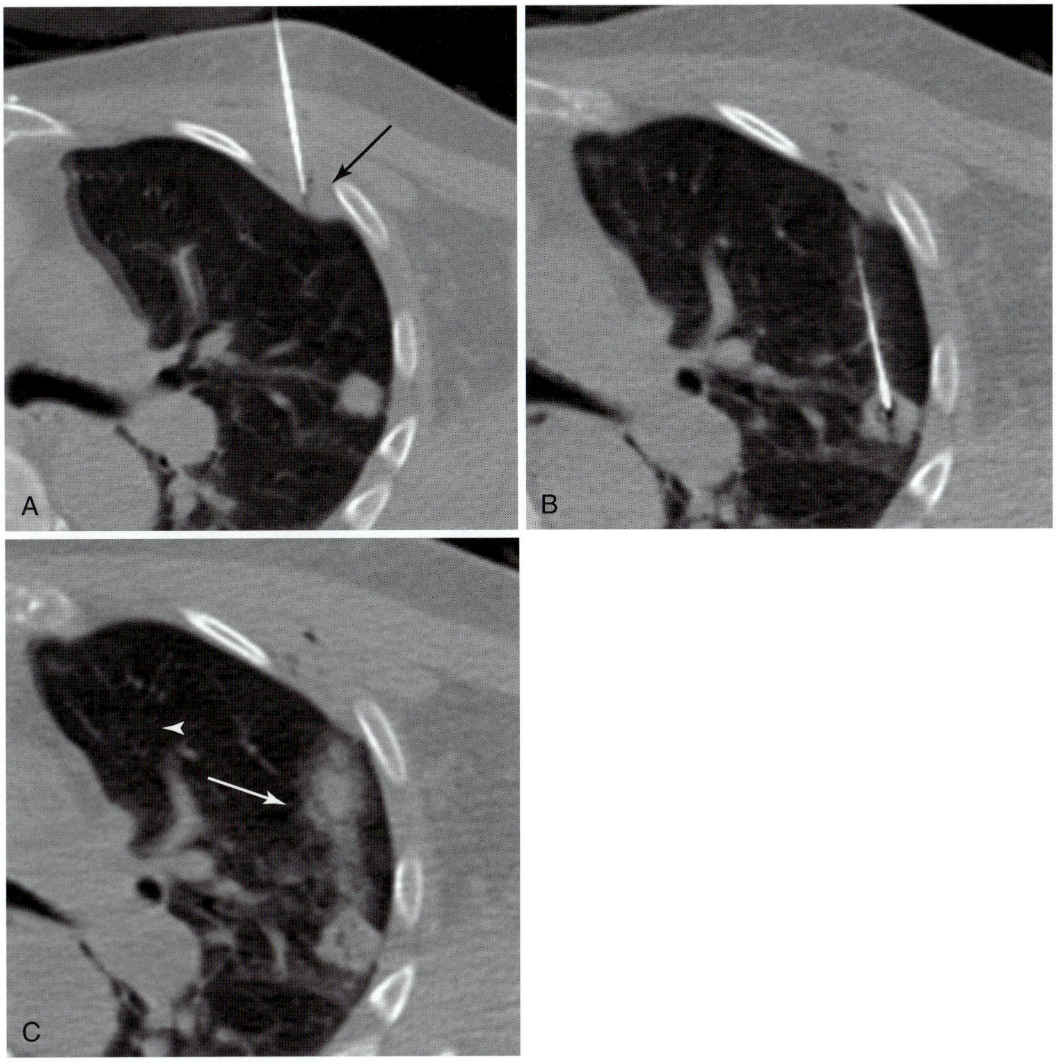

Figure 24-1 Biopsy of peripherally located left upper lobe mass. A 19-guage coaxial needle was advance beyond the internal thoracic fascia into the extrapleural space. Lidocaine was administered to achieve pleural anesthesia. A pleural wheel (*black arrow*) is present (A). The coaxial needle was then advanced into the mass using a tangential approach parallel to the pleural surface (B). On needle removal, a blood patch (*white arrow*) was placed (C).

directional correction is possible, as the density of the chest wall soft tissues maintains the needle in its extrapulmonary trajectory.

The coaxial needle is then advanced into the lung. A brisk jab should be used to traverse the pleura to ensure that the lung is appropriately entered; slower pushing movement will tend to displace the lung away and possibly result in a pneumothorax. Roughly 2 cm of lung tissue must be entered to ensure that the needle does not retract intermittently into the pleural space.

The needle is then guided into the target lesion using intermittent CT. Care is taken to avoid traversing major vascular structures and airways. Fine adjustments in needle trajectory are often required to achieve this goal. The needle is advanced to the near-edge of the target. When possible, it is advisable to imbed the needle into the target to ensure appropriate sampling (Figure 24-1, *B*). This may not be possible with small pulmonary nodules less than 6 mm in diameter.

Core biopsy samples are then obtained using a 20-gauge cutting needle placed through the outer cannula of the coaxial needle. Several samples should be obtained in order to obtain adequate tissue for a diagnosis, and therefore minimize the risk of a false-negative biopsy. In our institution, a touch imprint of the first core biopsy sample is evaluated by a cytotechnologist, who is able to confirm cellularity of the specimen. The remaining cores are then placed directly into formalin. If a lymphoproliferative disorder, most commonly lymphoma, is suspected, the cores are placed into a medium from which flow cytometry can be performed (ex RPMI [Roswell Park Memorial Institute] medium). When lymphoma is suspected, larger cores may be required. Lymphoproliferative masses requiring traversal of lung tissue for biopsy are sampled with a smaller system, as the use of larger coaxial needles has been shown to lead to a higher rate of pneumothorax.[39] Cores should be sent for culture if infection is a possibility.

As the needle is removed, a blood patch may be placed by injecting a suspension of reconstituted blood at a rate of 1 mL/cm to the level of the pleura. This blood should be obtained at the time of laboratory blood draw. The goal of the blood patch is to prevent pneumothorax by occupying airspaces along the needle tract (Figure 24-1, *C*). Since initial description by McCartney,[40] several studies have evaluated the efficacy of blood patch. The results have been mixed. Lang showed decreased occurrence of pneumothorax when a blood patch was applied.[41] Other studies have failed to find a benefit.[42,43]

A postprocedure CT is performed to ensure no immediate event occurs requiring intervention. The field of view is increased to maximize the evaluation, and should include the heart. Specific attention should be made to evaluate for pneumothorax, hemorrhage, and air embolism. More regarding the management of these adverse events will be discussed in a subsequent section.

The patient is then placed in the decubitus with the biopsied lung in a dependent position to minimize lung excursion, a further effort to prevent development of a pneumothorax. Oxygen is continued via nasal cannula. The patient is transferred to the postprocedure unit and observed for 3 hours. Two portable upright radiographs are obtained with an identical technique, at 1 and 3 hours, to evaluate for delayed or increasing pneumothorax. In the absence of significant or enlarging pneumothorax, the patient may be discharged with instructions to return to the emergency department for increasing shortness of breath, chest pain, or hemoptysis. We prescribe codeine elixir to limit cough in the days following the procedure.

Targeting and Trajectory

There are several considerations when choosing a trajectory of a percutaneous chest intervention, including the motion of the chest wall and lung during respiration, as well as the orientation of pleural interfaces, blood vessels, and airways. Preprocedure planning to account for each of these variables is essential for a successful and safe intervention.

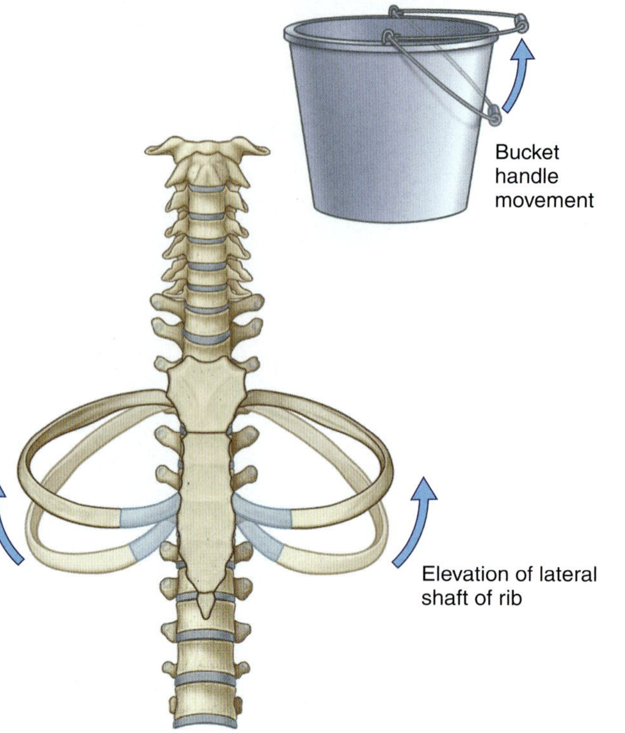

Figure 24-2 Rib motion during respiration. The ribs move in an up-and-out bucket handle fashion during inspiration, making lateral approaches to lung procedures unfavorable. *From Drake R, Wayne Vogl A, Mitchell Adam WM:* Gray's Basic Anatomy, *Philadelphia, 2012, Churchill Livingstone; Figure 3.28B.*

CHEST WALL MOTION

Although the shortest skin to target approach is often appealing on a static image, it can prove quite frustrating in practice. Significant motion of the chest wall occurs with normal respiration, which can result in considerable movement of the needle or probe, which both decreases targeting, and increases the chance of a complication.

The chest wall and ribs move in an up-and-out bucket handle direction during inspiration, with most motion occurring laterally (Figure 24-2). A lateral intercostal approach should be avoided when possible to avoid considerable needle motion and redirection by moving ribs. The preferred access into the thorax is from close to either the anterior or posterior midline, as there is relatively little motion of the intercostal space at the costovertebral and costochondral junctions (see Figure 24-1, *A*).

PERIPHERAL LESIONS AND THE TANGENTIAL APPROACH

Similarly, the lungs move considerably during the respiratory cycle, which is particularly problematic when targeting peripheral lesions. If such a lesion is targeted in a direct manner perpendicular to the chest wall, the tip of the needle has the tendency to retract to the level of the pleura during inspiration, particularly if the needle is being held firmly by the chest wall soft tissues. As a result, targeting is made more difficult, and there is increased risk of multiple pleural punctures (Figure 24-3).

A tangential approach to peripheral lung lesions is quite useful. The tangential approach utilizes a shallow, elongated, intrapulmonary course in parallel to the pleura, directed toward the lesion (see Figure 24-1, *B*). Targeting is aided as the needle and lesion move in tandem with each other. The lung tissue itself acts as a stabilizer of the needle, and there is little chance of the needle backing itself out of the lung. Finally, the tangential approach is essential in many thermal ablations of peripheral lesions in order to limit backward thermal injury of the pleura and chest wall.

CENTRAL LESIONS AND THE AXIAL APPROACH

The bronchovascular architecture of the lung originates in the hilum and fans out toward the periphery. Centrally located lesions are therefore in closer proximity to a number of blood vessels and airways, adding to the technical difficulty of intervention. These lesions can be targeted successfully, and safely, by using an axial approach. The needle or probe is placed in parallel to the bronchovascular structures, which minimizes the need to traverse large vessels and airways. The final position of the needle at the time of biopsy or ablation will likewise be directed in parallel to these structures, and thereby limit the chance of inadvertent laceration (Figure 24-4, *B–D*).

Similarly, it is advisable to use a parallel approach when a target lesion is located in proximity to critical, pulsating central structures, including the aorta, pulmonary arteries and veins, and heart and pericardium (Figure 24-5). These structures have significant excursion during systole, which is not captured on static CT images. Puncture injuries can occur when the needle is directed perpendicular to these structures, which may result in severe blood loss, cardiac tamponade, and death.[44]

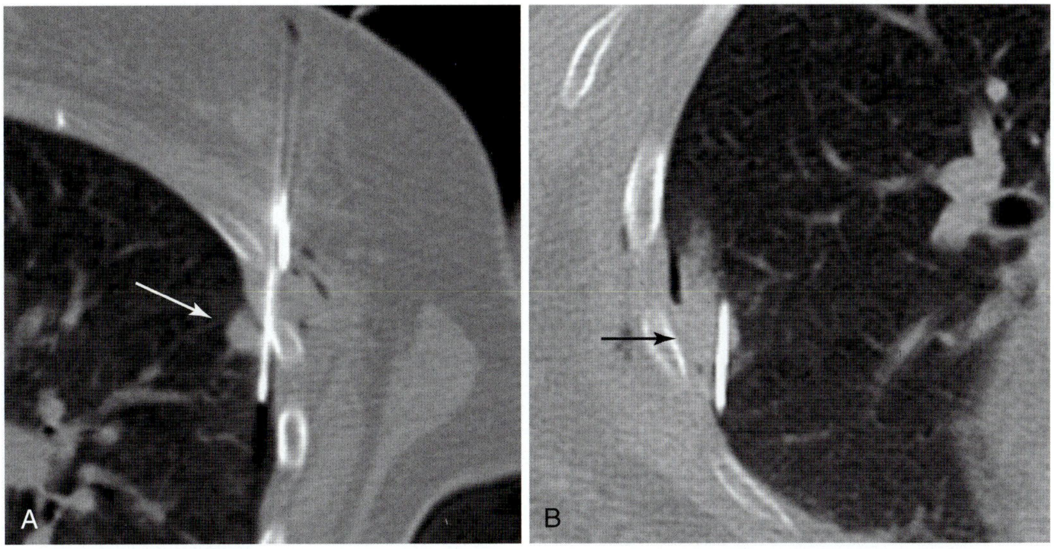

Figure 24-3 Approach to peripheral lesions. This patient previously had a right pneumonectomy for NSCLC, presenting with a new left upper lobe nodule. Initial biopsy from a lateral approach (*white arrow*) was difficult secondary to motion of the nodule (A). The patient has subsequent MWA of the nodule performed via a tangential approach (*black arrow*) with more ease (B).

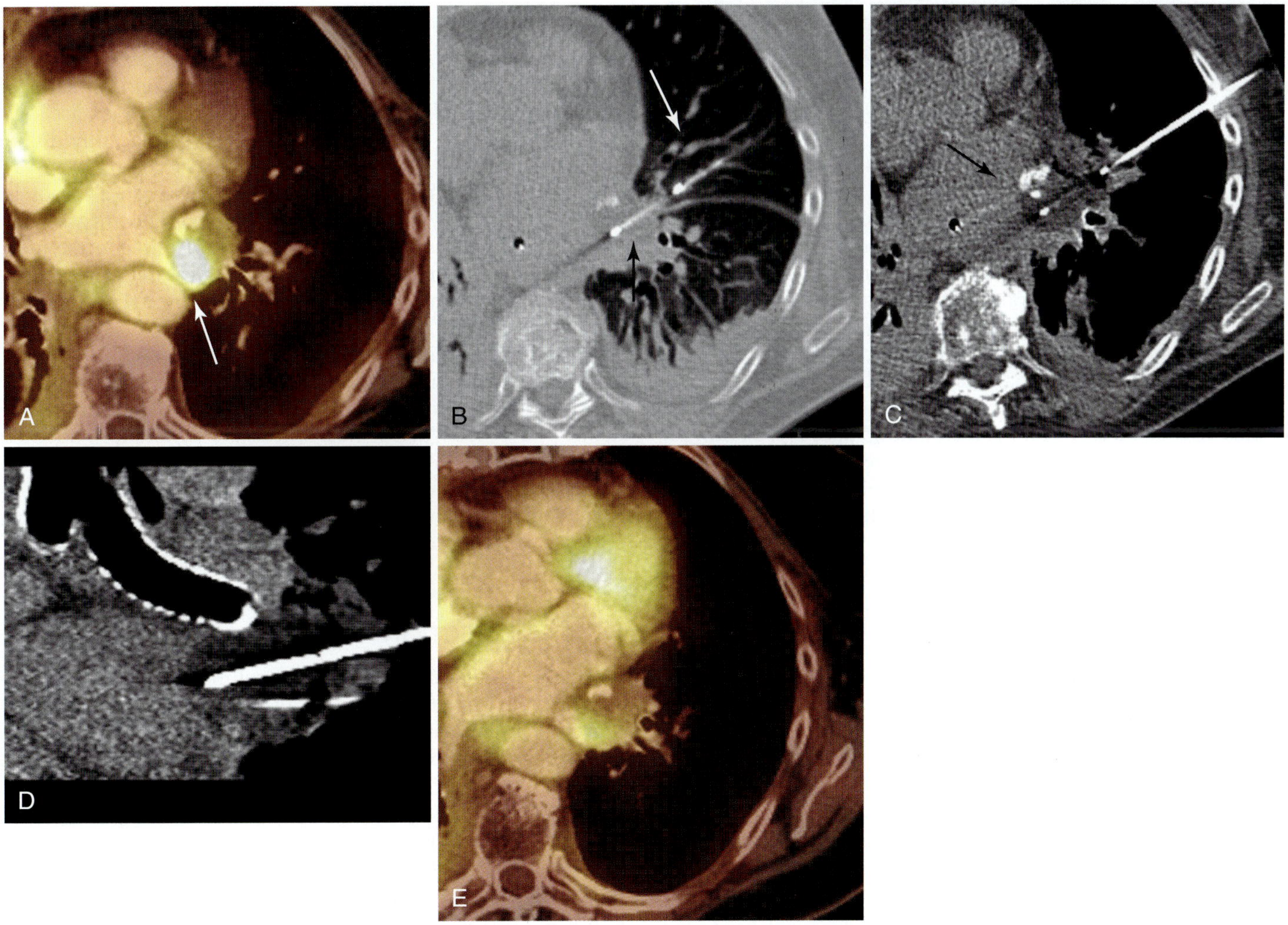

Figure 24-4 Cryoablation of central pulmonary mass using axial approach. Patient with recurrent mesothelioma in the left infrahilar region compressing the left inferior pulmonary vein (*white arrow*) (A). Two Perc-24 cryoablation probes (*black arrow*) were placed into the mass using an axial technique parallel to the bronchovascular (*white arrow*) structures (B). The edge of the ice conforms to the left atrium (*black arrow*) and left inferior pulmonary vein (*white arrow*) because of heat-sink effect (C). Coronal images demonstrate the extent of ice formation (D). Postprocedure PET/CT demonstrated a small amount of residual PET activity along the tumor margin bordering the pulmonary vein (E). This remained stable for 12 months, but ultimately progressed.

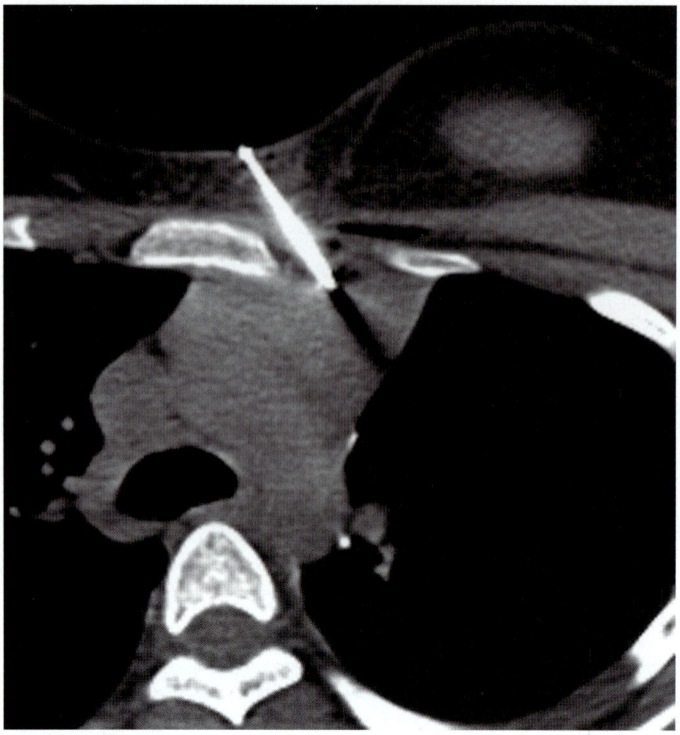

Figure 24-5 Biopsy of mediastinal mass tangential to aorta.

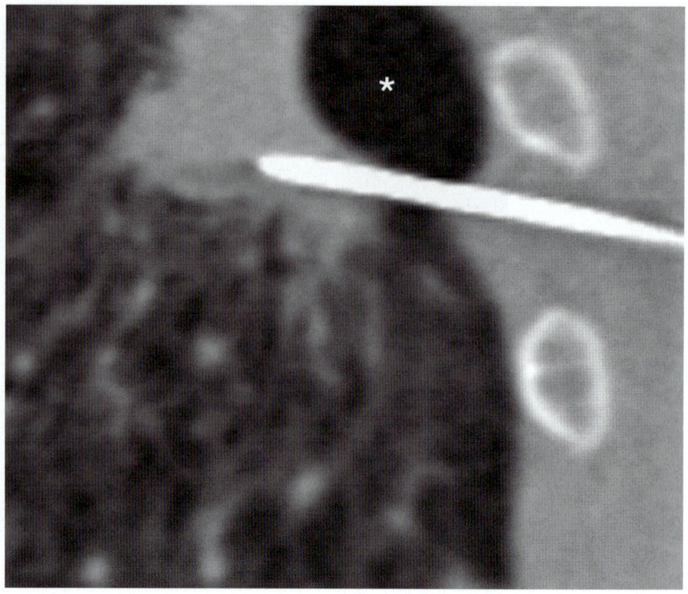

Figure 24-6 Biopsy of left upper lobe mass, avoiding adjacent bulla (asterisk).

PLEURAL INTERFACES

Violation of the visceral pleura when accessing the lung provides a potential communication between the alveolar sacs and the pleural space, and as such, is the primary risk factor for developing a pneumothorax. The visceral pleura should be crossed as little as possible during a procedure, preferably no more than once with a given needle, as each crossing would be expected to add proportionate risk of a subsequent air leak.

Pulmonary fissures are formed from a double layer of infolded visceral pleura, with the intervening space representing a continuity of the pleural space. The fissures should not be traversed during intervention, unless absolutely necessary, as crossing a single fissure results in two holes in the visceral pleura.

ENLARGED AIRSPACES

Many patients presenting for lung intervention will have enlarged airspaces. Causes include bullae and architectural destruction in emphysema, and airspace dilation in airways disease or in the presence of prior lung resection. The decreased density of pulmonary parenchyma results in increased risk of both pneumothorax and significant hemorrhage due to the relative lack of ability to tamponade the hole.[45] Attempts should be made to traverse regions of normal lung architecture to minimize risk (Figure 24-6).

Thermal Ablation

OVERVIEW

The delivery of cytotoxic thermal energy in the form of heat (RFA and MWA) and cold (PCT) has been well established as an effective means for treating localized primary and secondary tumors of the thorax. Thermal ablation has likewise been used to treat residual or recurrent disease at the margins of surgical resections and radiation fields. All three modalities are well tolerated and safe, with complications not significantly different from percutaneous core-needle biopsy.

All modalities aim to deliver thermal energy to a tumor in order to create a cytotoxic ablation zone that encompasses the entirety of the visualized tumor along with a disease-free margin, theoretically equivalent to that of surgical wedge resection. In general, there is an overlap in selection of one ablative modality over another when treating most thoracic neoplasms. A learning curve exists for each device—comfort with the device is of the upmost importance in achieving an effective ablation.

Although no direct comparison studies of the ablative modalities have been performed, important differences do exist between RFA, MWA, and PCT that can lead to a more effective, better tolerated, and safer ablation on a case-by-case basis. The following sections will provide a general discussion of patient selection for thermal ablation and the thoracic application of each modality.

PATIENT SELECTION

In general, ablation of a primary lung neoplasm is only appropriate for early-stage, localized disease. It is essential that all patients referred for thermal ablation be well integrated into a multidisciplinary lung cancer team that includes thoracic surgeons, medical oncologists, radiation oncologists, and intervention radiologists. A determination as to whether the patient has surgically resectable disease needs to be made. The patient also requires evaluation by the medical oncologist to ensure appropriate postintervention care and possibly adjuvant chemotherapy.

Most patients who are referred for ablation will have stage I or II disease, and medical comorbidities that preclude surgery. Another subset of patients includes those who have previously had surgical resection or radiation therapy, but have local disease progression. Patients with synchronous or metachronous primary lung cancers may be referred for combined treatment with other modalities, in order to preserve lung volume. This is particularly true for the significant number of patients with preexisting lung compromise secondary to emphysema. Finally, some patients prefer a nonsurgical management of the tumor, in particular for radiologically detected adenocarcinoma in situ or minimally invasive adenocarcinoma.

A decision regarding preferred ablation modality is usually made based on the size, location, and proximity of the tumor to vital structures (Table 24-2). Complete ablations can be compromised by the heat sink effect when the lesion borders blood vessels measuring greater than 3 mm.[46]

The relative contraindications to lung ablation are similar to those of surgical resection. Patients with decreased pulmonary functional reserve, including those with severe emphysema, airways disease, prior lung resection, and pulmonary arterial hypertension, are at increased risk. Likewise, patients with coronary artery disease, valvular heart disease, and arrhythmia are at increased risk for anesthesia. Although ablation is typically performed with conscious sedation, assistance of an anesthesiologist may be indicated in these cases.

Thermal ablation has been shown to be safe in patients with a cardiac pacemaker or AICD[47]; however, RFA can disrupt the function of the device. MWA likely has less effect on pacing devices than RFA. It is our practice to obtain a cardiac consultation prior to and following heat-based ablation to ensure appropriate device function. PCT is safe to use with cardiac devices, and obviates cardiology consultation, although patients with cardiac disease taking blood thinners, including warfarin, require bridging with short-acting anticoagulants, such as enoxaparin, prior to the procedure.

POSTABLATION CARE

Following ablation, patients are instructed to not exert themselves for several days. It is common to have a small amount of blood-tinged sputum, which should resolve after a day or two. Mild chest discomfort is expected, but severe chest pain or shortness of breath are not and may indicate a pneumothorax or increasing pleural effusion.

TABLE 24-2 Preferred Choice of Ablative Zone

Parameters	Radiofrequency	Microwave	Cryoablation
Size <3 cm	±	±	±
Size >3 cm	±	+	±
Thermal sink	−	+	±
Peripheral	−	±	+
Border mediastinum	±	−	+
Border large airways	−	−	+
Hemorrhage	±	±	−
Ablation zone visibility	±	±	+
Pacemaker	−	±	+
Time	±	+	−
Pneumothorax	±	−	+
Pleural effusion	±	±	−

The modalities are rated as + (adequate), ++ (has advantages), and – (has deficiencies) for lesions with several characteristics.

It is common to experience a flulike "postablation" syndrome following RFA and MWA, which is characterized by low-grade fever, malaise and myalgias, and may last up to 2 weeks. PCT is not associated with development of postablation syndrome.

Clinical follow-up is essential. We attempt to see the patient within 1 week if he or she is not already consulting another clinician. Initial imaging follow-up is in 1 month, with subsequent imaging at 3, 6, 9, 12, 18, and 24 months. Yearly imaging is subsequently obtained for stable disease.

Radiofrequency Ablation

MECHANICS

Radiofrequency ablation employs thermal energy, delivered via needle electrodes conducting high-frequency alternating current (460–500 kHz or radio waves) from the radiofrequency generator to local tissues, causing tissue destruction by controlled heating. The operator uses CT image guidance to confirm electrode placement within the target tumor. The RF current released at the noninsulated tip of the electrode is grounded by one of two methods: a monopolar system in which grounding pads are placed on the patient's thighs or a bipolar system in which the operator places a grounding electrode to reabsorb current. The RF current produced at the noninsulated tip of the electrode agitates ionic dipolar molecules, causing the frictional heating of the surrounding tissues and fluids.[48] Tumor ablation tissue temperatures typically range from 60°C to 100°C, which is sufficiently high to cause coagulative necrosis of surrounding tissues.[48,49] The operator can achieve ablation zones of varying size and shape depending on the number of electrodes utilized, duration of ablation, generator used, and specific guidelines of the manufacturer.

Because aerated lung parenchyma acts as an insulator for thermal energy applied to a tumor, lung cancer is well suited to treatment using thermal energy. In general, in the thorax, lower energies (than used in the liver) result in effective ablation. This is commonly referred to as the "oven" effect.[50] Tissue temperatures in excess of 105°C–115°C can cause carbonization of tissue and gas formation, insulating the residual tumor from thermal energy, resulting in incomplete ablation.[51] Conversely, many ablative scenarios consist of the lesion in contact with tissue other than aerated lung. In such scenarios, additional energy is required to ablate the same volume of tumor because of greater heat dissipation through tissue. When a tumor is situated adjacent to a blood vessel, and to lesser extent large airways, a "heat-sink effect" can readily dissipate heat, resulting in higher energy demands to achieve tissue necrosis. Lastly, at the margins, the high impedance of normal lung parenchyma inhibits thermal energy from effectively heating a 1-cm surgical margin around the lesion.[52]

TECHNIQUE

Prior to needle placement, dispersive grounding pad placement should be carefully chosen, avoiding bony prominences. The operator should periodically check the pads during the procedure to ensure close contact. Failure to properly ground the current can result in heat buildup and serious skin burn injuries.[53,54]

The first technical steps are identical to percutaneous core-needle biopsy. Following administration of pleural anesthesia, one or more RFA electrode probes are advanced into the target mass under intermittent CT guidance. The device-specific prospectus for anticipated ablation zones guide decisions regarding the number of probes required for a complete treatment. The ablation zone should be planned to extend at least 6 mm beyond the radiologic edge of the tumor. This is to engulf microscopic tumor that is not detected by CT, but exists at the periphery of the tumor.[55]

Once the RF electrode is in place, energy is applied, leading to coagulative necrosis of the tumor and surrounding margin. Impedance, duration of ablation, and temperature primarily determine the end points for a given ablation.[52] Lung RFA at a single station is typically performed for 12–15 minutes. An initial power of 10 W is used, which is slowly ramped up to 100 W over 5 minutes to prevent tissue charring. Increased impedance and cycling of the control-box between on and off positions indicate that the ablation has reached its maximum extent at a given position. Intraprocedural imaging aids the determination of ablation adequacy. A circumferential zone of ground-glass attenuation measuring at least 1 cm around the ablated lesion is desired.

IMAGING APPEARANCE

Imaging follow-up of the ablation zone is divided into early (<1 week), intermediate (>1 week–2 months), and late (>2 months) phases.[56] CT is most commonly used in follow-up. Contrast-enhanced CT, CT densitometry, and PET/CT have all demonstrated utility while monitoring the ablation zone.

Early Phase (<1 Week)

Achieving adequate imaging to confirm the complete and uniform coagulation necrosis of a given RFA target can be a challenge. Although inferences can be drawn from CT scans as a guide for adequacy of tumor ablation, adequacy of treatment can only be confirmed by extended follow-up imaging.

Immediately following treatment, an ablation zone has a characteristic light bulb appearance with alternating attenuated tissue. The innermost layer is dense, representing coagulation necrosis of the tumor. The surrounding ground glass represents a combination of coagulation necrosis and alveolar effusion[57] (Figure 24-7).

The development of ground-glass opacity in the surrounding lung can be an indication of thermal energy sufficient for cell necrosis outside of the area of tumor. The “ground glass” should optimally surround the tumor by 10–15 mm, roughly providing a 1-cm “surgical margin.” Animal studies indicate that ground-glass attenuation overestimate the area of true coagulative necrosis by up to 4.1 mm.[57] At the completion of the procedure, the electrode tract can be cauterized during needle removal. Cauterization theoretically reduces the risk of

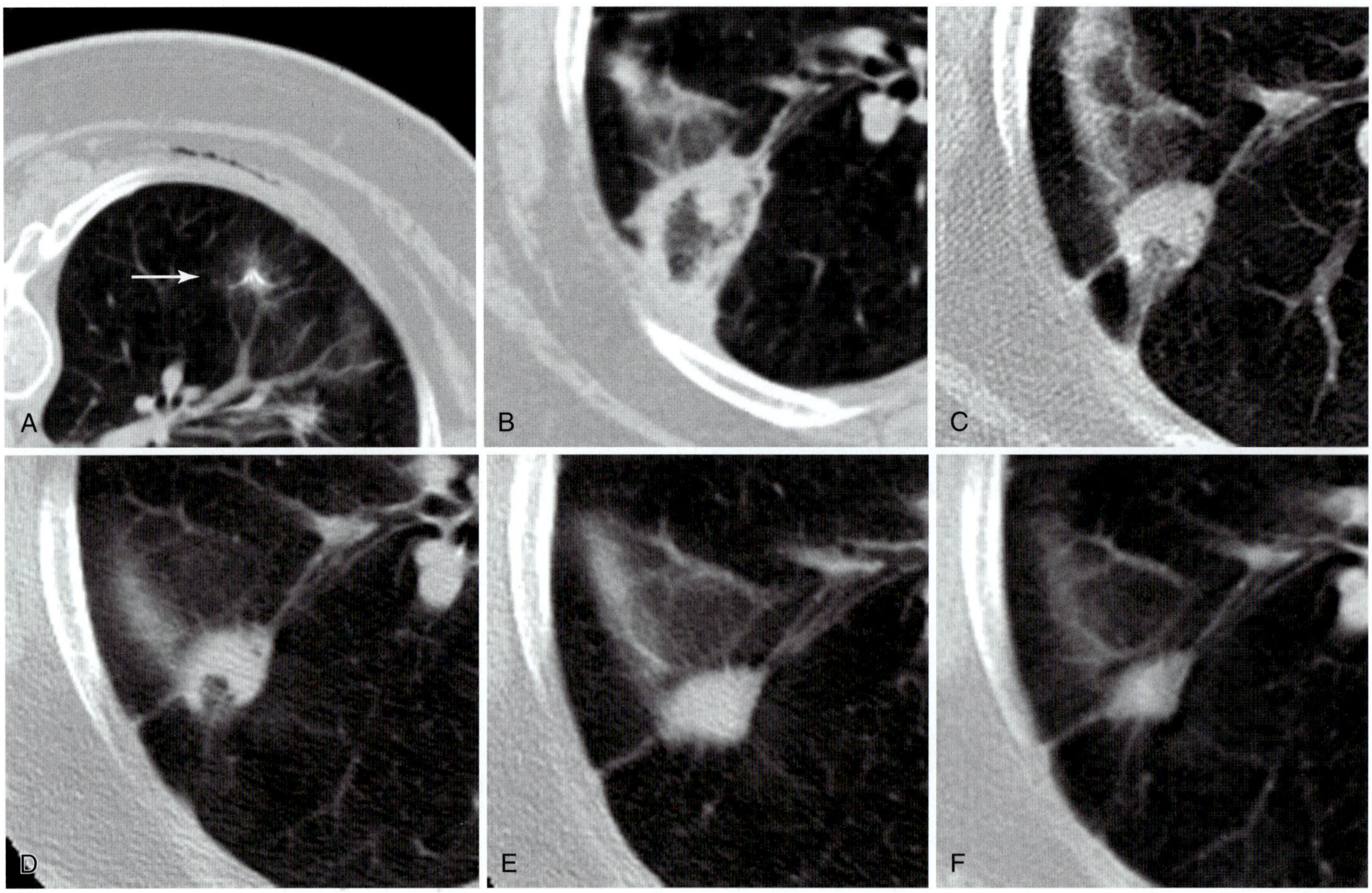

Figure 24-7 Imaging follow-up following lung RFA. The patient had RFA performed for a biopsy-proven right lower lobe NSCLC. Imaging during the procedure (A) demonstrates ground-glass attenuation develop around the nodule (*white arrow*). The ablation zone has expanded at 30 days (B), and then subsequently involutes at 3 months (C), 6 months (D), 1 year (E), and 2 years (F). By 6 months, the size of the ablation zone had returned to the size that was present at the completion of the ablation.

hemorrhage, pneumothorax, and tumor seeding. Following removal of the electrode, a postprocedure CT scan is performed to assess for procedure-related complications.

A second described postablation pattern is the *cockade phenomenon* of five concentric rings of alternative attenuation. Zone A is small and hypoattenuated and correlates with the electrode tract. Zone B is dense, coagulated tumor. Zone C is ground-glass attenuated coagulation necrosis of the pulmonary parenchyma. Zone D is dense tissue consisting of pulmonary coagulation necrosis combined with hemorrhage. Zone E is ground-glass attenuated inflammation (Figure 24-8).

The size of the ablation zone is larger than the treated tumor as it includes a margin of ground glass corresponding to cell death and inflammation. The size of the ablation actually increases over the course of the first week following treatment, as hemorrhage and inflammation ensue.

Intermediate (>1 Week–2 Months)

Ground-glass opacity has resolved by this point. The ablation zone continues to remain larger than the treated mass, but should show involution in comparison to prior scans (see Figure 24-7, *C*). Some lesions may cavitate, which has been used as a positive predictor of treatment response. Cavitation is more common in small lesions (<2-cm) and when the ablation zone is greater than 200% the size of the tumor (Figure 24-9).[58-60]

Late (>2 Months)

The ablation zone continues to involute for up to 6 months. Cavitations may take longer, up to a year, to resolve. As the ablation zone scars, there is localized architectural distortion and traction on adjacent structures, including the pleura and airways. By 6 months, the ablation zone is smaller than the treated lesion (see Figure 24-7, *D*).

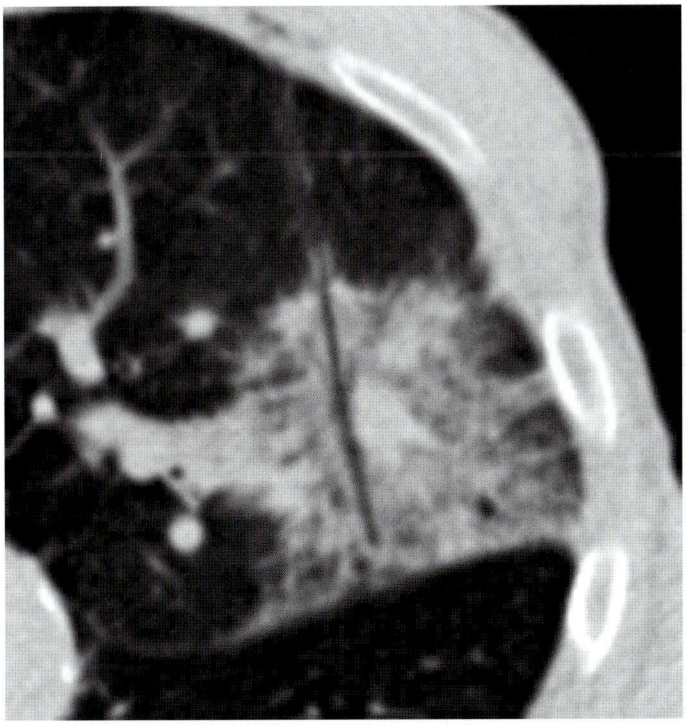

Figure 24-8 Cockade appearance post microwave ablation. Patient with NSCLC was treated with three microwave antennae. The postablation appearance demonstrates the "Cockade" appearance of alternating bands of attenuation. Margins extend circumferentially around the mass.

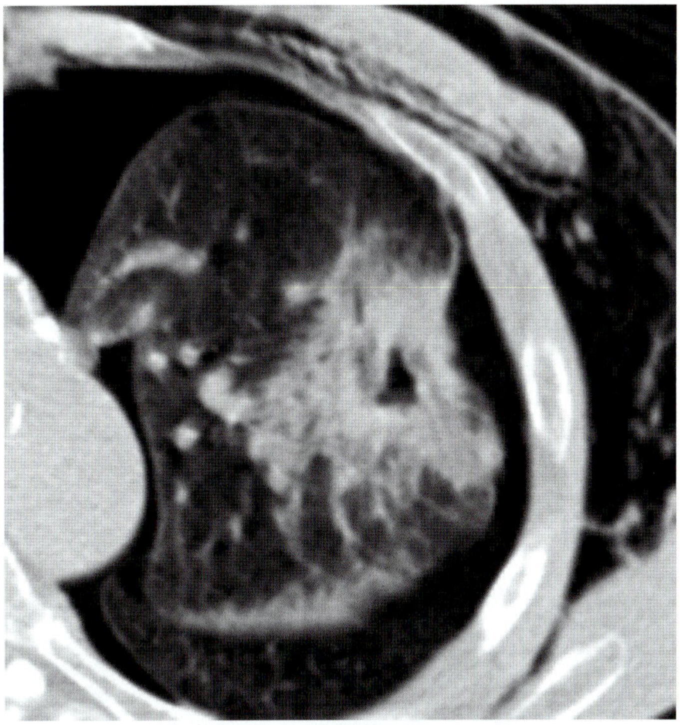

Figure 24-9 Cavitation of mass post microwave ablation. Same patient as in Figure 24-8. This patient developed mass cavitation and pneumothorax at the completion of the procedure, requiring chest tube placement.

Any growth of tissue after 3 months should raise the possibility of residual disease. Other features of recurrence include eccentric nodular growth (Figure 24-10 F), or eccentric focal enhancement of the postablation lesion on CT. There may be corresponding eccentric activity on the PET scan at this time, although evaluation may be difficult. In suspicious cases, close interval follow-up contrast-enhanced chest CT is helpful to document the focal increase in size or enhancement. In equivocal cases, CT-guide biopsy can also be performed.[56]

PITFALLS

Treatment of peripheral lesions may result in the undesired complication of pneumothorax and skin burn. A tangential approach should be used for needle placement, which provides for an elongated path through the lung parenchyma and, thereby, prevents backward burning along the needle into the pleura, subcutaneous soft tissues, and skin.

In general, a consideration of adjacent structures must be made when performing an ablation. Injury to the recurrent laryngeal, phrenic, intercostal, and brachial plexus nerves have been reported.[61,62] Vascular pseudoaneurysm, hemorrhage, and death have also been reported.

RESULTS

Numerous case series have demonstrated the safety and efficacy of RFA.[63-72] Although there are minor differences in reported survival following RFA between these studies, two of the largest studies have reported 1-year survival of 70%–78% and 2-year

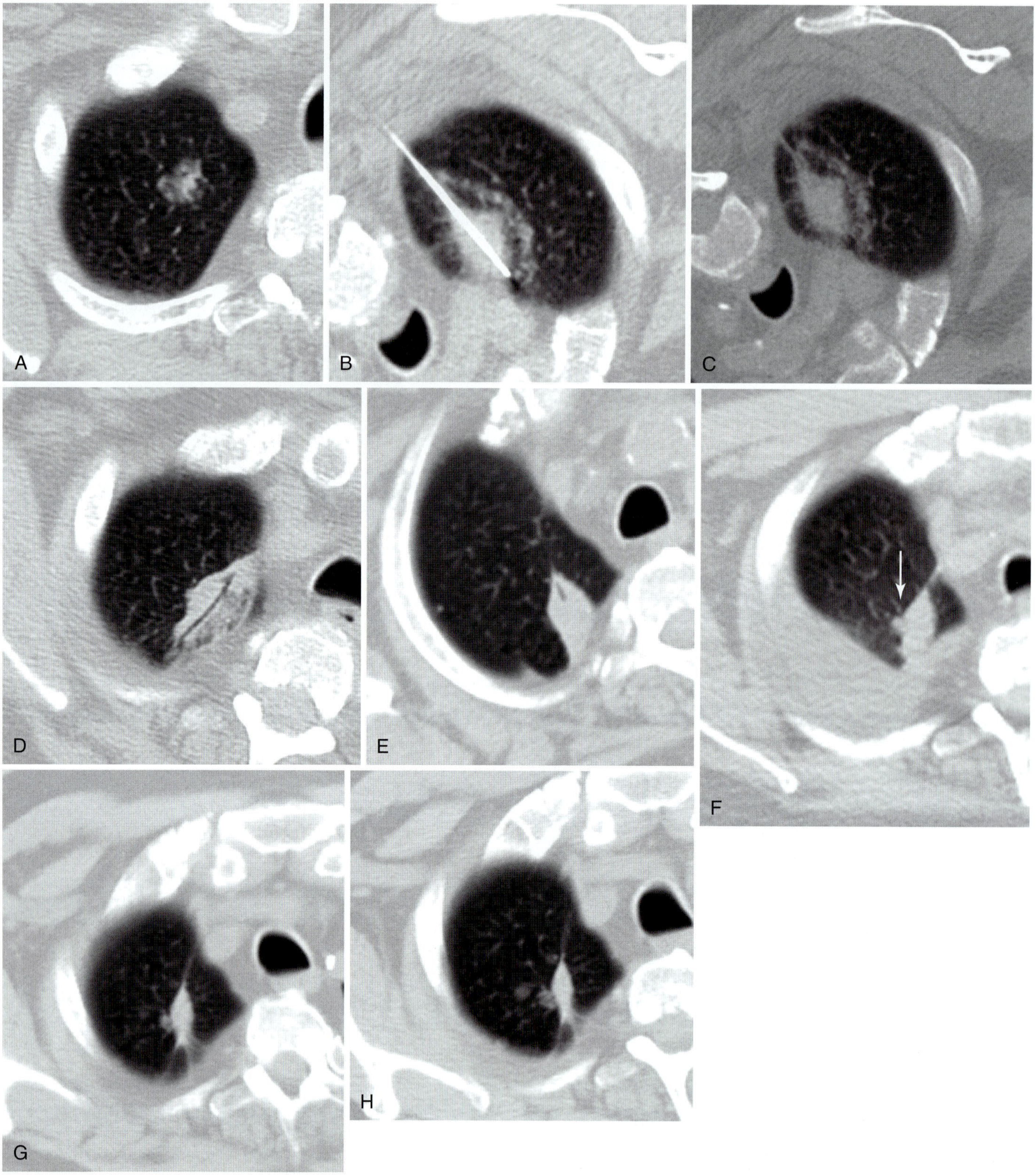

Figure 24-10 Recurrent tumor following RFA. The solid nodule (A) was targeted with a single Cool-tip RF probe (Covidien, Inc.), and ablation was performed for 12 minutes (B). Final measured temperatures were cytotoxic and the probe was removed with tract ablation. The postablation CT (C) demonstrates a "light bulb" appearance of alternating attenuation with margins extending beyond the original tumor. Initial scans at 3 weeks (D) and 2 months (E) demonstrate appropriate retraction of the ablation zone. Nodular growth (*white arrow*) appeared along the lateral margin of the ablation zone at 5 months (F), and showed growth at 13 months (G). By 17 months, there was multifocal tumor recurrence at the margins of the ablation zone (H).

survival of 48%–57%. The rate of tumor progression has been reported at 31.5% for stage 1 NSCLC treated with ablation.[73]

Numerous predictors of local recurrence have been reported. Although RFA has been shown to be effective for lung tumors less than 3 cm in diameter, there is increased marginal recurrence in larger masses. Difficulties with ablation size and margin are compounded when blood vessels larger than 3 mm border the targeted tumor, a particular issue with central lesions (Figure 24-11). The ablation provided by a single electrode is oblong in shape with the length of ablation being largest along the length of the electrode shaft. Multiple clustered electrodes can contribute to a larger, more spherical ablation zone that may be required. No direct comparison study between RFA and either wedge resection or SBRT has been performed.

Microwave Ablation

MECHANICS

Microwave uses electromagnetic waves with frequencies of 915 MHz to 2.45 GHz to excite water molecules in adjacent tissue, which results in frictional heating and cell death. In comparison with RFA, MWA has the advantage of achieving higher temperatures with larger ablations zones in a shorter period of time.[74] Temperatures reaching up to 150°C have been recorded. As opposed to radiofrequency ablation in which electrical current is directed through the patient, no grounding pads are required with MWA. The size of the MWA is not limited by tissue charring, which can lead to a more robust volume of the ablation zone. Although large tumors can be successfully treated, as with RFA, the success

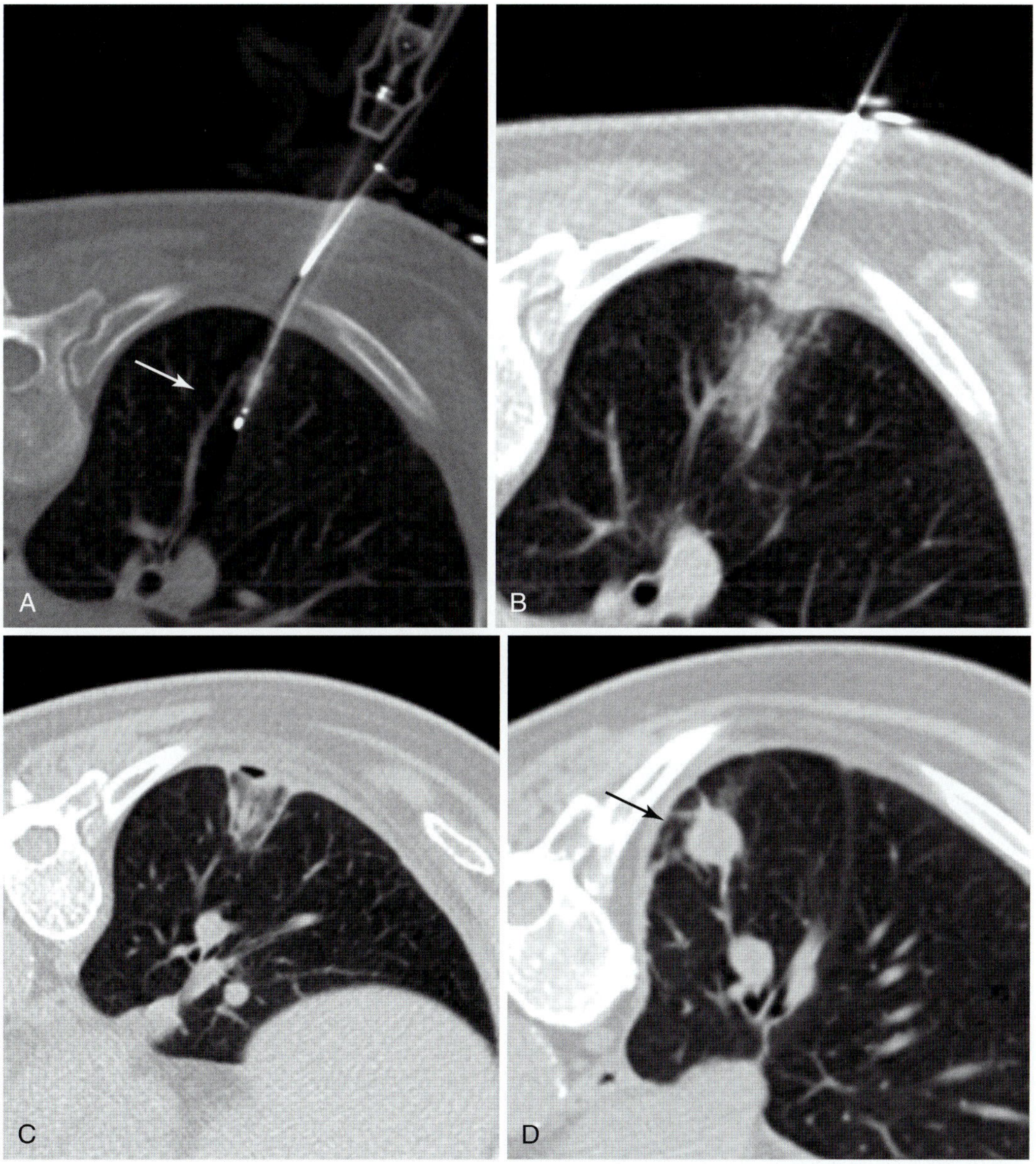

Figure 24-11 Tumor recurrence secondary to heat sink. A patient with biopsy-proven invasive adenocarcinoma presented for radiofrequency ablation of a right lower lobe nodule adjacent to a 3-mm blood vessel (*white arrow*). A single Cool-tip RF probe was used (A). The medial margin was small because of the heat-sink effect of the adjacent blood vessel (B). Follow-up CT at 8 months (D) demonstrated localized tumor recurrence (*black arrow*), most likely due to suboptimal cytotoxic effect at the margin of the blood vessel.

of treatment is less with lesions measuring greater than 3 cm.[75] Pain is less an issue with MWA in comparison to RFA.

PATIENT SELECTION

MWA is favored over RFA under several circumstances. Although study results are variable, MWA is favored when treating lesions larger than 3 cm because of larger ablation size.[76] Likewise, MWA is favored by some for peripheral lesions, as it induces less pain than is generated by the electrical current of RFA when it is used in the vicinity of intercostal nerves. MWA is more effective in treating central lesions adjacent to large blood vessels, as the robust ablation appears to overcome some effects of the heat sink. Contraindications do not differ from RFA.

TECHNIQUE

Placement of MWA antennae is essentially identical to RFA. However, some of the MW systems require placement of the antenna with the tip well beyond the edge of the tumor (Figure 24-12). After one or more antennae are positioned, the microwave system is activated. Multiple antennae can be used to concurrently heat tissue. The power that can be supplied depends on the system and number of antennae used, ranging from 30 to 200 W.

Currently six microwave systems are commercially available in the United States (Tyco Healthcare Group, Boulder, CO; MicrothermX, BSD Medical, Salt Lake City, UT; Avecure, Medwaves, San Diego, CA; Certus 140, Neuwave, Madison, WI; Amica, Hospital Service, Rome, Italy; Acculis MTA, Microsulis Medical, Hampshire, United Kingdom). Although the principle used to obtain cell death is the same, the technology differs and the operators need to understand the technical parameters dictating the optimum location of the antenna and hence the end point of ablation for each system. An estimation of the intended ablation zone is made based on the device prospectus provided by the device manufacturer. Intermittent CT monitoring is performed during the procedure to establish adequacy of the ablation, which mirrors that for RFA. The size of MWA can at times be less predictable than that of RFA, which necessitates close monitoring, typically every 2 minutes.

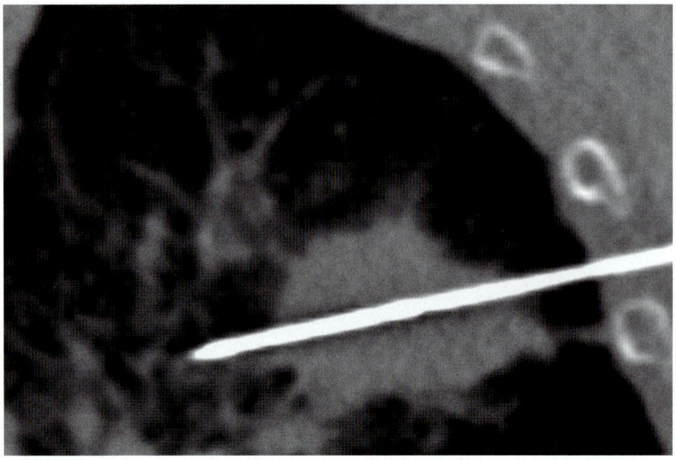

Figure 24-12 Microwave ablation of NSCLC. A Neuwave LN15 antenna is advance 1 cm beyond the mass to maximize tumor heating.

Ablation time varies based on lesion size, but is typically 7–10 minutes. As with RFA, a margin of ground-glass attenuation around the tumor of 10–15 mm is used to establish an adequate margin (see Figure 24-8). The antenna is removed with or without tract ablation, and an immediate postprocedure CT is performed to ensure no complications occur, specifically pneumothorax and hemorrhage.

IMAGING

Imaging features following MWA are similar to those of RFA, and can be followed by imaging in the same manner.

PITFALLS

Immediately following ablation, there is frequently greater retraction of the central portion of the ablation zone, because of tissue desiccation from rapid heating. When the zone is peripheral and adjacent to the pleura, this retraction can lead to the development of pneumothorax (see Figure 24-9). During intermediate imaging, pleural thickening is often noted adjacent to the ablation zone.

Cavitation of the ablated lesion is more frequent with MWA (see Figure 24-9). This has been shown to be a positive predictor of adequate treatment, but can lead to the development of pneumothorax. Infection of the cavity has likewise been described.

Soft tissue and skin burns may be more likely with MWA. The postablation syndrome is less frequent than with RFA.

RESULTS

Fewer studies of lung MWA exist than lung RFA. Indications are that MWA performs on par with RFA, with possible ability to extend the ablation zone to larger lesions. Wolf and colleagues reported their results of MWA in 82 lung tumors of 50 patients. Local control at 1 year was seen in 67%. Unlike RFA, the index tumor size of larger than 3 cm did not affect patients' actuarial survival or cancer- specific mortality. However, patients with an index tumor size >3 cm were significantly more likely to have recurrent disease at the ablation site (3 cm vs. >3 cm, $P = 0.01$).[75]

Cryoablation

Mechanics

Percutaneous cryoablation therapy utilizes subzero temperatures to freeze tissue and cause necrosis. It has a long history of use surgically, and has recently emerged as a reliable option for percutaneous thermal ablation. Current PCT systems make use of the Joules-Thompson effect in which liquid argon is allowed to expand into a gas, thereby lowering the temperature of the probe and surrounding tissues to lethal temperatures. Imaging during cryoablation demonstrates iceball formation to a zero degree isotherm at the iceball periphery. Helium is subsequently used to heat the probe during tissue thaw.

Cold-based tumor ablation achieves a zone of tissue death via both direct and indirect mechanisms.[77,78] Instantaneous cell death in the lung is caused by temperatures of less than $-40°C$. Prolonged freezing at the $-20°C$ isotherm leads to extracellular ice formation, resulting in a fluid shift from cells to the extracellular matrix, causing intracellular hyperosmolality. Upon thawing, fluid from the extracellular matrix returns into cells, leading to cell swelling and ultimate lysis. The completeness of necrosis within the ablation zone is proportional to the length of time that cells spend at lethal isotherms. The damaging effects of cellular fluid shifts are most important at the periphery of the ablation zone.

The indirect mechanisms of PCT-induced cell death are from small vessel vascular injury from in situ vessel thrombosis and vasoconstriction, which cause a zone of tissue ischemia. Emerging evidence indicates that cryoablation may induce an immunological cascade that leads to a systemic antitumoral effect following treatment.[79]

PATIENT SELECTION

PCT is reasonable for most cases being considered for ablation. In comparison to the heat-based ablative modalities, PCT is associated with less pain when treating peripheral lesions. Many patients experience an analgesic effect from the treatment, making PCT an excellent ablative modality in the treatment of painful malignancies.

As opposed to RFA and MWA, the ability to visualize the extent of the ablation zone intraoperatively, as marked by ice-ball formation, allows for a more precise ablation when treating tumors adjacent to critical structures, such as the pericardium, esophagus, and large airways. Additionally, freezing preserves tissue architecture; hence, structural damage to tissue in the ablation zone is limited, and cryoablation can be used adjacent to tissues such as the tracheobronchial tree.[80] PCT does not utilize electromagnetic energy, and is therefore safe in patients with cardiac pacemakers.

The degree of hemorrhage can be significantly greater in PCT when compared with heat-based ablations (Figure 24-13). PCT is less favorable for patients who are coagulopathic and thrombocytopenic. Patients with enlarged airspaces, primarily from emphysema, are more at risk for uncontrolled periablation hemorrhage; RFA and MWA are favored in these patients because of their cauterizing effect.

TECHNIQUE

Probe selection and number are based on the prospectus provided by the device manufacturer, which are typically based on in vitro models that do not account for differences in tissue architecture and the temperature-dissipating effect of blood vessels. These maps can be used to predict the extent of ice ball formation and planning ablation (see Figure 2-18). A common early error is underablation. Probes must provide ice-coverage that extends beyond the margin of the tumor in order to ensure that the tumor itself is at least treated to −20°C. The edge of the ice marks the 0°C isotherm and does not lead to complete tissue necrosis.

Ice shape varies between probes, but all are elliptical with the long axis along the shaft of the probe. As such, the tumor is skewered along its long axis when possible, to maximize ice coverage. A close evaluation of proximity to medium- and large-sized blood vessels is made, as incomplete ablation is common when vessels measuring greater than 3 mm in diameter are present at a margin of the tumor because of cold sink effects, which are similar to heat sink effects in that the vessel warms nearby tissue, preventing lethal ice formation. This may lead to an incomplete ablation (Figure 24-14) and may necessitate placement of additional probes to achieve an adequate ablation. The stick-function or 10% freeze function of cryoprobes, which freezes the probe in position to −10°C, is used to keep the probes in tissue and maintain needle position before ablation and is frequently used when multiple probes are placed.

Multiple freeze–thaw cycle protocols have been reported. In our practice, pulmonary neoplasms are typically treated with freeze cycles of 3, 7, and 10 minutes with intervening passive thaw cycles of not more than 3 minutes, with probes turned off, not actively thawed. The initial freeze and thaw incites a small amount of pulmonary hemorrhage, which acts to extend the ablation zone and allows the border of ice to be well visualized. Active, extended thaw cycles are avoided to prevent procedure limiting pulmonary hemorrhage. Intermittent CT monitoring

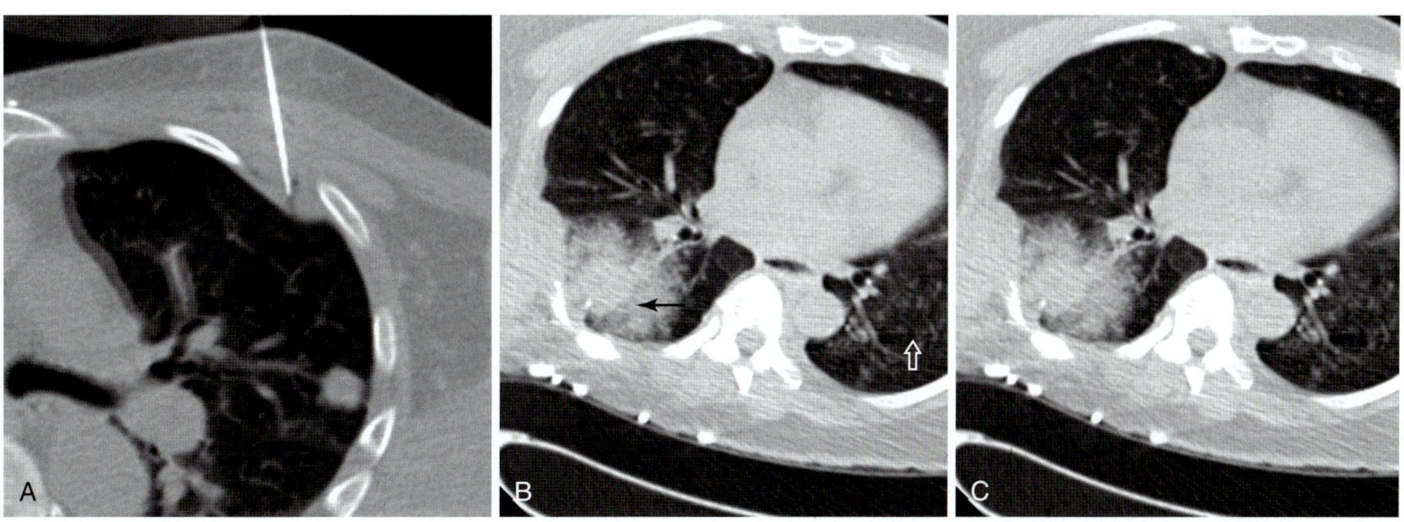

Figure 24-13 Pulmonary hemorrhage following cryoablation. Woman with breast carcinoma and a solitary right lower lobe lung metastasis. (A) Cryoablation was performed with two Perc-24 cryoprobes (Endocare) placed from a posterior approach. Freeze cycles of 3, 7, and 10 minutes were used at a single probe position. After probe removal, the patient was placed in supine position. (B) The postprocedure CT demonstrates a large amount of pulmonary hemorrhage in the right lower lobe (*solid arrow*), and endobronchial spread of blood to the contralateral left lung (*open arrow*). (C). The patient was placed in right lateral decubitus position to prevent endobronchial propagation of hemorrhage. Postprocedure chest radiograph demonstrated no further expansion of the hemorrhage.

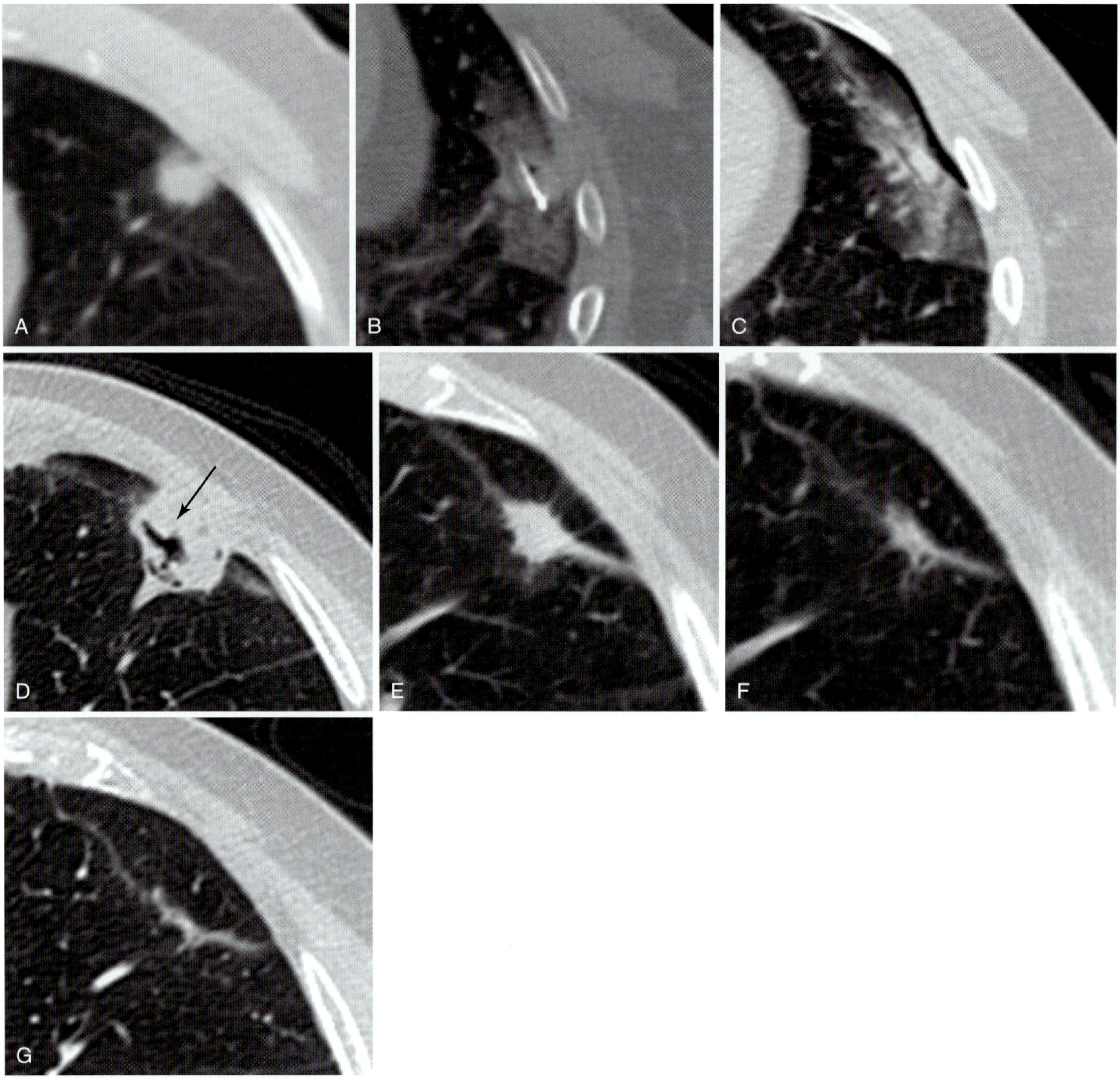

Figure 24-14 Imaging follow-up following cryoablation. Patient with NSCLC undergoing cryoablation of peripheral lingula nodule. Imaging before (A), during (B), and immediately following ablation (C) demonstrates development of ground glass around the target nodule. At 30 days (D), the ablation zone has expanded and cavitated (*black arrow*). The ablation zone is subsequently shown to involute at 3 months (E), 5 months (F), and 8 months (G). By 8 months, the zone has completely scarred.

is performed roughly every 3 minutes. Following the final freeze, each probe is actively thawed and removed once the probe thermocouple measures 20°C, or the probe is freed from the ice ball. The access site is immediately cleaned, a sterile dressing is applied, and the patient is turned with treated lung in a dependent position to protect the contralateral lung from spill of pulmonary hemorrhage via the bronchial tree as the ice melts. As a rule, the patient should be positioned in this fashion within 3 minutes of probe removal. Finally, a postprocedure CT is performed to ensure no early complication occurs, specifically no extensive hemorrhage or pneumothorax.

The freeze–thaw cycle is different for treating soft tissue neoplasms outside of the lung. The initial 3-minute freeze is foregone, as it is not necessary to incite pulmonary hemorrhage to extend the ablation zone. We typically use two freeze cycles when treating these tumors, often extending the second freeze to 12 minutes.

IMAGING

Early (<1 Week)

The immediate appearance of the ablation zone prior to ice melting is development of decreased density of the tumor and a surrounding rim of hypoattenuation representing the ice ball itself. This area of hypoattenuation represents a zone of cryonecrosis consisting of trapped air and necrotic tissue. At the periphery is a zone of hyperattenuation, representing a combination of necrotic tissue and hemorrhage. This zone of hemorrhage can be extensive. On melting of the ice, the entirety of the ablation zone is hyperattenuated because of hemorrhage (Figure 24-14C). The initial postablation hemorrhage should subside quickly, and within 24 hours a hyperdense postablation zone larger than the original tumor should be present.

Intermediate (1 Week–2 Months)

By 1 week, much of the surrounding hemorrhage has resolved. The remaining area of consolidation represents the extent of the ablation zone. As opposed to heat-based treatment, the ablation zone does not continue to enlarge following PCT.

Early tumor cavitation may be present (Figure 24-14, *D*), but typically resolves by 3 months. It is more common with PCT to have a reactive pleural effusion that appears in the days following treatment, and typically resolves within a month. Care should be taken to recognize progressive symptomatic effusions, which are managed with drainage or short-term chest tube placement. A residual of pleural thickening may remain following effusion resolution.

Late (>2 Months)

The ablation zone should progressively decrease in size following PCT. Any increase in size after 2 months suggests the presence of residual tumor. Presence of enhancing pulmonary nodules, irregular rim enhancement at the periphery of cryozone, and development of hypermetabolic activity on PET raise the possibility of recurrence.

PITFALLS

Hemorrhage is the primary risk of cryoablation in comparison to the heat-based modalities. Cryoablation is avoided in patients with borderline coagulation status. Again, the treated lung must be placed in a dependent position following treatment to prevent extension of the expected periprocedural hemorrhage into the contralateral lung via the bronchial tree.

A reactive pleural effusion is common, particularly when treating peripheral lesions. At times, a thoracentesis must be performed several days following ablation for symptomatic relief. In our experience, administering intravenous ketorolac at the time of procedure, followed by 3 days' treatment with oral antiinflammatory agent, limits effusion development.

Many cryoprobes are of larger caliber than RFA or MWA ablation probes, making skewering small nodules difficult. In these cases, two probes should be placed around the tumor, which we have been termed loosely the "chopstick" approach (Figure 24-15).

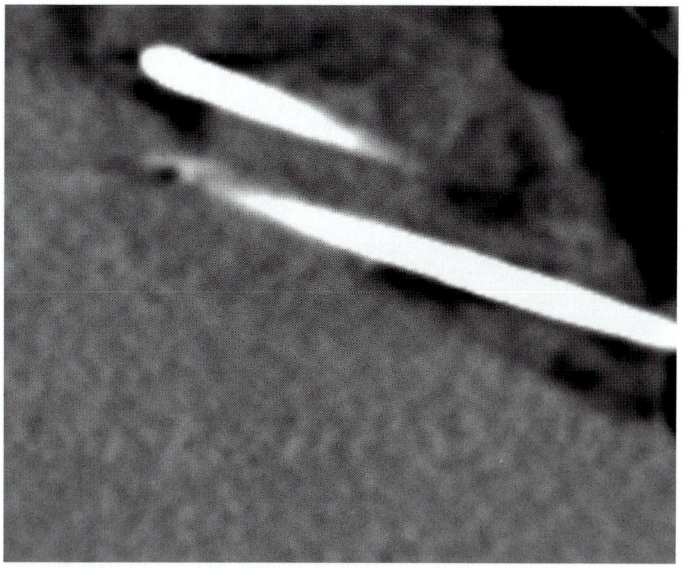

Figure 24-15 Chopstick configuration of PCT ablation probes while treating a right lower lobe nodule secondary to metastatic chordoma.

Advanced Ablation Techniques

Many target tumors border critical structures, such as nerves (phrenic and laryngeal), pericardium, esophagus, and trachea. Methods to displace the tumor away from these structures, or to monitor for ablative injury, can be employed to perform a safe ablation.

ARTIFICIAL PNEUMOTHORAX

Pulmonary tumors that are positioned adjacent to mediastinal structures can be displaced away by induction of an artificial pneumothorax. This can be safely performed by introducing a coaxial, Chiba, or Veress needle into the pleural space, and introducing room air or CO_2 (Figure 24-16). The Veress needle is spring-loaded with a blunted tip, which allows the visceral pleura to be displaced from the parietal pleura to create a potential space for air introduction.

An alternative method for tissue displacement is hydrodissection. This method is useful when ablating tumors bordering critical structures, particularly those that invade the pleura and are, therefore, resistant to displacement by pneumothorax. A 22-guage Chiba needle is advanced into the tissues surrounding the tumor and fluid is instilled. When using RFA, D5W is instilled to avoid theoretical ion excitation and extension of tissue heating. This method is frequently employed in our practice when treating soft tissue malignancies with cryoablation, to protect the skin from frostbite.

DIRECT TEMPERATURE MONITORING

With the notable exception of PCT (in which ice ball formation can be seen on imaging), the borders of ablation zones are not precisely visualized during the ablation. Thermocouples can be introduced along the margin of the ablation zone in the region of critical structures to actively monitor tissue temperature. An alternative is placement of an intraluminal thermocouple, such as an esophageal temperature probe. Esophageal probes have the added benefit of precisely marking the esophagus, which is normally obscured by adjacent mediastinal structures.

Adverse Events: Prevention and Management

Lung biopsy and ablation are safe procedures, particularly when compared with surgical alternatives. Despite efforts at minimizing risk, adverse events are expected. The majority of instances

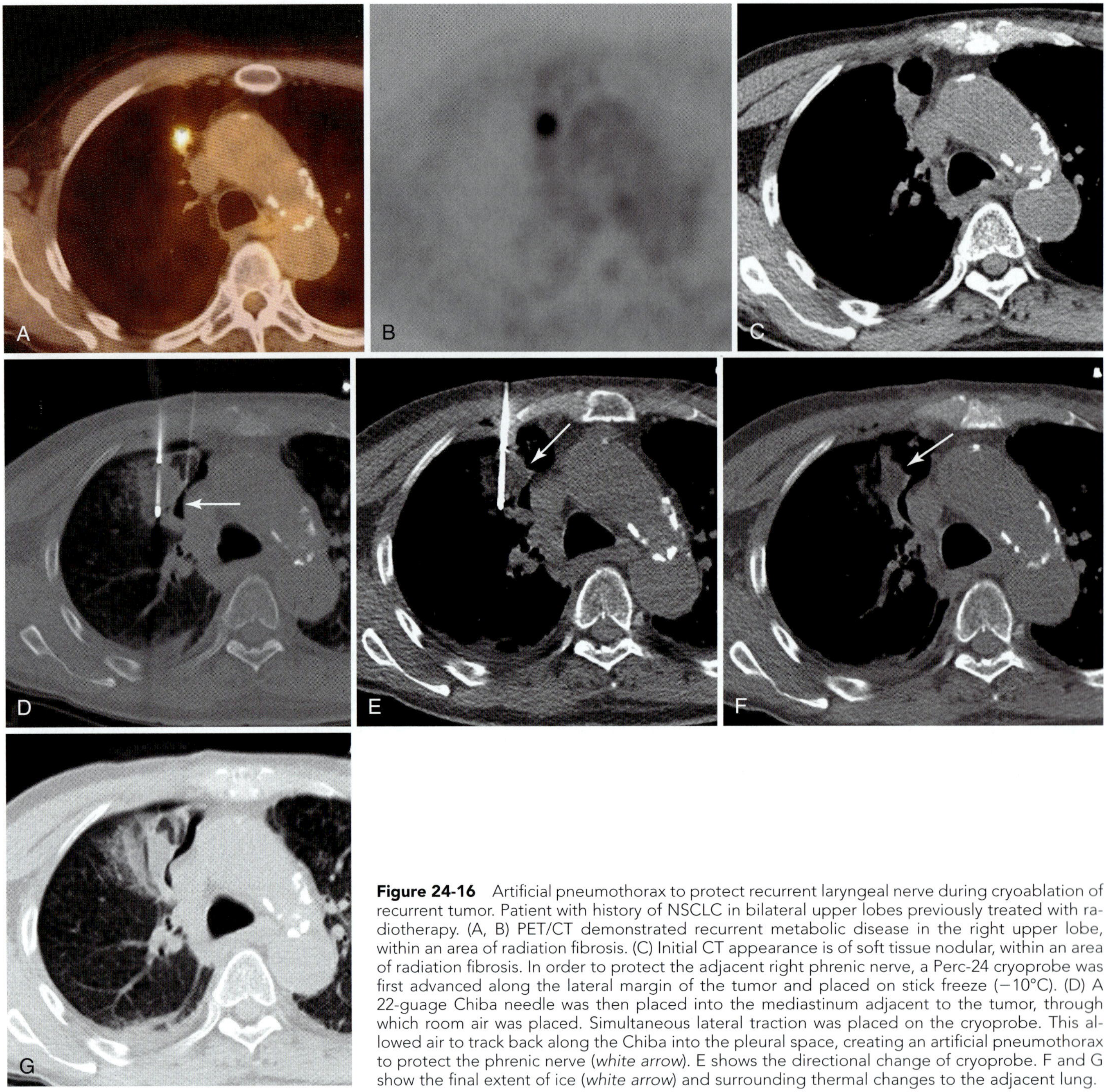

Figure 24-16 Artificial pneumothorax to protect recurrent laryngeal nerve during cryoablation of recurrent tumor. Patient with history of NSCLC in bilateral upper lobes previously treated with radiotherapy. (A, B) PET/CT demonstrated recurrent metabolic disease in the right upper lobe, within an area of radiation fibrosis. (C) Initial CT appearance is of soft tissue nodular, within an area of radiation fibrosis. In order to protect the adjacent right phrenic nerve, a Perc-24 cryoprobe was first advanced along the lateral margin of the tumor and placed on stick freeze (−10°C). (D) A 22-guage Chiba needle was then placed into the mediastinum adjacent to the tumor, through which room air was placed. Simultaneous lateral traction was placed on the cryoprobe. This allowed air to track back along the Chiba into the pleural space, creating an artificial pneumothorax to protect the phrenic nerve (*white arrow*). E shows the directional change of cryoprobe. F and G show the final extent of ice (*white arrow*) and surrounding thermal changes to the adjacent lung.

are without consequence when treated promptly. An understanding of prevention and management of pneumothorax, hemorrhage, and air embolism are essential for all thoracic interventionalists.

PNEUMOTHORAX

Pneumothorax is by far the most frequent anticipated adverse event of thoracic interventions, occurring in up to 30% of cases. Most pneumothoraces are asymptomatic and require no intervention beyond a period of monitoring to ensure that there is no delayed enlargement. When a pneumothorax is identified during or at the completion of a procedure, it is typically observed on subsequent imaging to evaluate for stability. A sliver of pleural air is the norm, and requires no intervention.

When a pneumothorax develops, the first steps should be to maintain the patient on oxygen and position them with the effected thorax in a dependent position.[81] Oxygen has been shown to improve resolution of pneumothoraces. The dependent position of the affected thorax helps both by tamponading the puncture site, and by decreasing lung excursion and air flow on the affected side.

Approximately 7% of pneumothoraces will ultimately require intervention including chest tube[82] placement, although we find that in practice, this is only necessary following 1%–2% of lung interventions. Our indications for placement of a chest tube is a pneumothorax that radiographically continues to expand temporally, causes greater than 30% atelectasis of the lung, or is symptomatic (decreased oxygen saturation, shortness of breath, and/or chest pain).

When placing a chest tube following lung intervention, attempt is made to place the side holes close to the pleural puncture, to promote apposition of the visceral and parietal pleura and arrest the leak at the site. At times, a large pneumothorax requires aspiration despite demonstrating stability over time. In this case, a needle with stylet is placed into the pleural space to perform the aspiration, and subsequently removed.

The pneumothorax is aspirated to completion on the table and then the tube is left closed.[83] A delayed CT is obtained after several minutes, which often shows resolution of the air leak, allowing removal of the tube on the table. For patients with a persistent leak, the tube is connected to a Hemilich® valve or Pleur-evac® and either placed to water seal or wall suction based on the vigor of the air leak. Most pneumothoraces resolve within days, but on occasion, surgical intervention is required to treat a bronchopleural fistula. This typically involves video-assisted thoracoscopic surgery with pleurodesis or wedge resection, and sometimes both.

Again, certain patients are at increased risk for pneumothorax, particularly those with emphysema, air-trapping, or hyperinflation secondary to prior lung resection. An extreme example of patients at risk from the consequences of pneumothorax are those status postpneumonectomy, and requiring intervention in the remaining lung. When treating these patients, a chest tube is kept open on the table for rapid deployment in the event of a pneumothorax. Aggressive treatment of even small pneumothoraces is typically indicated in this patient group.

Coughing increases the potential for pneumothorax via increased thoracic pressure and alveolar rupture. The cough reflex is stimulated by pulmonary hemorrhage. When hemorrhage is noted during the procedure, the patient is encouraged not to cough. Further antitussive control is achieved by the administration of morphine as a part of the conscious sedation regimen.

HEMORRHAGE

All patients undergoing elective biopsy and ablation should be optimized with regard to platelets, coagulation factors, and anticoagulant/antiplatelet medications prior to the procedure to minimize risk of major hemorrhage. Although minor hemoptysis is a common occurrence, risk of life-threatening hemorrhage is low. A thorough understanding of the vascular anatomy of the thorax allows interventions to be performed in a manner that further decreases this risk.

Procedure-related hemorrhage in the thorax is divided into intra- and extrapulmonary types. Preventable causes of extrapulmonary hemorrhage typically involve injury to intercostal or internal mammary vessels (Figure 24-17). The intercostal arteries and veins run in parallel with the intercostal nerves along the undersurface of the ribs. Needles should either be placed in the center of the intercostal space or over the superior margin of a rib. Attention to the internal mammary artery is necessary for all anterior, parasternal interventions.

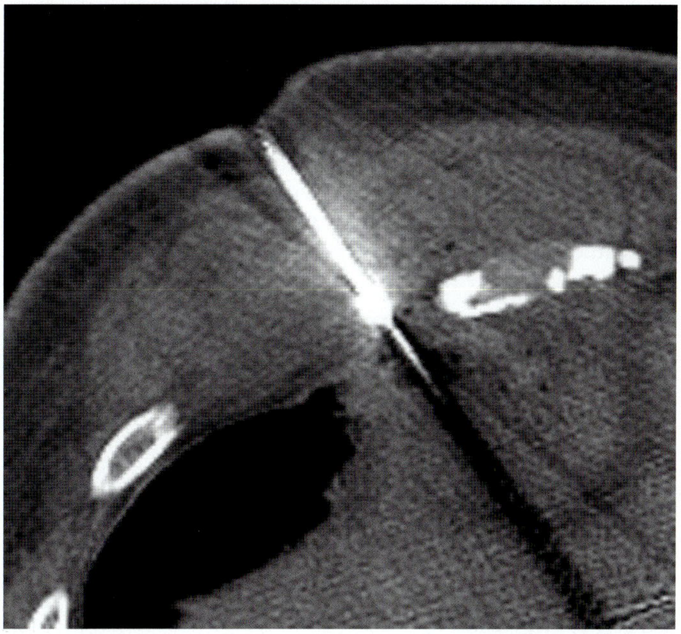

Figure 24-17 Anterior chest wall hemorrhage during cryoablation. The bleeding likely resulted from traversing an intercostal artery or vein. It stopped spontaneously.

Intrapulmonary hemorrhage results from injury of small and medium-sized pulmonary vessels. Pulmonary hemorrhage presents clinically as coughing and hemoptysis. This is associated with ground-glass and more consolidated airspace opacification on CT (see Figure 24-13, *B*).

When discovered during the procedure, hemorrhage should be closely monitored for evidence of expansion. The vast majority of pulmonary hemorrhage stops rapidly. If the hemorrhage continues to expand, measures should be taken to protect the remaining aerated lung from further contamination. The most important step is to prevent overflow of blood into the contralateral lung via central bronchi by placing the affected injured lung in a dependent position, thus confining the hemorrhage to one lung (see Figure 24-13, *C*). A single aerated lung will allow most patients to ventilate adequately. Continued unrelenting hemorrhage may require surgery or endovascular embolization.

Patients with emphysema, cystic lung disease, and obstructive pulmonary disease are at increased risk for pulmonary hemorrhage because of decreased pulmonary parenchymal density, which limits internal compression of injured vessels. Blood is able to fill these expanded airspaces, and tends to be more extensive than in normal lung.

Of all ablative techniques, cryoablation is most associated with hemorrhage. A small amount of hemorrhage is in fact expected as the ice ball melts, and is typically self-limited. Cryoablation is generally avoided in patients with severe emphysema, and those with decreased platelet and coagulation function. Such patients are more safely treated with heat-based ablation, which cauterizes the treated tissue.

AIR EMBOLISM

The most feared, and fortunately rare, adverse event of thoracic intervention is air embolism into the systemic circulation via the pulmonary veins. This can result in obstruction of the coronary and cerebral arteries, with disastrous consequences. Clinically, air embolism presents with sudden alteration of mental status, sense of doom, cardiopulmonary arrest, and death.[84,85] All post-procedure CTs should be extended into the left heart to exclude the presence of intracardiac air. When air is identified in the systemic circulation of asymptomatic patients, steps can be taken to prevent an adverse clinical outcome (Figure 24-18).

Risk factors for development of air embolism are not defined—a testament to its infrequent occurrence. We generally avoid traversing dilated air spaces (such as in emphysema and cystic lung disease) and visible bronchi in order to limit exposure of the pulmonary venous circulation to air flow. Additionally, we advise breathholding and minimizing the time that coaxial biopsy systems are left open when performing lung biopsy.

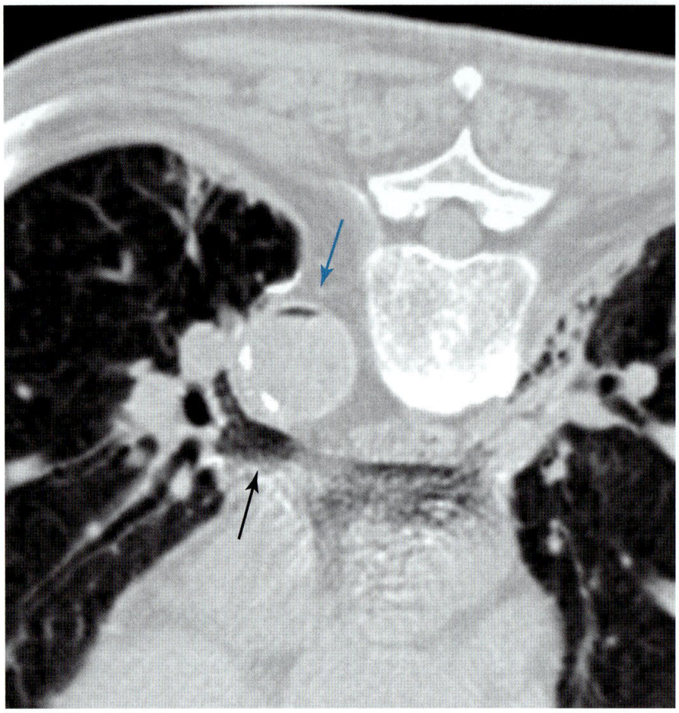

Figure 24-18 Air embolism following lung biopsy. Immediate postprocedure CT following lung biopsy demonstrates a large amount of intravascular air in the systemic circulation. The pulmonary veins (*black arrow*), left atrium, and aorta (*blue arrow*) all contain air. The patient was left in prone position and placed on 100% oxygen via face mask. A delayed scan after 15 minutes demonstrated resolution of the intravascular air.

When air is identified in the left atrium or ventricle during a procedure, it is important to take several steps to minimize the chances of systemic propagation of air. The patient should be placed on 100% oxygen face mask to promote reabsorption of room air. The patient should be positioned in the supine or Trendelenberg position to trap air within the heart. When air is confined to the left atrium, the patient may be placed in left lateral decubitus position to trap air within the atrium. Under no circumstances should the patient be allowed to lift his or her chest or head into an elevated position, as this will allow air to ascend to the cerebral circulation.

Conclusion

Interventional radiologists are now essential in the diagnosis and management of primary lung carcinomas. Thermal ablation of lung cancers has become established as an effective primary local treatment for patients with a contraindication to or preference against surgical resection. Ablation also has a role in management of local and distant recurrent disease. Allowing for limitations in establishing clear surgical margins, ablation has the advantage of being less invasive than surgical resection, which has expanded the spectrum of patients who can be treated.

The basic technique and management of patients undergoing biopsy and ablation is similar. An understanding of risk, along with prevention and management of potential adverse events, allows these procedures to be performed safely and effectively.

REFERENCES

The complete reference list is available online at www.expertconsult.com.

25

Metastatic Disease

QUAZI ZUBAIR AL-TARIQ | SCOTT GENSHAFT | STEPHEN T. KEE

KEY POINTS

- Interventional management of thoracic metastases involves careful consideration not only of parenchymal lesions, but also pleural and chest wall disease.
- Management of parenchymal metastases is similar to that of primary neoplasms, with the same technical considerations applying.
- Malignant effusion is the most common manifestation of pleural metastases that the interventionalist will be called upon to treat. This is largely accomplished through the use of temporary or indwelling drainage catheters with or without administration of a sclerosing agent to achieve pleurodesis.
- Painful osseous metastases may be treated with ablative therapies. Although much of the recent literature supports the use of RFA for this indication, cryoablation offers certain unique advantages, such as direct visualization of the ablation zone. This is especially helpful when ablating near critical structures.

Introduction

The thorax is a common site of metastatic disease, with frequent involvement of the lungs, pleura, osseous structures, and regional lymph nodes. Interventional radiologists are integral to the confirmation of thoracic involvement of malignancy via tissue sampling. There is growing support for the role of image-guided interventions in treating the manifestations of thoracic metastatic disease. This includes thermal ablation of metastatic disease to the lungs and pleura, catheter placement and sclerosis of malignant pleural effusions, and palliative pain management for osseous and soft-tissue metastases.

Techniques for percutaneous biopsy and thermal ablation of lung and bone neoplasms have been discussed in other chapters in this textbook. The first portion of this chapter will focus on patient selection for thermal ablation of discrete lung and pleural metastases. The second section will discuss management of malignant pleural effusion. The chapter will conclude with a section discussing the palliative management of painful osseous and soft tissue metastases with thermal ablation.

Lung Metastases

The lung is one of the most common sites of metastatic disease. Lung metastases are present in up to 30% of patients dying from all cancer types[1] (Figures 25-1 and 25-2). The surgical literature has demonstrated that metastasectomy offers improved survival for patients presenting with a limited number of lung metastases.[2] Many of these patients have medical comorbidities, which make them poor surgical candidates. These patients can benefit from alternate forms of therapy, including external beam radiation as well as image-guided thermal ablation.

RATIONALE FOR ABLATION OF LUNG METASTASES

Patients are referred for thermal ablation of lung metastases with the intent to either cure localized disease or to decrease tumor burden for palliative reasons. The basis for treatment of lung metastases is found in the surgical literature, where a survival benefit of metastasectomy for patients with limited pulmonary tumor burden has been demonstrated. The safety and efficacy of thermal ablation of primary and secondary lung neoplasms has been well established.

General surgical selection criteria necessitate that the primary tumor be controlled; there should be no or few extrathoracic metastasis, with the exception of liver; the metastases are in locations that make them amenable to surgically resection; and the patient's overall status and pulmonary function must be able to tolerate the procedure. When the above criteria can be met, the survival outcomes are generally good, with a 5-year survival rate that ranges between 30% and 50% in several retrospective studies.[3] Furthermore, Yamamoto et al. showed the potential for complete cure following metastasectomy of pulmonary colorectal carcinoma metastases of 17%.[4] Although the lack of randomized controlled studies makes it difficult to conclude that the survival benefit is due to the surgery itself, the data that have been presented in case series has allowed pulmonary metastasectomy to become well established as a treatment of localized metastatic disease.

The recurrence of disease following metastasectomy is quite high. According to the International Registry of Lung Metastases, the recurrence rate for all patients undergoing complete resection is 53%.[5] Rates of recurrence tend to be higher with certain primaries, such as sarcoma and melanoma. In many series, these patients have been treated with repeat resection.[6] More recently, data have emerged to support nonsurgical management of oligometastatic pulmonary disease, including thermal ablation and stereotactic body radiation therapy.[7,8]

A considerable amount of data has been reported over the past decade to support the safety and efficacy of thermal ablation in the treatment of localized metastatic disease. As in the surgical literature, many of the studies have consisted primarily of colorectal carcinoma, renal cell carcinoma, and sarcomas. The unifying characteristic of each of these malignancies is the occasional presentation of discrete oligometastatic pulmonary disease. The main objective of ablation therapy is eradication of tumor cells within a finite volume of lung so as to not significantly disrupt the overall functional reserve. This is particularly important in patients with limited baseline pulmonary function, such as those with fibrosis or emphysema. In comparison to surgical resection, presumed benefits from thermal ablative therapies include more targeted therapy with greater sparing of functional lung tissue in patients with suboptimal pulmonary function, lower costs, repeatability, and decreased morbidity and mortality[9] (Figure 25-3).

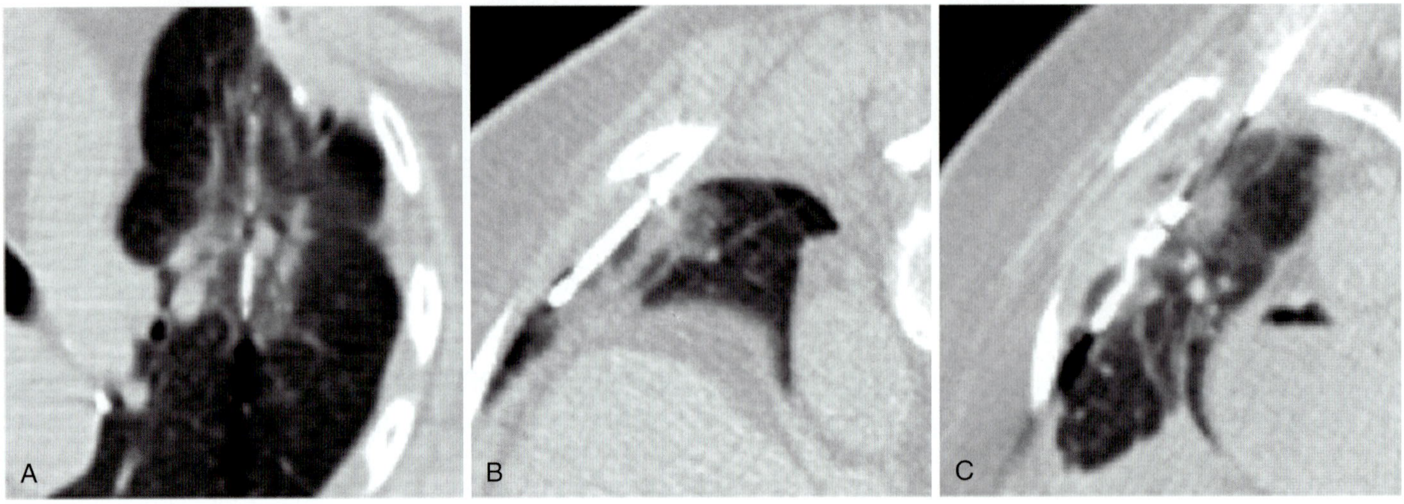

Figure 25-1 Multiple ablations performed at various time points using cryoablation (A, B) and microwave (C) in patient with oligometastatic renal cell carcinoma.

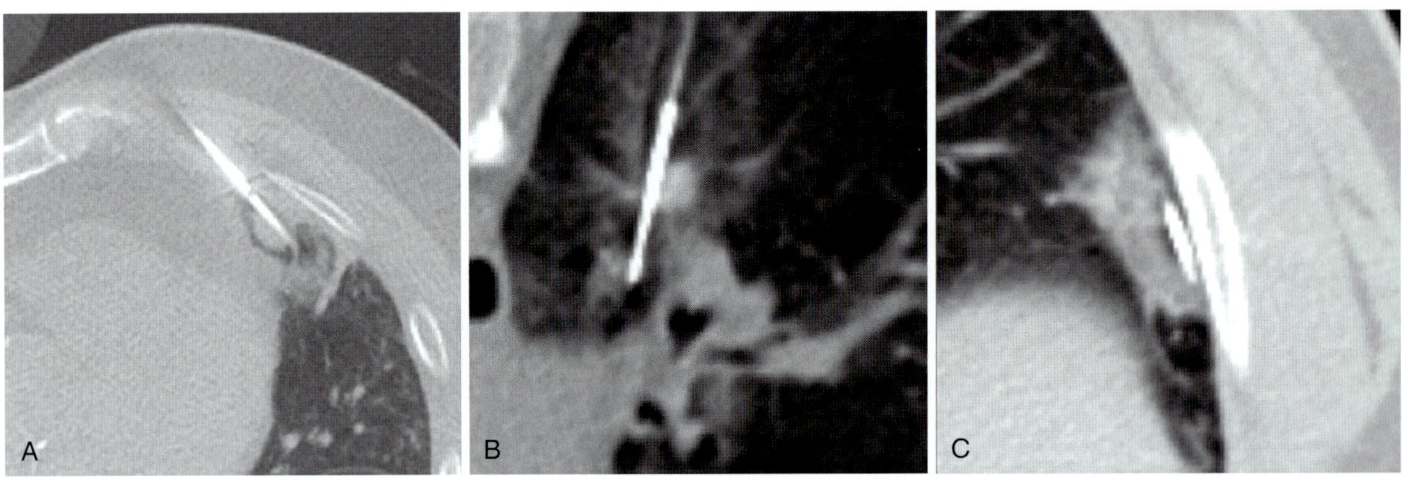

Figure 25-2 Multiple cryoablations (A, B, C) performed on different lesions in same patient with oligometastatic disease from tracheal adenoid cystic primary.

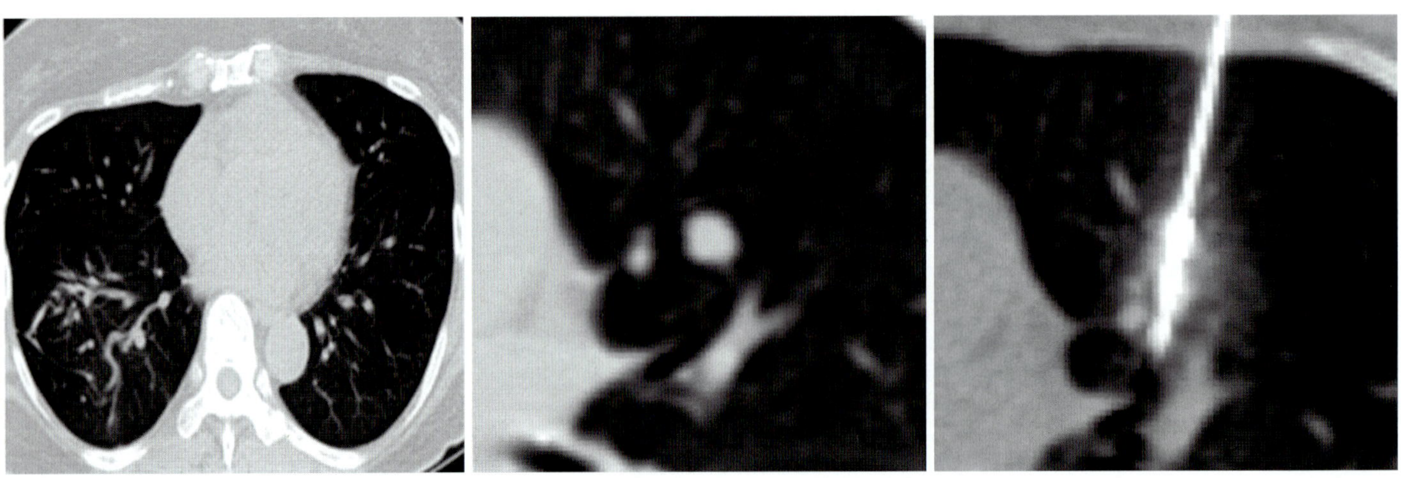

Figure 25-3 Patient with oligometastatic leiomyosarcoma initially underwent right lower lobe sublobar resection/metastasectomy. She subsequently developed another metastatic focus in the lingula. To avoid further loss of parenchyma, a decision was made to treat with RF ablation.

Much of the outcomes data reported have used RFA as the ablative modality. This is not surprising, as RFA was the earliest thermal ablation technique to be adopted for use in the lungs.[10] Studies looking at long-term survival demonstrated 5-year survival rates of approximately 27%, which is comparable to some of the numbers quoted for metastasectomy in the surgical literature.[4] A study that looked at 3-year cancer-specific survival demonstrated percentages of 90.6 for sublobar resection, 87.5 for RFA, and 90.2 for cryoablation.[11]

Some patients with more extensive metastatic disease may be candidates for percutaneous thermal ablation when the bulk of disease is stable, but a select number of metastases display aggressive growth. These lesions may be targeted to prevent complications, particularly airway or vascular compression, which could potentially cause increased symptoms or possibly death. Although cytoreduction is not an indication that is well established in the literature, it is a selection criterion that we have used for treating a select group of patients.

PATIENT SELECTION

Patients who may benefit from treatment of lung and pleural metastases have a countable number of discrete lesions that are limited to the lung or pleural surfaces. Several cancers that commonly present with oligometastatic thoracic disease include colorectal and renal cell carcinoma, osseous and soft tissue sarcomas, and tracheal adenoid cystic carcinoma. Various numbers have been used to quantify "oligometastatic" disease. In general, we will consider patients with five or fewer metastases, but we have treated patients with a larger number of lesions when the metastases have shown stability for 6 months or longer. The extent of disease should ideally be limited to the thorax, but again, exceptions are sometimes made when discrete treatable lesions are present elsewhere, such as in the liver.

Patients should only be considered after appropriate consultation with a medical oncologist. Thermal ablation is often used concurrently with system chemotherapy. The rationale is that chemotherapy may be more effective for small, microscopic metastatic implants, and may incompletely resolve larger metastases.

Although some groups treat multiple lesions, including those in both lungs, during a single session, we advocate treating a single lesion during each session. This is for several reasons. Each ablation should be performed with ideal patient positioning, whether prone, supine, or oblique. Placement of multiple probes increases the risks of the procedure, including the development of hemorrhage and pneumothorax.[12] This is particularly true when lesions are present in both lungs. Most patients can tolerate a degree of respiratory compromise from pneumothorax or hemorrhage into a single lung, but the possibility of compromise of the function of both lungs must be considered prior to performing a bilateral lung ablation.

When treating a patient with multiple metastases, a decision as to the order of treatment must be made prior to commencing. Lung ablations are performed with conscious sedation. Patient cooperation with breath holding and remaining stationary is essential. We advise performing a technically simple ablation during the first procedure to allow the patient to get accustomed to the experience. This allows treatment of more difficult lesions during subsequent procedures. It is best not to delay treating lesions that may be more problematic in the future, such as one that is encroaching upon a major vessel that could function as a heat sink (Figure 25-4).

Patients will typically require 1–2 weeks to recover after lung ablation. It is reasonable to schedule a patient for weekly procedures if they are doing well clinically. The goal should be to complete a set of treatments within 2 months. The patient should then undergo active surveillance, both to evaluate for treatment failure and to monitor for disease progression. If disease progression in the form of new lesions is discovered during a set of treatments, it signifies disseminated disease that is unlikely to be controlled via local therapy. Consultation with the patient's medical oncologist is required.

PROCEDURE AND FOLLOW-UP

Perioperative management and technical factors for performing a successful percutaneous lung ablation were discussed in the previous chapter. Radiofrequency ablation (RFA), microwave ablation (MWA), and percutaneous cryotherapy (PCT) can be used interchangeably for ablative procedures of lung metastases. The use of one modality over the other is based primarily on operator preference, with the individual modalities having particular strengths and weaknesses (Figure 25-5).

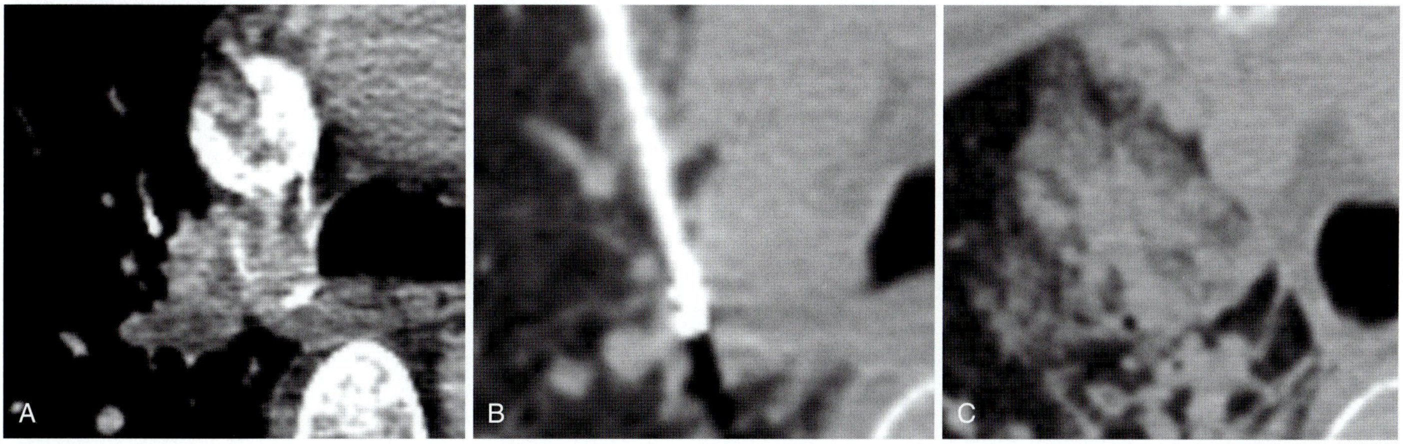

Figure 25-4 RF ablation performed in patient with renal cell carcinoma metastasis to the right perihilar region (A). Despite proximity to adjacent vascular structures (potential heat sinks), adequate ablation zone was achieved (B, C).

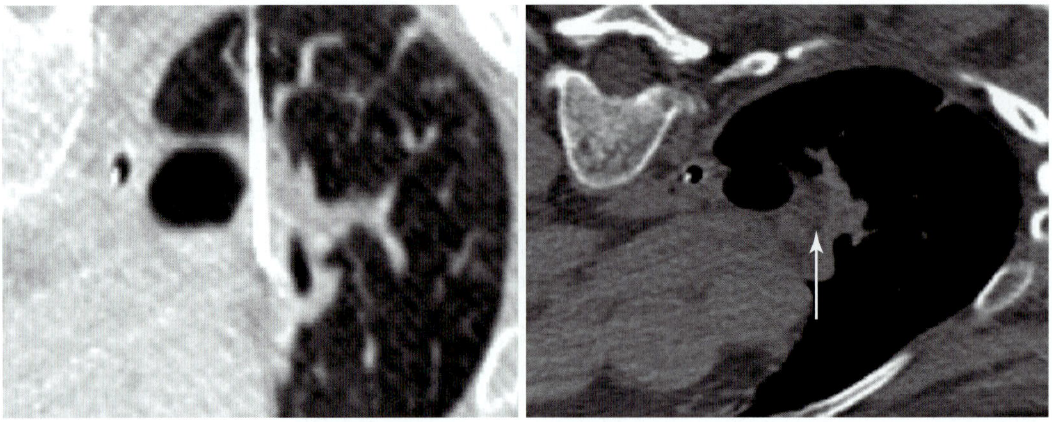

Figure 25-5 Cryoablation performed on chondrosarcoma metastasis located immediately adjacent to the left mainstem bronchus. Note ice ball at target location (*arrow*). The integrity of the adjacent bronchus is preserved. Safety profile of cryoablation for lesions near airways and large vessels was the justification for using the technique in this instance.

Safety considerations prior to ablation include management of coagulation status, and sedation risk. Most lung ablations are performed with conscious sedation, and therefore, some of the risks of anesthesia are minimized. Additionally, as opposed to ablation of primary lung carcinomas, many patients undergoing ablation of metastatic lung disease have normal pulmonary function.

Technical considerations for safe thermal ablation are identical to those used for treatment of primary lung carcinoma. These include use of tangential approach for peripheral lesions (Figure 25-6) and the axial approach for central lesions (Figure 25-7). Care should be taken to not cross major vascular and airway structures during needle placement, as well as avoiding a needle position with the tip pointed toward a major vascular structure. In order to obtain a complete ablation, the interventionalist must be aware of the device-specific expected ablation zone. Multiple probes may be required to fully treat the target lesion. Heat sinks are a major factor that can limit the extent of an ablation.

Potential complications include pneumothorax, hemorrhage, and air embolism. The prevention and management of these complications were discussed in Chapter 24 (Figure 25-8).

The imaging follow-up is identical to that described after ablation of primary lung cancer as described in Chapter 24. It should be coordinated with the patient's medical oncologist, given that the nature of the disease is by definition, systemic.

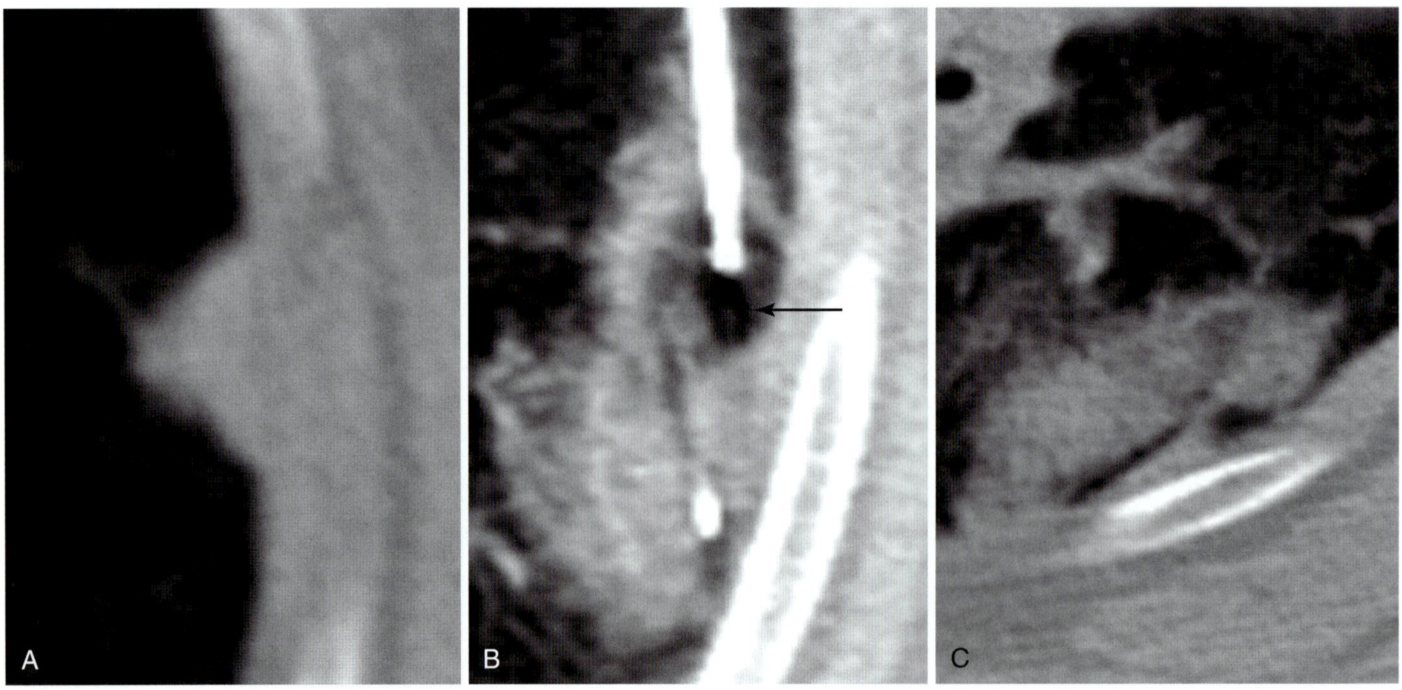

Figure 25-6 (A–C) Cryoablation performed using tangential approach on a peripherally located metastasis from renal cell primary. Note ice ball formation, seen as a rounded hypodensity, at the target location (*arrow*) (B).

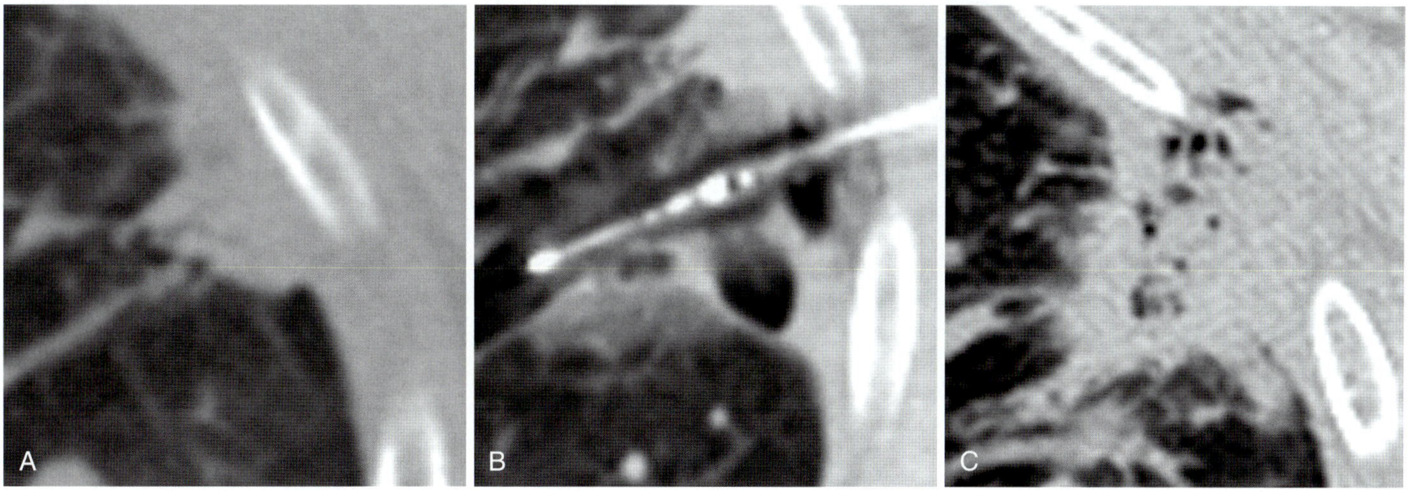

Figure 25-7 (A–C) MW ablation performed in patient with peripheral metastatic focus from tracheal adenoid cystic carcinoma using axial approach.

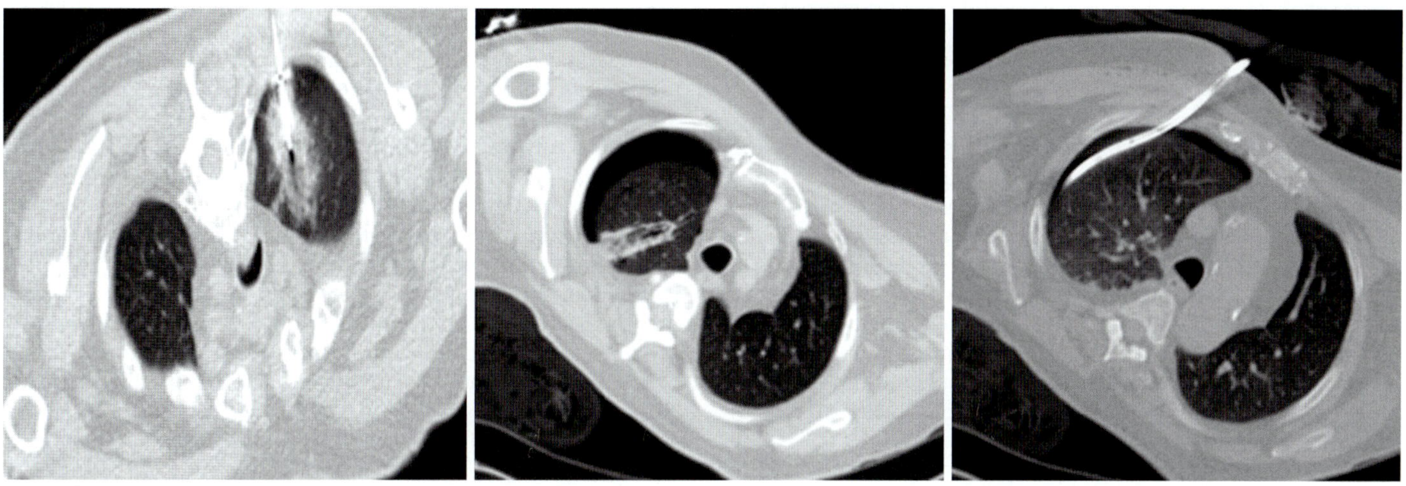

Figure 25-8 Patient developed moderate-sized pneumothorax following cryoablation of right upper lobe nodule. The pneumothorax was large enough to necessitate chest tube placement.

Pleural Disease

When a tumor, whether primary or secondary, invades the pleural space, it disrupts the capillary endothelium and obstructs lymphatic drainage. Together, these factors lead to the formation of malignant effusions. Malignant pleural disease accounts for half of all exudative effusions that present for thoracentesis.[13] Lung and breast cancer, along with lymphoma, account for up to 75% of malignant effusions.[13]

Patients with malignant pleural effusions suffer significant morbidity, including dyspnea, cough, and repeated thoracentesis. Patients with refractory malignant effusions requiring frequent (monthly) large-volume thoracentesis may benefit from procedures aimed at diverting the accumulating fluid, or those that obliterate the pleural space, and thereby, prevent fluid accumulation.

Traditional surgical treatment options include pleuroperitoneal shunting and video-assisted thoracoscopic surgery (VATS) with talc pleurodesis.[14] Although these methods have a long successful history of clinical implementation, they are associated with prolonged hospital stay and significant financial cost. Furthermore, there has been some concern that talc may in some cases cause an acute respiratory distress syndrome–like syndrome.[15]

Both of these surgical options are increasingly being replaced by image-guided tunneled catheter placement into the pleural space, with or without intrapleural administration of sclerosing agents. Tunneled pleural catheters, for example PleurX® (Figure 25-9), allow self-drainage of pleural fluid and have been shown to provide a high rate of pleurodesis and the potential for tube removal.[16] Direct comparison studies of talc pleurodesis versus indwelling tunneled pleural catheter (PleurX) have demonstrated both to be equally effective at relieving symptoms such as dyspnea.[17] A benefit of PleurX is that in can be placed in an outpatient setting, whereas talc pleurodesis requires hospital admission for up to 4 days. The cost was comparable for patients with a prognosis of 6 months or less. In cases where prognosis is less than 6 weeks, PleurX catheter treatment is generally preferred.[18]

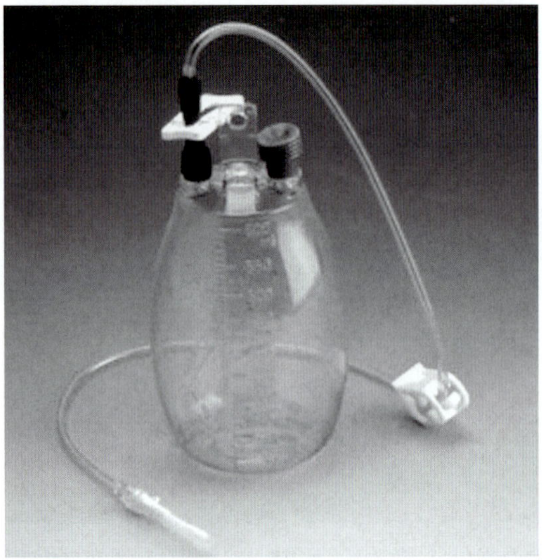

Figure 25-9 PleurX drainage catheter system demonstrates cuffed catheter and vacuum drainage catheters. *From Pollak JS, Burdge CM, Rosenblatt M, Houston JP, Hwu WJ, Murren J: Treatment of malignant pleural effusions with tunneled long-term drainage catheters,* J Vasc Interv Radiol. *12(2):201-208, 2001; Figure 1B.*

Warren et al. have shown a high rate of pleurodesis following tunneled pleural catheter placement. Overall, 58.6% of patients had pleural catheter removal, which was performed, on average, 29.4 days following placement. Only 2.9% of these patients had subsequent reaccumulation of fluid to the point of having dyspnea. It should be noted that this group reported aggressive catheter drainage, including 1500 mL at the time of placement, 600 mL every other day for 1 week, and then continued drainage every other day. This maintenance of low pleural fluid volume most certainly contributed to the high rate of pleurodesis with subsequent catheter removal (Figure 25-10).

A low rate of complications has been reported, including catheter blockage, cellulitis, empyema, and tumor infiltration through the catheter site. Several factors have been shown to be negative predictors of successful pleurodesis, including trapped lung and prior irradiation. Interestingly, patients with malignant pleural fluid cytology have a higher rate of pleurodesis than those who did not.[16]

TUNNELED PLEURAL CATHETER PLACEMENT

The PleurX catheter is a 15.5-French soft catheter with multiple side holes within the pleural portion of the tubing. The catheter is tunneled subcutaneously prior to entering the pleural space. This provides for both security of adhesion and prevents infections. A one-way valve is present on the back end of the catheter, which is opened when proprietary vacutainer bottles are attached for drainage.

Standard labs, including CBC, platelets, and coagulation panel should be obtained prior to placement. The procedure should generally not be performed if INR >1.5, platelets $<50{,}000$, or if the patient is actively being treated with an anticoagulant or antiplatelet agent. Although catheter placement can be performed with local anesthesia, conscious sedation is typically utilized for patient comfort. There are no data to support or refute the use of periprocedural antibiotics at the time of catheter placement. The low rate of catheter-related infection that has been reported suggests that antibiotics are not necessary, but many interventionalists will choose to administer an agent with coverage of skin flora, such as Cefazolin or Clindamycin.

Pleural effusions are most easily accessed with the aid of ultrasound guidance; fluoroscopic or CT guidance is generally reserved for patients who are unable to sit upright. The catheter is placed using the Seldinger technique. Access is in a low intercostal space, in the midaxillary line. The site of access is dilated to 16-French and a peel-away sheath is used for catheter placement. A subcutaneous tunnel approximately 2 cm in length is created with the included tunneling device. The tunnel should be created within the same intercostal space as the access site for patient comfort (Figure 25-11).

The catheter is placed so that the polyester cuff is just inside the skin opening. This cuff promotes adhesion of the catheter, and must be dissected free during catheter removal. It is important to confirm that all side-holes for the catheter are within the pleural space, which can be an issue in obese patients or if the

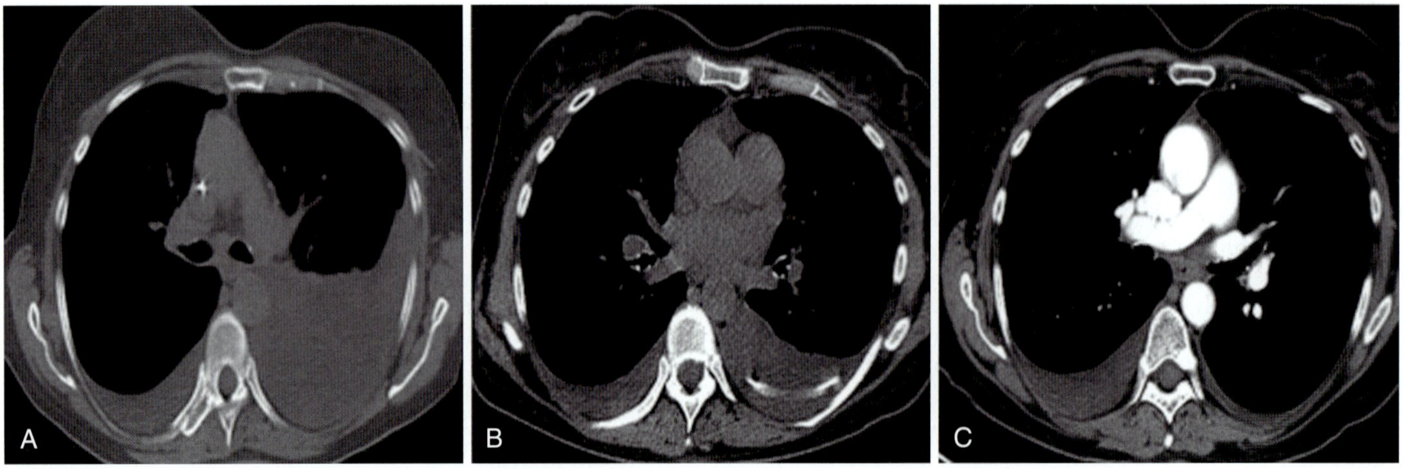

Figure 25-10 (A) Patient with malignant effusion related to breast carcinoma. (B) Reduction in size of effusion following placement of PleurX catheter. (C) Spontaneous pleurodesis which persisted following PleurX removal

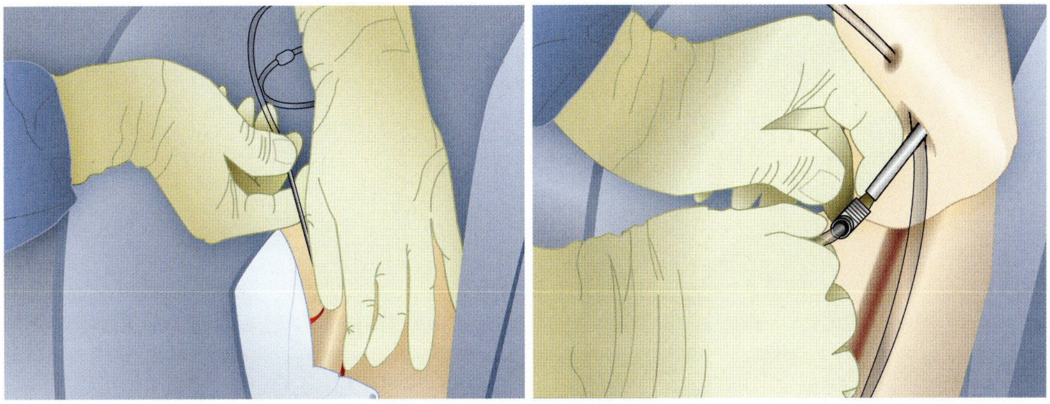

Figure 25-11 During the placement of the pleurX catheter, the tunneler is directed posterolaterally toward the access site (approximately 5 cm away). Once the cuff is secure, the proximal end of the catheter may be advanced through the peel-away.

tract is excessively long. Side-holes that course through the subcutaneous soft tissues will allow soft tissue fluid accumulation.

Following tube placement, a complete thoracentesis, up to 1500 mL, is performed to ensure appropriate catheter function. A sterile dressing is included in the catheter kit. The patient is instructed to perform home drainage once every other day, up to 1000 mL per drainage. The drainage kits come with 1000-mL and 500-mL bottles, which are discarded following use.

For patients who have already had placement of nontunneled thoracostomy tubes, we recommend removal of the tube for a week or two prior to placement of a tunneled catheter. During this time, the effusion is managed with therapeutic thoracentesis.[19,20]

PleurX catheters may be left in place and are typically not removed unless drainage is less than 50 mL/day. Even though the catheters may be left in place for an extended time, the reported rate of associated infection is low. In one large study, only 5 of 231 patients developed an infection, with 4 of the infections occurring at the insertion site.[21] Localized infections can be treated with antibiotics. Empyema requires tube removal, aggressive intravenous antibiotics, and possible surgical washout versus decortication.

CATHETER-DIRECTED PLEURODESIS

A minimally invasive interventional alternative to placement of a tunneled pleural catheter is chemical pleurodesis through small-bore catheters (8–12 Fr). To avoid reexpansion edema within the adjacent lung, generally no more than 1.5 L are initially withdrawn.

For successful pleurodesis, there must be reexpansion of the lung and complete evacuation of the effusion, resulting in apposition of the parietal and visceral layers of pleura. Resolution may be determined through the use of serial radiographs or when daily catheter output falls below 100 mL. Once the above criteria are met, a sclerosing agent can be directly administered into the pleural space. Talc suspension has the highest overall success rate (93%–95%) and is the preferred agent of choice.[22] Other available options include doxycycline, minocycline, and bleomycin.

When performing the pleurodesis, the sclerosing agent is typically mixed with lidocaine and then injected through the catheter. Following injection, the catheter is clamped and the patient is rotated to ensure that the agent coats the entire pleural surface. The catheter is then unclamped and placed to suction, usually for 1 day before being removed.

Failed pleurodesis is defined by symptomatic reaccumulation of malignant effusion within 1 month of the procedure. Complications of the procedure include infection and pneumothorax. Pleurodesis should not be performed in patients unlikely to reexpand their lungs. Contraindications include trapped lung, a thick pleural peel, endobronchial obstruction, or underlying restrictive lung disease.

Palliative Ablation for Painful Chest Wall and Osseous Metastases

Osseous metastases account for the most common cause of cancer-related pain and can prove a management dilemma. Combinations of analgesia, chemotherapy, and external beam irradiation are used with mixed results. Ablative therapies may be used as an alternative for patients who fail to reach adequate levels of pain control with other regimens.

Recent studies have demonstrated that thermal ablation provides significant pain relief in the majority of patients and that there may be a synergistic effect with external beam irradiation when both therapies are used within 90 days of one another. The same study also showed that patients who experienced pain relief with ablation generally lived slightly longer than those who did not respond (11.2 months vs. 4.3 months). Although the majority of ablations performed for this indication were done using radiofrequency ablation, chest wall lesions were also treated with microwave and cryoablation techniques. The procedure has a favorable safety profile, with the most common adverse effects being pain flare. Patients with preexisting brachial neuropathy may have an exacerbation of symptoms.[23]

In our own practice, our preferred modality for treatment of painful bone and soft tissue metastases is with cryoablation (Figure 25-12). This use of cryoablation has advantages over heat-based modalities in several respects. Most important is the rapid analgesic effect of cold. Patients typically report an initial sense of discomfort as freezing commences, which rapidly decreases after approximately 1 minute, as adjacent nerve fibers are stunned or destroyed. The heat-based modalities, in particular RFA, tend to cause severe nerve irritation during the procedure prior to definitive nerve injury, to the extent that general anesthesia is often required. Cryoablation of bone and

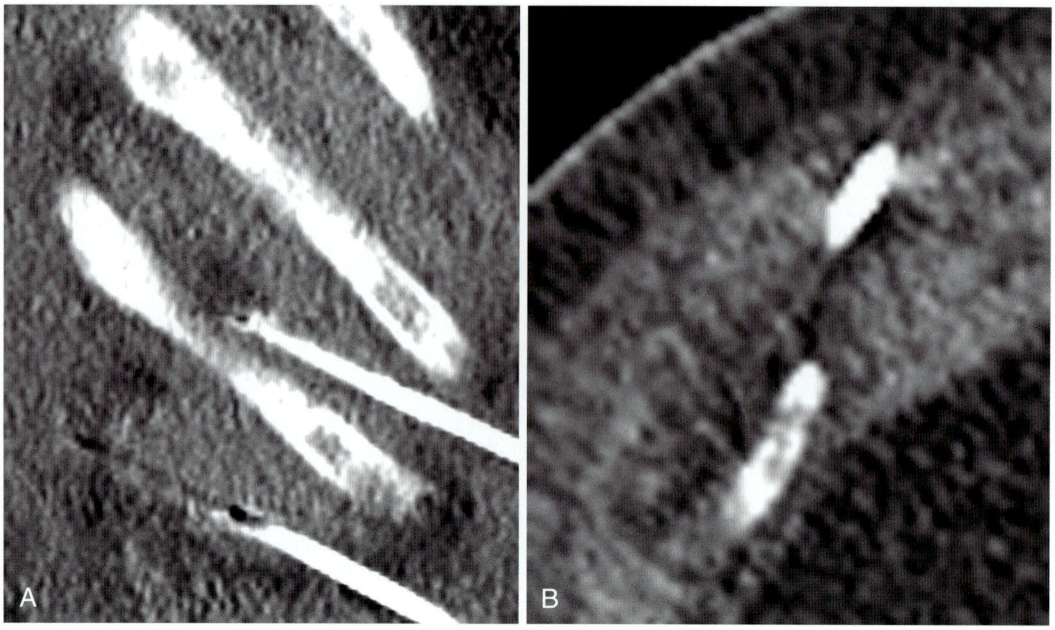

Figure 25-12 Cryoablation may also be used for the treatment of extrapleural disease as demonstrated in A and B in which a chest wall metastasis from mesothelioma is being treated.

soft tissue lesions can typically be performed with conscious sedation, unless the ablation is extensive or adjacent to a critical area, such as the spine, for which absolute absence of motion is required.

The second advantage of cryoablation is the ability to see the extent of the ablation zone during the procedure, because of the low attenuation of the ice that is formed. This ensures adequate coverage of the target. It should be noted, however, that visualization of ice within dense bone is difficult, and cannot be relied on to accurately track the extent of ablation. This is an important consideration when ablating adjacent to a critical structure, such as the spine.

Finally, there are concerns that the use of heat-based ablations, particularly RFA, may allow backward heating along the shaft of the coaxial bone introducer needle. In our practice, this has not been an issue with cryoablation.

Although guidance may be achieved with ultrasound, CT is generally recommended to confirm complete coverage of the target mass. Soft tissue ablations can typically be performed following direct introduction of the ablation probe into the target mass. When ablating bone lesions or sclerotic metastases, coaxial techniques involving an intraosseous trocar needle and guiding cannula (i.e., Kyphon® needle) can be employed. Ablation probes are fragile and will break if attempts are made to forcibly place them within a bone mass, unless the lesion is predominantly lytic and there is no intervening cortex (Figure 25-13). The needle should be at least 16 G in order to create a tract that can accommodate most ablation probes. The needle can usually be advanced using manual pressure when the cortex is soft and thin. In instances where the overlying cortex is thick, a hand-held drill may be employed. Once the needle has been placed in the target lesion, a biopsy of

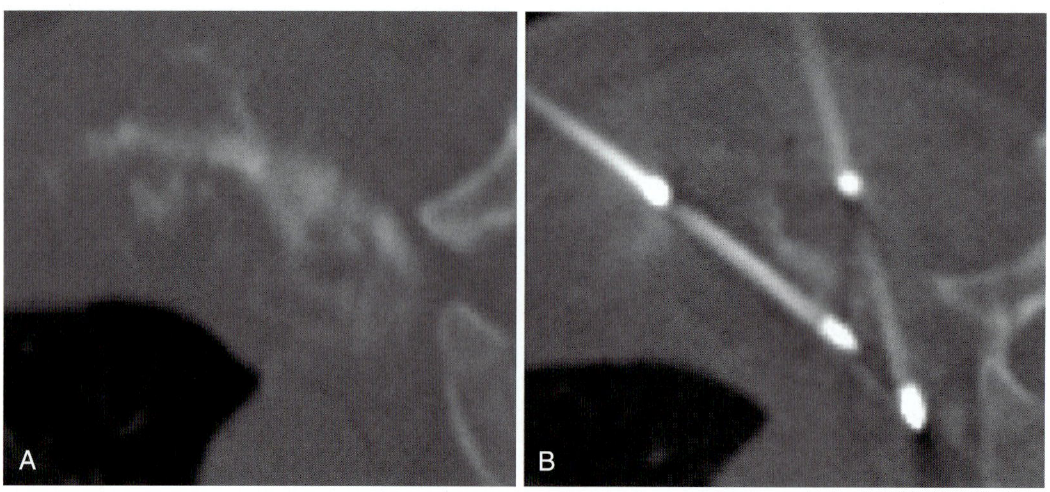

Figure 25-13 Multiple techniques may be used for palliation in patients with bony metastasis. In this case of colon cancer metastasis (A), two cryoprobes are placed directly within the lesion (B). The patient reported significant reduction in pain postprocedure.

the lesion may be performed if it is necessary to confirm malignancy.

As with ablations performed elsewhere, the size of the lesion should determine the size of the probe used. The largest currently available probes can be used for lesions up to 5 cm in size. For bone ablations, the ablation zone should extend to the cortex, as cortical bone destruction and irritation of the periosteal nerves typically contributes significantly to the patient's pain.

When using a coaxial technique with an osseous trocar, the trocar must be completely retracted away from the active portion of the ablation device after probe placement, so that the entire extent of the active probe is exposed. Long-length probes are required for most bone introducer needles to allow this exposure.

Immediately following the conclusion of ablation, the lesion may be injected with a mixture of polymethacrylate and tantalum powder for radiopacity under CT or fluoroscopic guidance for the purposes of protecting against pathologic fracture. This has also been demonstrated to provide pain relief for patients.[24] Some authors promote the use of tract ablation at the conclusion of the procedure to prevent tumor seeding of the tract.

Adjunctive techniques to improve ablation zones include preprocedural transarterial embolization, with the goal of reducing local heat sink effects.[25] This, however, may lead to uneven ablation zones with increased risk of thermal injury to adjacent tissues and should thus be performed selectively. The use of self-cooled electrodes can also improve ablation size by reducing tissue charring at the probe tip.

REFERENCES

The complete reference list is available online at www.expertconsult.com.

PART
6

Musculoskeletal Oncology

ALDA L. TAM

26

Percutaneous Musculoskeletal Biopsy

COLETTE SHAW | ADAM ZOGA

KEY POINTS

- Percutaneous musculoskeletal biopsy planning should involve multidisciplinary collaboration
- Recognize common "pseudotumors" and "don't-touch lesions"
- A solitary bone lesion of unknown etiology is a primary tumor until proven otherwise
- Perform the biopsy with imaging modality that best demonstrates the lesion
- The biopsy needle path should:
  - Be aligned with the proposed surgical incision
  - Be confined to the anatomic compartment involved
  - Not cross joint spaces, tendons, ligaments, or neurovascular structures

Background

Percutaneous, image-guided musculoskeletal biopsy (PMB) is a well-established, safe, and accurate procedure.[1-4] It has significantly reduced the need for open surgical biopsy—a more invasive and less cost-effective procedure that is associated with a higher complication rate, longer recovery time, and longer time to initiation of therapy. Historically, clinicians have been reluctant to refer their patients for image-guided percutaneous biopsy following reports of diagnostic errors, complications, and unnecessary amputations, particularly if biopsies were performed at centers not specialized in orthopedic oncology.[5] It is now widely accepted that the assessment and biopsy of musculoskeletal lesions should be performed at the institution where the lesion can be definitively managed. Unlike other percutaneous biopsies performed by radiologists, the approach used for biopsy of musculoskeletal lesions, particularly those in the extremities, needs to be closely aligned with the planned surgical approach.

An additional challenge relates to the ever-increasing demand for high-quality tissue samples.[6] Targeted drug therapy for each unique genetic profile is one of the primary goals of a personalized model of patient care.[7] The histologic and biologic heterogeneity of tumors has significant implications for the molecular profiling of cancers, including the ability to identify specific tumor markers and predict the response to targeted therapies. Changes in tumor biology during therapy need to be characterized in patients with disease progression prior to commencing second- and third-line agents. In those with metastatic disease, treatment should be based on the "metastatic" tumor biology, rather than that of the initial diagnostic specimen from the primary lesion. Communication between the interventional radiologist and the orthopedic pathologist is essential to ensure that the appropriate types, quantity, and quality of samples are acquired.

This chapter reviews the approach to percutaneous image-guided biopsy of musculoskeletal lesions. The various techniques and devices are outlined, and the merits, limitations, and complications of each are discussed.

Indications and Contraindications

The most common reason to perform musculoskeletal biopsy is to diagnose malignancy or infection (Table 26-1). Solitary bone lesions that are not clearly benign should be regarded as sarcomas until proven otherwise. There are no absolute contraindications to percutaneous biopsy (Table 26-2); however, not all lesions identified by imaging warrant biopsy.[8] A plain-film radiograph or CT of a classic osteoid osteoma does not require biopsy prior to percutaneous ablative therapy (Figure 26-1). Lesions identified incidentally and believed to be latent or active but nonprogressive may be observed, for example, nonossifying fibroma or enchondroma (Figure 26-2). Familiarity with common pseudotumors is essential to avoid unnecessary and possibly hazardous interventions. Lesions that can mimic a tumor include those related to soft tissues and bony structures.[9-12] Trauma, overuse, infection and symptomatic normal variants are the primary causes of pseudotumors. Many magnetic

TABLE 26-1 Indications for Percutaneous Musculoskeletal Biopsy

1. Determine the benign or malignant nature of a lesion
2. Confirm and characterize metastatic disease in a patient with one or more existing primary tumors
3. Evaluate tumor response to chemotherapy or radiotherapy
4. Characterize the nature and extent of a benign systemic process
5. Obtain material for microbiology analysis in a patient with suspected infection

TABLE 26-2 Relative Contraindications to Percutaneous Musculoskeletal Biopsy

1. "Don't-touch lesions"
2. Uncorrectable coagulopathy
3. Inability of the patient to cooperate or to be positioned for the procedure.
4. Systemic infection or infection involving the overlying soft tissues
5. Lack of a safe pathway to the lesion, for example, C1 and the odontoid process of C2 lesions

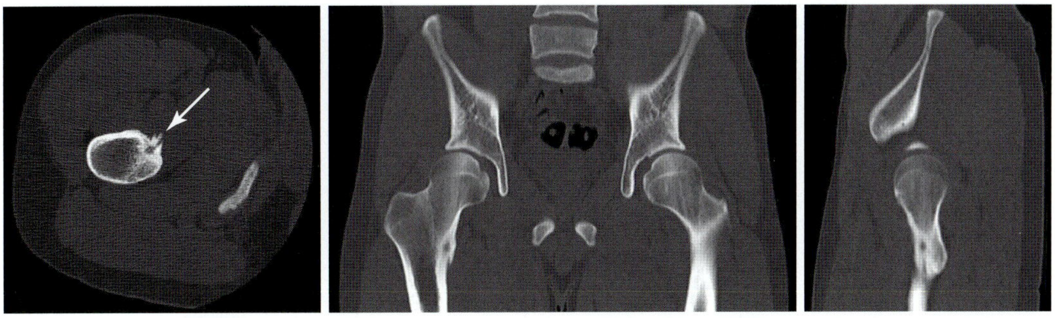

Figure 26-1 Osteoid osteoma. CT right hip axial coronal and sagittal images in a 20-year-old male with chronic right hip pain. The study demonstrates a 9-mm lucent lesion at the medial cortex of the right femoral neck with a central calcification (nidus) and surrounding cortical thickening. Bone proliferation is noted at the insertion of the iliopsoas tendon (*arrow*).

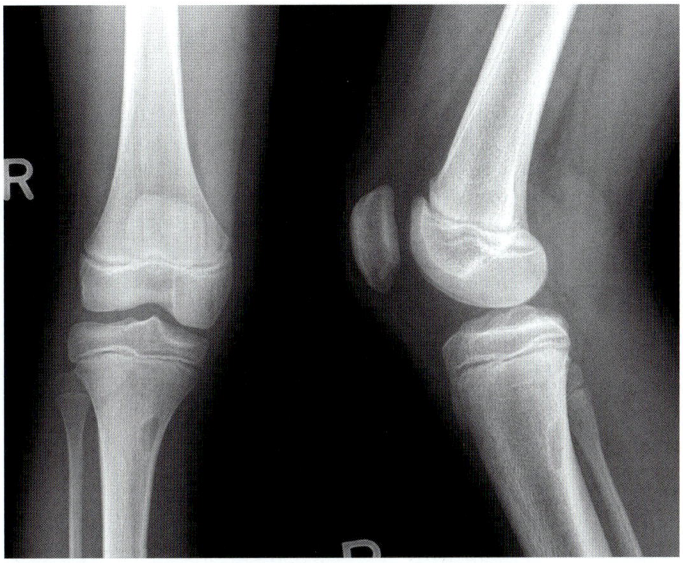

Figure 26-2 Nonossifying fibroma. Plain-film radiographs, AP and lateral projections, of the right knee in an 11-year-old. An eccentric lucency in the metaphysis of the tibia with a thin sclerotic margin is characteristic of nonossifying fibroma. No further imaging or intervention was indicated.

resonance imaging (MRI)-detected abnormalities and mass-like lesions may have characteristic appearances on plain-film radiography or computed tomography (CT) that enable diagnosis.[12] Examples of pseudotumors include the peripheral calcific rim of myositis ossificans, retained radiopaque foreign bodies, stress fracture of bone, and hydroxyapatite deposition within tendons. In myositis ossificans, biopsy during the early phase of development can give a false-positive diagnosis of osteosarcoma because of the intense osteoblastic activity. The diagnosis may be evident some weeks later when a peripheral rim of calcification might be seen on radiographs or CT imaging.[13] Soft tissue hematomas may be associated with trauma or coagulation disorders, for example, hemophilia or anticoagulant therapy (Figure 26-3). Complex MRI findings can result from repeated hemorrhage into the soft tissues confounded by muscle movement and time elapsed since the bleeding event. A simple hematoma can sometimes be difficult to distinguish from hemorrhage into a tumor.[9] Diabetic myonecrosis is a myopathy associated with poorly controlled diabetes mellitus that may be associated with an intramuscular soft tissue mass (Figure 26-4). Normal variants and their overuse can lead to symptoms and the appearance of a mass on MRI, for example, supernumerary bones,[14] tarsal coalition, and accessory soleus muscle. A ruptured Baker's cyst may present as a mass in the medial calf on MRI. Extension to the posteromedial knee should enable a diagnosis to be made. Similarly, bursitis tends to occur at reproducible locations around joints and can present as a mass. Metabolic disorders including amyloid deposition and hyperparathyroidism can also be associated with MRI pseudotumors. Brown tumors are a feature of secondary hyperparathyroidism and are frequently nonspecific on MRI (Figure 26-5). The findings may be correlated with hypercalcemia, hypophosphatemia, and high serum parathormone level.

The biopsy of certain lesions needs to be approached with caution (Figure 26-6). Hypervascular masses may be associated with significant morbidity particularly if they are located within a confined space, for example, a limb or the spinal canal. Hemorrhage into a limb compartment may predispose to compartment syndrome. Hemorrhage within the spinal canal may result in cord or nerve root compression. The proximity of vessels and nerves in the neck increases the complication risk for cervical spine biopsy compared with thoracic and

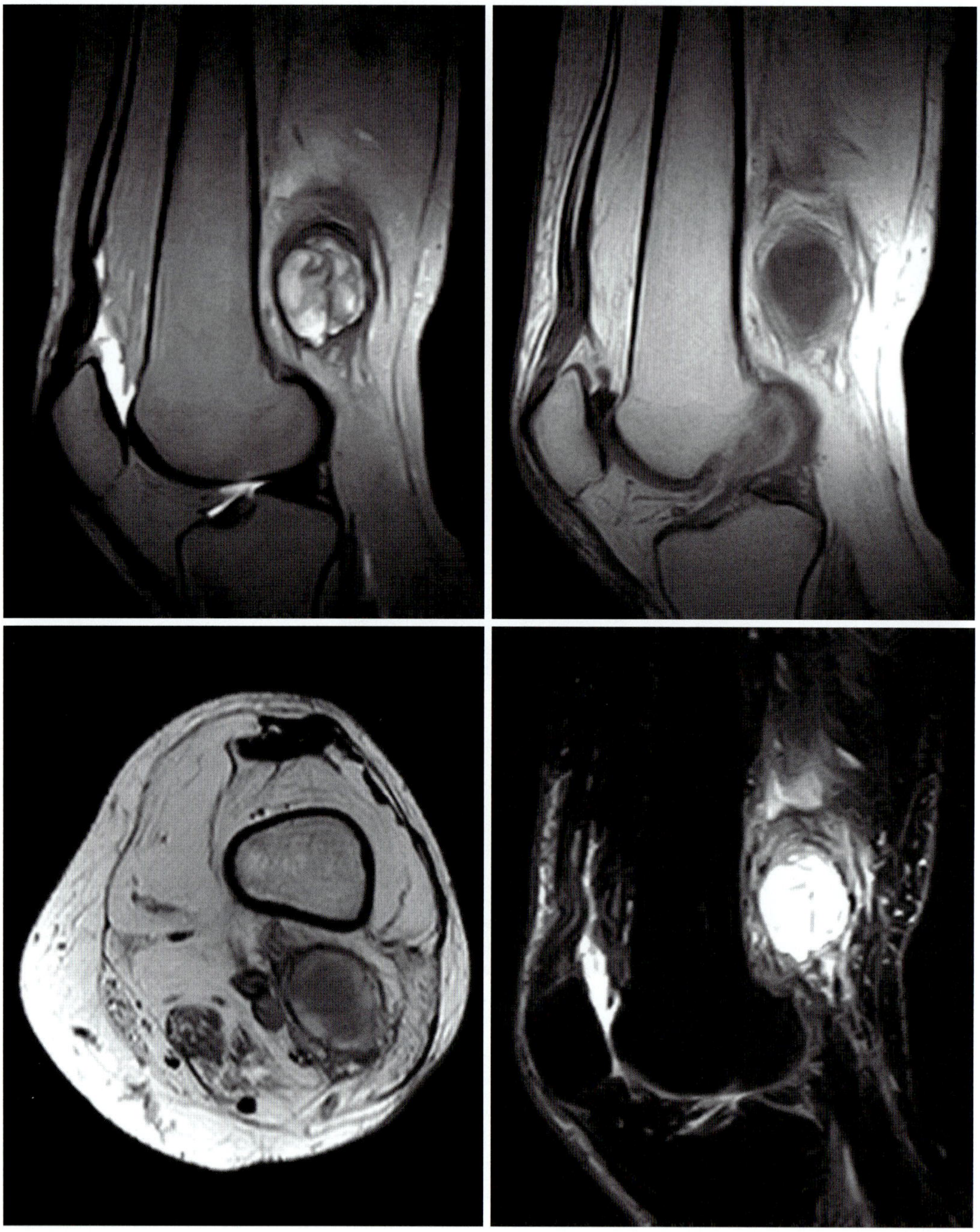

Figure 26-3 Hematoma left thigh. (*left* to *right*): MRI T2-weighted sequence sagittal projection, T1-weighted sequence sagittal and axial projections, T2-weighted sequence with fat saturation sagittal projection demonstrate a well-circumscribed complex intramuscular mass centered on the biceps femoris muscle. High signal intensity consistent with fluid is noted on the T2 fat-saturated sequence. These findings and a history of trauma were consistent with hematoma.

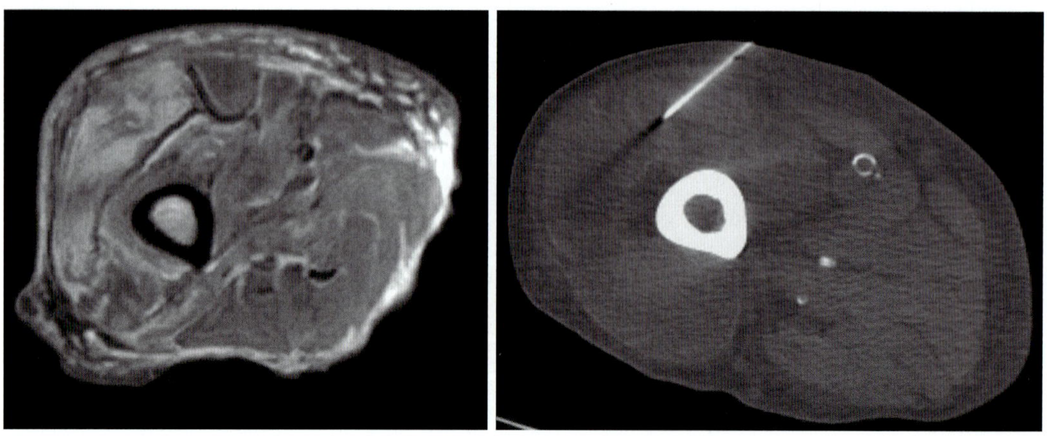

Figure 26-4 Diabetic myonecrosis. CT axial image of the right thigh shows needle sampling of an edematous vastus lateralis muscle (*right*). MRI of the right thigh, T2-weighted sequence axial projection shows diffused hyperintensity in the vastus lateralis muscle with preservation of surrounding tissue planes (*left*). Differential diagnosis included pyomyositis and necrotizing fasciitis.

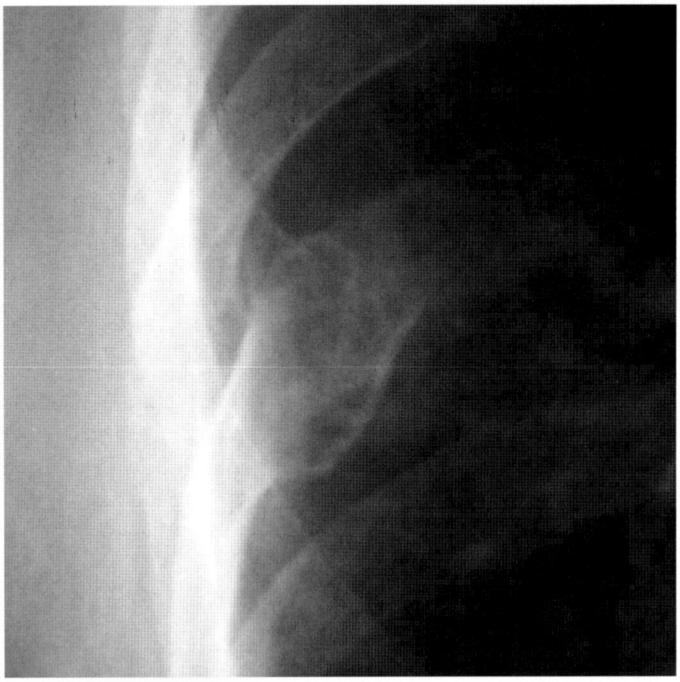

Figure 26-5 Brown tumor. Plain-film radiograph of the ribs demonstrates a purely lytic expansile rib lesion associated with thinning of the cortex in a patient with secondary hyperparathyroidism.

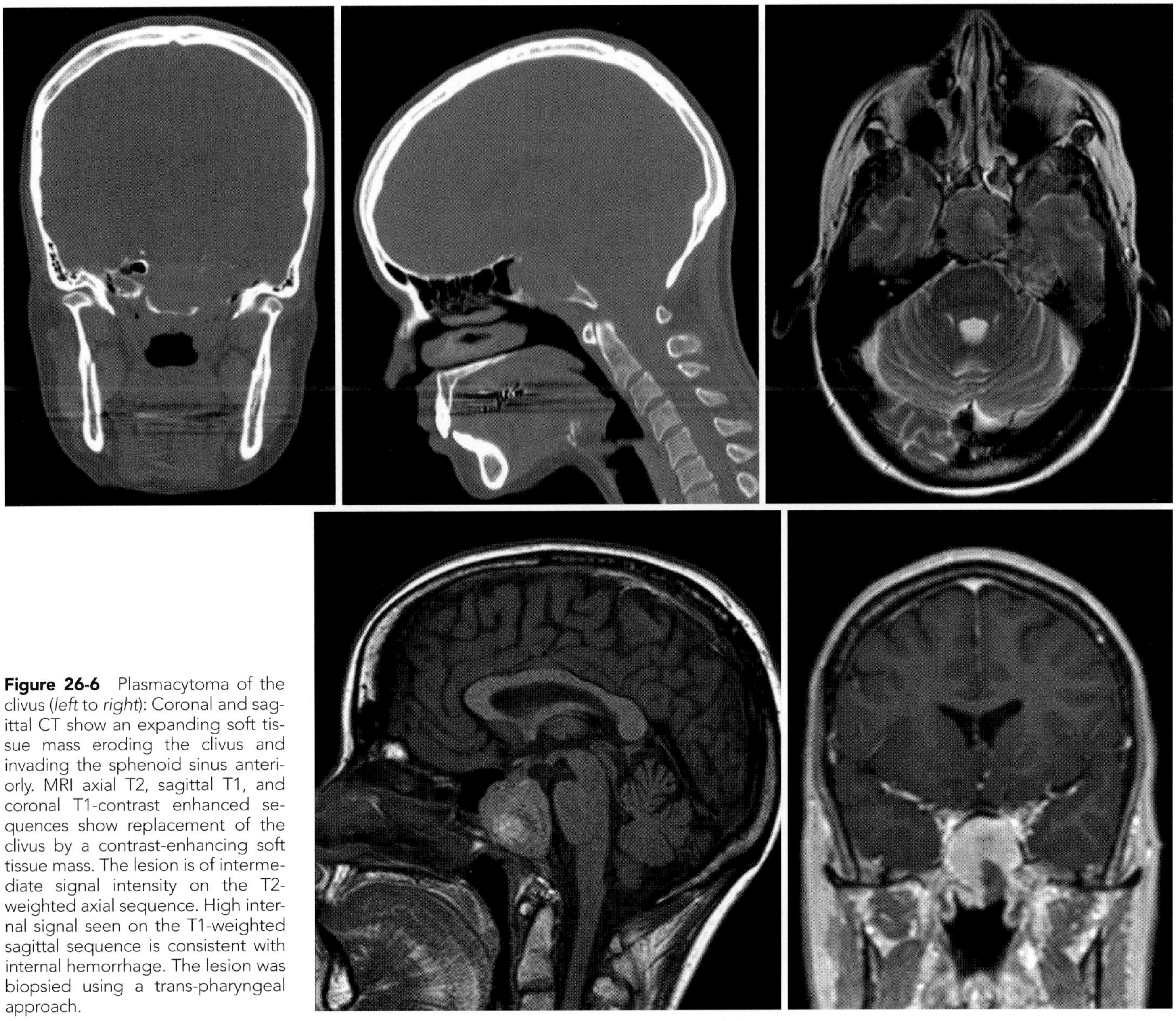

Figure 26-6 Plasmacytoma of the clivus (*left* to *right*): Coronal and sagittal CT show an expanding soft tissue mass eroding the clivus and invading the sphenoid sinus anteriorly. MRI axial T2, sagittal T1, and coronal T1-contrast enhanced sequences show replacement of the clivus by a contrast-enhancing soft tissue mass. The lesion is of intermediate signal intensity on the T2-weighted axial sequence. High internal signal seen on the T1-weighted sagittal sequence is consistent with internal hemorrhage. The lesion was biopsied using a trans-pharyngeal approach.

lumbar spine biopsies. A safer route for biopsy of lesions involving the odontoid or the dens may be a transpharyngeal approach. Bone biopsy should be avoided whenever possible in the presence of local soft tissue infection.

Patient Selection and Procedure Planning

Preprocedure planning includes a review of the patient's clinical history, physical examination, and a thorough evaluation of all available imaging studies (Figure 26-7). With a differential diagnosis in mind, the radiologist must determine whether a diagnosis can be made with the information available, confirmed by less invasive means, or that a biopsy is indeed indicated. The technical feasibility of a percutaneous biopsy is determined from a focused clinical examination and review of cross-sectional imaging studies. Planning of the percutaneous biopsy and subsequent surgical resection should then be performed in tandem, particularly if primary malignancy is a consideration and curative surgical intervention a possibility.[15] The local extent of the lesion including proximity to the skin, neurovascular structures, joint capsule, and muscle invasion should be documented. Proximity to scar tissue and graft material from previous surgical procedures should be noted. An approach in which the risk of tumor dissemination is minimized or where the track can be resected with the lesion should be identified.[16,17] The needle path should be confined to the anatomic compartment involved, avoid neurovascular bundles, and should not cross joint spaces, bursae, tendon, or ligamentous insertions.[18] This is particularly important for limb salvage surgery. Local recurrence rates for sarcomas after open biopsy has been shown to increase from 7% to 38% when the biopsy tract is not excised with the surgical specimen.[19] In patients with Ewing sarcoma, local recurrence is associated with a 5-year overall survival of only 29%.[20] Mankin et al. reported a compromised surgical procedure in 10% and unnecessary amputation in 5% of cases following a poorly planned surgical biopsy.[5] When multiple lesions exist, the biopsy should be taken from the largest and/or most accessible lesion. Maximum yield of viable tissue may be obtained by targeting areas of increased metabolic activity seen on PET CT studies or regions that demonstrate contrast enhancement on CT and MRI scans.

The patient should be informed and educated about the procedure, its benefits, and risks. If pleural transgression is a possibility, for example, paraspinal biopsy, written informed consent should include the possibility of chest-tube placement. A history of anticoagulation therapy and antiplatelet agents should be obtained. Antiplatelet agents should be withheld 5 days before a procedure. Patients receiving low-molecular-weight heparin should have one dose held prior to the procedure. Commonly used laboratory criteria for biopsy include a platelet count greater than 50,000/μL and an internationalized normalized ratio of less than 1.5.[21] Platelet transfusion is recommended for patients with a platelet count less than 50,000/μL. Patient comfort and cooperation may be optimized with the use of conscious sedation, including intravenous midazolam

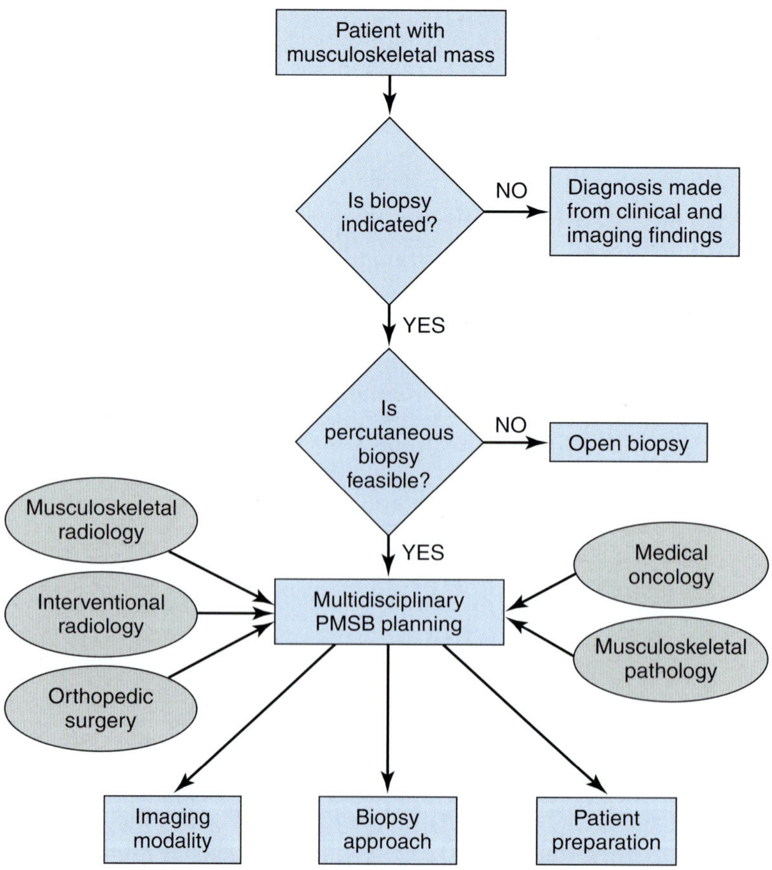

Figure 26-7 Algorithm for the evaluation of musculoskeletal lesions.

and fentanyl citrate administered by dedicated nursing staff with continuous pulse oximetry and noninvasive blood pressure monitoring. Respiratory compromise, decompensated cardiac failure, morbid obesity and diagnosed sleep apnea, pregnancy, pediatric patient status, and an inability to lie in the required position for the procedure are among the reasons that a referral to anesthesia may be required. Patient cooperation may be required for lesions close to neurologic structures in order to elicit symptoms of nerve impingement—in these cases, local anesthesia alone may be indicated. If infection is a consideration, the radiologic findings should be correlated with the white cell count, C-reactive protein level, and erythrocyte sedimentation rate. Antibiotic therapy, if already started, should be stopped for 24 to 48 hours before biopsy in order to optimize the yield of the microorganism to be sent for culture.[22]

Technique

IMAGING MODALITY

PMB can be performed with one of a number of imaging modalities: conventional fluoroscopy, CT and/or CT fluoroscopy, ultrasound, or MRI. Ideally the biopsy should be performed in the modality in which the lesion is best visualized. Other modalities may be used as an indirect guide, for example, a lesion to be biopsied using CT or CT fluoroscopy may require correlation with MRI to identify and avoid the adjacent neurovascular structures, or ultrasound to enable tissue sampling from the solid component of the lesion. Other factors that may influence the choice of imaging used include the location of the lesion, operator expertise, and the availability of imaging modalities (Table 26-3).

CT and CT Fluoroscopy

CT and CT Fluoroscopy are the modalities most frequently used for PMB. CT provides high spatial and contrast resolution and excellent delineation of intervening structures, such as vessels and bowel, thus enabling accurate needle localization. Cortical bone destruction, bone erosion, and calcified tumor matrix are best visualized with CT. The operator can easily correlate the findings on CT and functional imaging (e.g., positron emission tomography [PET]) to target the appropriate part of the mass for biopsy and to avoid areas of necrosis.[23] Standard CT acquisition parameters for musculoskeletal biopsies are 3–5-mm-thick contiguous transverse sections. CT fluoroscopy combines the advantages of the high-resolution imaging of CT with the real-time imaging of fluoroscopy. When using this modality, the operator should be aware of the available techniques to reduce radiation exposure for both the operator and the patient, including dedicated needle holders to keep the operator's hand away from the gantry, using a low tube potential and current, and using CT fluoroscopy intermittently during needle advancement instead of continuously. Angulation of the gantry and/or the use of stereotactic needle guide devices may be useful when an oblique needle trajectory is required.

Fluoroscopy

Conventional fluoroscopy is widely available, is inexpensive, and enables real-time visualization of the needle during placement and tissue sampling. It delivers a lower radiation dose than CT for the same duration of exposure.[24] It is best used for large, superficial lesions and/or appendicular lesions that are visible radiographically. Although lumbar vertebral lesions may be safely biopsied using fluoroscopic guidance, the margin for error is considerably less with thoracic and cervical spine biopsy, in which case CT guidance is advised. The low-contrast resolution of fluoroscopy limits its use in the setting of complex bone lesions.

Ultrasonography

Ultrasonography may be used to biopsy a range of relatively superficial soft-tissue lesions and guide bone biopsy if cortical destruction is present (Figure 26-8).[25-27] Necrotic or cystic components of a lesion can be aspirated and samples sent for cytology and culture. Application of transducer pressure can displace and compress overlying fat, thus reducing the needle-path distance. In cervical spine biopsies, real-time imaging of the needle tip, the ability of color Doppler to delineate major vascular structures in and around the target lesion, and the capacity to identify alternative, oblique access routes to the target lesion reduce the risk of injury to vital structures in the neck.[25,28] Other advantages include lack of exposure to ionizing radiation, decreased procedure time, and lower cost. In the thoracic and lumbar spine regions, ultrasound guided biopsy is usually confined to posterior element lesions. A sonographic-guided anterior approach is limited by pulmonary air in the thorax and bowel gas in the abdomen that obscures the view of the lesion and overlying critical structures. The major drawback of ultrasound-guided biopsy is the fact that it is an operator-dependent method and thus may have low reproducibility. For those less experienced in ultrasound-guided interventions, a needle guide can facilitate visualization of the needle and reduce the time spent searching for the needle tip. This technique also ensures that the sampling is limited to the lesion. Lesion interpretation and the ability to target viable tumor is central to attaining high-quality diagnostic tissue samples. This is particularly challenging when dealing with heterogeneous soft tissue sarcomas. It is recommended that a standardized prebiopsy ultrasonography be performed including color Doppler and spectral wave analysis. Preliminary studies using contrast-enhanced ultrasound to delineate tumor vascularity and identify the representative areas for sampling may improve sonographic targeting of inhomogeneous soft tissue sarcomas.[29,30]

TABLE 26-3 Choosing an Imaging Modality for Percutaneous Musculoskeletal Biopsy

1. Ultrasound
   a. Superficial soft tissue lesions
   b. Lytic bone lesion with cortical destruction
2. Fluoroscopy
   a. Appendicular bone lesions
   b. Superficial bone lesions
3. CT
   a. Smaller lesions
   b. Lesions close to critical structures
   c. Complex lesions
4. MRI
   a. Lesions not visualized using other modalities
   b. Subtle marrow lesions
   c. Pregnant patient or children

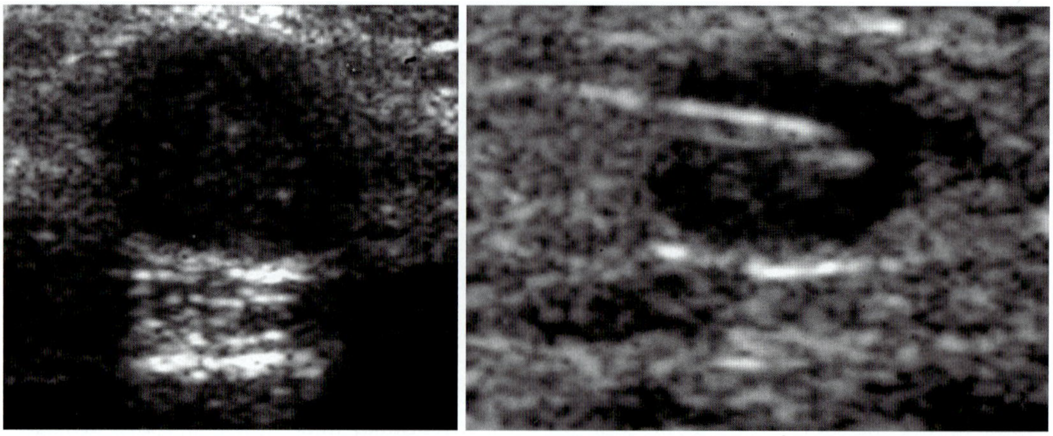

Figure 26-8 Melanoma soft tissue metastases. Ultrasound demonstrates hypoechoic mass in the superficial soft tissues (*left*). Ultrasound-guided percutaneous needle biopsy of the lesion (*right*).

Magnetic Resonance Imaging

The superb soft tissue contrast resolution achieved with MRI makes it a useful tool for localizing, staging, and sampling musculoskeletal tumors. MRI provides superior delineation of the internal composition of a lesion compared with noncontrast CT and thus can facilitate targeted needle biopsy of complex inhomogeneous sarcomas. Fluid-sensitive sequences are sensitive to marrow abnormalities that are often imperceptible using other imaging modalities (Figure 26-9).[31,32] Image resolution (spatial, temporal, and contrast), and rapid image acquisition are the primary yet conflicting goals of an interventional MRI sequence. This is best achieved using true Fast Imaging with Steady State Precession (FISP) type sequences.[33] Tissue contrast resolution can be further enhanced with breath-holds and contrast medium–enhanced sequences. Needle localization is achieved indirectly through susceptibility artifact or virtually visualized using optical tracking devices (Figure 26-10).[34] The size of the needle artifact is dependent on the strength of the magnetic field, needle position with respect to the magnetic field, needle material, the sequence used, and the frequency and phase encoding directions. MRI guided PMB is becoming more popular with the advent of new open-configuration MRI systems,[35,36] continuing development in the field of MRI-compatible instruments, and ultrafast MRI sequences that allow real-time imaging. Other advantages of MRI include its multiplanar capabilities, the lack of ionizing radiation, and its ability to visualize vessels without a contrast agent. These features make it particularly suitable for biopsy of lesions in children and the pregnant patient. Multi-planar imaging allows the radiologist to identify the safest trajectory for biopsy and maintain continuous visualization of the needle trajectory in that plane throughout the procedure. This is particularly relevant for spinal lesions or lesions adjacent to vital structures. Unfortunately, the cost of installing and maintaining an interventional MRI suite, and the cost of MR-compatible instruments has limited its availability. There are also less needle choices available for MR-guided interventions. Among the trephine needles used for osseous biopsies, the titanium needles are not as strong as the steel needles used in other modalities and thus can break or bend when used in thick sclerotic bone. MRI is contraindicated in patients with pacemakers or other ferromagnetic material adjacent to critical structures.

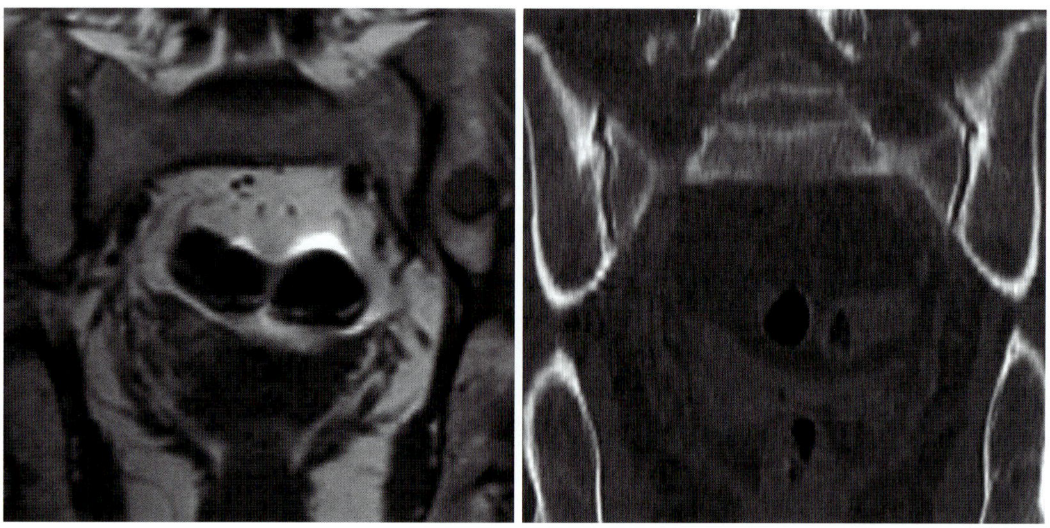

Figure 26-9 Choosing an imaging modality for guidance during biopsy. MRI T1-weighted sequence of the pelvis coronal projection: A well-circumscribed hypointense mass in the left posterior ileum is shown (*left*). The lesion is not apparent on the CT of the pelvis coronal reconstruction (*right*).

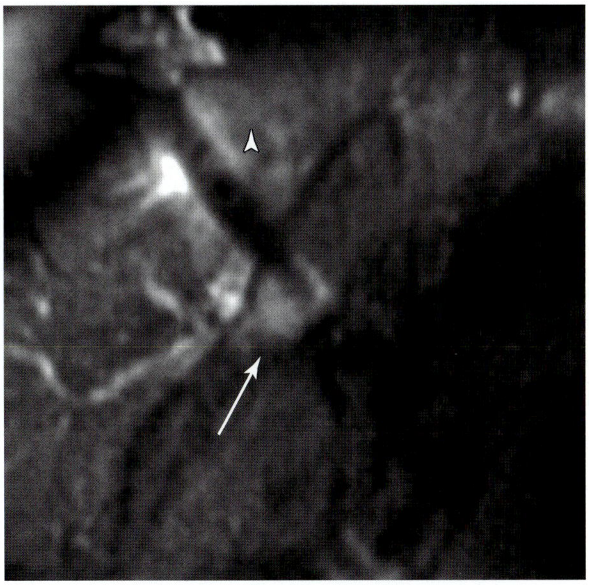

Figure 26-10 MRI-guided bone biopsy. MRI STIR sequence. The course of the biopsy needle is visualized using susceptibility artifact.

BIOPSY TECHNIQUES

The aim of percutaneous biopsy is to maximize the diagnostic tissue yield and keep complications including contamination of adjacent tissues to a minimum. PMB can be performed using single needle, tandem, or coaxial techniques.[17] One of the challenges for PMB is in accessing the lesion. In order to traverse corticated bone or access a sclerotic lesion, drill devices and/or larger bore needles (10–14-gauge) are required. With this in mind, the coaxial technique is best suited to PMB. It involves image-guided placement of an outer guide needle in or close to the lesion. A second biopsy needle is then placed through the guide needle to obtain samples. This method enables multiple samples to be acquired without having to reaccess the lesion each time. It also reduces the risk of tumor seeding or disseminating infection along the tract. The technique can be used with all imaging modalities. The tandem technique involves placement of a small needle, for example, 20–22 gauge in the periphery of the lesion under image guidance. This needle serves as a guide for placing the biopsy needle and is also used to administer local anesthetic to the subcutaneous tissues and the periosteum. The biopsy needle is then advanced parallel to the initial needle and to the same depth. Once the correct position is achieved the smaller needle can be removed. This method requires a new puncture for each sample obtained. The single needle technique involves a single needle placed under image guidance for each pass. It is associated with an increased risk of complications, increased radiation dose, and prolonged procedure time.

BIOPSY DEVICES

Closed biopsy of musculoskeletal lesions can be performed using fine-needle aspiration (FNA) with a small 18- to 23-gauge needle, core-needle biopsy (CNB) with a cannulated, cutting trocar system to obtain a core of tissue, or a trephine system using a stout, sharp bone-cutting tool. The needles chosen to obtain a specimen are determined by user preference, the site and appearance of the lesion, whether it is soft tissue or bone, and the volume of tissue that is likely to be required for an accurate diagnosis. The bore size of a biopsy needle is inversely related to gauge; thus, a smaller-gauge needle will yield a larger specimen. FNA and CNB are appropriate for soft tissue masses, bone tumors with a soft tissue component, or primarily lytic bone lesions. These needles cannot penetrate intact bone. Spinal needles, Chiba needles (Cook Medical, Bloomington, IN), and E-Z-EM needles (E-Z-EM, Lake Success, NY) are thin-walled 20- to 23-gauge needles with bevel angulations at the tip and are suitable for aspirating fluid, cytology of soft tissue lesions, and microbiologic sampling (Figure 26-11). These smaller needles carry a lower risk of hemorrhage and tract seeding than the cutting and trephine needles. Cores of tissue may be obtained with small-bore fine needles such as the Franseen (16–25 gauge) (Cook Medical), Greene (22 gauge) (Cook Medical), Rotex (19–21 gauge) (Havel's Inc, Cincinnati, OH), and Westcott (20–22 gauge) (Becton, Dickinson, and Company; Franklin Lakes, NJ) needles (Figure 26-12). These needles have circumferentially sharpened tips to optimize the yield of cytologic aspirates and histologic core specimens. In addition, semiautomated and automated core biopsy devices (14–20 gauge), such as the Tru-Cut needle (Baxter Healthcare Corp,

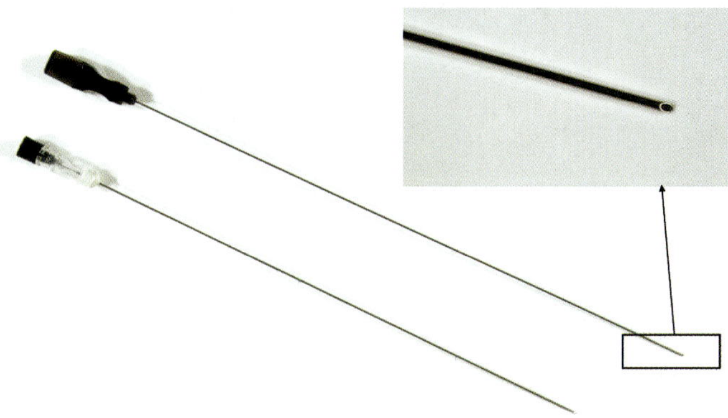

Figure 26-11 Biopsy devices. Chiba needle (Cook Medical) (*top*) and Spinal Needle (BD Medical) (*bottom*) with beveled tips are used for aspiration biopsy.

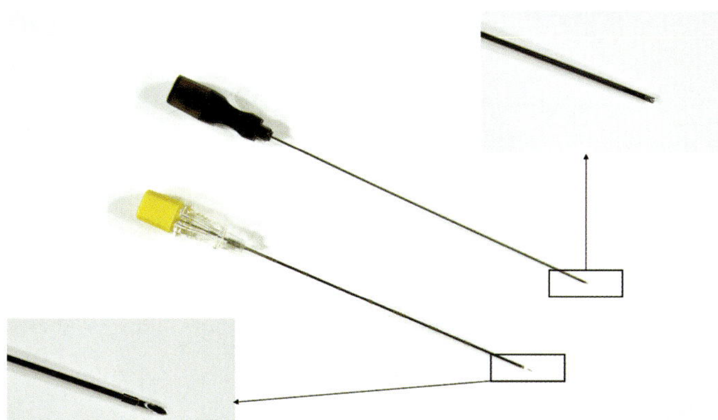

Figure 26-12 Biopsy devices. Franseen needle (Cook Medical) (*top*). The aspiration cannula has a serrated edge for cutting tissue specimens. Westcott needle (Angiotech) has a slotted opening measuring 2.2 mm in length approximately 3 mm from the needle tip (*bottom*). This creates a second cutting edge, in addition to the tip of the needle and enables aspiration of larger amounts of material.

Deerfield, IL), Quick-core (Cook Medical), and Temno (Bauer Medical, Clearwater, Florida) can be used to obtain slices of tissue for analysis (Figure 26-13). The fine needles can be inserted directly into the lesion if there is a soft tissue component or frank cortical destruction. In the majority of cases, a coaxial approach is used.

Trephine biopsy needles can penetrate intact bone and thus are the needle of choice for sclerotic bone lesions or lesions that lie deep to a thick intact cortex (Figures 26-14 through 26-19). These biopsies are considerably more painful and require conscious sedation. Trephine needles may be placed using a coaxial Seldinger technique or directly. Needles placed using a Seldinger technique are used for deep bone lesions, for example, vertebral biopsy. Seldinger technique allows coaxial placement of an external biopsy cannula and trephine needle in the same track as the thin anesthetic needle using a blunt guidewire. This reduces the risk of injuring the anatomic structures with the large trephine needle. Direct needle placement is simpler and more convenient for superficial bone biopsy or biopsy in anatomic structures remote from vital structures. Most trephine systems consist of an external cannula that remains in place whereas the trephine needle is withdrawn with the sample. Some bone needles have a special cutting tip designed to penetrate hard cortical bone or sclerotic bone. The Ostycut needle (Bard) is a trephine-type needle with screw threads that allows easy advancement with a turning motion. It consists of an outer trocar that remains fixed in the lesion and allows the removal of more tissue without the need for repositioning (see Figure 26-14). Although the system is limited by lack of a coaxial design, a fine cutting needle can then be passed in a coaxial fashion through the trocar needle to obtain material for histopathology. The Elson/Ackerman bone biopsy needle (Cook Medical) is a reusable coaxial system. It includes an outer cannula with either a hollow or solid stylet, a 22-gauge introducer needle with removable hub (VanSonnenberg needle), and the biopsy needle with a serrated tip (see Figures 26-15 and 26-16).

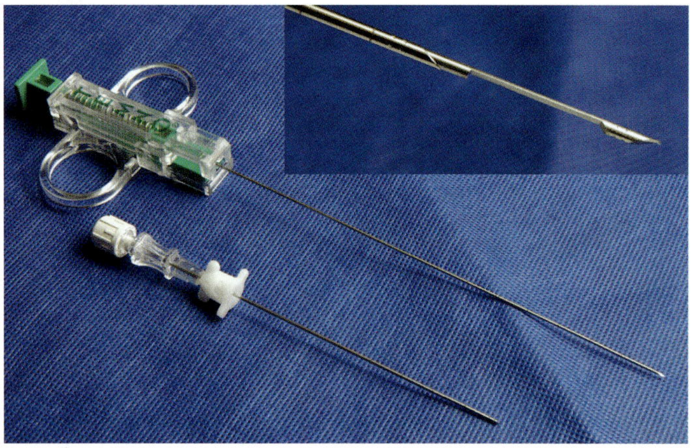

Figure 26-13 Core-needle biopsy devices. The Temno biopsy system includes a coxial introducer needle that facilitates multiple sampling from one percutaneous puncture. The biopsy needle is spring loaded. The sheath is retracted to expose the specimen collection chamber (*upper right*).

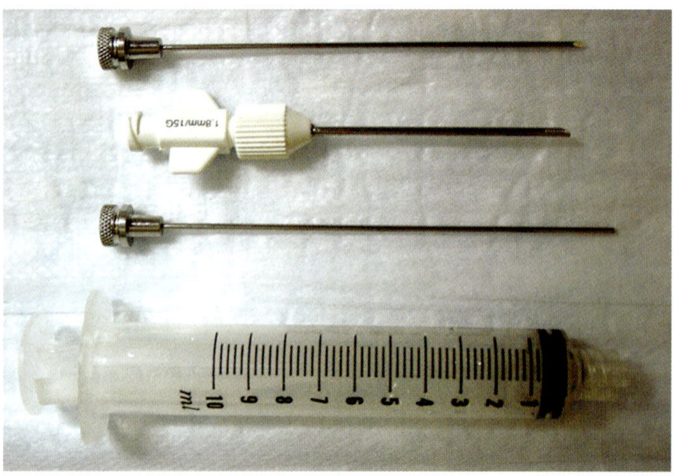

Figure 26-14 Trephine biopsy devices. The Ostycut needle (Bard) (14–17 gauge, 5–15 cm) features a stylet, an outer trocar needle with a threaded tip and an obturator. The cannula is advanced using a push-and-turn continuous clockwise motion. *(Image courtesy Catherine Roberts, MD, Scottsdale, AZ.)*

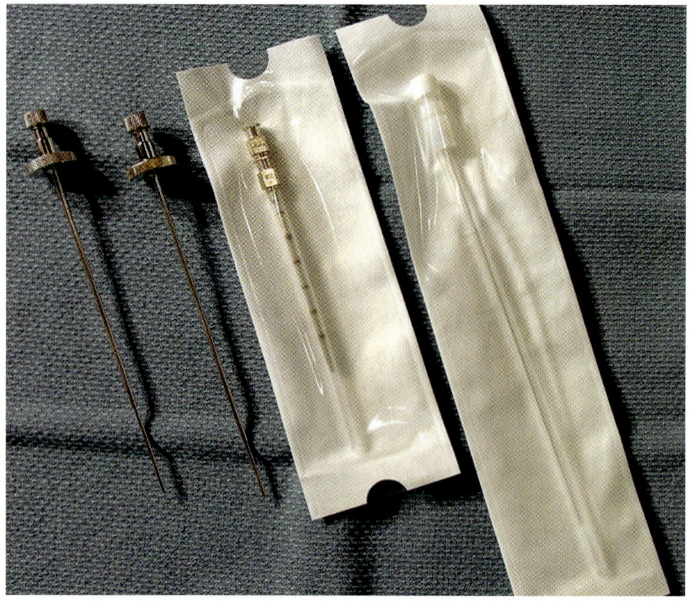

Figure 26-15 Trephine biopsy devices. The Elson/Ackerman needle coaxial system (Cook) consists of a sheath with hollow or solid stylet (12-gauge), a biopsy needle with a serrated tip and obturators (14-gauge, 9.6–18.3 cm), and a 22-gauge introducer needle with a removable hub. *(Image courtesy Catherine Roberts, MD, Scottsdale, AZ.)*

APPROACH AND RELEVANT ANATOMY

Spine Biopsy

Percutaneous spine biopsies may be from the vertebral body, posterior elements, disc, and paraspinal or epidural tissue and are most commonly performed using CT guidance.[28,37,38] Given the complexity of the neck anatomy, a contrast-enhanced CT is advocated to guide the approach to cervical spine biopsies. The trajectory used depends on the location and size of the lesion. An anterolateral approach is used primarily for accessing cervical spine lesions, for which patients are positioned supine. Posterior approaches may be posterolateral, transpedicular, or transcostovertebral, for which the patient is positioned prone. The posterolateral approach can be used for accessing paraspinal soft tissue lesions, laterally located vertebral body masses, and disc lesions in the lumbar and thoracic

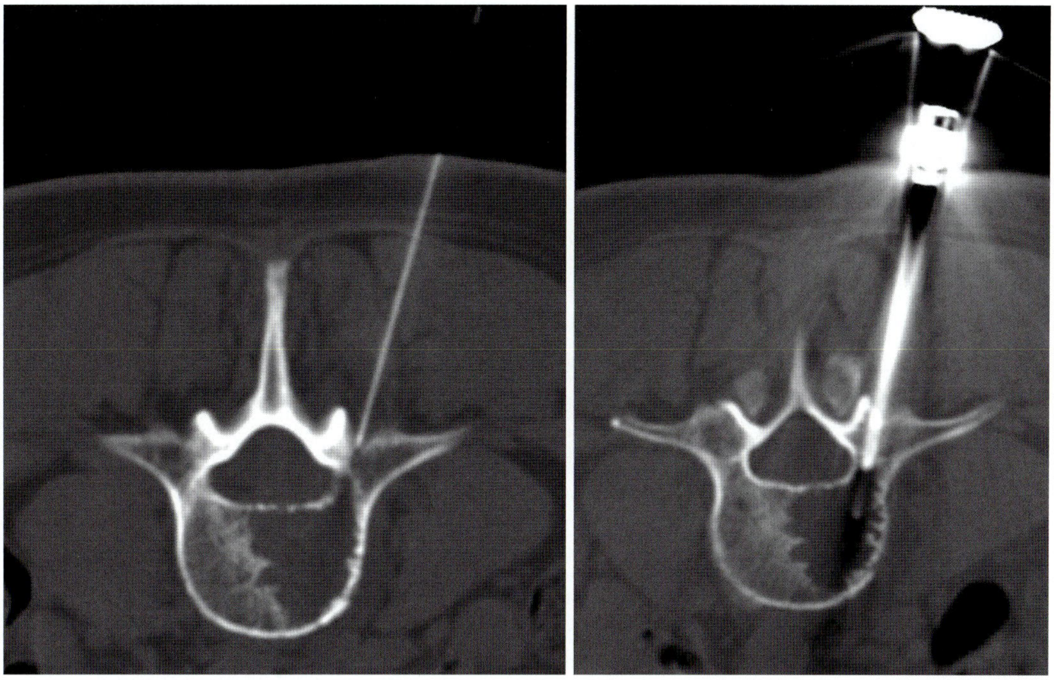

Figure 26-16 Spine biopsy. Transpedicular biopsy of a lumbar vertebra using Elson/Ackerman coaxial system. The lesion is localized with a 22-gauge VonSonnenberg needle and the hub is then removed (*left*). The sheath with hollow stylet is then placed over the hub-less localizer needle (*right*). Advancement of the sheath may be facilitated by a deep fasciotomy performed with a scalpel in advance.

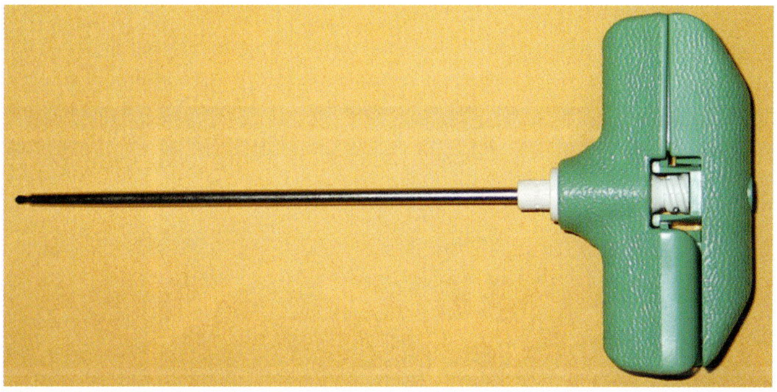

Figure 26-17 Trephine biopsy devices. T-handle Jamshidi bone marrow biopsy needle (8–13 gauge) (Carefusion) features a trocar-tapered stylet point and a triple-crown cannula tip that provides a sharp cutting edge for cortical penetration and medullary advancement.

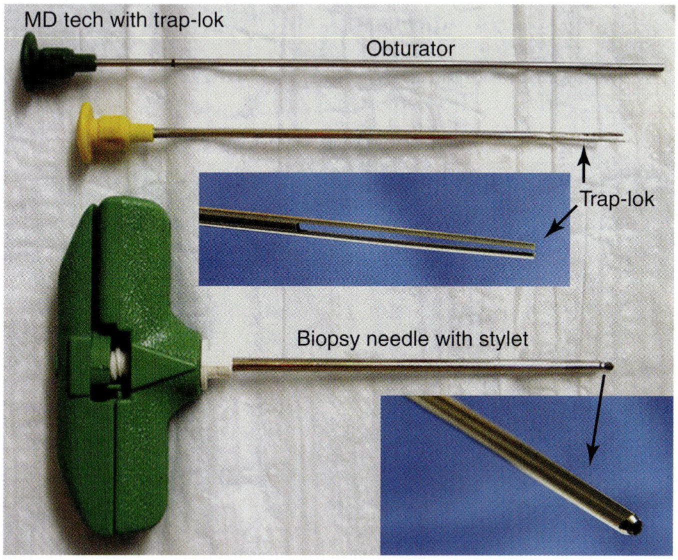

Figure 26-18 Trephine biopsy devices. T-Lok Bone Marrow Biopsy System (Angiotech) includes a T-Lok biopsy needle, an extraction cannula, and a marked obturator. The extraction cannula is aimed at ensuring a superior quality biopsy by entrapping bone marrow in the needle without altering the sample's architecture. The tapered tip of the biopsy needle is intended to cut the sample and reduce crush artifact. *(Image courtesy Catherine Roberts, MD, Scottsdale, AZ.)*

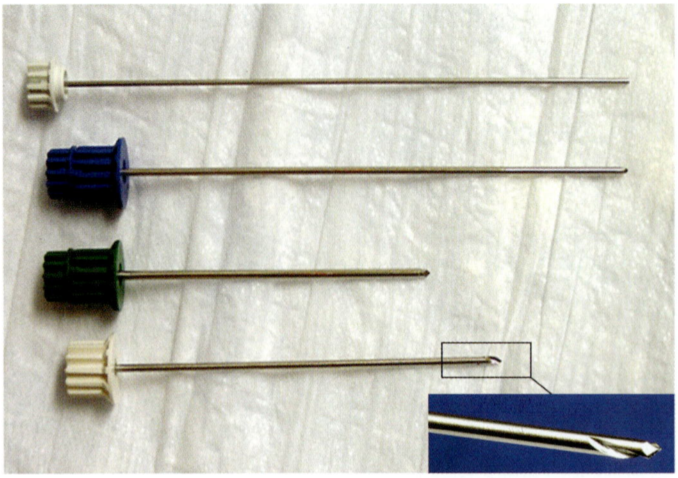

Figure 26-19 Trephine biopsy devices. The Bonopty Bone Biopsy system (Apriomed, Londonderry, NH) is a coaxial system that consists of a penetration set (12- to 14-gauge, 10 cm), a biopsy set and an extended drill (15-gauge). It is ideally suited for penetrating thick cortex. *(Image courtesy Catherine Roberts, MD, Scottsdale, AZ.)*

spine. A transpedicular approach is used to biopsy centrally located thoracic and lumbar vertebral lesions. The transcostovertebral trajectory can be used for thoracic disc, laterally located thoracic vertebral body masses, or thoracic paraspinal lesions.

Soft Tissue Masses

Paraspinal masses lie anterolateral to the vertebral body. The patient can be placed in the prone, prone-oblique, or lateral decubitus positions. The needle is advanced immediately lateral to the vertebral body. In the thorax, the plane lies between the endothoracic fascia and the parietal pleura. The needle should be placed above the rib to avoid injury to the intercostal bundle. If the paravertebral, extrapleural space is not wide enough to allow safe needle biopsy, saline solution may be injected to displace the mediastinal parietal pleura laterally (Figure 26-20).[39] The azygous vein, esophagus, nerves, and the vertebral vessels are also displaced by the saline injection, thereby reducing the risk of inadvertent injury to these structures. CT biopsies are usually performed using a 16- to 18-gauge guide needle, for example, Chiba, through which fine-needle aspirates and core biopsies may be obtained. Epidural mass biopsy carries a significant risk of morbidity should hemorrhage occur. Such lesions should only be biopsied if no other accessible lesions can be identified, and the risks and benefits have been discussed with the clinician and patient. The biopsy should be performed with a small-caliber needle. Aspirates obtained with a fine needle are usually sufficient (Figure 26-21).

Posterior Elements

The biopsy of the posterior arch elements in the cervical thoracic and lumbar spine requires precision and should be performed with CT guidance. The neural structures need to

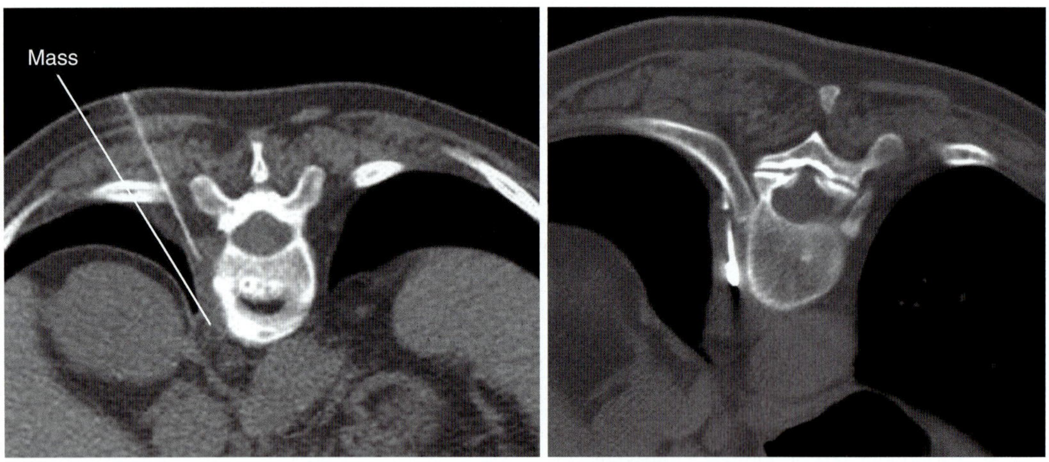

Figure 26-20 Injection of saline to decrease the risk of pneumothorax during biopsy. CT-guided biopsy of an isolated paraspinal soft tissue mass. Saline is injected in the subpleural space using a 22-gauge needle to displace the pleura laterally (*left*). Biopsy was then performed using a coaxial technique (*right*). Histology was consistent with lymphoma.

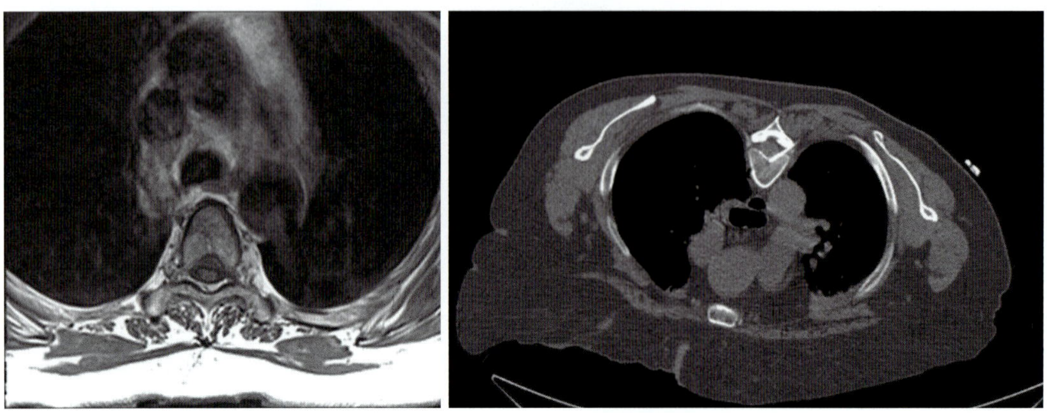

Figure 26-21 Epidural mass biopsy. MRI T1-weighted sequence axial projection shows a soft tissue mass in the anterior epidural space (*left*). Fine-needle aspirates acquired using CT guidance (*right*). Histology was consistent with lymphoma.

be identified and a tangential approach used to avoid injury to the cord, spinal nerve roots, and epidural space (Figure 26-22).

Cervical Vertebra and Disc

The third to seventh cervical vertebrae are usually biopsied using an anterolateral approach (Figure 26-23).[28] Access to the upper cervical spine may not be technically feasible or safe using a percutaneous approach, in which case a transoral route should be considered. Critical structures to be avoided include the carotid space structures, the oropharynx, hypopharynx, thyroid gland, esophagus, trachea, and the apex of the lungs. The carotid artery and internal jugular vein should be identified on a contrast-enhanced CT and a route that avoids these structures, either anterior or posterior to this space, should be used for needle placement. An alternative method and one traditionally used with fluoroscopic-guided biopsy of the cervical spine, is to manually displace the vessel posteriorly while advancing a small-caliber needle through the anterior sternocleidomastoid muscle beyond the vessel (Figure 26-24). Once past the vessel, a coaxial technique can be used, for example, a 16- to 18-gauge Chiba needle.

Thoracic and Lumbar Vertebra

The thoracic and lumbar vertebrae may be biopsied using transosseous (transpedicular) or extraosseous (posterolateral or

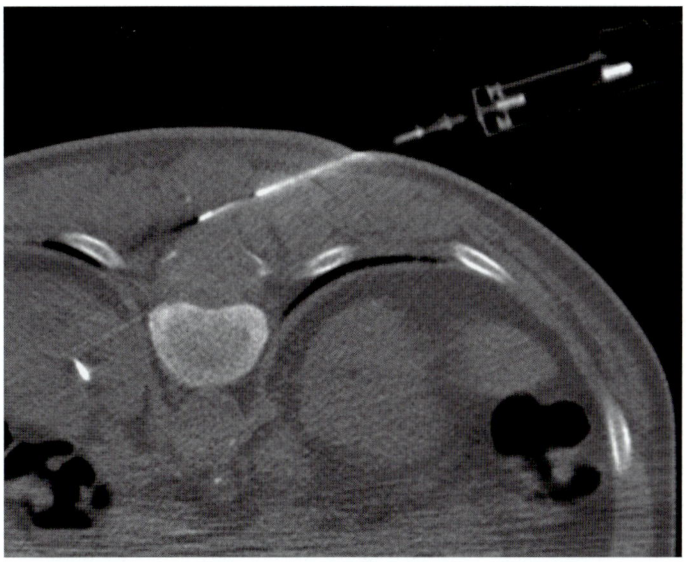

Figure 26-22 Biopsy of spinous process. CT-guided biopsy of soft tissue mass involving the spinous process. A spring-loaded core biopsy needle is used to acquire samples using a tangential approach. Histology was consistent with metastatic disease.

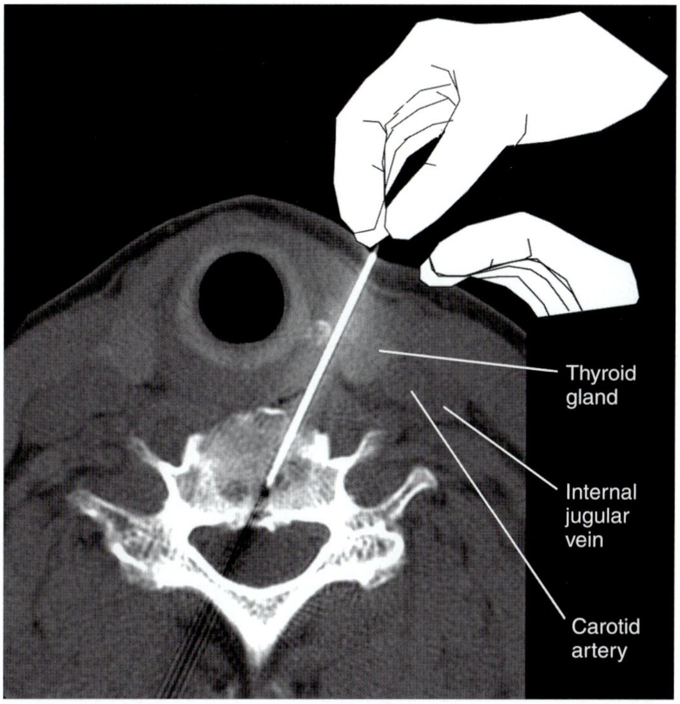

Figure 26-24 Tampieri biopsy technique for the cervical spine. CT-guided biopsy of a cervical vertebral body using a trans-thyroid anterolateral approach. To avoid the carotid artery, the fingers of one hand palpate and laterally deflect the vessel while the needle is directed through the thyroid gland (Tampieri technique).

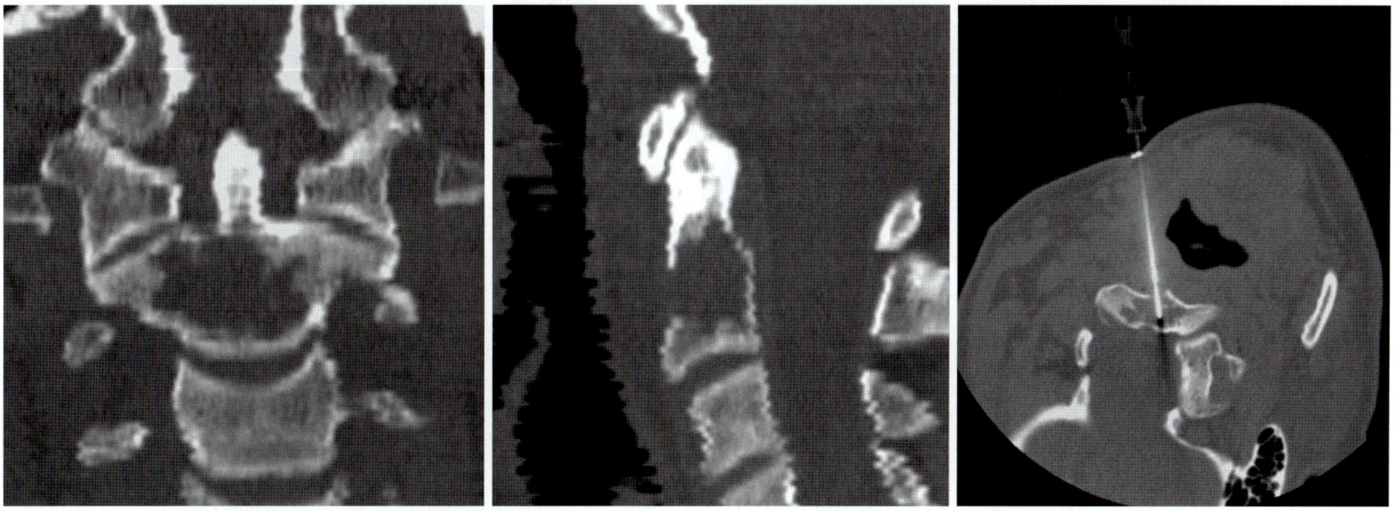

Figure 26-23 Biopsy of C2 vertebral body. CT coronal and sagittal reconstructions (bone window) demonstrate lytic lesion associated with cortical erosion involving the body of C2 (*left* and *middle*). The lesion is biopsied using an anterolateral approach and coaxial technique (*right*). Histology was compatible with Langerhans cell histiocytosis.

transcostovertebral) approaches. The transosseous approach should be used if surgical resection of a potentially malignant lesion is being considered. It is best suited to the biopsy of large vertebral lesions or lesions close to the pedicle (Figure 26-25). Although transpedicular biopsies can be performed using either CT or fluoroscopic guidance, the thoracic pedicles are relatively small and require more precise needle positioning; thus, CT is the preferred imaging modality in the thorax (Figure 26-26). For fluoroscopic-guided biopsy, the patient is positioned prone (Figure 26-27). The vertebral level is localized in the lateral projection. The pedicle is identified in the anteroposterior (AP) projection or oblique "Scotty dog" projection. If an AP approach is used, the skin is marked approximately 4 cm lateral to the ring of the pedicle. The needle is advanced into the pedicle through the skin mark keeping the needle tip between the medial and lateral walls of the pedicle at all times. Needle position is monitored intermittently using both AP and lateral views. Once the posterior wall of the vertebral body is traversed, the needle position can be monitored in the lateral projection only. If the oblique "Scotty dog" trajectory is preferred, the beam is rotated approximately 40° until the pedicle represented by the dog's eye is identified. The skin is

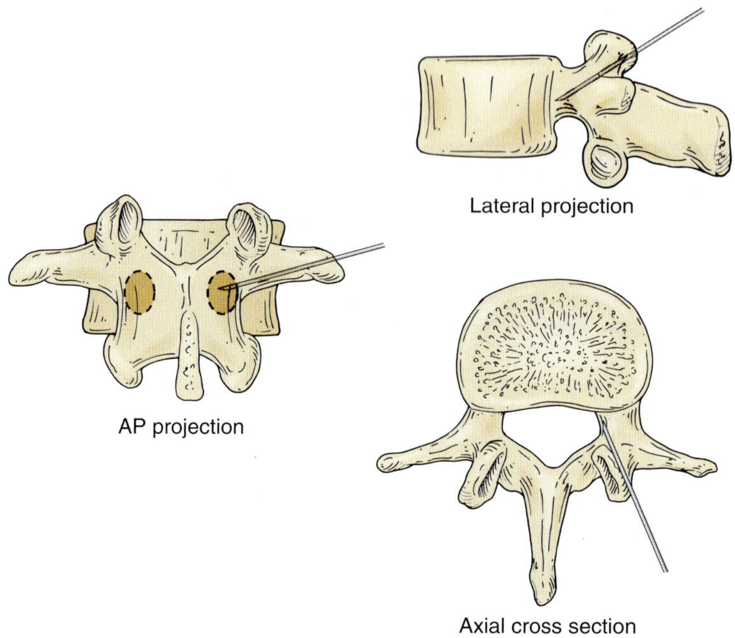

Figure 26-25 Transpedicular biopsy of a vertebral body. The schematic illustrates the fluoroscopic projections and appearance of landmarks that are using during transpedicular access of a vertebral body.

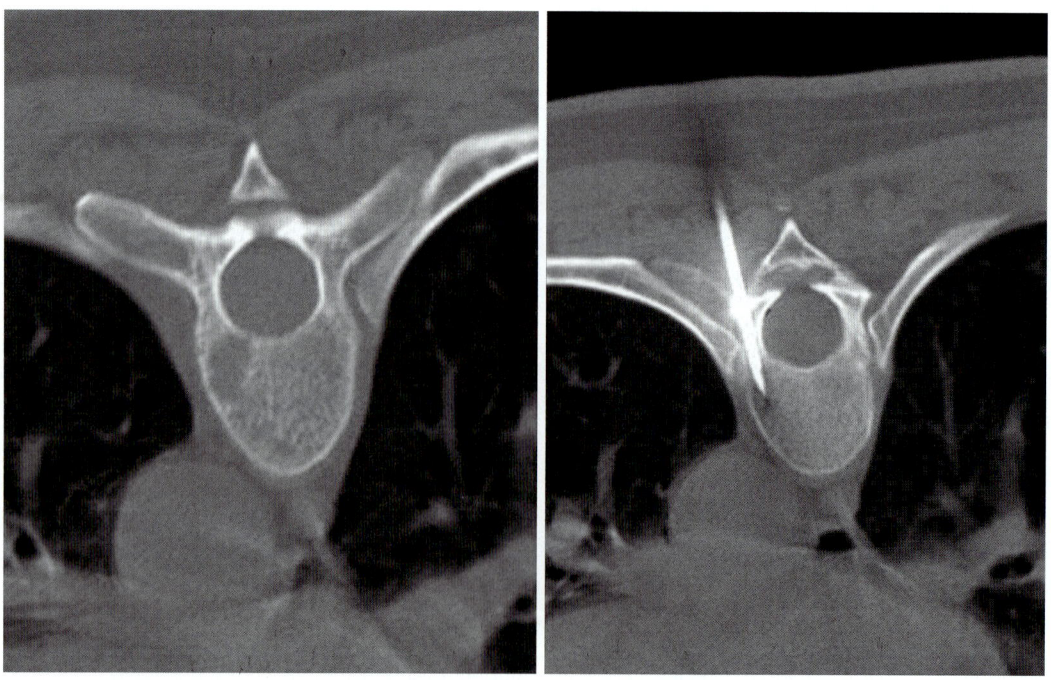

Figure 26-26 CT-guided transpedicular biopsy of a lytic thoracic vertebral body lesion.

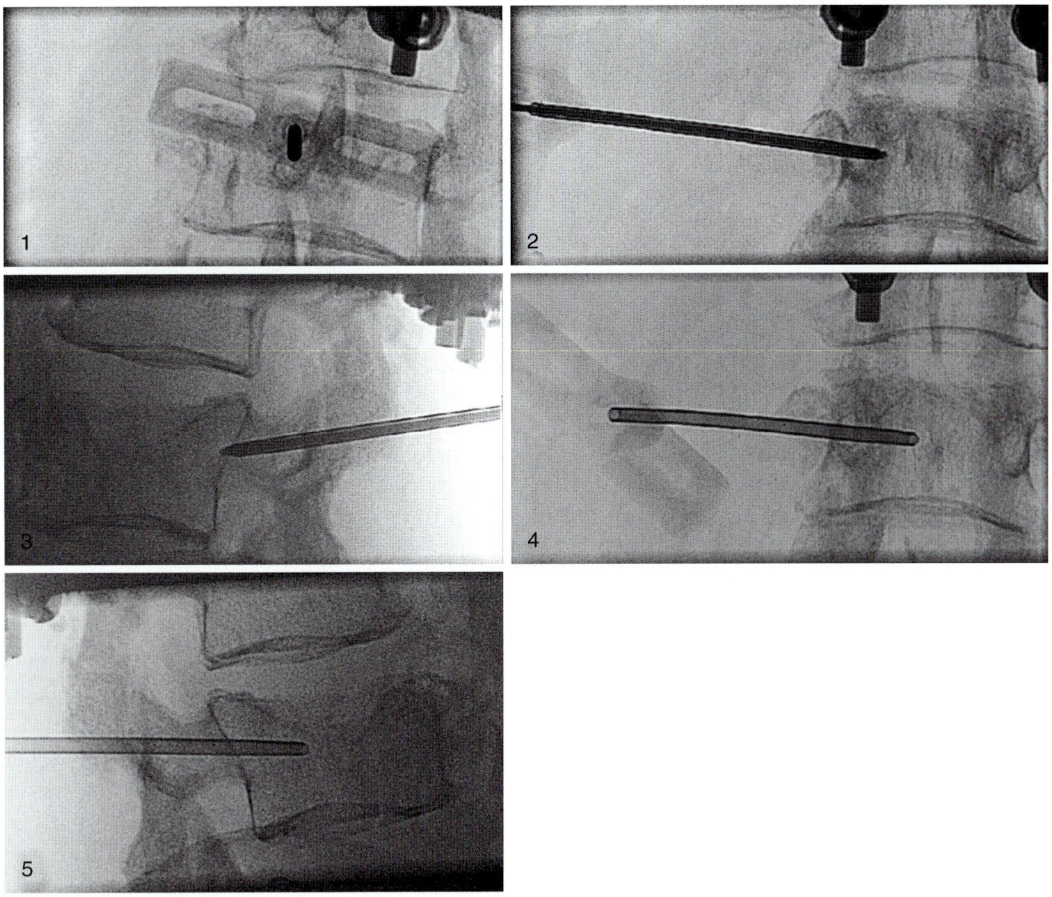

Figure 26-27 Fluoroscopic-guided transpedicular biopsy of a lumbar vertebral body lesion. The needle skin entry site is marked over the pedicle or "eye of the Scotty dog." This is identified in the oblique projection (1). The needle tip must be maintained between the medial and lateral walls of the pedicle until the posterior wall of the vertebra is traversed (2–4). Once within the vertebral body, the needle tip position can be monitored in the lateral projection only (5).

marked over the eye and the needle advanced from this angle. This oblique trajectory is associated with an increased risk of cortical and canal penetration. Using CT guidance, the vertebral level is determined from a topogram. A radiopaque grid is placed over the level of the lesion and a limited noncontrast study performed. The gantry may need to be angled in order to visualize the entire needle trajectory on the same slice. The needle is then introduced under CT or CT fluoroscopic guidance. The pedicle is accessed at the junction between the transverse process and the adjacent facet joint (see Figure 26-26).

The extraosseous approach is usually performed for laterally located focal lesions in the lumbar spine and is the preferred approach in the thoracic spine for all lesions. The thoracic and lumbar posterolateral approach is similar (Figure 26-28).

Figure 26-28 CT-guided biopsy of a lumbar vertebral body using a paravertebal approach. This approach enables biopsy of central lesions that can be challenging from a transpedicular trajectory.

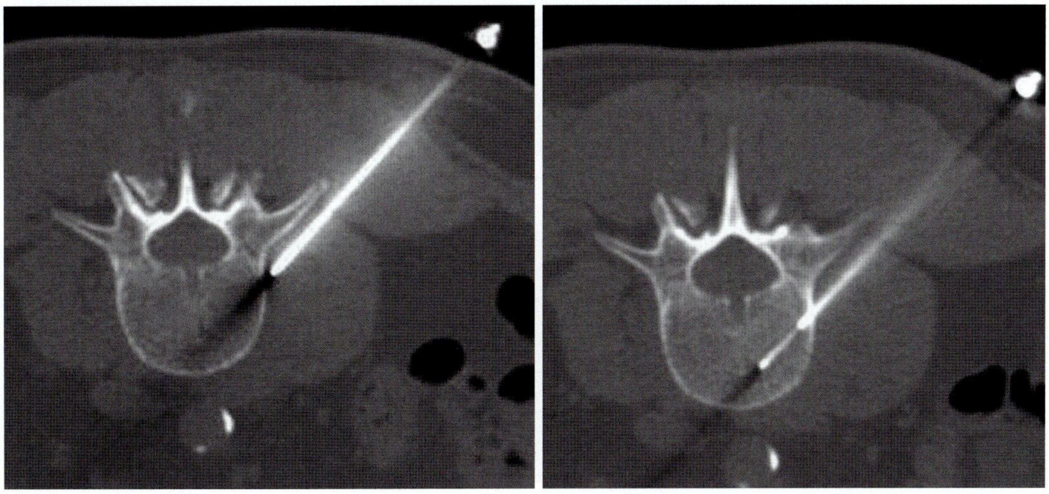

It involves a longer and more oblique trajectory than that used with a transosseous biopsy. The tangential needle trajectory requires greater effort to penetrate the bone and is thus associated with an increased risk of shearing. Close communication with the patient is required to avoid injuring the spinal nerve root at that level. The costovertebral approach is the trajectory of choice for all thoracic lesions (Figure 26-29). It can be performed with CT or fluoroscopic guidance. Like other extraosseous routes, the approach is longer and more oblique than the transpedicular approach. Using fluoroscopic guidance, the beam is rotated until the ring of the pedicle and the articular processes projected over the mid-disc space are visualized. The needle is advanced between the head of the rib and the pedicle inferior to the transverse process, and medial to the pleural reflection. Once the vertebra is reached, the needle tip is monitored in the AP and lateral projections. With CT guidance, the vertebral level is localized with the topogram. A noncontrast CT and radiopaque grid placed over the region of concern enable the skin entry site and the target to be marked and the trajectory can then be delineated. Once again, the gantry may be angulated to facilitate visualization of the entire trajectory on a single slice. The needle must remain medial to the pleural line, and its position is monitored with intermittent CT imaging until the target is reached. The costotransverse trajectory is an alternative approach to thoracic vertebral biopsy that involves an oblique needle path between the transverse process and the posterior part of the adjacent rib. Because the risk of pneumothorax is significantly greater, the biopsy should be performed only with CT guidance. The needle tip is monitored with intermittent CT or CT fluoroscopy.

Disc Biopsies

An anterolateral approach similar to that for vertebral biopsy is used in the cervical spine. Thoracic and lumbar discs are sampled via posterolateral or costovertebral approaches using CT or conventional fluoroscopic guidance. Every effort should be made to avoid injury to the nerve root at that level by aligning the needle as close as possible to the posterior articular processes. The trajectory used with CT guidance should be parallel to the disc, and extend from the skin to the center of the disc, tangential to the posterior articular processes. This may require angulation of the gantry particularly at the lumbosacral junction. In the thoracic spine, the trajectory is costovertebral, in which the needle passes between the posterior articular process and the head of the adjacent rib. With conventional fluoroscopy, the level is determined from the lateral projection. In the lumbar spine, the c-arm is rotated until the "ear of the Scotty Dog" (inferior articular process of the vertebra above) lies at the center of the disc to be sampled (Figures 26-30 and 26-31). The needle is aligned with the inferior articular process and once the posterior joint is reached, the needle is angled craniocaudally to facilitate sampling of both the disc and the subchondral bone. In the thoracic spine, the disc is sampled using a costovertebral approach. The c-arm is rotated until the articular processes are projected over the center of the disc. The needle is advanced between the superior articular process and the adjacent rib. AP and lateral projections are used to monitor the needle tip. Anterior and posterior aspects of the disc can be selectively sampled by rotating the c-arm and aligning the inferior articular

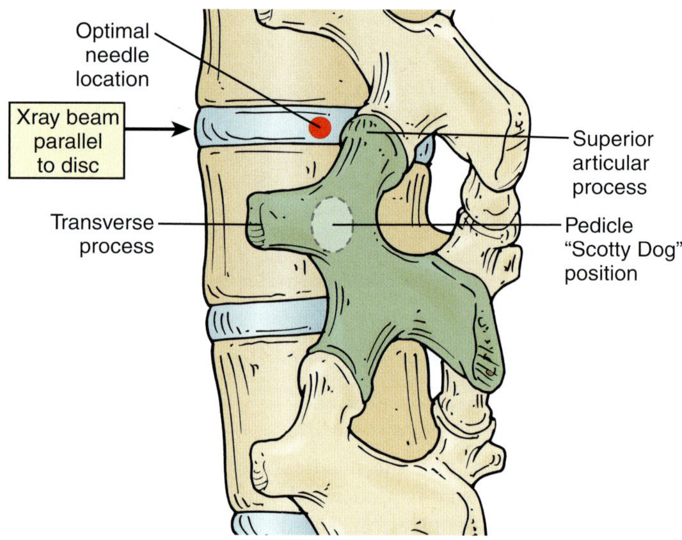

Figure 26-30 Anatomic landmarks seen on fluoroscopy during disc aspiration or endplate biopsy.

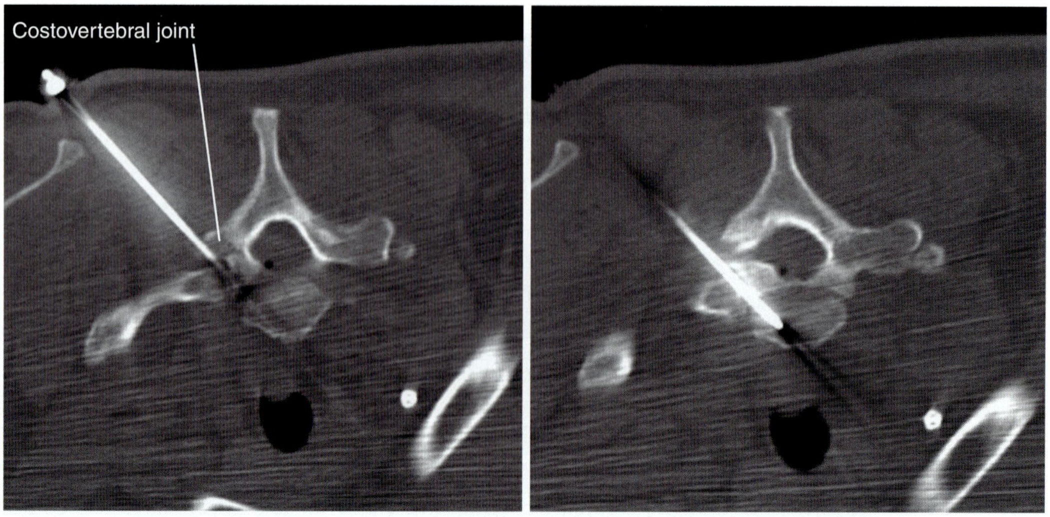

Figure 26-29 CT-guided biopsy of an upper thoracic vertebral body using an extraosseous costovertebral approach.

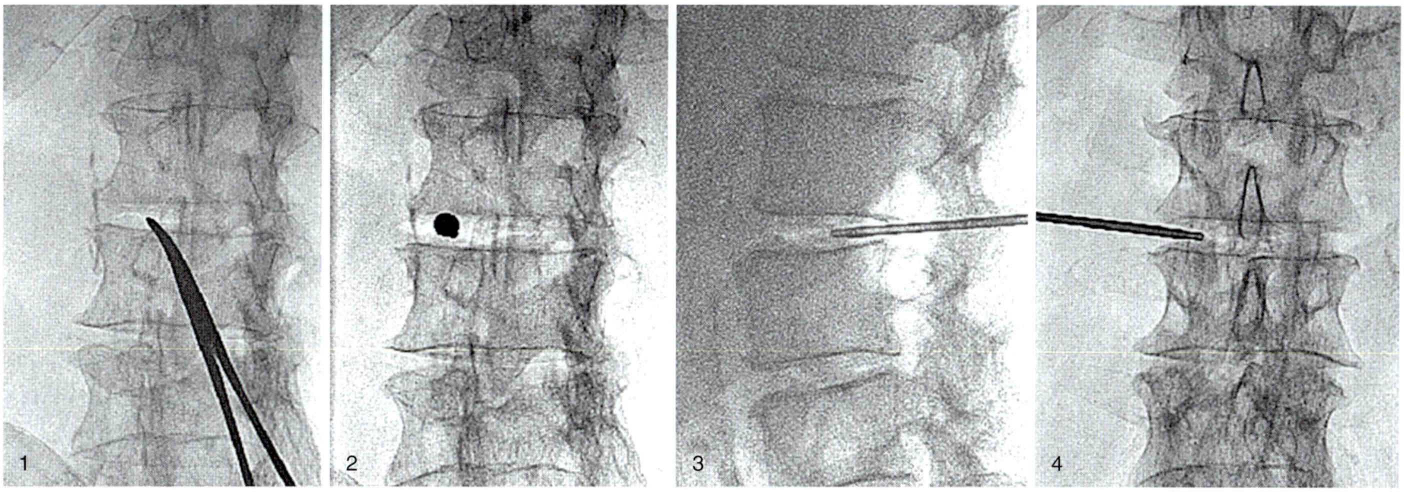

Figure 26-31 Fluoroscopic-guided lumbar disc aspiration. The x-ray beam is angled craniocaudally to visualize the target disc space and then mediolaterally until the superior articular process lies halfway between the anterior and posterior wall of the vertebral body (1 and 2). The biopsy needle is advanced toward the disc just anterior to the superior articular process, checking position periodically on the AP view. At the margin of the disc, the biopsy needle stylet is removed and a long 18-gauge needle is advanced coaxially into the disc for aspiration (3 and 4).

process with the junction of the anterior third and posterior two-thirds, or the posterior third and anterior two-thirds of the disc space. The disc alone can be biopsied using a 16- to 18-gauge coaxial system. If the bone is to be biopsied as well as the disc, the access needle should be at least 14 gauge.

Flat Bones

The superficial flat bones, for example, ribs, scapula, and clavicle, can be biopsied using fluoroscopic or CT guidance. An oblique trajectory is recommended for flat bone biopsies to minimize the risk of injuring underlying structures (Figure 26-32). A posterior oblique approach can be used for most sacral and iliac bone biopsies (Figures 26-33 and 26-34). Acetabular lesions can be biopsied from a direct anterior or posterior approach. Skull biopsies should be performed with CT guidance to enable visualization of the needle tip and its location with respect to the epidural space (Figure 26-35).

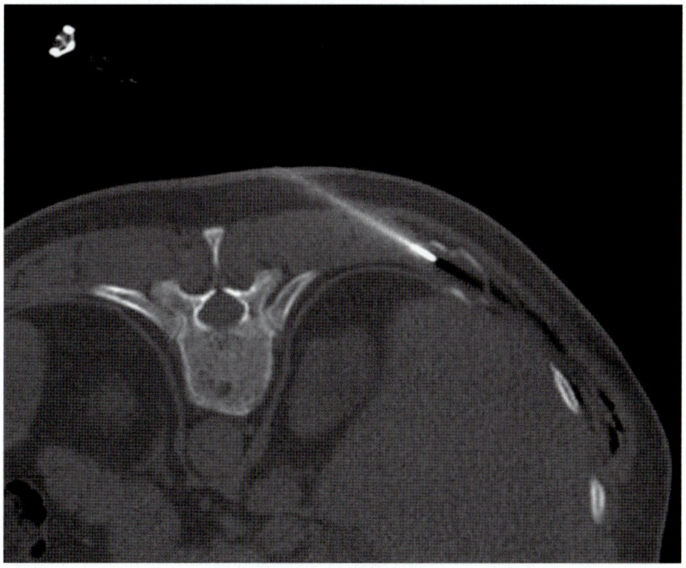

Figure 26-32 CT-guided biopsy of an expansile lytic posterior rib lesion. The biopsy is performed using a tangential approach to avoid injury to the liver.

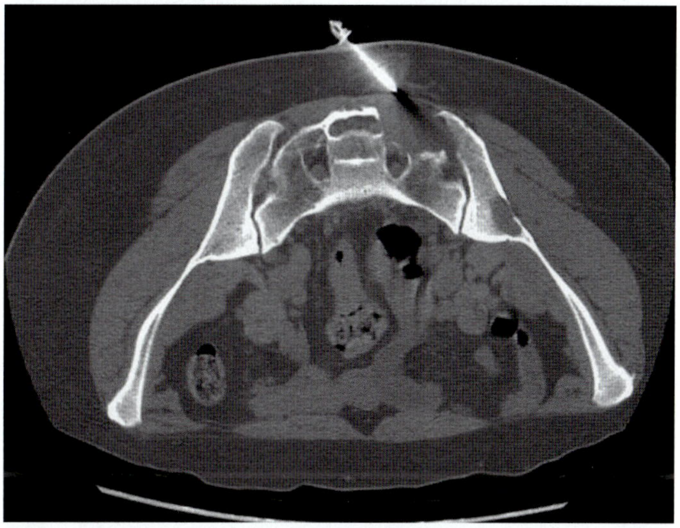

Figure 26-33 CT-guided biopsy of lytic process involving the right sacroiliac bone using a posterolateral approach.

Upper and Lower Limbs

Anatomically based guidelines for needle biopsy of long bone tumors have been compiled by Liu et al., and are based on the surgical approaches used for limb-sparing surgery (Tables 26-4 through 26-13) (Figures 26-36 and 26-37). Although some variability exists, it is advised that the radiologist discuss the imaging studies and the biopsy approach with the surgeon in advance. Once the segment of bone to be biopsied and the planned surgical approach are determined, the radiologist must identify the structures to be avoided at that level. The patients should be positioned so that the biopsy site faces upwards. Every effort should be made to limit the biopsy path to a single muscle compartment, and neurovascular bundles should be identified and avoided. When possible, articular surfaces should also be spared from the biopsy path and the joint cavity should not be violated for extraarticular lesions. Larger, deeper bones such as the femur, tibia, and humerus are generally best accessed with a coaxial system

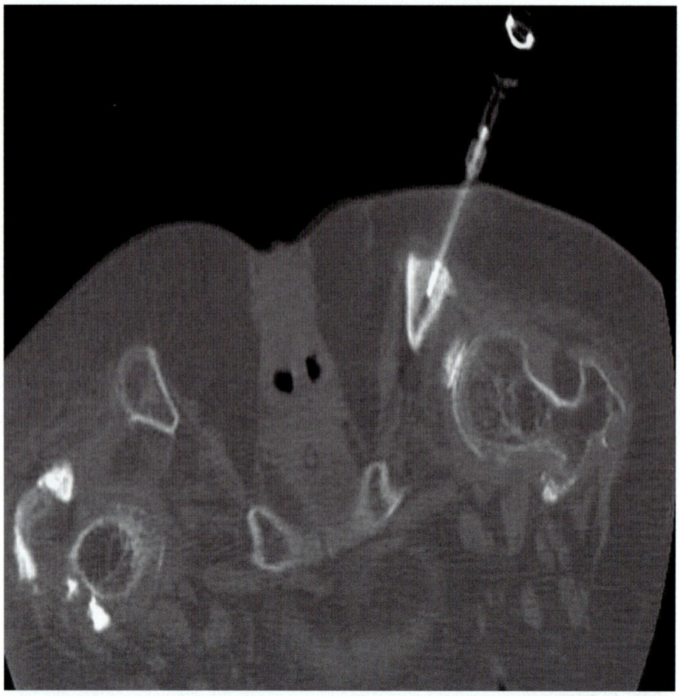

Figure 26-34 CT-guided biopsy of a sclerotic lesion in the right ischial tuberosity performed using a posterior approach.

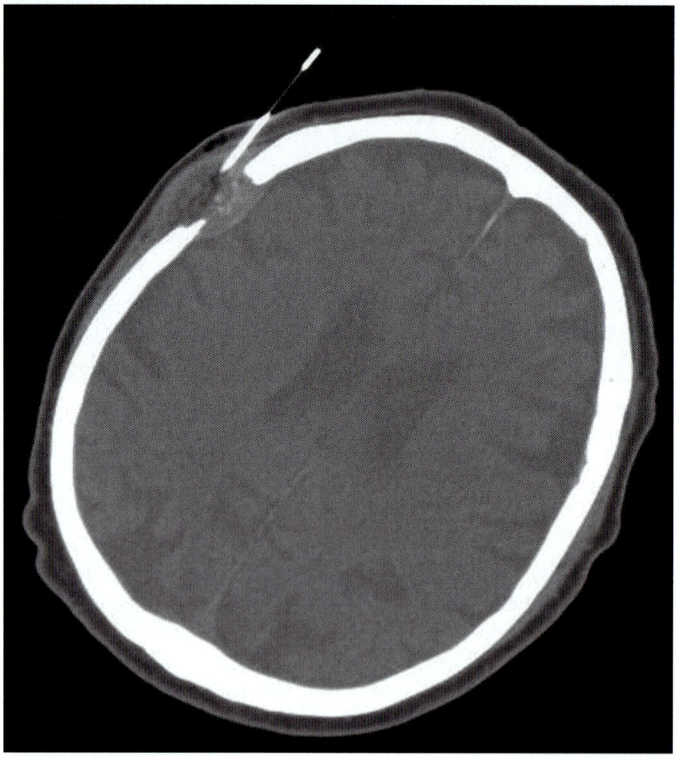

Figure 26-35 CT-guided biopsy of a skull lesion performed using a tangential approach. Histology was compatible with metastatic disease.

whereas a single-pass trephine-type device may be advantageous for more superficial osseous structures such as the metatarsals. For long bones, a direct approach, perpendicular to the diaphysis can help prevent soft tissue damage, which may occur when a device placed orthogonal to the bone slips during an attempt to anchor it into the cortex. Systems with an external drill are particularly useful in long bones with a thick cortex.

TABLE 26-4 Approach to Biopsy of the Shoulder

Patient Position	Supine
Arm position	External rotation to displace long head of biceps laterally
Biopsy approach	Lateral to the cephalic vein through the anterior third of the deltoid muscle
Structures to avoid	Cephalic vein Long head of biceps Radial nerve

TABLE 26-5 Approach to Biopsy of the Humeral Shaft

Patient Position	Supine
Arm position	Internal rotation
Biopsy approach	Posterior to biceps muscle and cephalic vein through the distal part of the deltoid and brachialis muscle
Structures to avoid	Cephalic vein Radial nerve Radial collateral artery

TABLE 26-6 Approach to Biopsy of the Distal Humerus

Patient Position	Supine
Arm position	Internally or externally rotated
Biopsy approach	Anterolateral approach through brachialis
Structures to avoid	Recurrent radial artery Radial nerve

TABLE 26-7 Approach to Biopsy of the Radius

Patient Position	Variable
Arm position	Rotate to place needle entry site facing upward
Biopsy approach	Radial head and neck: posterolateral approach Radial shaft: Medial approach Distal radius: Direct lateral
Structures to avoid	Radial nerve Radial artery Median nerve

TABLE 26-8 Approach to Biopsy of the Ulna

Patient position	Variable
Arm position	Rotate to place needle entry site facing upward
Biopsy approach	Olecranon: Posterior Ulnar shaft: Posteromedial through flexor digitorum profundus Distal ulna: Direct medial
Structures to avoid	Extensor pollicis brevis Abductor pollicis longus Extensor carpi ulnaris

TABLE 26-9 Approach to Biopsy of the Femur

Patient Position	Decubitus
Leg position	Target leg nondependent with hip partially abducted and femoral neck aligned with the scanner gantry plane
Biopsy approach	Inferolateral to superomedial
Structures to avoid	Greater trochanter bursa Femoral neurovascular bundle anterior to the femoral neck Lateral femoral circumflex artery (transverse branch)

TABLE 26-10 Approach to Biopsy of the Femoral Shaft

Patient Position	Prone or Prone Oblique
Leg Position	Externally rotated
Biopsy Approach	Posterolateral, anterior to the lateral intramuscular septum
Structures to Avoid	Anterior quadriceps muscle Sciatic nerve Profunda femoris artery

TABLE 26-11 Approach to Biopsy of the Distal Femur

Patient Position	Supine
Leg position	Internal or external rotation
Biopsy approach	Lateral approach—anterior to the lateral intramuscular septum, lateral to knee joint capsule Medial approach—through the postero-medial part of the vastus medialis muscle
Structures to avoid	Superficial femoral neurovascular bundle in the adductor canal Popliteal neurovascular bundle in the popliteal fossa Knee joint capsule Medial and lateral superior genicular arteries

TABLE 26-12 Approach to Biopsy of the Tibia

Patient Position	Supine
Leg position	Internal or external rotation
Biopsy approach	Anteromedial longitudinal approach overlying the anteromedial tibial cortex
Structures to avoid	Tibial tubercle Anterior and posterior tibial neurovascular bundles Peroneal neurovascular bundle Deep peroneal nerve

TABLE 26-13 Approach to Biopsy of the Fibula

Patient Position	Supine
Leg position	Internal rotation
Biopsy approach	Proximal and distal ends: directly into the fibula Fibular shaft: anterior to the posterior intramuscular septum through the posterior border of the peroneus longus muscle
Structures to avoid	Common peroneal nerve around the neck of the fibula

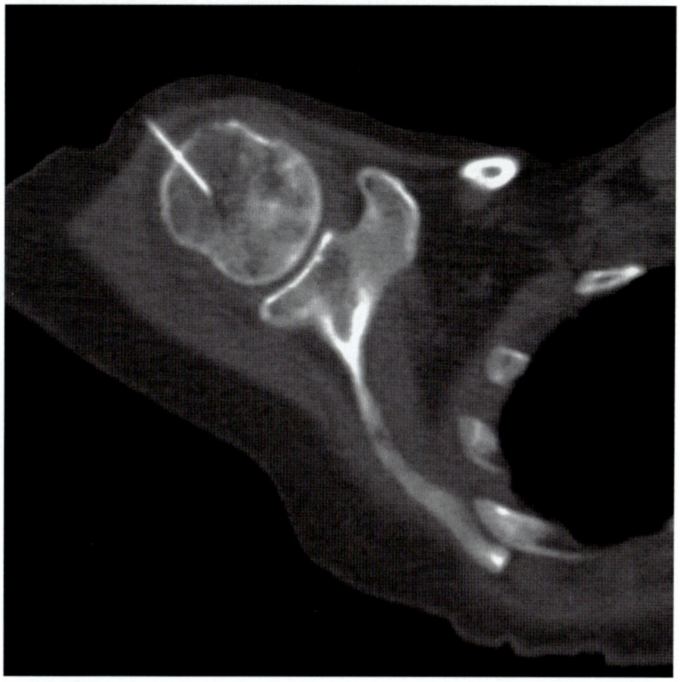

Figure 26-36 CT-guided biopsy of a chondroid lesion in the right shoulder using a lateral approach.

Complications and Management

Patients are observed for a minimum of 30 minutes and for up to 2 hours after the procedure to ensure that they recover from the sedation and that no delayed complications develop. Patients who have received intravenous sedation must be accompanied home by another adult. Appropriate postprocedure instructions should be given in relation to driving or operation of other machinery, resumption of anticoagulation or antiplatelet therapy, the symptoms and signs of postbiopsy emergencies, for example, compartment syndrome, spinal cord compression, or pneumothorax.

The complication rate for PMB is reported between 0% and 10% (<1% severe).[1,12,40] This compares with a 16% risk of adverse event following open musculoskeletal biopsy.[5,18,41] The most common complications include pain, bleeding, infection, bone fracture, neurologic injury, and pneumothorax. Hematoma is usually identified during the postprocedure observation period and in the majority of cases can be successfully managed with manual compression. In the event where significant bleeding occurs and the hematoma cannot be controlled with direct compression, angiography and embolization may be required.

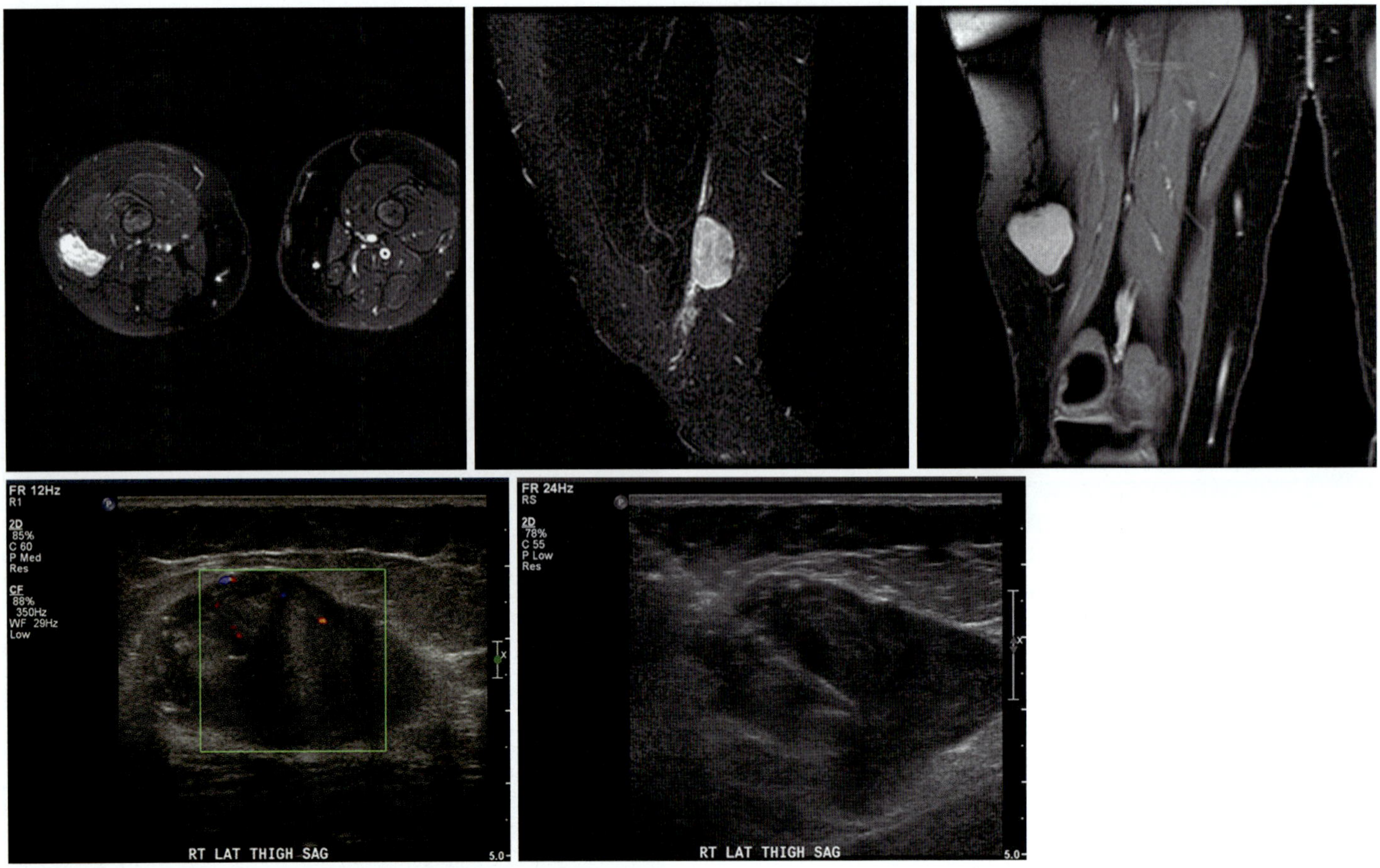

Figure 26-37 MRI of right thigh in female patient aged 17 years (*left to right*): T2-weighted fat-saturated sequence axial and sagittal projections, T1-weighted fat-saturated sequence postcontrast coronal projection demonstrate a hyperintense lobulated mass approximately 10 cm proximal to the knee joint in the lateral aspect of the right thigh. The lesion is centered in the subcutaneous tissues but intimately related to the superficial fascia of the tensor fascia lata. There is no deep muscle invasion. Ultrasound right thigh demonstrates a relatively nonvascular lobulated mass in the subcutaneous tissues of the right thigh. Ultrasound-guided biopsy was performed using a coaxial technique from a lateral approach. Histology was consistent with a synovial sarcoma.

Patients who undergo biopsy of an extremity need to be advised of the symptoms of compartment syndrome should significant bleeding only become evident after discharge. A neurologic injury can occur if the biopsy needle traverses a nerve bundle en route to the lesion. Prolonged paresis can occur if local anesthetic is infiltrated in the vicinity of nerves. Neurologic symptoms may also relate to cord compression by a postbiopsy hematoma. The greatest risk is with hypervascular vertebral lesions such as renal cell carcinoma. Thoracic spine biopsies are associated with pneumothorax in 4%–11% of cases.[24] The estimated risk of tumor seeding by FNA is 3 to 9 cases per 100,000 biopsies.[24] In the case of primary bone sarcomas, the needle entry site should be marked with indelible ink so that the tract can be excised when the patient undergoes definitive surgery. Diagnostic errors may be related to sampling, tumor type, sample fixation or handling methods, and pathologist experience.

Outcomes and Results

The SIR quality improvement guidelines for percutaneous image-guided biopsy define success as the procurement of adequate tissue for pathologic diagnosis or guidance of appropriate patient management. The reported success rate for PMB has been 76%–93%.[8] Several factors including the type of tissue, its location and radiologic appearance, the experience of the operator, and the modality used can influence the accuracy of PMB.[42] The sensitivity of PMB for metastatic lesions is superior to that reported for primary bone lesions: 82%–100% versus 74%–93%, respectively.[43-49] The radiologic appearance can have a significant bearing on the outcome from percutaneous biopsy of a bone lesion. Lower diagnostic rates have been reported for sclerotic lesions and vertebral compression fractures compared with lytic lesions.[44,50-52] A mass containing fluid or necrosis is more likely to give a false negative result.[51] The histologic yield from lesions with an osseous matrix is superior to those with a cartilaginous matrix. Poorer outcomes for hematologic conditions including lymphoma have been attributed to necrosis, failure to biopsy the medullary component of the bone, and destruction of the membrane antigens (required for phenotyping of the tumor) during the decortication process.[53] Contrast-enhanced CT and MRI and PET CT can help identify solid areas and metabolically active areas of the tumor, thus avoiding regions of necrosis.[54,55]

PMB outcomes for primary malignant bone and soft tissue lesions are not significantly different[4,42,56]; however, the diagnostic yield from soft tissue tumors is dependent on the histologic tumor type. Heterogeneous tumors with mixed cell types including angiosarcomas, liposarcomas, synovial cell sarcomas, hemangiomas, and schwannomas are associated with lower diagnostic rates from PMB.[57-59] These tumors can contain different cell types of different grade in different parts of the mass;

thus, PMB samples are often not reflective of the entire lesion.[58-60] The diagnosis of sarcoma is primarily dependent on cytologic analysis of fine-needle aspirates from which the malignant nature of the disease and its grade can be determined. Although this may be sufficient for surgical resection of these lesions, histologic subtyping necessitating core biopsy is required for radiotherapy and/or chemotherapy.[61]

FNA is best used to confirm the benign or malignant nature of a lesion, identify whether the lesion is a primary bone lesion or metastatic disease, confirm recurrent disease and for microbial analysis in the setting of infection. The more homogeneous the lesion, the more likely FNA will be diagnostic. A number of studies have reported greater diagnostic accuracy with core biopsy compared with FNA for bone and soft tissue lesi ons.[49,56,62,63] Schweitzer et al. recommended a complementary role for aspiration and core biopsy of skeletal lesions following a prospective evaluation of PMB in 138 patients. The diagnosis was made by core alone in 17, by aspiration alone in 11, and by both core and aspiration in 28. Neither core nor aspiration were diagnostic in 40.[64] Wu et al. recommended a minimum of three specimens in bone lesions and four specimens in soft-tissue lesions to optimize diagnostic yield from image-guided core biopsy of musculoskeletal lesions.[60]

PMB is 70% to 100% successful at confirming an infectious etiology.[65-67] Both histologic and microbiologic assessment is advised given that negative cultures are obtained in 40%–60% of cases.[67-69] Diagnostic accuracy is greater with core biopsy than with FNA; thus, sampling using both techniques is recommended.[8,24,68] The accuracy of percutaneous disc biopsy has been reported as low as 47% for spondylodiscitis. Because hematogenous spondylodiscitis originates in the subchondral bone, samples should be acquired from both disc and bone.[24,68]

Summary

Musculoskeletal pathology encompasses a vast range of disease entities that may be the manifestation of a local or systemic process. While the diagnosis of characteristic lesions can be readily made from the clinical findings together with the appropriate imaging study, many are atypical and require percutaneous biopsy for diagnosis. It is important that such cases are reviewed in a multidisciplinary setting. The issues surrounding PMB and the subsequent management of the lesion, whether it be the technical challenge for the individual performing the biopsy, the need for adequate high-quality tissue samples so the pathologist can correctly classify and grade a sarcoma, or the surgeon's plan to definitively resect the lesion while preserving musculoskeletal function, must be clearly understood by all involved.

REFERENCES

The complete reference list is available online at www.expertconsult.com.

27

Musculoskeletal Interventions for Benign Bone Lesions

SEAN M. TUTTON | RODRICK C. ZVAVANJANJA | ALDA L. TAM

KEY POINTS

- Radiofrequency ablation is now the standard of care for the treatment of osteoid osteoma.
- Surgical treatments carry significant morbidity and recovery times. Improved image guidance techniques drive the increased use of ablation options in treatment of benign bone tumors.
- A familiarity with bone biopsy needles, mallets, and drills are needed when performing bone interventions.
- Neuroprotective measures including hydrodissection, CO_2 insulation, and nerve monitoring are important adjuncts when ablating near neurovascular bundle or viscera.

Background

Benign bone tumors predominantly affect young patients,[1] and the majority of patients present with symptoms of pain and/or pathologic fracture secondary to the abnormal bone matrix in and around the bone lesion. Surgical resection and stabilization of the bone have served as the time-honored standard of care; however, although complete resection can be achieved in many situations, it is not without morbidity, which can be significant if the tumor to be resected is adjacent to vital structures or requires violation of a joint and the supporting musculotendinous architecture. Furthermore, the integrity of the cortex may be compromised after surgery if hardware for fixation has been inserted or if a prolonged non-weight-bearing status is prescribed. Therefore, balancing the benefits of a complete resection with these risks of the surgical approach is paramount when developing a plan of care for the patient. Over the past two decades, minimally invasive image-guided interventions for benign bone tumors have emerged that can leave the joint and the structural integrity of the underlying bone less disturbed. Thermal ablative techniques have been at the vanguard of these new minimally invasive techniques,[2,3] with radiofrequency ablation (RFA)[4] or laser ablation[5] now recognized as the treatments of choice for osteoid osteoma. The application of these techniques to other small, painful, focal bone lesions are emerging (Table 27-1).[6-11]

This chapter discusses the use of ablative techniques in the management of osteoid osteoma and other benign bone lesions, presents unique strategies for tackling challenging cases and lesions in difficult locations, and reviews the percutaneous interventions used in the management of unicameral and aneurysmal bone cysts.

Patient Selection

The accurate diagnosis of benign bone lesions is important in determining the appropriate management. The diagnosis is mainly based on the patient's age, clinical presentation, imaging features, and histology.[1,12,13] For bone lesions, multiplanar, cross-sectional CT imaging is preferred for lesion characterization and procedural planning. The diagnostic imaging will also reveal the presence of an impending fracture, pathologic fracture, or signs of arthritis. Radiography may also be useful as it allows for an accurate determination of the aggressiveness of the lesion and is a better modality for the evaluation of the bony matrix, if present, within a lesion. Additional imaging in the form of radionuclide bone scan and gadolinium-enhanced magnetic resonance imaging (MRI) may be helpful in the workup of equivocal cases.[14-16]

Although the lesions may be benign, the underlying pathophysiology plays an important role in determining treatment strategies and goals. For example, osteoid osteoma secretes high concentrations of prostaglandins and contains sensory nerve fibers, both of which are felt to be responsible for the characteristic severe pain. However, ablation of the nidus of the osteoid osteoma is sufficient for pain relief and is considered curative treatment. Other tumors, such as hemangioma, manifest rich networks of vascular channels resulting in pain-inducing pressure–volume effects and bone reabsorption. Treatment of these lesions needs to include management of the structural compromise because of the bone reabsorption. Giant cell tumors manifest high concentrations of unopposed osteoclasts at the bone–tumor interface resulting in pain and structural compromise. These lesions can be locally aggressive, infiltrating neurovascular structures and excluding the opportunity for cure by complete surgical resection or thermal ablation. In these cases, palliation and local control become the principal goals, and multimodality therapy involving a combination of medications, embolization, ablation, and structural reinforcement with osteoplasty or surgery is often required. As with all successful outcomes in neoplasm management, a multidisciplinary approach, involving the primary care physician, orthopedic surgeon, neurosurgeon, medical and radiation oncologist, and the interventional radiologist, is the cornerstone of good patient care.

A preprocedural clinical visit is essential and gives the interventional radiologist the opportunity to discuss the procedure, review patient expectations, and define realistic goals for treatment and recovery during the informed consent process. A focused history and physical examination are required. Physical exam findings of neural compromise (either sensory or motor), scoliosis, abnormalities of range of motion or limb length discrepancy should be documented. The findings on

TABLE 27-1 Summary of Benign Bone Tumors and Tumor Like Conditions Amenable to Image-Guided Interventions

Bone Forming Lesions
Osteoid osteoma
Osteoblastoma
Lesions of Cartilaginous Origin
Enchondroma
Chondroblastoma
Chondromyxoid fibroma
Fibrous, Fibroosseous, and Fibrohistiocytic Lesion
Fibrous cortical defect
Fibrous dysplasia
Desmoplastic fibroma
Miscellaneous Lesions
Giant cell tumor
Unicameral bone cyst
Aneurysmal bone cyst
Hemangioma
Eosinophilic granuloma
Paget disease
Oncogenic osteomalacia
Brown tumor of hyperparathyroidism

physical examination should be correlated with a recent multiplanar, cross-sectional (CT or MRI) imaging study to localize the pain to the lesion site. It is helpful to establish a baseline pain and disability score, objective criteria, which can be monitored following the procedure to determine treatment efficacy. Examples of pain scoring systems that are commonly used include the visual analog scale (VAS) or brief pain inventory (BPI). For lesions in the spine and pelvis causing back pain, the Roland Morris Disability Questionnaire (RMDQ) or Oswestry Disability Index (ODI) can also be used.

The patient's current medications should be reviewed and anticoagulation medications should be optimized prior to the procedure. Frequently, patients seeking treatment for benign bone lesions are younger and routine preprocedure labs may be unnecessary. In older patients, the Society of Interventional Radiology or American Society of Anesthesia (ASA) guidelines should be followed, and platelet count, prothrombin time, and partial thromboplastin time should be ordered to assess bleeding risk.[17]

Counseling of the patient and family are essential to provide education on expected outcomes, postprocedure pain related to flair response, potential complications, recovery time, and restrictions on activities during the recovery phase. When the lesion involves a weight-bearing long bone, the risk of impeding fracture must be discussed. Although fracture following thermal ablation is uncommon, a few cases have been reported in the literature following radiofrequency ablation (RFA).[18,19] In these cases, it may be appropriate to follow the ablation with a cementoplasty procedure to provide structural support; however, the need for possible surgical intervention to stabilize a postablation fracture should always be discussed. When the lesion to be treated abuts an articular surface, the risk of thermal damage to the cartilage, resulting in early-onset arthritis, is a risk that needs to be addressed.

There are a few absolute contraindications to thermal ablation. Lesions less than 1 cm away from a critical structure where hydrodissection, or carbon dioxide insulation cannot be performed (e.g., osteoid osteoma in vertebral body adjacent to spinal cord, lesions adjacent to major motor nerves or the artery of Adamkiewicz) are not suitable for thermal ablation.[20] Patients with skin infection or breakdown in continuity with the bone lesion or those with severe, uncorrectable coagulopathy are not candidates for ablation.

Technique

ABLATIVE MODALITIES

Thermal ablation of tumors either involves heating the tumor tissue to temperatures of 50°C–100°C or freezing the tumor tissue to temperatures below −40°C to induce cell death.[21,22] RFA and cryoablation are the most commonly used thermal ablation techniques. Other heat-based thermal ablation modalities include microwave ablation, high-intensity ultrasound (US), and laser photocoagulation.

RFA uses a high-frequency alternating current (460–500 kHz) to deposit thermal energy into tissue, resulting in ionic agitation, frictional heating, and coagulative necrosis. Current RFA generators in the United States are capable of delivering 200–250 W via RF electrodes of varying configurations and sizes (usually 14- to 17-gauge).[21] Three commercially available, FDA-approved, monopolar RF devices are available in the United States: Boston Scientific "LeVeen" (RF 3000, Boston Scientific, Natick, MA); Angiodynamics RITA (Model 1500X, RITA Medical Systems, Mountain View, CA); and, the Covidien Cool-Tip (Boulder, CO) RF ablation systems. The type of RF electrode and the size of the active tip will determine the size and extent of the ablation zone; however, for small, focal bone lesions, a rod electrode is usually sufficient. An initial low wattage between 4 and 10 W depending on lesion size is selected and ablation is carried out based on a manufacturer-prescribed time algorithm or impedance changes in the lesion. For osteoid osteoma treatment, lesions are heated up to 90°C for 6 minutes[4] (Figure 27-1). If there is high impedance during the ablation, the active tip may be buried in the bone, and withdrawing the electrode into the nidus will result in a drop in impedance.

During cryoablation, the delivery of argon gas through a segmentally insulated probe and the rapid expansion of the gas results in rapid cooling (Thompson-Joule effect) with tissue temperatures dropping to below −100°C within seconds. The characteristic properties of the cryoablation zone ("ice ball"), with its changes in intra- and extracellular water composition, allow for visualization using CT imaging and the ice ball appears as an oval or spherical zone of hypoattenuation (see Figure 27-5). The outer edge of the ice ball corresponds to 0°C and review of the isotherms of the ice ball is critical to defining the area that falls within the −40°C or below zone. There are two commercially available cryoablation systems available in the United States: Percryo (Healthronics, Austin, TX) and Galil Medical (Galil Medical, Arden Hills, MN). The probe sizes range from 14.7 to 24 mm in diameter. For many authors, cryoablation is the preferred ablation modality for large malignant or benign tumors. The ability to utilize as multiple probes simultaneously allows for the creation of very large ablation zones and nonspherical configurations tailored to the lesion size and location (Figure 27-2). Several published reports have demonstrated the safety and efficacy of cryoablation in benign and malignant tumors.[23-25]

Interstitial laser photocoagulation is widely performed in Europe and is shown to be safe for the treatment of osteoid

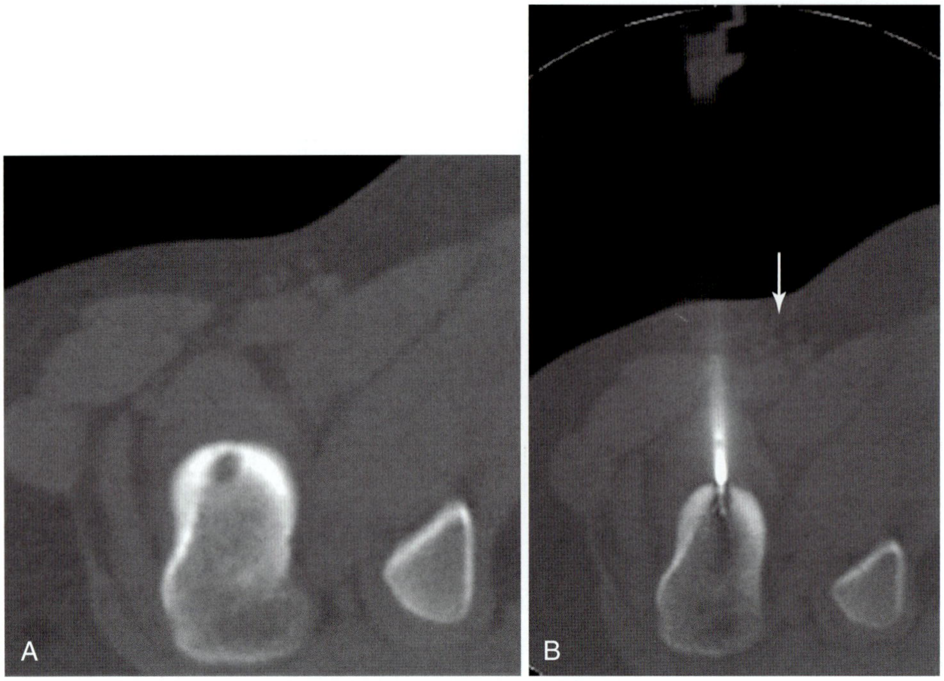

Figure 27-1 An 8-year-old boy with hip pain who was no longer participating in physical education class. (A) Axial image from a noncontrast CT shows a focal lytic lesion in the proximal femur representing an osteoid osteoma. (B) Axial image from a noncontrast CT after a multitined RFA probe has been introduced into the nidus. Note that the percutaneous access tract to the osteoid osteoma avoids the neurovascular bundle, which is located medially (*arrow*).

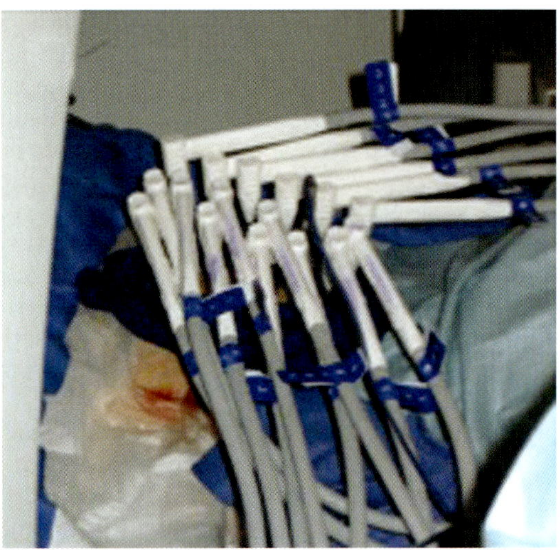

Figure 27-2 Fifteen cryoprobes were used to treat a large retroperitoneal tumor (not shown) and illustrate how cryoablation can be used to create a specific geometrical ablation zone.

osteoma.[5,26-28] In this technique, flexible, optical fibers are inserted into the lesion and transmit infrared light energy at low power (typically 2–4 W) to produce heat and coagulative necrosis.[29] The ability of the laser to deliver a fixed energy precisely to a target has made it useful in the treatment of small, focal bone lesions.[26] Other ablative technologies such as microwave, MR-guided high-intensity ultrasonography, and irreversible electroporation are at various stages of development and maturation and have yet to be commonly used in the ablation of benign bone lesion.

CEMENTOPLASTY

Cementoplasty, also called osteoplasty or vertebroplasty when performed in the spine, involves the injection of polymethylmethacrylate into the bone to provide structural support and reduce the risk of pathologic fracture. It has been used as a stand-alone or adjunctive procedure in the treatment of benign[30,31] and malignant bone tumors.[32,33] Because of the direct cytotoxic and thermal effects on tumor cells and sensory nerves, the injection of polymethylmethacrylate has also been shown to provide pain relief. Cementoplasty is a percutaneous technique that is being used increasingly in bone interventions and a familiarity with this procedure is necessary for interventional radiologists who manage bone lesions.

EQUIPMENT

Percutaneous ablation procedures can be performed using moderate sedation in adults[32]; however, for children or adolescents, general, spinal, or epidural anesthesia may be preferable both to eliminate anxiety associated with the procedure and voluntary patient movement during the course of target access.[34] Many authors believe CT imaging for procedural guidance is the best because it provides fast imaging acquisition, superior anatomic resolution of bone tissue, and is compatible with various ablative devices.[34,35] The initial preprocedure imaging needs to be adequate to cover the cranial and caudal extent of the lesion for assessment of lesion volume, configuration, and to plan an approach for access. Section thickness of 2–3 mm is recommended for best visualization.[34] As most are pediatric patients, it is important to minimize radiation dose exposure; and, once the lesion has been localized, intraprocedural images acquired during lesion targeting can be obtained with reduced x-ray tube current (often half of even less of the recommended dose by the CT manufacturer).[34]

Performing preprocedural biopsy of the lesion before RFA is controversial with inconclusive biopsy results varying from 27% to 64% in clinically and morphologically unequivocal osteoid osteoma[3,32,36]; however, Laredo et al.[36] have argued that histopathologic confirmation of the diagnosis may help, especially in cases of treatment failure or disease recurrence. There is really no disadvantage to performing a biopsy: tissue sampling can be achieved during lesion access and no additional time or complexity is added to the procedure.[34]

Frequently, there is no thinning or weakening of the overlying cortical bone, which can be quite hard in children and young adults, and access becomes the most challenging aspect of the procedure. Ablation probes are not designed to be hammered, screwed, or muscled into the bone and will break relatively easily; therefore, the interventional radiologist must become comfortable with several techniques and tools to gain access to the bone lesion safely. Sturdy bone biopsy needles (14-gauge Bonopty needle [Apriomed, Uppsala, Sweden], Laurane biopsy needle [Laurane Medical, Saint-Arnoult, France], or 13- or 11-gauge Osteosite M2 bone biopsy needle [Cook Medical, Bloomington, IN]) can be used in conjunction with mallets, hand drills, or a Stryker 4200 cordless drill (Stryker Instruments, Kalamazoo, MI) with Steinmann pins to create an osteotomy to gain access to the lesion.[36] Once an osteotomy has been made, a coaxial technique can be used to exchange the access needle for the ablation probe (Figure 27-3).

TECHNICAL CHALLENGES AND ADJUNCT MANEUVERS

A bone or soft tissue lesion will often be in proximity to a critical structure such as a major neurovascular bundle, spinal cord, bladder, or bowel. As a general rule, if the intended ablation zone is to be within 1 cm of a vital structure, additional measures and precautions are necessary to prevent collateral damage. The placement of a thermocouple next to a critical structure can be used for real-time temperature monitoring during the ablation (Figure 27-4). The temperature of the nontarget critical structure should not exceed 45°C in RFA cases or fall below 8°C in cryoablation cases.[19,37] Various thermal insulation techniques have been used to protect structures at risk for damage during percutaneous ablation procedures.[38] The instillation of carbon dioxide (CO_2) has been widely used as insulation technique in ablation.[20,37,39-41] CO_2 is highly soluble, nonallergenic, and lacks renal or hepatic toxicity. It is easily reabsorbed by vessels, eliminated by the respiratory system, and has low thermal conductivity. It can be injected through a 21-gauge spinal needle that is interposed between the lesion and the structure at risk (Figure 27-5), and volumes range from a few milliliters in the epidural space (Figure 27-6) to 1.5 L in the peritoneal cavity.[38] Because CO_2 can be absorbed, periodic evaluation with imaging is required to monitor the gas volume and determine the need for the injection of additional volume.

Hydrodissection can be performed to displace and insulate critical structures during ablation. In the abdomen and pelvis, the injection of fluid can be used to displace bowel away from the ablation zone and provide an added margin of safety when ablating liver, renal, or adrenal tumors. Fluid can also be injected

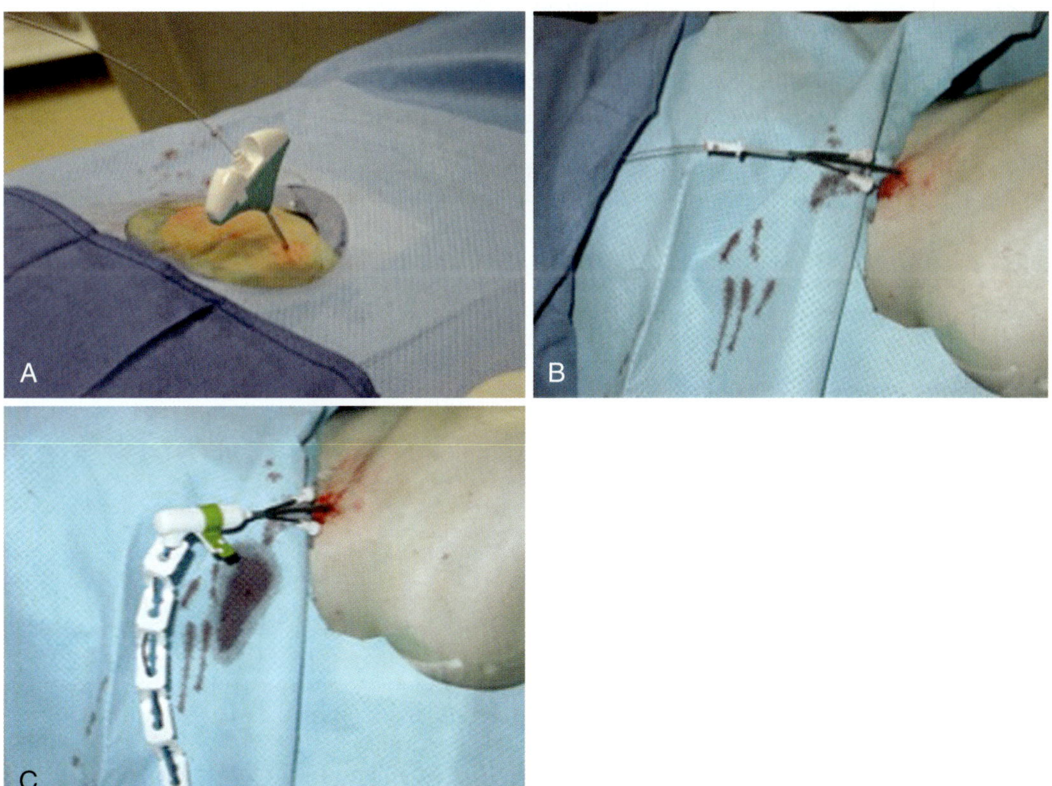

Figure 27-3 Coaxial exchange technique for placing the ablation probe through an existing osteotomy. (A) An osteotomy has been created using a 13- or 11-gauge bone biopsy needle and a 0.035-in. short wire is placed through the bone biopsy needle into the osteotomy. (B) The bone biopsy needle is exchanged over the wire for a 7- or 8-French peel-away sheath. The peel-away sheath should be telescoped up against the periosteum. This allows the probe to be guided into the osteotomy and has been useful in the authors' experience by obviating the need to "dig around" for the osteotomy. (C) With the RFA probe in place, the peel-away sheath must be retracted or removed (peeled away) before the ablation is performed to prevent melting or freezing of the plastic.

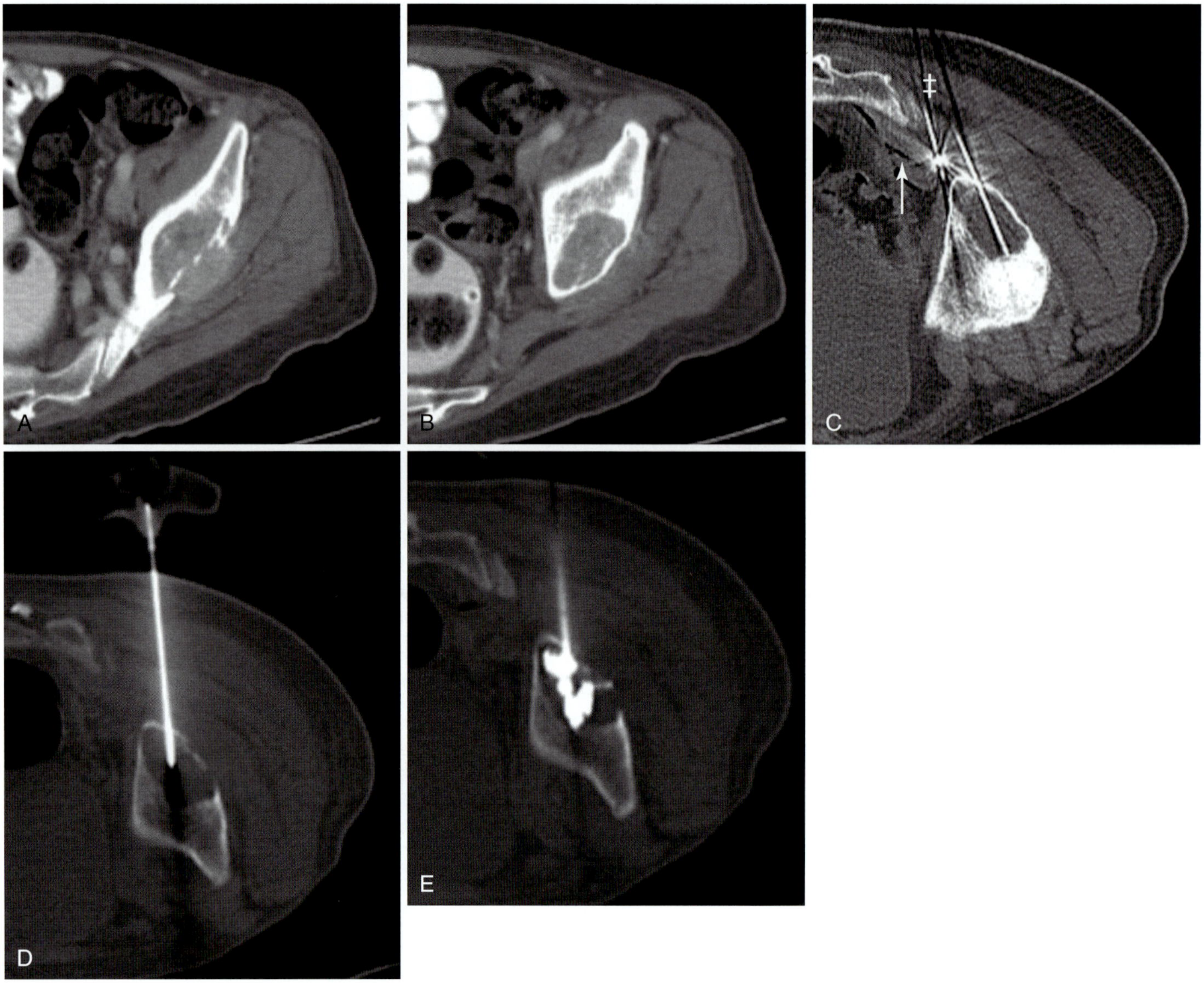

Figure 27-4 A 63-year-old man with metastatic renal cell carcinoma. The patient complains of excruciating left hip pain and cryoablation is requested for pain palliation. (A and B) Axial, contrast-enhanced images demonstrate a lytic lesion involving the left iliac bone and extending down into the acetabulum. Two 24-mm cryoprobes (HealthTronics, Inc., Austin, TX) were placed within the iliac bone, targeting the bone-soft tissue interface (not shown). A 17-mm cryoprobe (HealthTronics, Inc., Austin, TX) was placed within the acetabular portion of the lesion (C). Because of the proximity of the posterior border of the lesion to the sciatic notch, other protective techniques, in addition to routine CT monitoring of the ice ball progression, were used to monitor for potential injury to the left sciatic nerve. Sural nerve stimulation was performed throughout the procedure to assess the integrity of the sciatic nerve. A 21-gauge needle was used to inject CO_2 gas around the left sciatic nerve and this can be seen as air tracking along the fascial planes as denoted by the ↑ in (C). A 17-gauge thermocouple (HealthTronics, Inc., Austin, TX) marked as ‡ in (C) was placed adjacent to the left sciatic nerve. This provided real-time monitoring of the temperature near the nerve during cryoablation. As the lesion involved the acetabulum, cryoablation was followed by cementoplasty the next day to reduce the potential risk for fracture (D and E). Two 13-gauge vertebroplasty needles (Cook Inc., Bloomington, IN) were placed and a total of 5 mL of polymethylmethacrylate was injected into the acetabular roof under CT guidance. (*From Nazario J, Tam AL: Ablation of bone metastases,* Surg Oncol Clin N Am *20(2):355–368, ix, 2011; Review, Figure 5.)*

into the epidural space for use as a cooling method during thermal ablation of spinal tumors or injected into the joint space to protect the cartilage during thermal ablation of articular or juxtaarticular lesions[5,42,43] (Figure 27-7). Sterile saline or dextrose (5%) in water (D5W) for RFA procedures can be injected through a 21-gauge needle. The fluid injected can also be cooled or warmed to cool down or warm up the anatomic structures as risk. A dilute amount of contrast (20:1 in strength) can also be added to the fluid to improve visualization. Fluid injection may not be appropriate for use during cryoablation as the fluid may freeze on contact with the ice ball and increase the potential for thermal damage (Figure 27-8).

Skin injury in the form of burns or frostbite is a risk with any thermal ablation procedure. Placing a sterile glove filled with either warmed or cooled saline is often sufficient to protect the skin from thermal injury (Figure 27-9). The subdermal injection of sterile saline or lidocaine 1% to create a wheal of fluid under the skin at the site of ablation is commonly used to prevent skin injury during the treatment of superficial lesions (Figure 27-10).

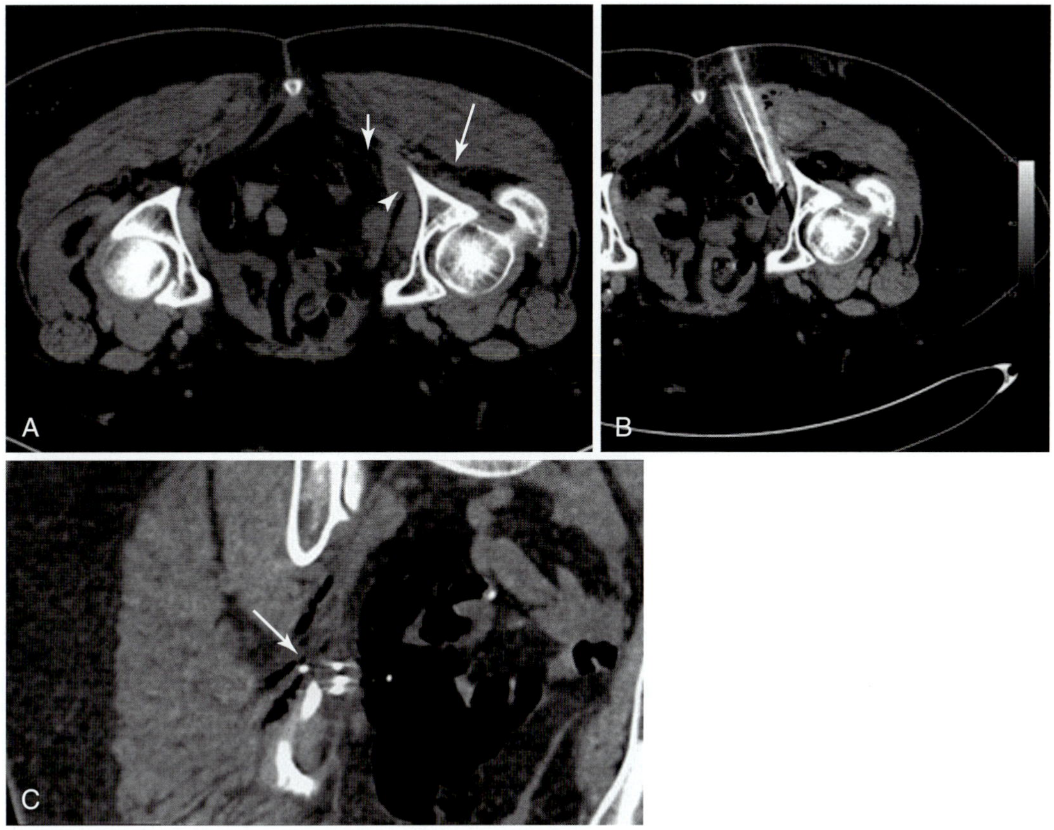

Figure 27-5 (A) Painful metastasis at the level of the ischial spine (arrowhead) adjacent to the sciatic nerve (*long arrow*) laterally, and the loop medially (*short arrow*). (B and C) CO_2 dissection was performed with a 21-gauge spinal needle medially (loop insulation) and an 18-gauge laterally (sciatic insulation), which also allowed the coaxial insertion of a thermocouple (*long arrow*) (temperature monitoring of the sciatic nerve). Note the satisfactory insulation of the loop and the sciatic nerve. *(From Tsoumakidou G, Buy X, Garnon J, et al: Percutaneous thermal ablation: how to protect the surrounding organs,* Tech Vasc Interv Radiol *14:170-176, 2011; Figure 1.)*

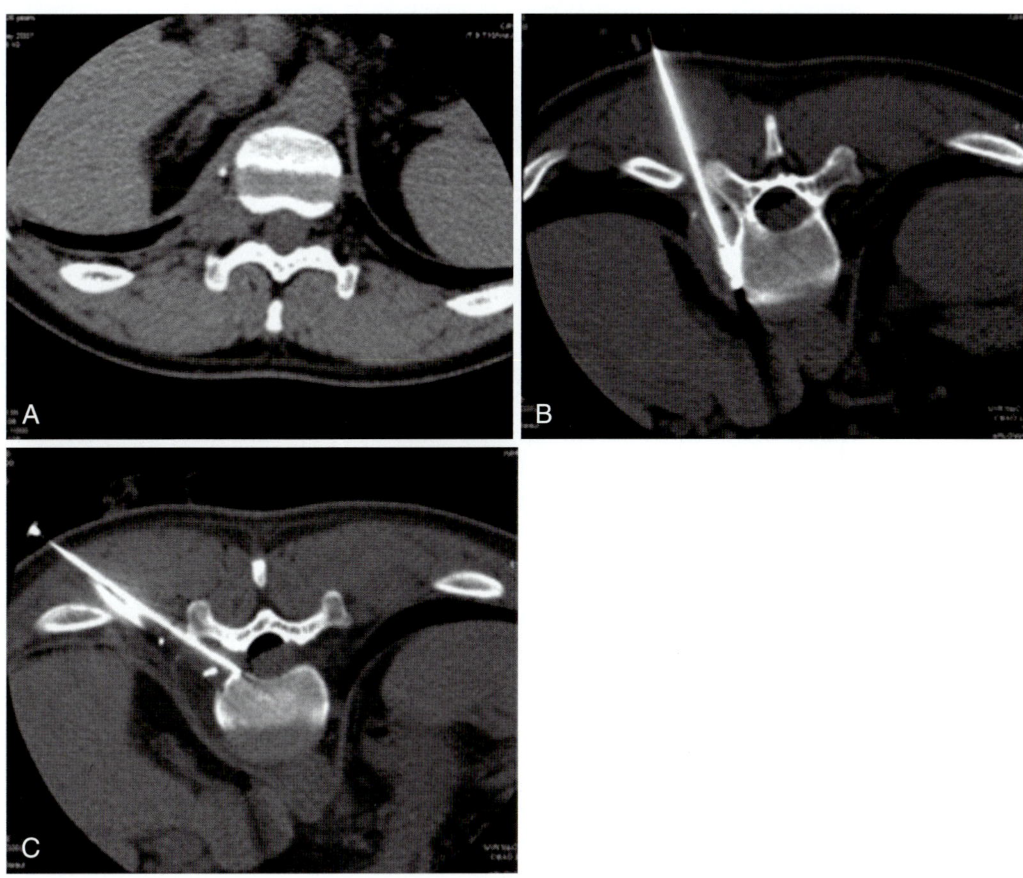

Figure 27-6 (A) Axial CT image of a painful paravertebral tumor (postsurgical recurrence of a metastasis of a testicular carcinoma). (B) Cryoprobe positioned in the tumor. In order to protect the dura, CO_2 was injected in the epidural space. (C) In addition, a thermocouple was positioned in the foramina. Note the CO_2 thermal blanket in the epidural space. *(From Tsoumakidou G, Buy X, Garnon J, et al: Percutaneous thermal ablation: how to protect the surrounding organs,* Tech Vasc Interv Radiol *14: 170-176, 2011; Figure 7.)*

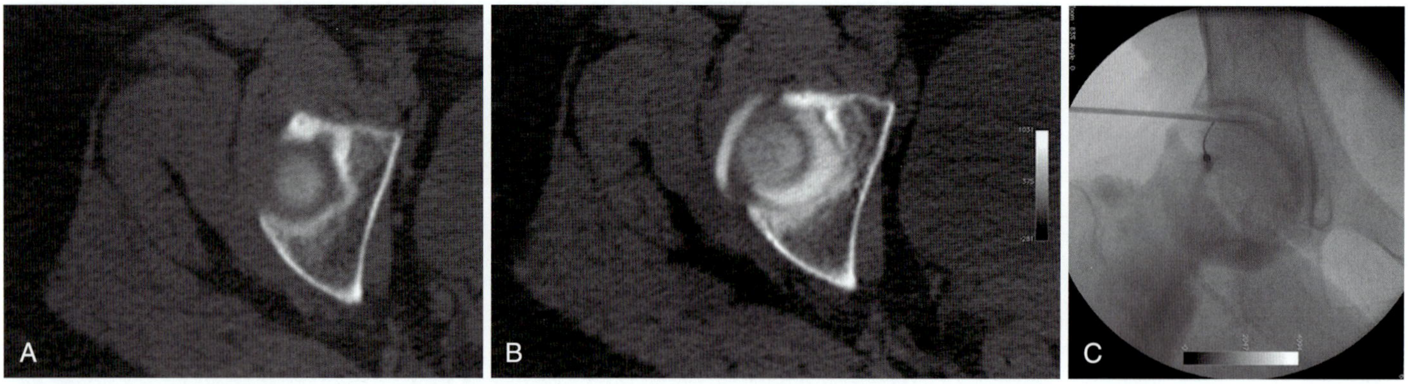

Figure 27-7 (A) Axial CT image of an osteoid osteoma of the acetabulum. (B) Axial CT image and (C) AP fluoroscopic image. Laser ablation of the tumor. To avoid cartilage damage of the femoral head, 20 mL of saline, opacified with contrast, were injected in the joint space, increasing the distance between the nidus and the cartilage. *(From Tsoumakidou G, Buy X, Garnon J, et al: Percutaneous thermal ablation: how to protect the surrounding organs,* Tech Vasc Interv Radiol *14:170-176, 2011; Figure 3.)*

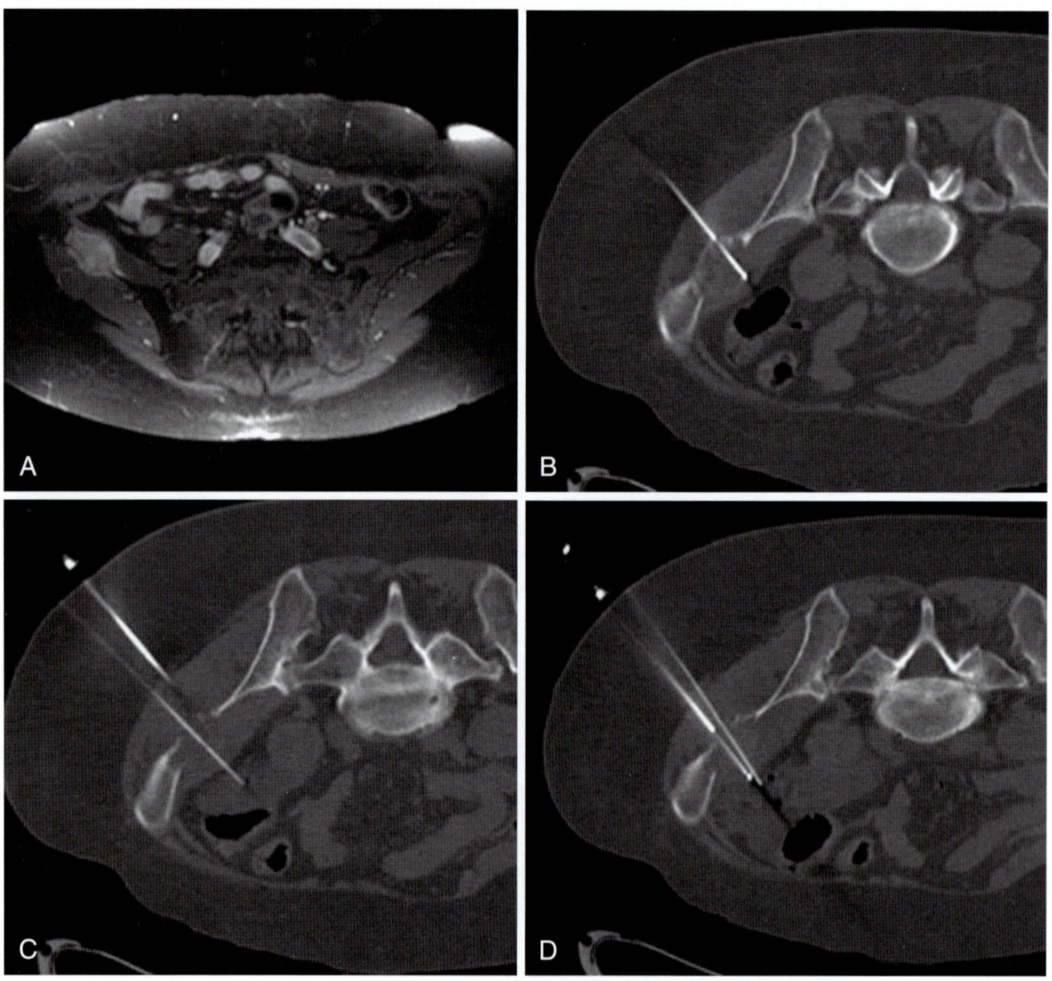

Figure 27-8 A 35-year-old woman with solitary bone metastasis from adrenal cortical adenocarcinoma. The bone metastasis was progressing despite radiation therapy and radiofrequency ablation was planned for local disease control. (A) Contrast enhanced T1-weighted MRI demonstrates an enhancing lesion involving the right iliac wing. (B) The patient was placed in a prone position during the procedure to try to displace the colon anteriorly with gravity; however, after placement of the initial RFA probe, the colon was noted to be quite close to the ablation zone. (C) An 18-gauge Hawkins needle (Cook Inc., Bloomington, IN) was introduced into the peritoneal cavity and D5W was injected to displace the colon. (D) Multiple overlapping RF ablations were performed with intermitting injection of D5W to keep the colon displaced.

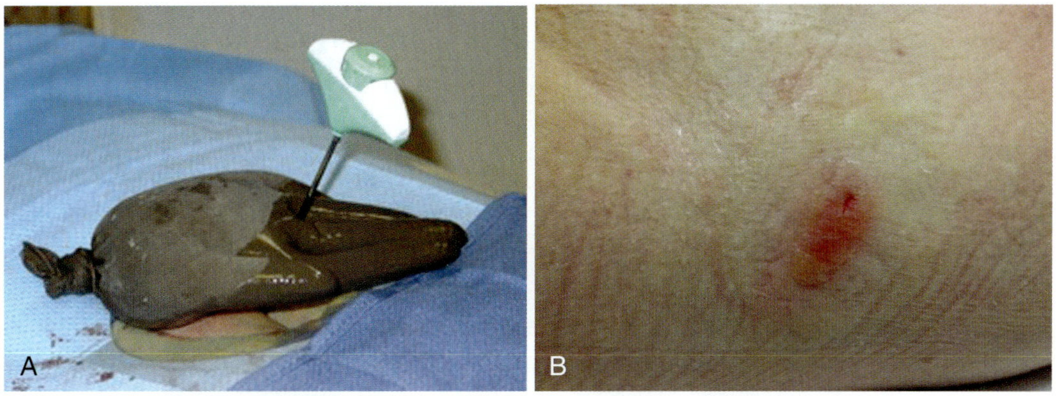

Figure 27-9 (A) A size 9 glove was filled with warm saline in preparation for cryoablation as a protective measure to prevent skin injury. As shown with the bone biopsy needle, the cryoprobe can be slotted through the fingers of the filled glove. (B) An example of mild skin injury with blister formation in the skin of the right axilla following lung cryoablation where the hub of the cryoprobe was in direct contact with the skin. This type of injury is usually self-limited and an antibiotic ointment can be applied until it heals.

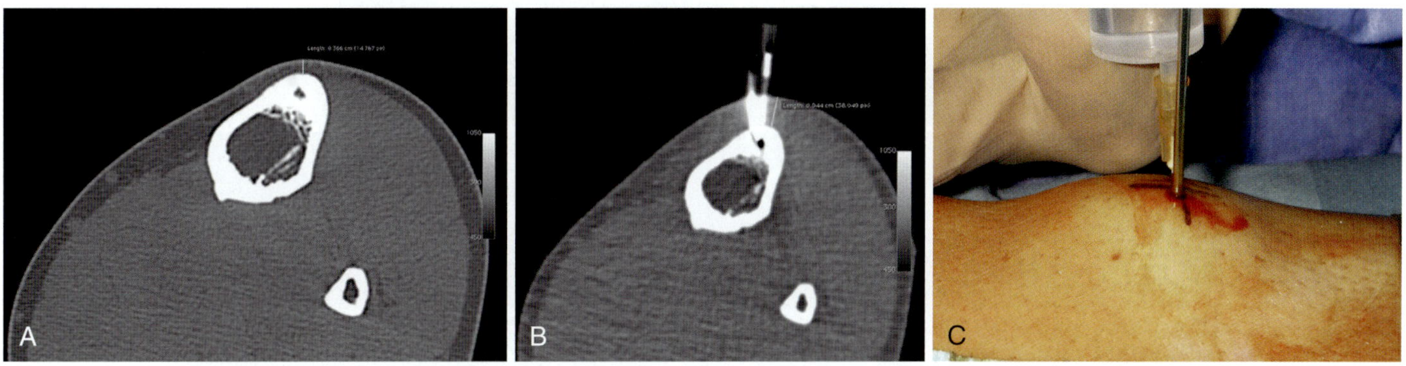

Figure 27-10 Laser ablation of a tibial osteoid osteoma. (A) Axial CT image showing the intracortical nidus. (B, C) To avoid skin burn subdermal injection of 20 mL of saline is administered. *(From Tsoumakidou G, Buy X, Garnon J, et al: Percutaneous thermal ablation: how to protect the surrounding organs,* Tech Vasc Interv Radiol *14:170-176, 2011; Figure 6.)*

NEUROLOGIC MONITORING

When ablating lesions in the cervical spine, near the brachial plexus, in the sacrum or near the sciatic notch, it can be useful to have continuous neural monitoring using somatosensory evoked potentials (SSEP).[44] SSEPs consist of a series of waves that reflect sequential activation of neural structures along the somatosensory pathways. A dedicated team is required to monitor the SEPs where peak latencies, wave amplitudes, and wave morphologies are evaluated. Changes to the parameters during an ablation procedure may indicate impending neural injury and give the interventional radiologist the opportunity to stop the ablation before causing further damage (Figure 27-11).

Complications

Complications related to percutaneous ablation of bone lesions are uncommon but include hemorrhage, infection, fracture, skin burns (both at electrode entry sites and at grounding pads), frostbite, incomplete hemiplegia, radiculopathy, and transient bowel or bladder dysfunction.[19,45,46] Because of the thickness of the cortex, care must be taken when accessing lesions and withdrawing instruments as there have been occasions in which a part of the needle has broken off in the bone.[18] Typically, the needle fragment can be left in the bone with no adverse sequelae; however, occasionally, surgical removal may be required (Figure 27-12). Some patients may have an acute flair response after treatment with increase in pain due to acute postablation edema and inflammation. This can be managed expectantly with supportive care or preprocedural steroids may be given to dampen the postprocedural inflammatory response.

Outcomes and Results

BONE FORMING LESIONS

Osteoid osteomas represent 10% of benign bone tumors.[13] They usually occur in patients between the ages of 10 and 35, with males more affected more frequently than females. Most osteoid osteomas are located in the long bones, typically in the femur or tibia, but as many as 20% may be within the spine.[47] Patients with symptomatic osteoid osteomas report the classic symptoms of pain that is present at rest, exacerbated by activity, worse at night, and responds to the use of nonsteroidal antiinflammatory medications. In addition to pain, osteoid osteomas have been known to cause growth disturbances

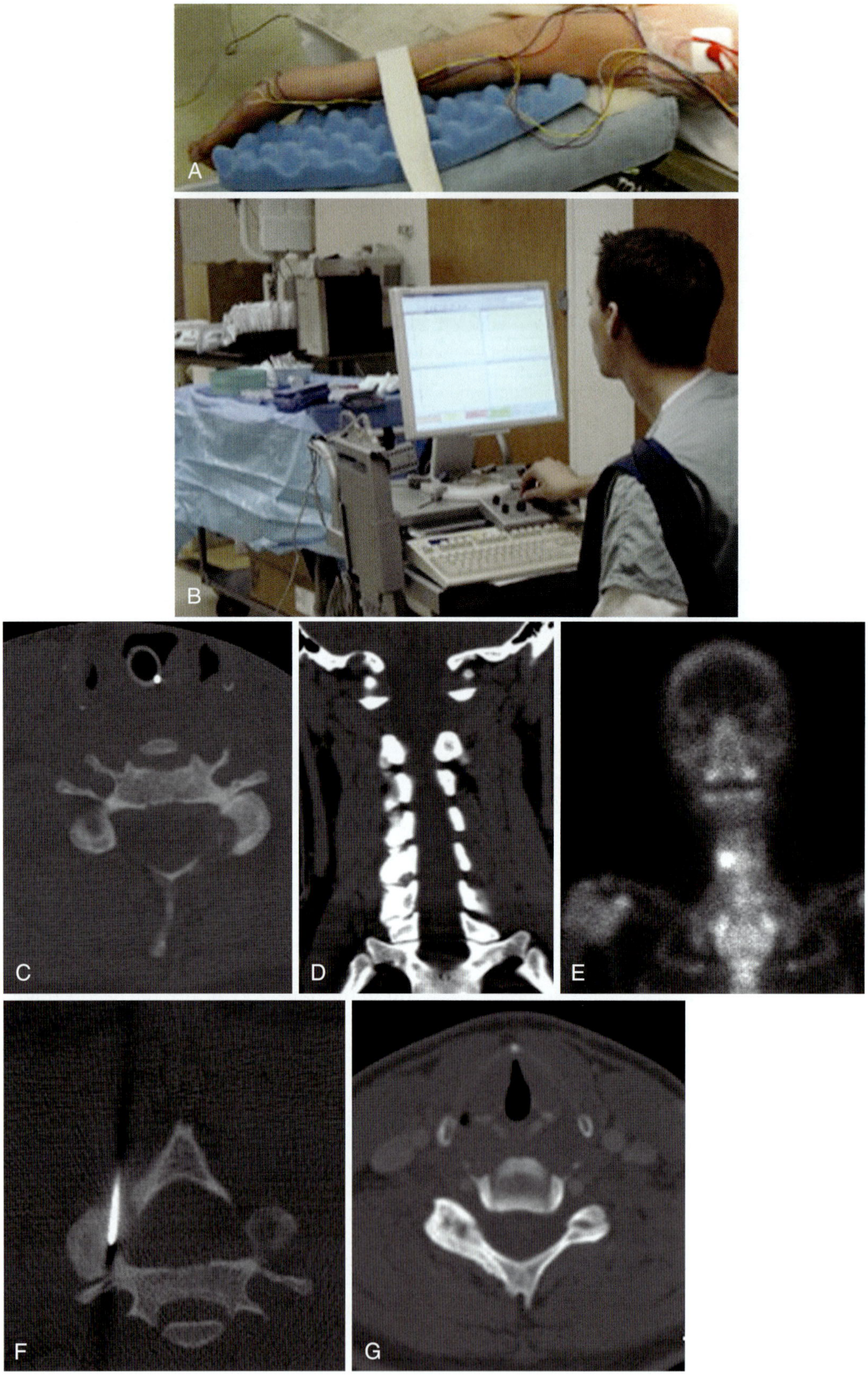

Figure 27-11 SSEP monitoring. A and B illustrate the neural monitoring and setup during an ablation of an osteoid osteoma of the C5-C6 facet in a 25-year-old right-handed engineer with right upper extremity pain and disability for greater than 1 year. A spine surgeon referred him for minimally invasive treatment because of unacceptable surgical morbidity. The proximity of this osteoid osteoma to the spinal cord and nerve roots required extra maneuvers to safely perform the procedure and continuous monitoring of the C5 and C6 nerve roots. (C and D) Axial and coronal CT image demonstrates a lytic lesion in the C5-C6 facet with a central nidus and surrounding reactive hyperostosis. (E) Bone scan demonstrates increased uptake in the lesion. (F) Axial CT image during RF ablation showing the probe in the nidus of the osteoid osteoma. (G) Axial CT image from a follow-up study obtained 6 months after RFA demonstrates healing and facet fusion. The patient had normal neurologic function.

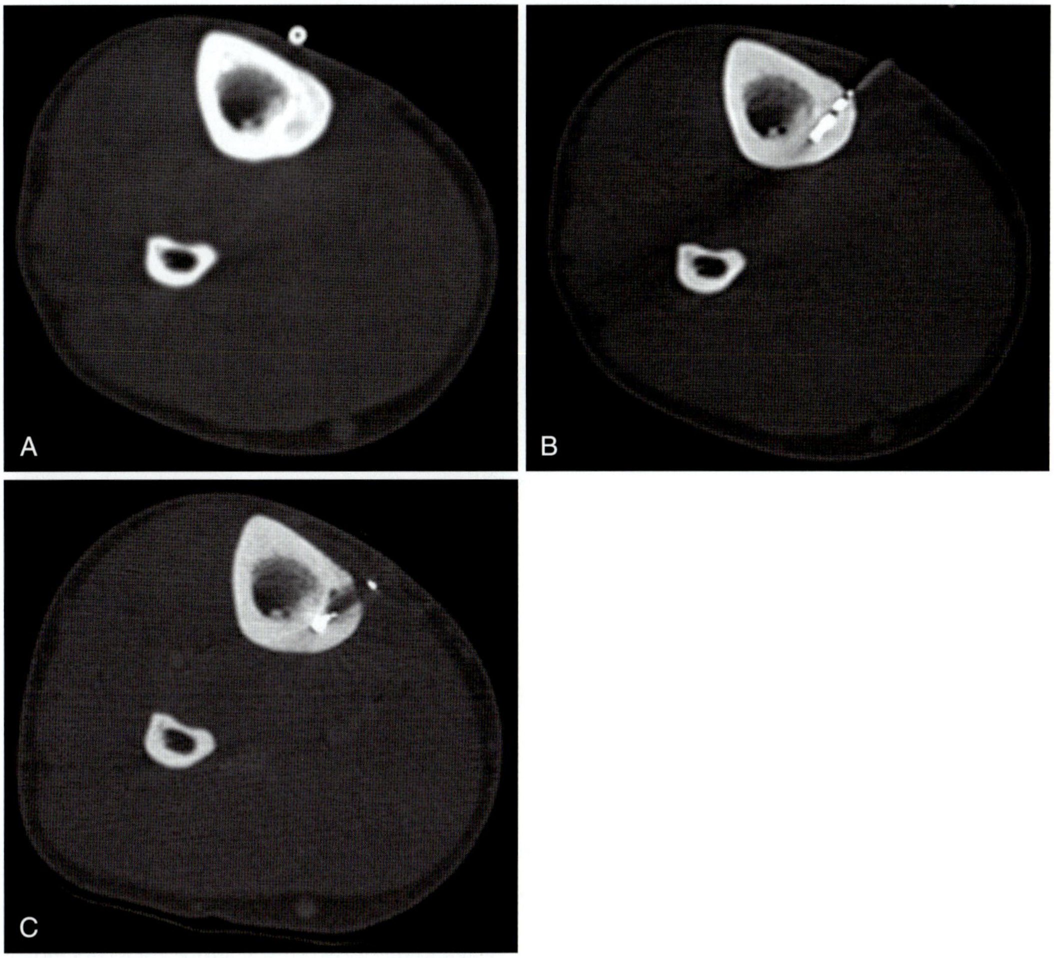

Figure 27-12 A 21-year-old man with osteoid osteoma of the right tibia that was treated with RFA. Six months after the initial treatment, the patient reported recurrence of right leg pain. (A) Axial CT image during second RF ablation demonstrates a small residual nidus with a thick overlying cortex. (B) Access to the lesion was difficult and had to be achieved with the aid of a hand-drill. The drill bit subsequently broke off within the cortex. The patient was discharged with antibiotics but returned 4 months later complaining of purulent drainage from the site. (C) Contrast-enhanced CT demonstrates the retained metallic drill bit with extrusion of a fragment that broke off. Changes in the bone indicated osteomyelitis, and the patient was taken to the operating room for incision and drainage as well as curettage of the right tibia.

if located close to an open growth plate, scoliosis, delayed-onset osteoarthritis, and severe muscle atrophy.[13,34,48] Imaging reveals a small, well-defined lesion that rarely exceeds 1.5 cm in diameter and is characterized by a nidus of osteoid tissue that may be purely radiolucent or have a sclerotic center. Edema may be present in the surrounding tissues and bone marrow and lesions within a joint may cause a joint effusion.

Minimally invasive image-guided treatment of osteoid osteoma is the most widely studied application of using percutaneous ablative techniques in benign bone tumors. The nature of this lesion, with its central nidus and surrounding sclerotic bone, provides an ideal scenario for the use of a thermal ablative technique. The thickened cortex serves as "insulation" effectively trapping heat and producing an oven effect that results in maximum kill of the nidus.[49] In 1998, Rosenthal et al. reported a 90% technical success rate, equivalent to that of surgical treatment, for radiofrequency ablation in treatment of osteoid osteomas.[50] In 2003, the same authors reported on their 11-year experience with using RFA to treat osteoid osteoma: 263 patients underwent 271 ablations, all of which were technically successful, with a 0.7% complication rate. Eighty-nine percent of patients experience a complete relief of symptoms and the aggregated recurrence rate is estimated to be 8% at 2 years, with the risk of recurrence being higher in lesions that have been previously surgically treated and those occurring in patients younger than age 5 years.[4,34] Additional data reported in the literature indicate that short-term (within 2 weeks) pain relief should be achieved in close to 100% of patients and durable relief from symptoms has been reported in 66%–96% of patients.[4,51-53] Most recurrences are a result of incomplete ablation of the nidus and usually present within 6 months of treatment. For these patients, retreatment with ablation is an option and is associated with similar success rates as the initial treatment.[54] Percutaneous ablation has now supplanted surgical resection as the standard of care in the treatment of osteoid osteoma[34,49]: percutaneous ablation is less invasive than surgery, results in less bone destruction, is associated with shorter hospitalization stay, and is equivalent in terms of safety and efficacy.[34]

Although some authors do not routinely recommend follow-up imaging,[34] preferring to rely on improvements in objective outcomes measures (pain scale) or patient reporting of recurrent symptoms to indicate treatment failure, others have used MRI to evaluate the treated lesion and for evidence of tumor regression either seen as a decrease in size or vascularity of the tumor or bone remodeling.[55]

Osteoblastomas are histologically similar to osteoid osteomas but are rare, representing 3% of benign bone tumors.[56] These tumors are often larger than 2 cm, may progress in size, and may behave aggressively.[18] Osteoblastomas are often found in the long bones and spine. They are almost always diagnosed before 30 years of age, and patients may be symptomatic or present with pain that does not respond readily to nonsteroidal antiinflammatory medications. Radiographically, these lesions may appear like a giant osteoid osteoma (>2 cm), an expansile lesion similar to the appearance of an aneurysmal bone cyst, an aggressive lesion mimicking a malignant tumor, or a periosteal lesion without perifocal bone sclerosis but with a shell of newly formed periosteal bone.[56] The standard treatment is surgical excision or curettage but recurrences are not uncommon.[57] In a few select cases, RFA has been used as a treatment alternative and the procedure is performed using electrodes with longer active tips and/or overlapping ablations to ensure the entire lesion is treated.[18,58]

LESIONS OF CARTILAGINOUS ORIGIN

Chondroblastomas, also known as Codman tumors, are benign cartilaginous lesions usually found in patients under the age of 20.[35] They occur in the immature skeleton in the epiphysis of long bones such as the humerus, femur, and tibia. In contrast to osteoid osteoma, chondroblastomas have a tendency to progress and their location near growth plates and joint spaces may hamper surgical removal, and recurrence rates have been reported to range from 5% to 20%.[6,18,34] Chondroblastomas tend to be painful and are discovered when small, making them suitable for percutaneous ablation therapy.[34] Radiographically, the lesions are usually located eccentrically, show a sclerotic border, and may demonstrate calcifications of the matrix.[59] The experience with using percutaneous ablation for the treatment of chondroblastoma is growing with evidence of sustained postprocedural pain control[6-9,11,18,35,60] (Figure 27-13). Cases of articular surface collapse and recurrence have been reported and some authors have described the avoidance of articular collapse by the combined use of RFA and bone grafting in conjunction with close follow-up to monitor outcome.[9,60]

Enchondromas represent about 10% of benign bone tumors and are characterized by the formation of mature hyaline cartilage.[59] Enchondromas are often asymptomatic but can present with pain if associated with a pathologic fracture. They are typically found in the short or long tubular bones and may undergo malignant transformation to chondrosarcoma. Only two cases of intracortical chondroma treated by percutaneous ablation have been reported in the literature[61] (Figure 27-14). One patient experienced pain relief following RFA but the other patient required surgery for definitive treatment. Chondromyxoid fibroma is another rare cartilaginous lesion seen in adolescents and young adults who may be amenable to percutaneous ablation. It is frequently located in the proximal tibia or distal femur and may range in size from 1 to 10 cm.[59] Chondromyxoid fibromas can be associated with symptoms of pain and swelling. Radiographically, they appear as eccentric, radiolucent lesions with a sclerotic, scalloped margin that may balloon out the cortex. Surgical curettage and bone graft may be associated with recurrence rates of 20% to 80%.[59]

FIBROUS, FIBROOSSEOUS, AND FIBROHISTIOCYTIC LESIONS

Fibrous cortical defects and non-ossifying fibromas are common fibrous lesions of bone seen in children and adolescents. They are seen more commonly in boys, located in the long bones, particularly of the lower extremity, and have a tendency to spontaneously involute.[62] These radiolucent lesions are elliptical and demonstrate a scalloped sclerotic border (Figure 27-15). Fibrous dysplasia, along with fibrous cortical defects and non-ossifying fibromas, is a fibroosseous lesion that is considered by some to be a developmental defect rather than a true neoplasm.[62] Fibrous dysplasia (FD) is characterized by the replacement of lamellar cancellous bone with abnormal fibrous tissue,

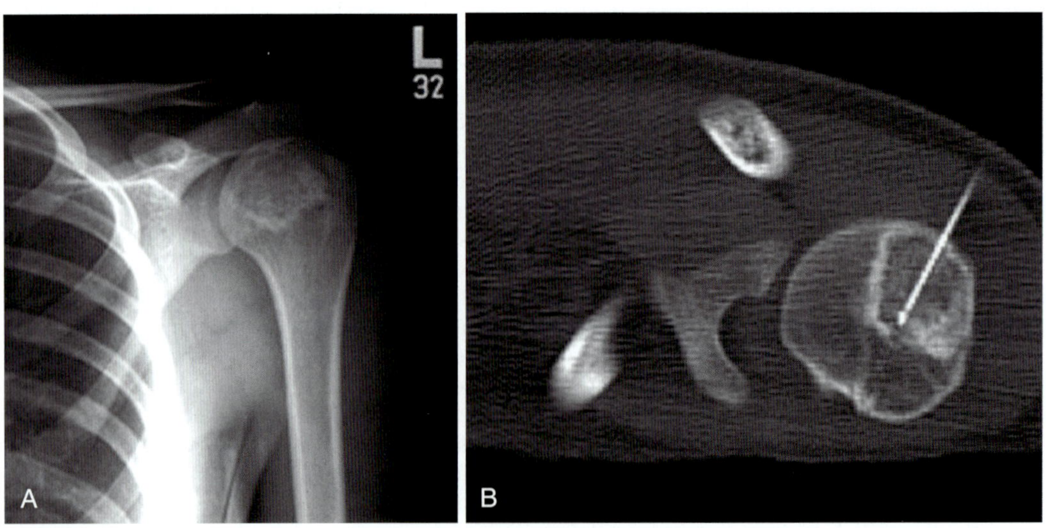

Figure 27-13 A 16-year-old right hand–dominant girl with left shoulder pain. (A) Radiograph shows a well-defined lesion with sclerotic margins within the humeral head. Calcified matrix is noted and chondroblastoma was suspected. (B) Axial CT image during RF ablation procedure. A biopsy of the lesion was taken prior to ablation and subsequently confirmed the lesion as chondroblastoma. Multiple overlapping ablations were performed using a Radionics ablation probe with a 2-cm active tip. The patient experience pain relief and was able to resume her regular activities.

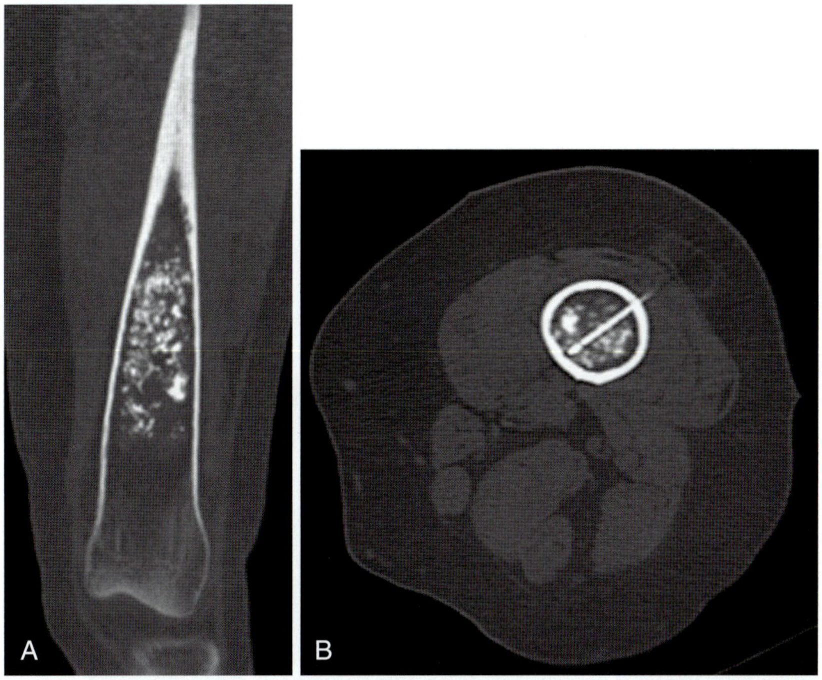

Figure 27-14 A 63-year-old woman with an enchondroma of the distal left femur. The patient complains of pain and was referred by the orthopaedic service for RFA. (A) Coronal reformat CT demonstrates an intramedullary lesion with a cartilaginous matrix consistent with an enchondroma. There is no evidence of malignant transformation. (B) Axial CT image demonstrates a Cool-Tip radiofrequency ablation probe with a 2-cm active tip within the medullary cavity. The access osteotomy was created using an 11-gauge vertebroplasty needle and multiple overlapping sites of ablation were performed. The patient experienced symptomatic relief after the procedure and was still pain free at 2-year follow-up.

and radiographically, it is described as having a "ground glass" appearance (Figure 27-16). Most of these lesions are asymptomatic but may become painful if associated with pathologic fracture. Sporadic cases of percutaneous ablation of these fibrous/fibroosseous lesions have been reported but the available data are insufficient to draw long-term conclusions regarding efficacy.[11] Surgical fixation is often required in FD; however, osteoplasty may be used in select cases to delay definitive surgical treatment (Figure 27-17).

MISCELLANEOUS LESIONS

Hemangiomas are common lesions found in the vertebral body that may, on occasion, extend into the pedicle and lamina. They represent 2%–3% of all spinal tumors with an incidence of 10%–12% in the general population; however, only 0.9%–1.2% of hemangiomas are symptomatic.[63] The incidence of hemangiomas increases with age and they are seen more often in women than men.[64] The lesion is composed of abnormal vascular channels and has a high concentration of osteoclasts at the bone–tumor interface. Radiographically, a hemangioma presents as a vertebral body with vertical striations on plain radiograph. On CT imaging, the vertical striations, representing reinforced vertical trabeculae of the cancellous bone, appear as multiple, coarse dots within the vertebral body. Patients with symptomatic hemangiomas present with mechanical back pain that may be associated with neurogenic pain when the hemangioma extends into the spinal canal or neural foramen.[63] A number of strategies have been used in the management of hemangiomas including preoperative embolization prior to surgical resection, embolization as a stand-alone therapy,[65] vertebroplasty,[30,31] and ablation (Figure 27-18). The most studied percutaneous intervention used in the management of hemangioma is vertebroplasty with pain relief reported in 80%–100% of cases. Complication rates range from 1% to 10%, and the most common complication is cement leakage.[30,63,66]

Giant cell tumors are locally aggressive lesions composed of richly vascularized tissue containing proliferating mononuclear stromal cells and numerous giant cells of osteoclast type.[64] Giant cell tumors represent 23% of benign bone tumors are found at the articular ends of long bones (proximal tibia, distal femur, distal radius, and proximal humerus) after skeletal maturity, and have a female predominance of 2:1.[64] Radiographically, it appears as a radiolucent lesion without sclerotic margins or periosteal reaction. Surgical treatment involves wide resection with stabilization or endoprosthesis implantation versus curettage and bone grafting. Radiation therapy has also been used but there is a risk for malignant transformation to fibrosarcoma, malignant fibrous histiocytoma, or osteosarcoma in recurrent lesions. The recurrence rate has been reported to be as high as 33% following surgical and radiation therapy.[67,68] Many now advocate a multidisciplinary approach for the management of these lesions. Medical therapy includes the use of bisphosphonates, calcitonin, and more recently, rank ligand inhibitors to attack the osteoclasts at the bone–tumor interface. Interventional radiologists may offer embolization and/or ablation therapies for pain palliation and local control in the form of growth arrest[35,67] (Figure 27-19).

Eosinophilic granuloma of bone is characterized by granulomatous proliferation of the reticulum cell and is considered a disorder of immune regulation rather than a neoplasm.[64] Lesions may be solitary or multiple, are usually seen in children

(Text continued on page 318)

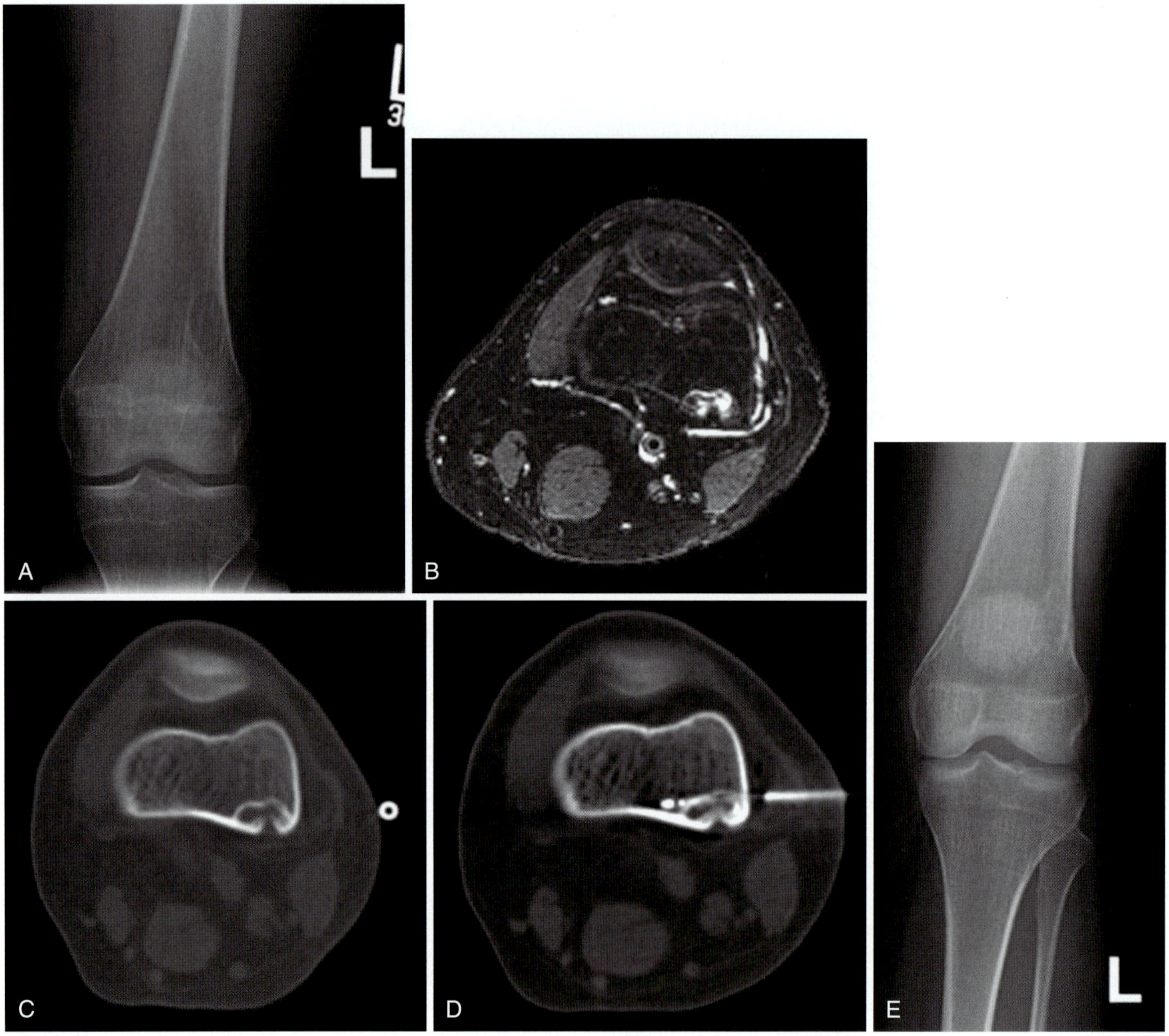

Figure 27-15 A 17-year-old girl with a history of neurofibromatosis type 1 and a painful lesion of her left femur. (A) Radiograph of the left femur reveals an intracortical, ovoid, lytic lesion in the distal metaphysis of the left femur that is a fibrous cortical defect or nonossifying fibroma. (B) Axial T2-weighted MRI of the left shows the lesion to have increased signal. (C and D) Axial CT images obtained during RF ablation demonstrate the well-defined borders of the lesion. Access through the cortex (not shown) was created using a Bonopty biopsy needle (Apriomed, Uppsala, Sweden). Two Cool-Tip radiofrequency ablation probes with a 1-cm active tip were inserted to ensure adequate coverage of the lesion (only one probe placement is shown). (E) The ablation relieved the patient's pain and she remains pain free at 1-year follow-up, with the follow-up radiograph demonstrating bone healing.

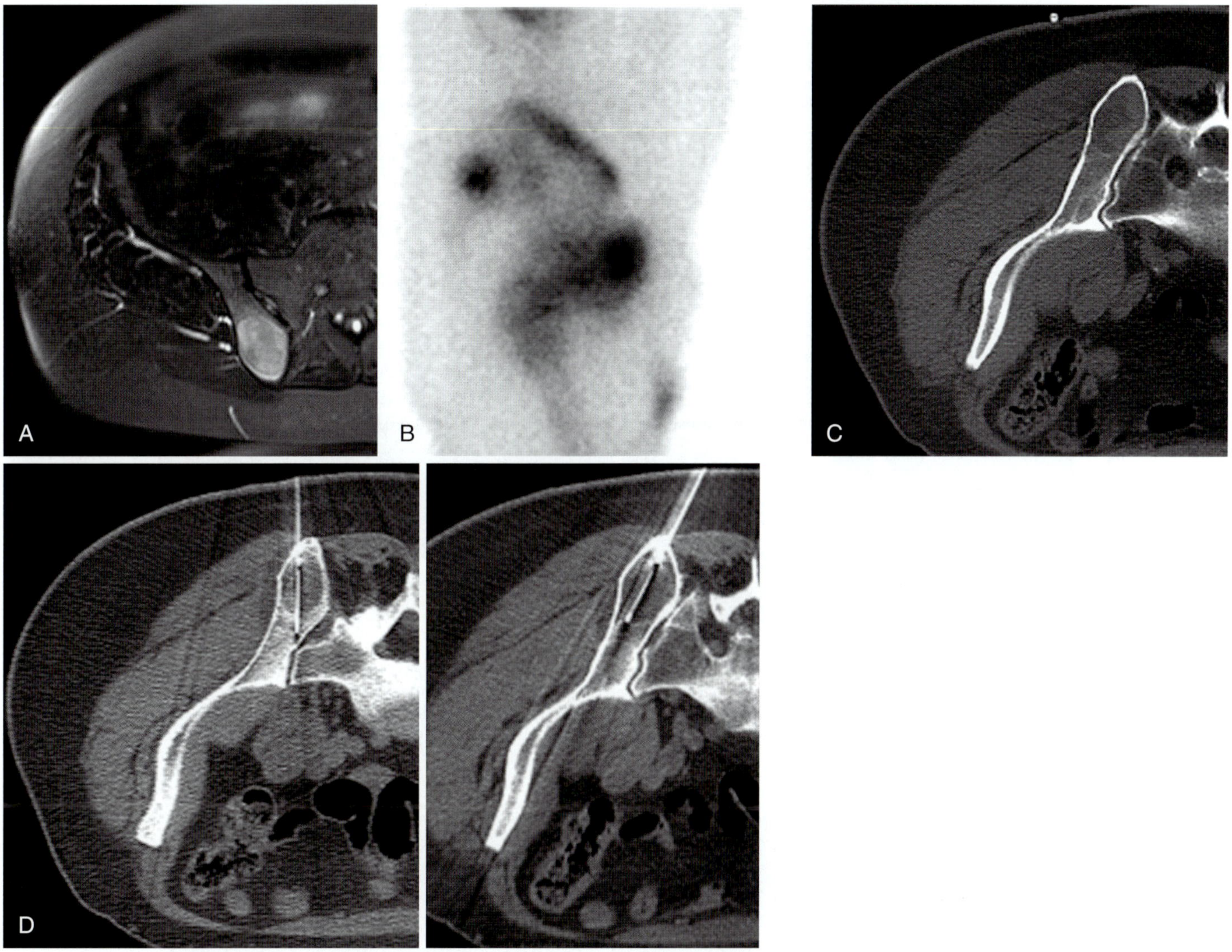

Figure 27-16 A 70-year-old man with a history of stage 3a renal cell cancer. The patient presented with pain in the right pelvis. (A) Axial T2-weighted MRI of the pelvis revealed a high-signal-intensity lesion in the posterior right iliac bone that corresponded to an area of increased uptake on bone scan (B). Based on these imaging findings, concern for a solitary bone metastasis was raised and the patient was referred for cryoablation for local control. (C) Axial CT image of the pelvis demonstrates the lesion to be lytic with the suggestion of internal matrix. (D) Two access sites into the bone were created using 13-gauge vertebroplasty needles and a 16-gauge bone biopsy needle was used to obtain specimen prior to ablation (not shown). Two Perc-17 cryoprobes (Healthtronics Inc., Austin, TX) were placed in the lesion and cryoablation was performed. Note the hypodense rim of ice extending beyond the cortex, into the gluteal muscles laterally. Final pathologic diagnosis was unclassified fibroosseous lesion. In some areas, the lesion exhibited woven bone formation within a bland spindle cell background reminiscent of fibrous dysplasia. In other areas, there was no bone formation, but rather a proliferation of spindle cells arranged in whorls and short fascicles with focal hemorrhage and aggregates of osteoclast-type giant cells resembling a solid aneurysmal bone cyst (ABC). The differential diagnosis included fibrous dysplasia with ABC-like changes, or less likely giant cell granuloma or giant cell tumor, among others. There was no evidence of involvement by renal cell carcinoma, as a pankeratin immunostain was negative. The patient's pain was relieved after the procedure.

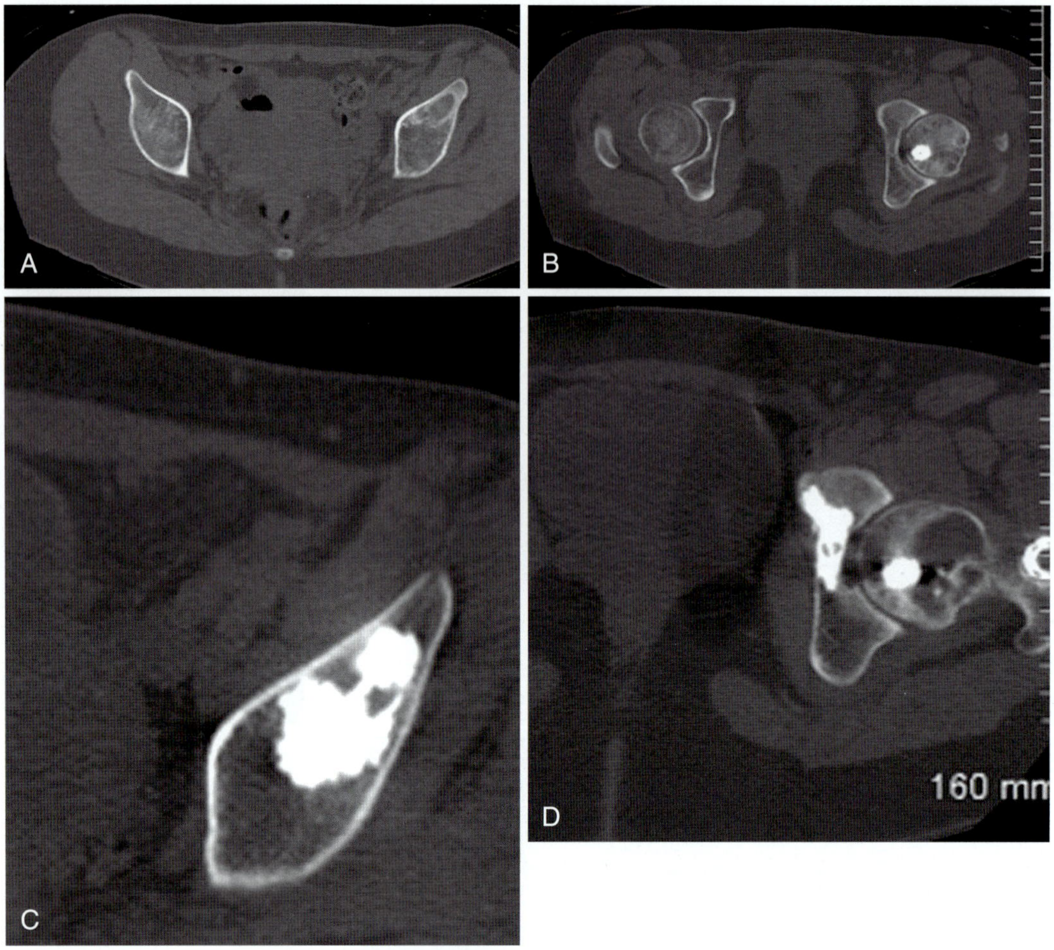

Figure 27-17 A 22-year-old active female with Fibrous Dysplasia of the left limb with prior surgical fixation of the femoral lesion and progressive involvement of the acetabulum and quadrilateral plate resulting in pain with jogging, and a feeling of instability. Total hip replacement was planned in the future, but due to academic commitments, the patient requested a minimally invasive option in the interim. (A, B) CT revealing ground glass appearance of lesions in the anterior acetabulum and quadrilateral plate respectively. (C, D) CT-guided osteoplasty for reinforcement of the cystic regions of the same lesions resulting in decreased pain and greater sense of stability stable at 12-month follow-up.

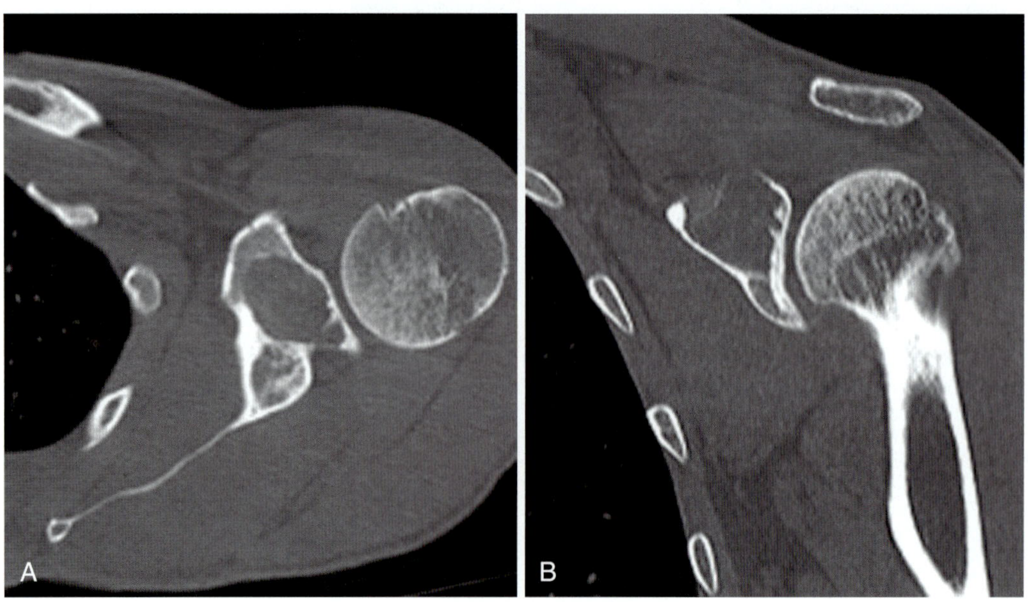

Figure 27-18 A 40-year-old avid golfer with progressive left shoulder pain during abduction. (A and B) Axial and coronal reformat CT images demonstrate a lytic lesion in the scapula with thickened trabeculae indicative of a hemangioma. There is cortical disruption superiorly. The surgical resection would have involved violation of the rotator cuff and the patient did not want to risk an injury that would prevent him from playing golf in the future. A treatment plan of ablation followed by cementoplasty was formed.

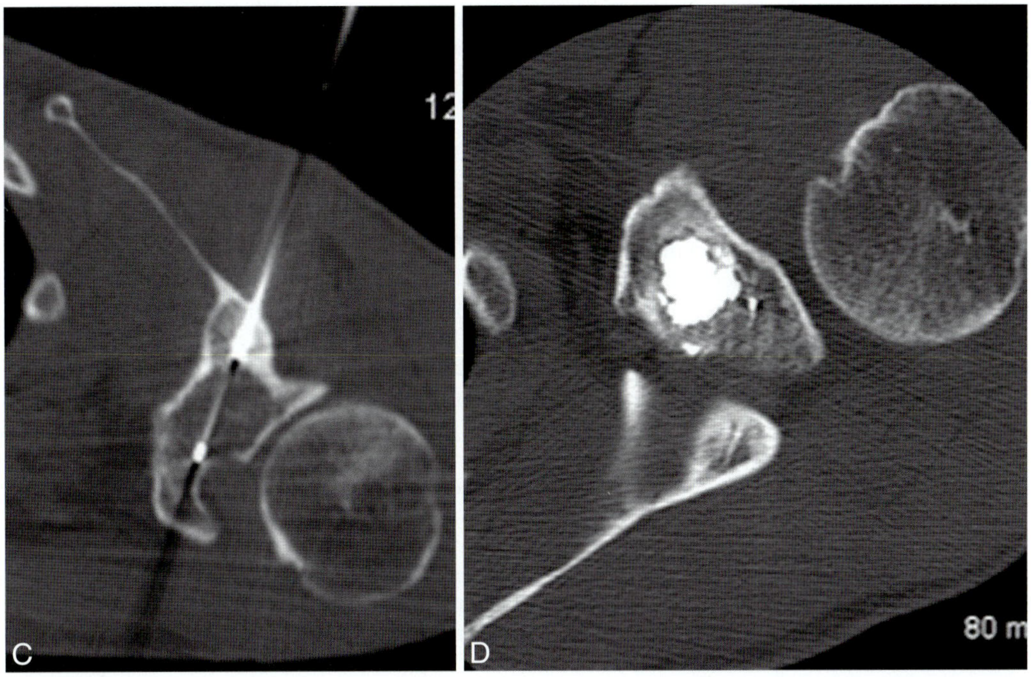

Figure 27-18, Cont'd (C) Axial CT image acquired during cryoablation. Note the posterior approach that avoids injury to the rotator cuff, vascular, and brachial plexus structures. (D) Axial CT image obtained postcryoablation and cementoplasty with evidence of new bone formation, which is evidence of healing.

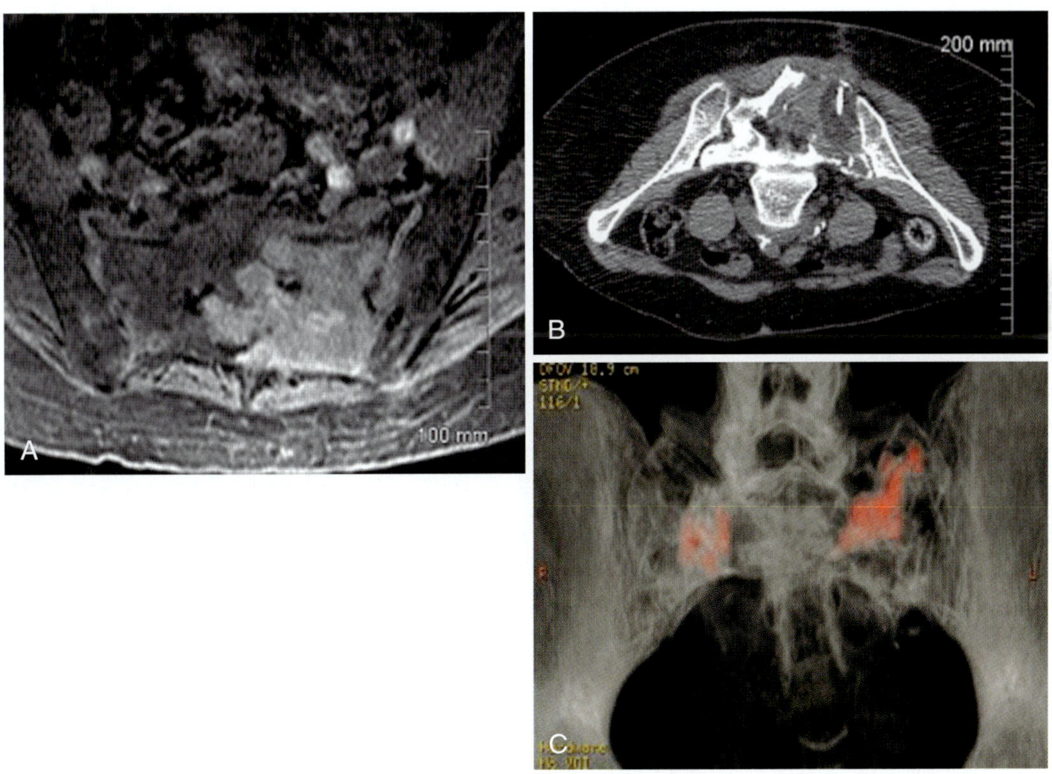

Figure 27-19 A 54-year-old woman with a biopsy-proven large, giant cell tumor of the left hemipelvis. Although neurologically intact, the patient was experiencing pain with ambulation. The surgical option that was offered was limb-sparing hemipelvectomy with a high risk of neurologic injury and permanent disability. Given the risks, the patient elected to try percutaneous ablation first. Because of the size of the tumor and its proximity to the neuroforamen in the sacrum, neuromonitoring during cryoablation was planned as a protective measure against injury to L5, S1, and S2. The degree of bone loss in the sacrum places the patient at risk for postablation fracture, and a postablation sacroplasty was also planned. (A) Axial image from a T2-weighted MRI reveals a high-signal, large, expansile lesion in the left sacrum consistent with the patient's known history of giant cell tumor. (B) Axial CT image obtained during cryoablation demonstrates the ice ball covering the bone–tumor interface of the lytic lesion in the left sacrum. (C) 3D CT with volumetric reconstruction shows bilateral sacroplasty with injection of polymethylmethacrylate. Following these interventions, the patient's symptoms completely resolved and she continues to be pain free at 2-year follow-up, with the MRI demonstrating stability of the lesion (not shown).

ranging in age from 1 to 15 years, and may be found in the skull, ribs, pelvis, spine, and long bones. Radiographically, eosinophilic granuloma of the long bones presents as radiolucent lesion associated with a lamellated periosteal reaction.[64] Clinical symptoms from eosinophilic granuloma include pain, restricted activity, growth disturbance, or pathologic fracture.[69] Recently, Corby et al. reported on the use of RFA to treat three cases of eosinophilic granuloma with prompt clinical response and no treatment-related complications.[10] Large eosinophilic granulomas may require treatment with multiple tined RFA probes or multiple overlapping ablations to ensure coverage of the entire lesion.[10] Lesions involving weight-bearing bones may require cementoplasty or surgical stabilization to prevent postablation fracture.[10,18]

BIOLOGICALLY ACTIVE TUMORS AND PARANEOPLASTIC SYNDROMES

Tumor-induced osteomalacia (TIO) is a paraneoplastic syndrome associated with various benign (giant cell tumor, ossifying fibroma, hemangiopericytoma, mesenchymal tumor of bone [phosphaturic variety]) and malignant tumors (sarcoma, prostate carcinoma, breast carcinoma, multiple myeloma, chronic lymphocytic leukemia, and small cell carcinoma) that secrete certain hormones. It is characterized by the overproduction of FGF 23, which is seen in rickets, and results in hypophosphatemia and low bone mineral density. Patients typically manifest with bone pain, fatigue, and fractures. The occult bone tumor may be difficult to find and whole body imaging (positron emission tomography, MRI, or octreotide scan) may be required for localization. This entity is rare and the literature is limited. Wide resection of the offending tumor is recommended in the largest series.[70] RFA ablation has been reported to be successful in treating one case of TIO.[71] (Figure 27-20)

Percutaneous Interventions for Unicameral or Aneurysmal Bone Cysts

ANEURYSMAL BONE CYSTS

An aneurysmal bone cyst (ABC) is a benign osteolytic lesion of probable vascular origin. Standard treatment involves curettage with bone grafting; however, associated risks include recurrence rate of up to 22%, severe bleeding, and damage to nearby nerve roots or growth plates in children.[72] As an ABC can be a challenging lesion to treat using a single modality, a number of minimally invasive, image-guided interventions have been used as adjuncts: arterial embolization, alcohol sclerosis, injection of phosphorus-32 chromic phosphate colloid, and injection of bone-inducing materials.[72-74] Small case series have demonstrated that each of the aforementioned image-guided interventions has had success in relieving pain, interrupting the growth of the lesion, and allowing for bone healing and reformation.

UNICAMERAL BONE CYSTS

A unicameral bone cyst (UBC) is a benign, fluid-containing lesion usually seen in children before skeletal maturity. Although many spontaneously resolve, the goals of management are to prevent pathologic fracture and control pain.[75] Percutaneous curettage remains the mainstay of treatment; however, percutaneous injection of autologous bone marrow or steroid has also

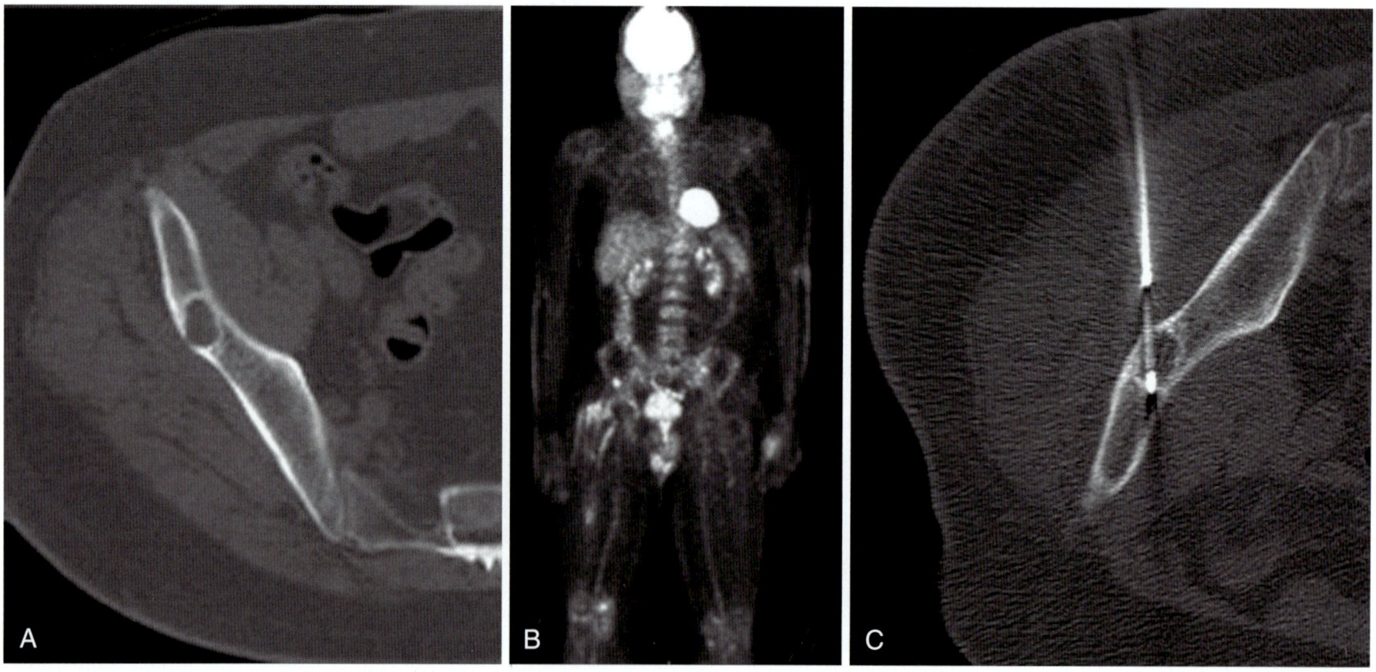

Figure 27-20 Oncogenic osteomalacia secondary to hemangiopericytoma. (A) Axial CT reveals a small, focal lytic lesion in the right iliac bone. This was biopsied and diagnosed as a hemangiopericytoma. (B) Bone scan with SPECT imaging demonstrates increased uptake in the right hip region related to the endoprosthesis placed for right hip fracture, a stress fracture in the right knee, and the hemangiopericytoma in the right iliac bone lesion. (C) Axial CT image shows a cryoprobe placed within the lesion. Cryoablation of the hemangiopericytoma resulted in normalization of the patient's phosphorus levels within 24 hours.

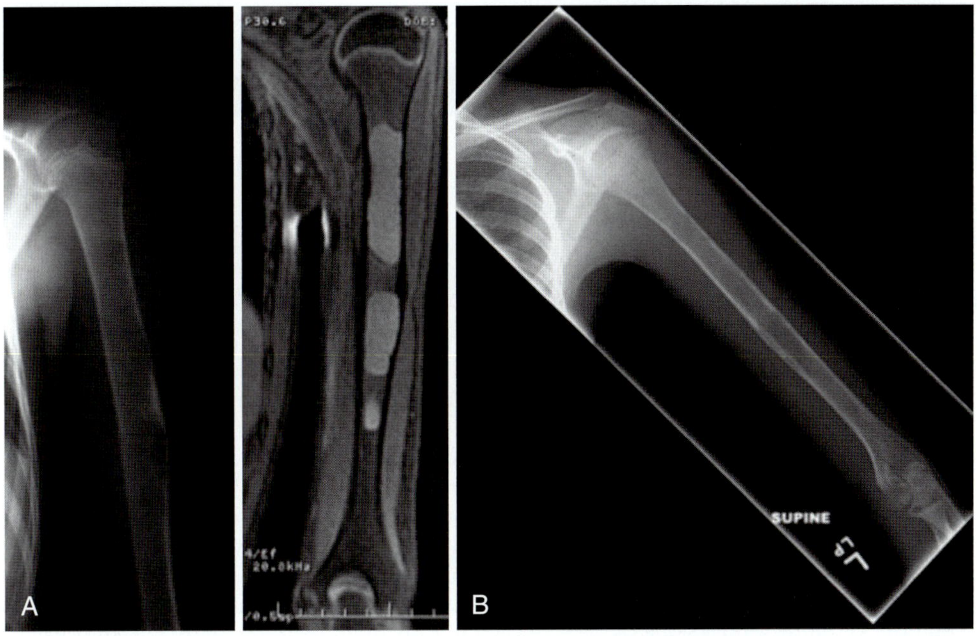

Figure 27-21 An 11-year-old girl with a unicameral bone cyst of the left humerus that was discovered after she sustained a fall and subsequent pathologic fracture. (A) Radiograph and coronal STIR image from MRI demonstrates a large lytic lesion involving the majority of the diaphysis of the left humerus. The patient was referred for steroid injection. (B) Two 16-gauge Hawkins needles (Cook, Inc., Bloomington, IN) were placed at the cephalad and caudal aspect of the lesion (not shown). Approximately 60 mL of serosanguineous cystic content was aspirated. The dose of methylprednisolone was calculated by determining the volume of the cyst based on the maximal width, length, and depth of the lesion on anteroposterior and lateral radiographs. A total of 90 mg of methylprednisolone (3 mg/mL) was injected into the lesion, with the dose split between the cephalad and caudal aspects of the cyst. (B) Follow-up radiograph obtained 1 year after the procedure demonstrates progressive sclerosis of the UBC. Since the procedure, the patient has been pain free and not had a recurrent pathologic fracture.

been used as management. Some studies have demonstrated that the injection of methylprednisolone is superior to bone marrow but the healing rate after injection treatment ranges from 21% to 41% versus up to 70% following curettage.[75] Serial injections of steroid or bone marrow may be necessary to treat the entire UBC (Figure 27-21).

Summary

Benign bone tumors are a frequent cause of bone pain and disability. Although surgery will often be the most reasonable treatment option to eradicate the tumor and alleviate symptoms, it can be associated with undesirable morbidity and may require significant recovery. Benign bone tumors lend themselves well to consideration for minimally invasive image-guided percutaneous interventions. The potential advantage of using a minimally invasive image-guided treatment approach is the ability to limit disturbance to the joint, cortical bone strength and musculotendinous apparatus, thus allowing for a more rapid recovery and return to normal function when compared to surgical resection with or without stabilization. Percutaneous ablation for the treatment of osteoid osteoma has become the standard of care; however, the application of minimally invasive image-guided interventions in the treatment of other benign bone tumors is in its infancy, and additional investigation to validate the safety and effectiveness of the technique in each disease entity is required prior to its incorporation into standard treatment algorithms.

REFERENCES

The complete reference list is available online at www.expertconsult.com.

28

Ablation of Musculoskeletal Metastatic Lesions Including Cementoplasty

ANIL NICHOLAS KURUP | MATTHEW R. CALLSTROM

KEY POINTS

- Percutaneous ablation of bone and soft tissue metastases may be performed for palliation of pain, prevention of complications due to progressive disease, and local disease control in nonsurgical patients.
- Patients treated for palliation of painful metastases should have at least moderate pain levels, pain referable to a limited number of metastatic lesions on imaging, and target lesions separated (or separable) from critical normal structures.
- Preablation workup should include laboratory assessment and correction of coagulation parameters and platelets, pain and quality of life assessments using standardized scales, and focused physical examination to enable correlation of painful site(s) with imaging findings. Preablation imaging should guide safe percutaneous access to the bone or soft tissue metastasis and assessment of nearby vital structures, particularly nerves, to be avoided or monitored during treatment.
- Ethanol ablation offers inexpensive, relatively effective treatment of painful lesions with the disadvantage of unpredictable diffusion of the ablative agent. Radiofrequency ablation offers fast, effective ablation with minimal bleeding risk; however, the procedure cannot be monitored easily, and patients often experience increased periprocedural pain. Cryoablation provides safe, effective ablation with easy monitoring of the ablation zone with CT or MRI, less periprocedural pain, and simultaneous activation of numerous applicators to treat large tumors; its disadvantages include larger applicator diameters, greater expense, and longer procedures. Microwave ablation, laser ablation, and high-intensity focused ultrasound are emerging ablation alternatives.
- Cementoplasty provides structural support to ablated metastases at risk for fracture. Although it is frequently used as an adjunct to ablation, it also provides an independent anesthetic effect.

Background

Percutaneous ablation of skeletal and soft tissue metastases has become increasingly common over the past several years. This rise reflects the clinical challenges multidisciplinary teams face in treating patients with metastatic disease. First, a large number of cancer patients have metastatic disease to bone, including up to 85% of patients with the three most common cancer types—lung, breast, and prostate.[1] Skeletal metastases remain an important source of morbidity for these patients, leading to pain, pathologic fracture, and neurovascular compromise. Additionally, bone-related cancer pain is frequently undertreated, with up to 79% of patients experiencing severe pain before adequate palliative efforts are initiated.[2] Patients with skeletal metastases have a poor prognosis in general, with median survival of less than 3 years and 5-year survival varying from 5% to 40% depending on tumor histology.[3,4] Treatment options facing oncology patients with musculoskeletal metastases and the multidisciplinary teams that care for them are numerous.

Most patients with diffuse metastatic disease are treated systemically. Chemotherapy, hormonal therapy, and biological agents may be administered, depending on tumor type. These agents are critical to attempt to limit metastatic progression and target micrometastatic disease. Oral analgesics, including opioids and nonsteroidal antiinflammatory drugs, provide sufficient pain relief for many patients with metastases to bone and soft tissue. In those with advanced malignancies, however, high-dose opioids may cause significant nausea, constipation, and sedation.[5] Bisphosphonate medications, which have an osteoclast-targeted effect, are increasingly employed to reduce the risk of skeletal-related events in patients with skeletal metastases.[6-10] Radiopharmaceuticals also play a role in the treatment of certain skeletal metastases.[11,12]

The standard of care treatment for patients with limited, painful skeletal metastases is external beam radiation therapy. The majority of patients experience a reduction in pain, but approximately 30% fail to experience pain relief, and those that respond to treatment have a median duration of response of 12–28 weeks.[13-20] Limitations in normal tissue tolerance prevent retreatment of painful metastases within previously irradiated fields.

Surgery for skeletal metastases is usually reserved for cases of impending fracture or after pathologic fracture.[21-23] Additionally, spinal metastases causing neurologic compromise due to spinal cord compression should be treated with surgical decompression and adjuvant radiotherapy.[24] Less commonly, surgical metastasectomy is performed in patients with limited metastatic disease to bone or soft tissue.[25,26] Comorbidities of patients with advanced malignancies make many patients poor surgical candidates. Furthermore, expected postoperative morbidity and recovery times may limit surgical approaches in these patients.

Given the limitations of the conventional therapies above for musculoskeletal metastases and successes of ablation in treating metastases in liver and lung, percutaneous ablative techniques have been applied to the treatment of bone and soft tissue metastases. Thermal device-based techniques, including radiofrequency ablation (RFA), cryoablation, microwave ablation, and laser ablation, have been used. In addition, chemical ablation with ethanol, noninvasive treatment with focused ultrasound, and bone consolidative treatment with cement instillation (cementoplasty and vertebroplasty) have also found a role in the treatment of these patients.

Indications and Contraindications

Percutaneous ablation of bone and soft tissue metastases is broadly used to treat four groups of patients (Table 28-1).[27] First, patients with limited painful metastases that are refractory to conventional therapy are well suited to palliative ablative therapy. Similarly, patients who refuse conventional therapy may benefit from ablation. Second, skeletal or soft tissue metastases that place patients at risk for future morbidity, either due to impending pathologic fracture or potential for direct invasion of an adjacent critical structure, are appropriate targets for ablation. Third, percutaneous ablation of limited metastatic disease to bone and soft tissue in patients who are nonsurgical candidates may be performed to obtain local control of all clinically detectable disease. Finally, ablation may be used to treat hormonally active or hemorrhagic symptomatic metastases.

Cementoplasty may be performed alone or in conjunction with tumor ablation. The cytotoxic effect of the cement polymer is limited, and cementoplasty should not be used with curative intent alone. It is indicated to provide pain relief and bone strengthening in painful, osteolytic metastases within the axial skeleton.[28] It may also be used in focal skeletal lesions or pathologic fracture sites due to hematologic malignancies, including lymphoma and multiple myeloma. The cement is resistant to compressive forces, as experienced by weight-bearing bones like vertebrae and acetabula, but of limited benefit for the mixed tension and torsion forces to which diaphyses of long bones are subjected.[29]

Percutaneous ablation of bone and soft tissue metastases has few, nonspecific absolute contraindications (Table 28-2). These include uncorrectable bleeding diathesis, intolerance of the level of anesthesia required for the procedure, and inability to access the targeted tumor safely from a percutaneous approach. Active infection is another contraindication to these sterile procedures. Furthermore, patients who have spinal metastases causing spinal cord compression with resultant neurologic compromise should be treated with surgical decompression and/or radiotherapy.

Relative contraindications include diffuse skeletal or soft tissue metastases for which systemic therapy would be more appropriate than a focal approach. Those patients with widespread skeletal metastases may be candidates for palliative ablation, however, if they have a limited number of target lesions that are particularly painful or at risk for causing significant morbidity because of their locations. In addition, musculoskeletal metastases causing only mild pain are usually not appropriate for ablation. Finally, tumors in proximity to critical structures that cannot be displaced or cannot be monitored sufficiently to allow safe tumor ablation may not be appropriate targets. Cementoplasty should be performed cautiously in osteolytic lesions with largely disrupted bony walls along the epidural space or a joint space.

A simple algorithm may be applied to the treatment decisions regarding skeletal metastases in most patients (Figure 28-1).

TABLE 28-1 Indications for Ablation of Bone and Soft Tissue Metastases

Indications
Palliation of painful metastases
Local control of oligometastatic disease
Prevention of complication from local progression
Fracture risk
Neurologic compromise
Palliation of hormonally active or hemorrhagic metastases

TABLE 28-2 Contraindications for Percutaneous Ablation of Bone and Soft Tissue Metastases

Contraindications
Absolute
Bleeding diathesis
Inability to tolerate anesthesia
No safe percutaneous access
Active infection
Relative
Widespread metastatic disease
Mildly painful metastases
Close proximity to vital structures

Patient Selection

Successful percutaneous treatment of metastases outside of lung and liver requires proper patient selection (Table 28-3). (Figure 28-2) The preablation workup should include a focused history and physical examination, limited laboratory assessment, and high-quality cross-sectional imaging.

HISTORY

Brief review of a patient's oncologic history, including previous local and systemic therapies and current disease burden, is critical in the evaluation of each patient considered for local tumor ablation. Prior consultation with an experienced oncologic surgeon avoids inappropriate application of ablation in surgical candidates. In patients referred for control of oligometastatic disease, assessment of a patient's disease-free interval prior to the development of metastases or rate of metastatic disease progression may offer some prognostic information and help set appropriate expectations for the patient and referring physician. In patients referred for palliation of painful metastatic disease, initial assessment of pain level is crucial. Patient pain levels should be recorded using a standardized visual analog scale, such as the Brief Pain Inventory (BPI) short form.[30,31] This includes patients' self-assessment of their best, worst, and average pain scores. Ablation should be performed on those patients with moderate to severe pain, meaning those with pain levels of 4 or greater on a 10-point scale. Ablation may not be as effective in those with mild pain levels, as they are difficult to improve on and are usually adequately controlled with oral analgesics. Similarly, patient assessment of quality of life parameters should be performed. These assessments should occur both before and serially in the months after ablation to measure the effectiveness of the procedure. Moreover, measurement of

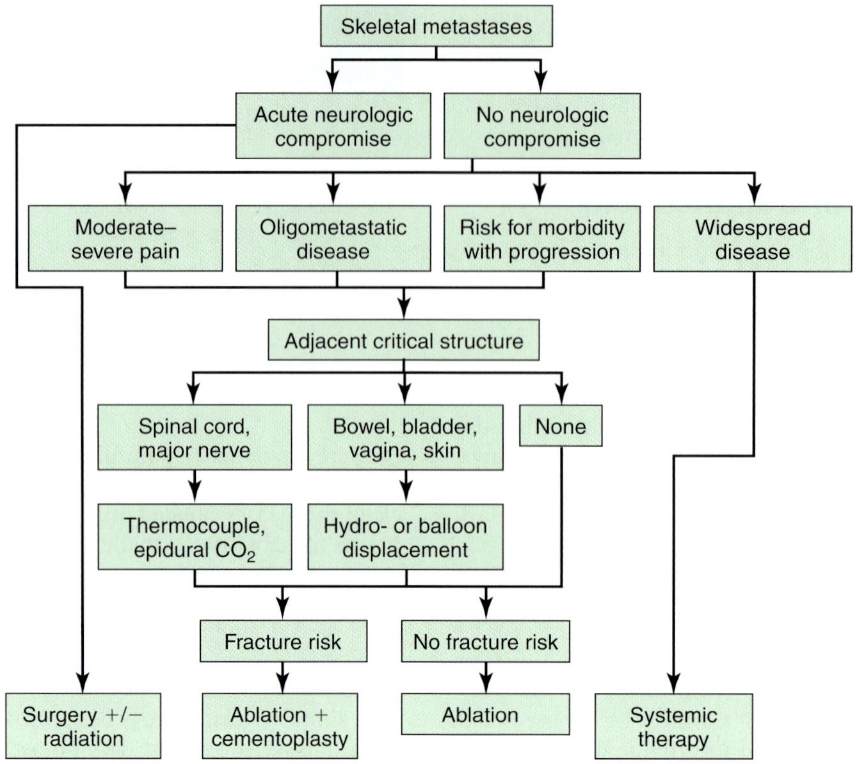

Figure 28-1 Algorithm for ablation of musculoskeletal metastases.

TABLE 28-3 Patient Selection Criteria for Percutaneous Ablation of Painful Bone and Soft Tissue Metastases

Selection criteria
Limited metastatic disease (1–3 sites)
Moderate pain (≥4 on 10-point scale)
Metastasis on imaging corresponding to painful site
Target lesion remote (or can be separated) from vital structures

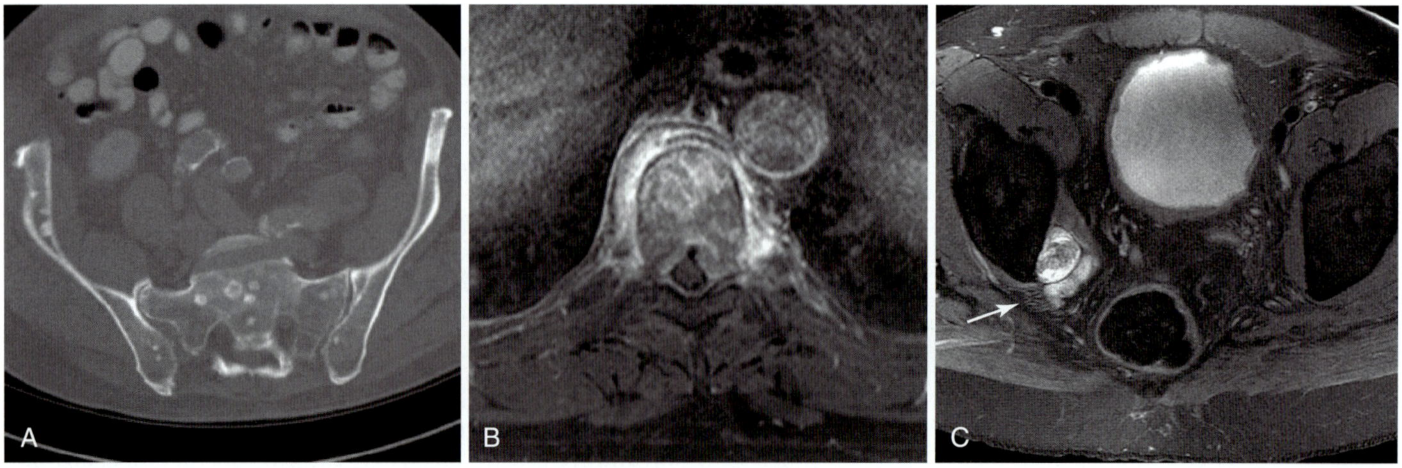

Figure 28-2 Poor candidates for percutaneous ablation of musculoskeletal metastases. (A) Diffuse osteoblastic prostate adenocarcinoma metastases in this 90-year-old man would be better treated systemically. Pain is usually difficult to localize to 1–3 metastases to target for local therapy in these patients. (B) A large T8 vertebral body metastasis has a significant epidural component compressing the spinal cord. Percutaneous ablation would carry significant risk of dural and spinal cord injury, and surgical decompression and stabilization are indicated. (C) A T2 hyperintense locally recurrent chordoma along the right pelvic side wall is in very close proximity to the sciatic nerve (*arrow*) as it passes through the sciatic notch in a 40-year-old man. This patient was treated with stereotactic body radiation therapy (SBRT) instead.

a patient's use of analgesics before and after ablation may demonstrate effectiveness of the procedure. Also, a patient's activity level may influence the decision of whether to perform adjunctive cementoplasty to consolidate ablated bone. Finally, a patient's medication list should be reviewed for drugs that increase bleeding risk.

PHYSICAL EXAMINATION

A focused physical examination should be performed prior to ablation of metastases, particularly when performed for palliation of painful metastases. In this context, the site of maximal pain or tenderness should correlate with the index lesion to be treated on cross-sectional imaging. In addition, assessment of neurologic deficits prior to the ablation should be performed. For tumors near motor nerves, frequently those located in the pelvis, preablation documentation of strength in the at-risk pathways may influence the decision to pursue ablation, alter the planned path to the target lesion, and/or improve informed consent to the risks involved in the procedure. Careful consideration of bowel and bladder continence may also be necessary to treat tumors in the pelvis (Figure 28-3).

LABORATORY STUDIES

Preablation workup should include limited laboratory studies typically performed before any nonsuperficial percutaneous intervention, including platelet count and coagulation parameters. In general, platelets should number 50,000 or greater, and international normalized ratio (INR) should be 1.5 or less. Preprocedural transfusion with blood products may be required to achieve these laboratory values and minimize the risk of hemorrhagic complications. Additional laboratory studies may be helpful, depending on the primary tumor histology and clinical scenario. For symptomatic, hormone-secreting tumors, such as neuroendocrine metastases, assessment of serum or urine hormone levels (e.g., catecholamines, serotonin, 5-HIAA) allows quantitative measurement of ablation effect (Figure 28-4). For tumors with elevated serum tumor markers, such as hepatocellular carcinoma (AFP), colon carcinoma (CEA), ovarian carcinoma (CA-125), or prostate carcinoma (PSA), measurement of these tumor markers before and after ablation allows assessment of the effect of the treatment and may improve detection of early tumor recurrence.

IMAGING ASSESSMENT

High-quality preablation cross-sectional imaging is essential for patient selection and treatment planning. The number of targeted metastases should be limited, typically between one and three lesions and very rarely greater than 5 lesions. Patients with more numerous metastases are more suitable for systemic, rather than focal, therapy, as it is difficult to localize symptoms with widespread disease. In patients referred for control of oligometastatic disease, patients should be adequately staged with imaging, often with CT of the entire torso or whole body positron emission tomography or computed tomography (PET/CT), to avoid unnecessary treatment of a few metastases in a background of additional untreated tumors. In patients referred for palliation of painful metastases, a metastasis should be present on imaging to correlate with the site of a patient's reported pain. All types of skeletal metastases may be treated with percutaneous ablation. However, osteolytic tumors, mixed osteolytic/osteoblastic tumors, and predominantly soft tissue tumors are more technically accessible, but when necessary, osteoblastic metastases may be treated with the use of bone biopsy or drill devices.

Assessment with the imaging modality to be used for intraprocedural guidance should be performed prior to the procedure to ensure adequate visualization. Imaging should guide safe percutaneous access to the metastasis and assess nearby vital structures, particularly nerves, to be avoided or monitored during treatment. A margin of 1–1.5 cm around the target lesion(s) without involving a critical structure is ideal. If the adjacent structure falls within this margin, adjunctive procedures to displace the structure from the tumor or to monitor the structure for collateral injury are often necessary. In cases in which the distance between a critical structure and the ablation zone is expected to be narrow, the risks and benefits of the procedure should be carefully considered. A combination of imaging modalities (e.g., ultrasonography and CT) may be required for initial assessment. Although MRI is not often used for intraprocedural guidance and monitoring in most centers, it may be valuable to define the local anatomy best and subsequently use landmarks on CT or fusion-imaging for intraprocedural guidance.

Technique

ANESTHESIA AND MEDICATIONS

Level of anesthesia for tumor ablation procedures depends on local preference and practice patterns and may be altered by

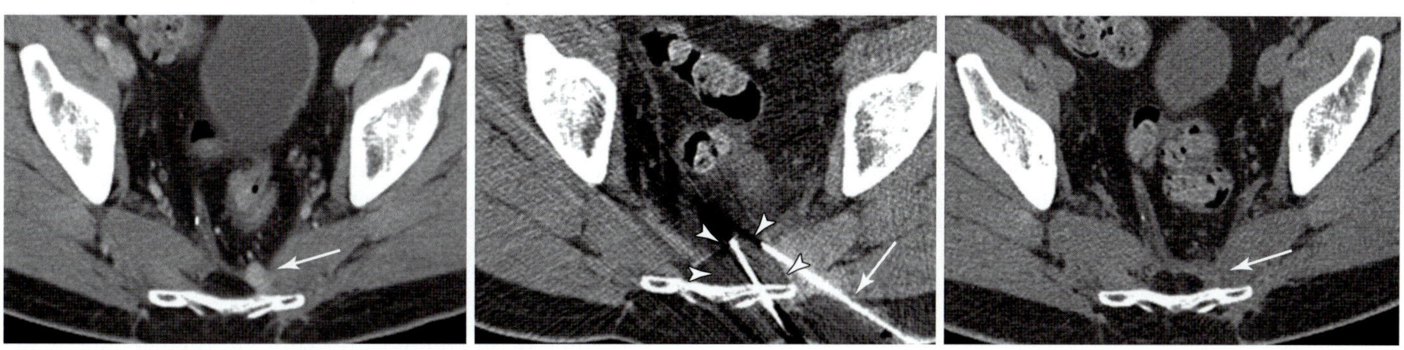

Figure 28-3 CT-guided cryoablation of perineural tumor in patient with preexisting neural deficits. (A) Enhancing recurrent myxopapillary ependymoma (*arrow*) anterior to S3-4 in a 32-year-old man with saddle anesthesia and neurogenic bowel and bladder due to partial sacrectomy performed 3 years earlier. (B) Ice ball (*arrowheads*) surrounding a cryoprobe covers the tumor. A spinal needle (*arrow*) was placed for hydrodissection to displace colon. The sacral nerve roots were previously sacrificed so ice ball encroachment on their expected local is inconsequential. (C) No enhancement is present at the ablation site (*arrow*) on 3-month follow-up CT.

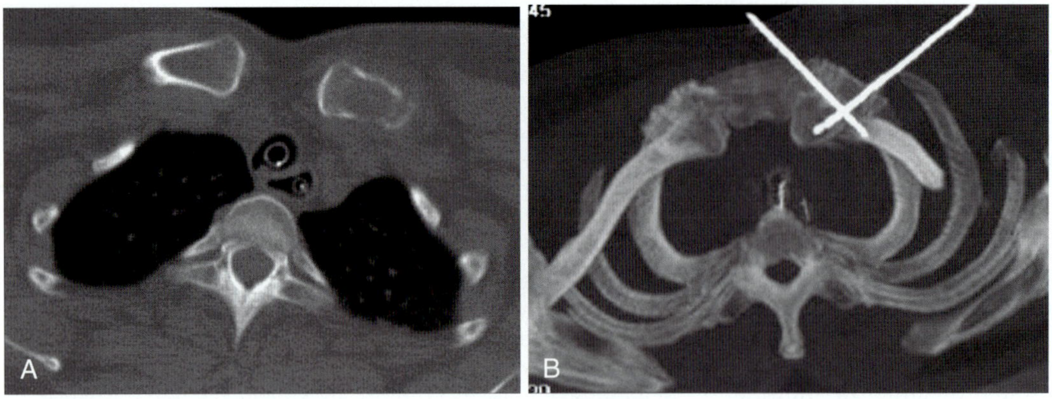

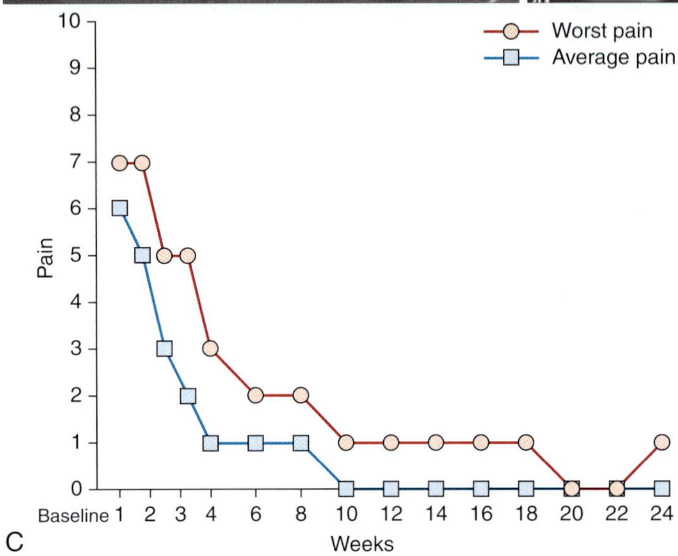

Figure 28-4 Metastatic paraganglioma involving the clavicular head treated with cryoablation. (A) Noncontrast CT demonstrates an osteolytic lesion involving the left clavicle. The lesion caused 7/10 worst pain in a 24-hour period prior to treatment. (B) 3D volumetric CT scan showing two cryoprobes placed into the lesion. (C) Worst and average pain scores over a 24-hour period at baseline and over a 2-year follow-up period. *(From Callstrom MR, Charboneau JW, Goetz MP, et al: Image-guided ablation of painful metastatic bone tumors: a new and effective approach to a difficult problem,* Skeletal Radiol *35(1):1-15, 2006; Figure 3.)*

patient preference. General anesthesia provides maximal control of a treated patient's airway, respiration, hemodynamics, and positioning and minimizes intraprocedural patient discomfort. Conscious sedation shortens procedure time and is less expensive. Minimal sedation levels allow focused neurologic physical examination during the procedure to serve as a method for monitoring of vulnerable neural structures. Cryoablation may be possible with lower levels of anesthesia than heat-based techniques because of the relative painlessness of ice formation within the body. Tumor size, location, accessibility, and proximity to critical structures all contribute to the complexity of each case and may dictate the level of anesthesia needed for successful treatment. Conscious sedation is usually sufficient for cementoplasty.

Long-acting local anesthetics (e.g., bupivacaine, ropivacaine) administered intraprocedurally along the periosteum are frequently helpful to diminish postprocedural pain. Intraprocedural intravenous prophylactic antibiotics covering skin flora (cephazolin, 1–2 g) are recommended for percutaneous vertebroplasty and frequently administered during other percutaneous interventions, although there is no clear consensus on the need for prophylactic antibiotics for tumor ablation.[32] In general, antiplatelet agents and anticoagulants should be held before these procedures and reinitiated 24–48 hours later.

IMAGING GUIDANCE AND MONITORING

Appropriate imaging guidance is required for percutaneous ablation of metastases to bone and soft tissue. The modality used to guide the procedure depends on its ability to visualize the tumor of interest and associated local anatomy for device positioning and ablation monitoring. Fluoroscopy offers high spatial and temporal resolution, relatively low expense, and lower radiation exposure than CT. It is frequently used to guide vertebroplasty procedures and may be used for ethanol ablation. However, it is not sufficient for thermal ablation techniques because of limited visualization of small skeletal or soft tissue metastases and inability to monitor the ablation zone. These limitations may not be present when using angiographic c-arms with flat panel detectors capable of producing cone beam three-dimensional CT scan reconstructions.[33,34]

Ultrasonography provides good spatial and excellent temporal resolution, is widely available, and is inexpensive. However, its use is restricted to visualization of superficial lesions with large soft tissue components. It cannot target deep lesions or those with overlying intact cortical bone, and the sound waves cannot penetrate the gas produced by heat-based techniques or ice produced during cryoablation. The gas seen during ablation does not reliably correlate with the size of the ablation zone, and only the superficial aspect of the ice ball is seen. Typically, ultrasonography is very effective as guidance during applicator placement, whereas CT and MRI are used for ablation monitoring (Figure 28-5).

CT, alone or in combination with ultrasonography, is the most commonly used imaging modality for musculoskeletal ablation procedures. Its strengths include wide availability, good spatial resolution of most bone and soft tissue tumors, excellent overview of the local tumor environment and access

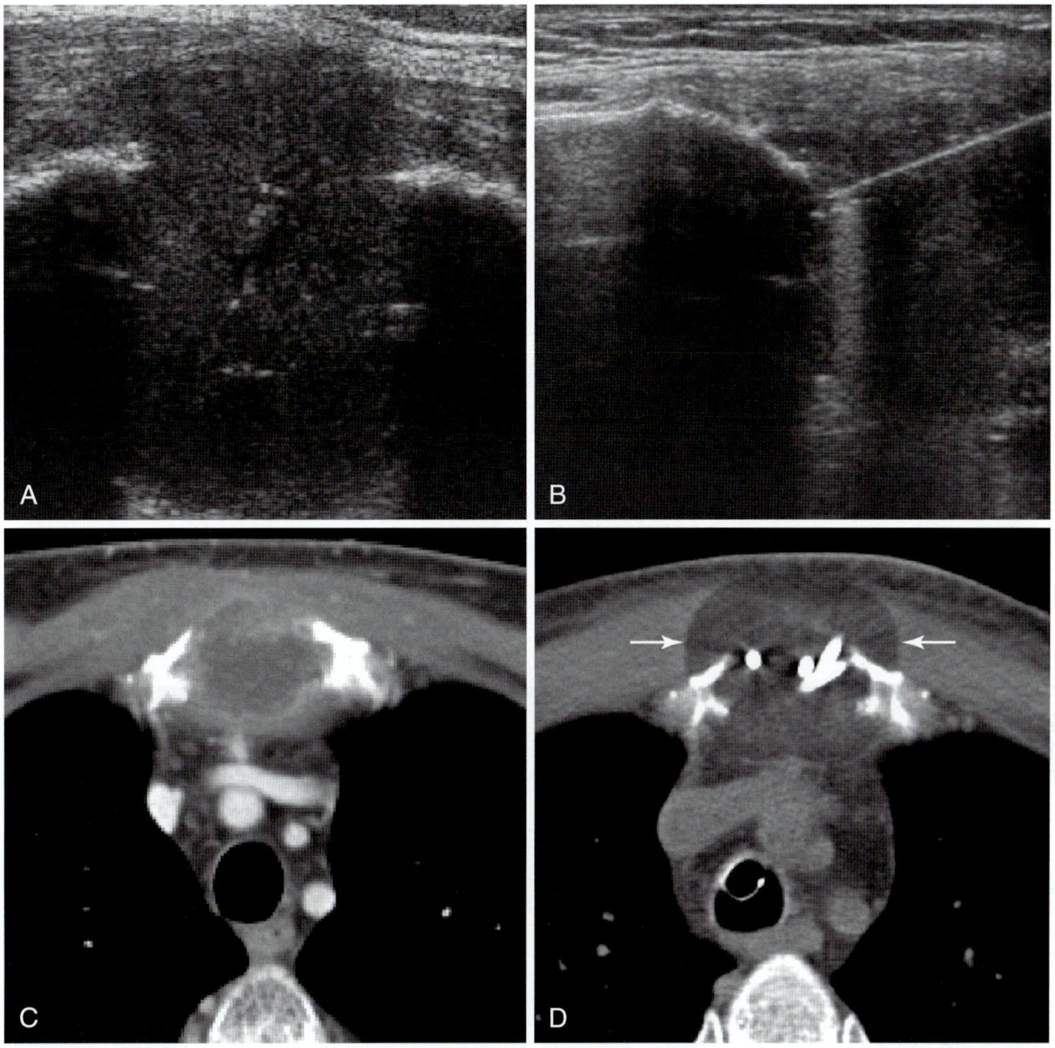

Figure 28-5 Ultrasound guidance for ablation of a skeletal metastasis. (A) Transaxial ultrasonographic image of a synchronous 3.6-cm sternal metastasis in a 46-year-old man with non–small cell lung carcinoma. This metastasis was painful despite prior radiation therapy. (B) Longitudinal ultrasonographic image shows placement of one of four 2.4-mm-diameter cryoprobes. High-frequency transducers were used for both images because of the superficial location of the metastasis. (C) Axial contrast-enhanced CT image shows the peripherally enhancing tumor before ablation. (D) Axial unenhanced CT image shows the ice ball (*arrows*) encompassing the tumor.

pathway, and good temporal resolution with continuous or intermittent CT fluoroscopy techniques. Multidetector CT scanners may rapidly reconstruct images to provide multiplanar evaluation for device placement and ablation zone coverage. During cryoablation procedures, intermittent unenhanced CT scanning, usually performed every 2–3 minutes during freeze cycles, allows visualization of the growing ice ball for accurate ablation zone monitoring.[35-38] Radiation exposure during CT-guided ablations should be controlled through careful dose reduction techniques.

MRI provides the highest bone and soft tissue contrast resolution. Near-real-time imaging sequences for device placement as well as temperature-sensitive sequences for thermal ablation monitoring are now available. MRI is the only imaging modality that can provide some accurate intraprocedural information regarding the volume treated with heat-based techniques. It may be used during cryoablation, showing the ice ball as an area of signal void, and is also used for guidance during focused ultrasonographic procedures (Figure 28-6). However, MRI-guided procedures are often time consuming. Moreover, MRI-compatible ablation equipment is limited, and MRI scanners are not available for interventional procedures in most clinical settings.

SPECIAL DEVICES

Bone Access

Percutaneous ablation applicators may be placed directly into metastases that are completely or predominantly composed of soft tissue, osteolytic metastases with disrupted or thin overlying cortical bone, or metastases within severely osteopenic bone. Special equipment may be required, however, to access sclerotic metastases or lesions deep to intact, thick healthy cortical bone for any percutaneous ablation procedure. Access may be obtained manually with the use of a bone biopsy kit or trocar. These are typically 10- to 14-gauge in diameter with sharply beveled or trephinated tips. Ablation device applicators may be placed in a coaxial fashion if they are of satisfactory length and diameter (Figure 28-7). An automatic bone drill with drill bits or Steinmann pins may be needed in cases in which manual pressure with a bone biopsy needle is insufficient.

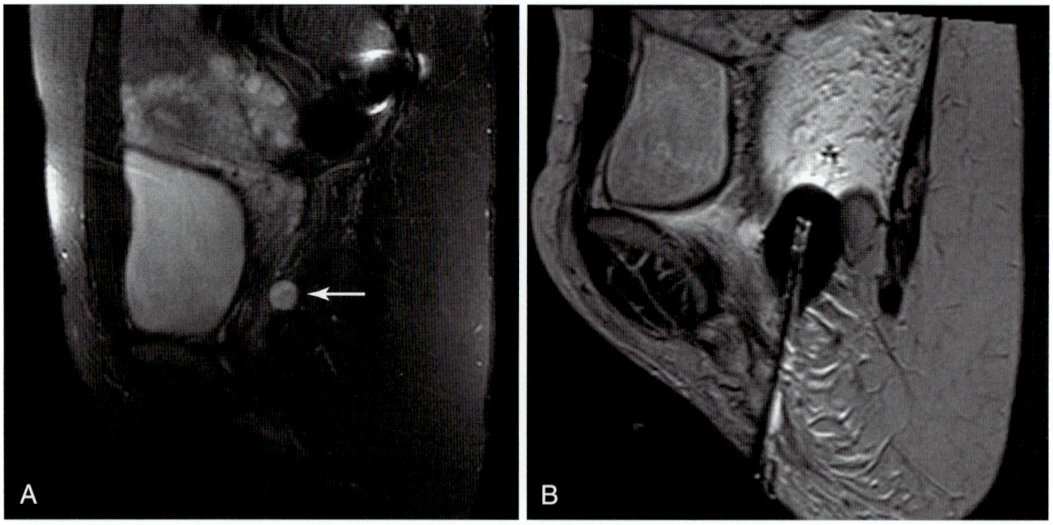

Figure 28-6 MRI guidance during cryoablation of locally recurrent chordoma in the pelvis in a 31-year-old woman. (A) Sagittal T2-weighted MR image with fat saturation shows a small nodular recurrence (*arrow*) adjacent to the vagina in the ischiorectal fossa. (B) Intraprocedural T2-weighted MR image without fat saturation shows the signal void of the ice ball surrounding the cryoprobe and encasing the tumor completely. Hydrodisplacement had been performed to displace the nodule from the vagina.

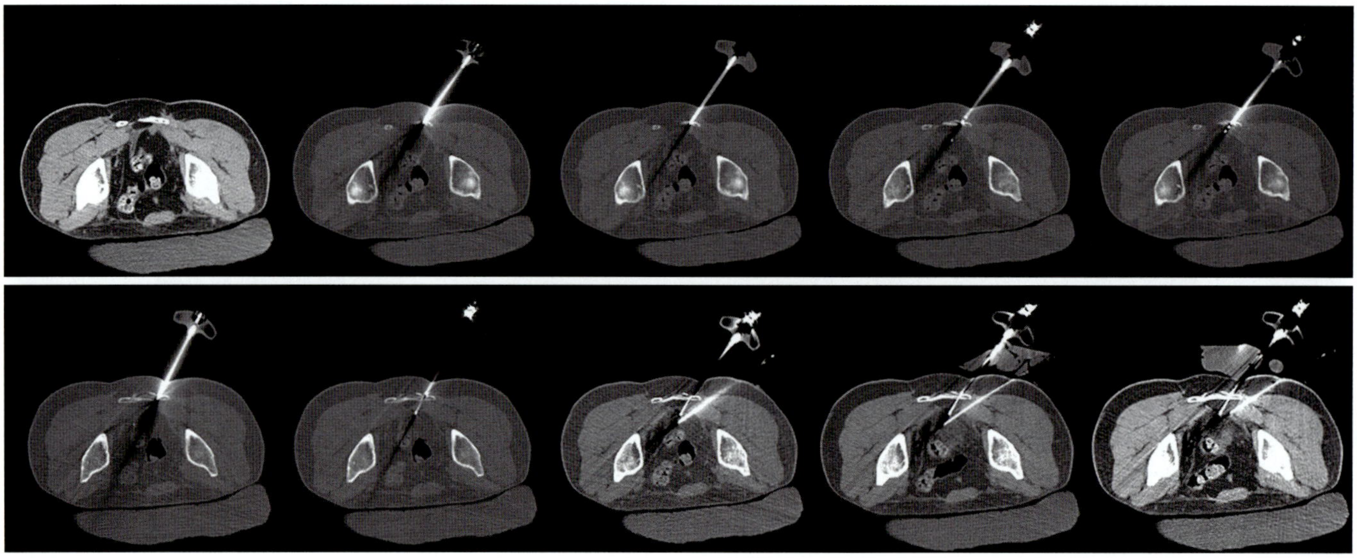

Figure 28-7 Placement of the two cryoprobes and hydrodisplacement for the case in Figure 28-2. (A) Axial CT image shows the presacral recurrent tumor before placement of the probes with the patient in prone position. (B) Access through the sacrum was achieved with an 11-gauge bone biopsy needle. (C) The inner stylet was removed. (D) The 15-mm-diameter cryoprobe is placed through the outer stylet in typical coaxial fashion. (E) The cryoprobes are extended into the soft tissue tumor. (F) To access the cephalad portion of this tumor, a second bone biopsy needle is advanced through the sacrum. (G) After removing the access needle, the 17-mm-diameter probe is placed into the tumor (noncoaxial technique). (H) Because of the proximity of colon, a 19-gauge needle was advanced near the tip of the cephalad cryoprobe. (I) Hydrodisplacement was performed with sterile saline. (J) Ice ball remains remote from colon.

Radiofrequency Ablation

Radiofrequency ablation (RFA) is the most widely used method of percutaneous tumor ablation. In bone, RFA was first applied to the treatment of osteoid osteomas and has become the standard of care for these benign tumors.[39,40] Application of RFA to the treatment of malignant bone tumors was originally reported in 1998 and is now routinely used.[41] High-frequency (450–600 kHz) alternating current is delivered through a needle applicator, producing focal ionic agitation in the intra- and extracellular spaces around the exposed tip.[42] This leads to heat generation up to lethal temperatures, between 60°C and 100°C. Protein denaturation, cell death, and coagulative necrosis occur locally. At greater temperatures, tissue carbonization and vaporization occurs, which can insulate electrical conduction and impair maximal treatment effect. To complete the electrical circuit and dissipate the deposited energy, grounding pads are placed on the skin surface, typically along the upper thighs. RF generators and applicators, called electrodes, are made by several different vendors. The electrodes are generally 17-gauge in caliber with uninsulated tips, which heat the tissue. Various strategies have been used to increase the volume of tissue ablated. Cluster electrodes, composed of three linear electrodes connected proximally, and expandable electrodes, which have multiple tines to be deployed to a varying degree by the operator, are shaped to allow larger burns (Figure 28-8). In addition, some electrodes are internally cooled with chilled water, while others perfuse the tips with saline into the tissue in an effort to prevent tissue charring and resultant insulation to RF energy. Once an impedance limit (for some systems) or a target temperature of 100°C is reached, the tumor is ablated for 5–15 minutes. Tumors ≤3 cm may be treated with a single ablation, whereas larger tumors are generally treated with multiple overlapping ablations. A maximum of three electrodes may be used simultaneously with a switching generator.[43]

Microwave Ablation

Microwave ablation is a similar, heat-based method, which causes oscillation of water molecules in tissue.[44] A few different vendors manufacture generators that operate at either 915 MHz or 2.45 GHz. Microwave applicators, termed antennae, are 17-gauge in caliber and linear in configuration. Systems generally allow up to three antennae. Microwave energy has several advantages over RF energy, including faster heating, larger volume of heated tissue, less susceptibility to perfusion-mediated tissue cooling (heat sink), and no requirement for grounding pads.[44] Multiple applicators may operate continuously, simultaneously, and synergistically, unlike the switching that occurs when multiple RF electrodes are used. Because of bone's low electrical and thermal conductivity compared to its relative permittivity, microwave energy may be more effective in treating skeletal tumors.[42]

Laser Ablation

Laser ablation, also called laser interstitial thermal therapy or interstitial laser photocoagulation, may be performed using small-caliber, flexible Nd-YAG or diode laser fibers, which are placed into tumor coaxially though an access needle. The access needle is then partially withdrawn to expose the tip of the laser fiber. These lasers use infrared photons, rather than electrical or microwave energy, to generate a burn, with lethal temperatures reached similar to other methods. Each laser fiber operating continuously at 2 W produces only a small volume burn of about 1.6 cm diameter in bone.[29]

Cryoablation

Modern cryoablation systems use room temperature, pressurized argon and helium gases for tissue freezing and heating, respectively. These systems allow either 8 or 25 cryoprobes to be used simultaneously. The expansion of argon gas within each cryoprobe leads to rapid cooling to −100°C within seconds (Joule–Thompson effect). The resultant ice ball along the uninsulated tip is visibly low attenuation on CT using standard body window/level and low signal on MRI (Figure 28-9). Complete tissue destruction occurs when temperatures reach −20°C to −40°C,

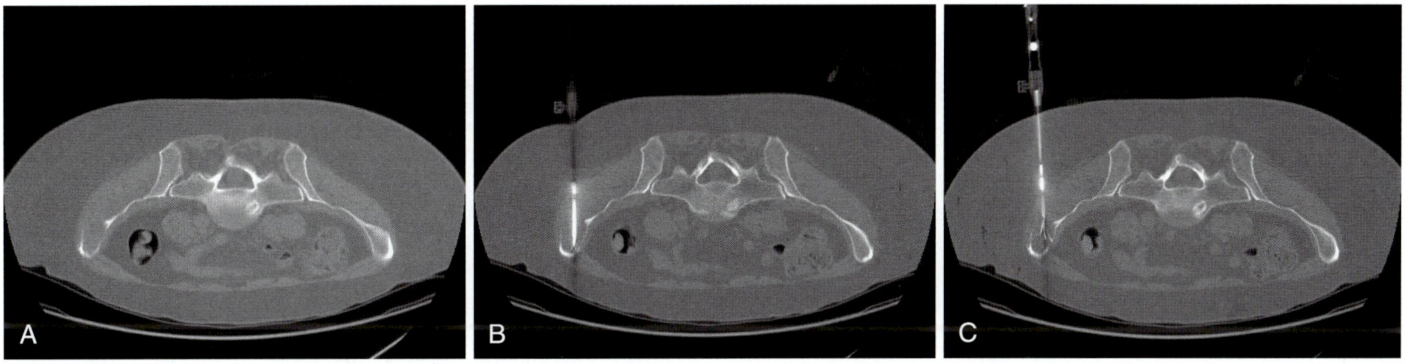

Figure 28-8 Radiofrequency ablation (RFA) of a painful iliac crest metastasis. (A) Axial CT image with the patient in prone position shows the osteolytic right iliac crest metastasis. (B) Multitined RFA electrode placed into the metastasis from a posterior approach. (C) Once deployed, the expandable tines extend into the periphery of the tumor to create a larger ablation zone.

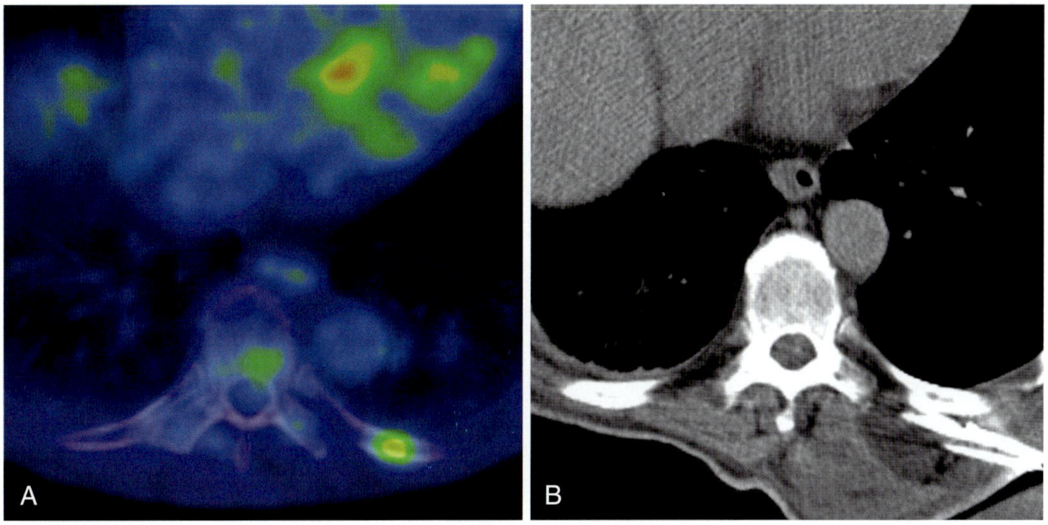

Figure 28-9 Cryoablation of a rib metastasis. (A) Axial fused PET/CT image shows a small FDG-avid melanoma metastasis in the posterior left 9th rib of a 71-year-old man. (B) Axial unenhanced CT image shows the cryoprobe placed alongside, rather than within, the rib. The low-attenuation ice ball encompasses the metastasis.

typically 3–5 mm deep to the 0°C ice ball margin.[35-38] Cell death occurs because of a combination of cell membrane rupture by ice crystals, cellular dehydration, and delayed vascular thrombosis and ischemia. Cryoprobes are 11- to 17-gauge in caliber and may produce ice balls measuring up to 3.5 cm in diameter and 5.5 cm in length when used alone. Probes are generally placed within 2 cm of each other and 1 cm of the tumor margin. Treatment usually consists of two freeze cycles of 10 minutes each separated by a 5-minute passive thaw, although cycle lengths may be varied to allow for adequate tumor coverage and avoidance of contiguous vital structures. Several minutes of helium-induced active thaw are required before cryoprobe removal. Cryoablation offers several advantages over heat-based technologies such as RFA in the treatment of bone and soft tissue metastases (Table 28-4).

Focused Ultrasound Ablation

Focused ultrasound (FUS) ablation, also known as high-intensity focused ultrasound (HIFU), is a noninvasive thermal ablation method. Focused ultrasound energy heats and destroys tissue without the need for percutaneous applicators. Bone has high acoustic absorption, making it a good target for this therapy.[45] The mechanism of pain relief is probably destruction of periosteal nerve fibers at the bone surface.[46,47] MRI guidance is usually used with FUS for tumor targeting and sonication (ablation) monitoring. This technique requires an acoustic window to the target lesion, which is placed on top of a coupling gel pad and positioned on the MRI table over a water bath containing the ultrasound transducer. Bowel or neurologic structures interposed between the skin surface and bone tumor may be injured. Skin temperature must be monitored.

Ethanol Ablation

Ethanol instillation or sclerotherapy produces cellular dehydration, vascular thrombosis, tissue ischemia, and necrosis. Simple and inexpensive, ethanol ablation does not require any specialized equipment. However, it is very painful, and adequate anesthesia is required. A combination of iodinated contrast media and local anesthetic is initially instilled into the tumor through a small caliber needle, typically 20- to 25-gauge.[28] The distribution of the contrast material demonstrated on CT or fluoroscopy is used to predict the eventual distribution of ethanol. If the fluid extends beyond the tumor boundaries to contiguous vulnerable structures, the procedure is terminated. If not, 3–30 mL of >95% ethanol is injected, depending on tumor size.[28] Ethanol should be immediately diluted with saline if it inadvertently contacts neurologic tissue. Multiple needle positions and injections may be required to achieve adequate distribution within the tumor.

Cementoplasty

Percutaneous injection of polymethylmethacrylate (PMMA) medical cement is termed cementoplasty or osteoplasty generally, or vertebroplasty when applied in the spine. This procedure decreases pain from metastases likely because of direct effect of the cement on nociceptors as well as stabilization of micro-fractures.[48] The cement polymer comes as a powder, which is activated when mixed with a monomer liquid under a ventilation hood and agitated to allow polymerization. Access to the ablation cavity or fracture site is obtained with a bone biopsy trocar as with any other percutaneous procedure. The PMMA is packaged with a cement delivery system, which is attached to the trocar after removing the stylet. It should be administered slowly under continuous or near-continuous monitoring with conventional or CT fluoroscopy with attention to concerning areas of potential extravasation, such as disrupted cortices, epidural and joint spaces, or along the access needle. The cement should be anchored to normal bone. The trocar needle should be withdrawn slowly to fill the cavity, and the stylet should be replaced prior to removal of the needle to avoid spillage of cement. Cementoplasty is usually performed the day after ablation (Figure 28-10). Patients may bear weight within a few hours after the procedure.

TABLE 28-4 Comparison of the Relative Strengths of Radiofrequency Ablation (RFA) and Cryoablation in the Treatment of Painful Bone and Soft Tissue Metastases

Issue	RFA	Cryoablation
Cost	✓	
Time	✓	
Applicator size	✓	
Large tumor		✓
Penetration of bone		✓
Adjacent critical structure		✓
CT or MRI monitoring		✓
Periprocedural pain		✓

APPROACH AND RELEVANT ANATOMY

For percutaneous ablation of bone and soft tissue metastases to be performed safely, interventional radiologists must have a solid understanding of the local anatomy surrounding the target lesions. Vital structures, which may be in proximity to these metastases and should be avoided, include the spinal cord, nerve roots, major peripheral nerves, artery of Adamkiewicz, bowel, bladder, and skin (Figure 28-11). As most skeletal metastases are in the spine and axial skeleton, the central and peripheral nervous system structures are of primary importance in most cases. Ideally, these structures may be visualized directly with CT or MRI. Intrathecal contrast administration immediately before the procedure and oblique planar imaging of the region of interest, using MRI or angulation of the CT gantry, may be helpful to image central neural structures (Figure 28-12).

Without adequate direct visualization, physiologic monitoring of the vulnerable neural structure may be warranted. In addition, thermal insulation or displacement of the structure from the ablative energy encompassing the metastasis may be necessary.[49] Preablation conventional, CT, or MR spinal angiography to define the origin of the artery of Adamkiewicz may be warranted in paraspinal lesions located between T5 and L3. Unfortunately, intact cortical bone provides variable protection against thermal injury to the central nervous system and may not even be present in some spinal metastases.[49-53] Although a 1–1.5 cm margin between target lesion and adjacent normal critical structure is a reasonable estimate for safe tumor ablation, in practice the permissible distance depends on the visibility of the tumor, critical structure, and ablation zone; use of temperature or physiologic monitoring equipment; indication for the procedure; and experience of the interventional radiologist.

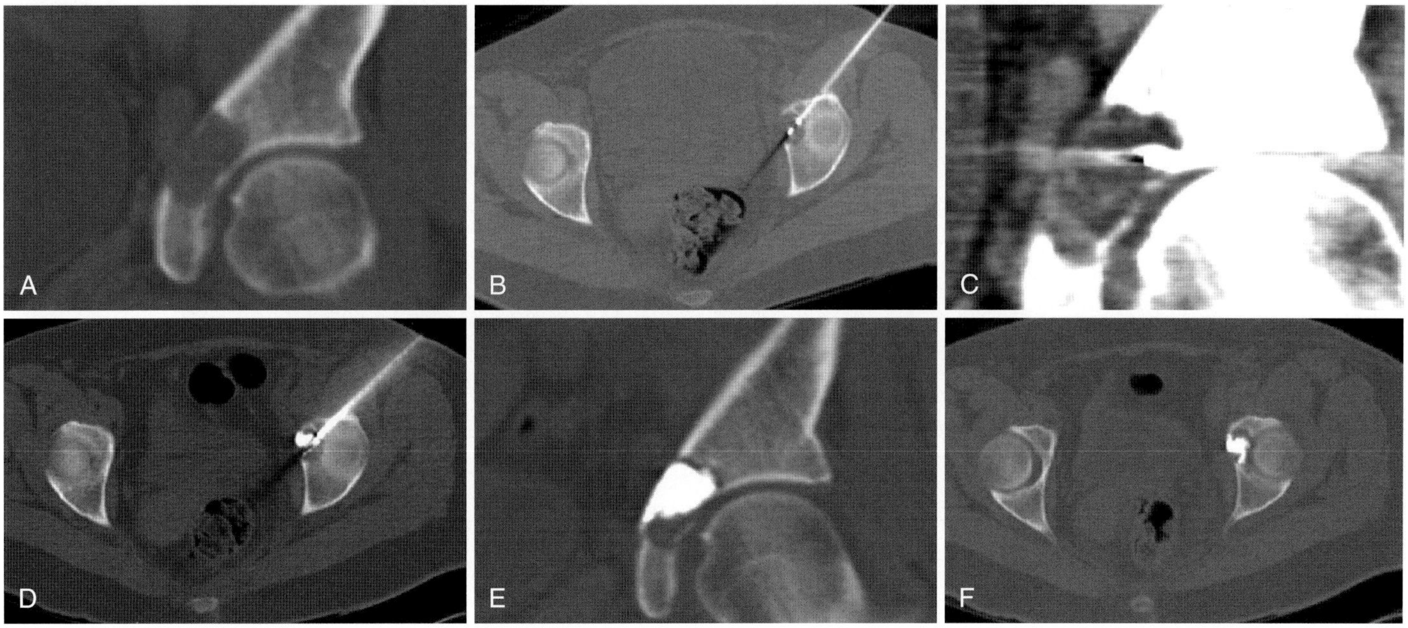

Figure 28-10 Combination cryoablation and cementoplasty. (A) Coronal reformatted CT image shows a left acetabular renal cell carcinoma metastasis at risk for fracture. (B) A single cryoprobe was placed in the metastasis. (C) Coronal image in soft tissue window and level shows the low attenuation ice ball. (D) The following day, cementoplasty was performed through a 13-gauge bone biopsy needle. Careful attention was paid to avoid injection of cement into the joint space. (E) Coronal and (F) axial CT images show the cement forming a nice bridge to provide structural support to this important weight-bearing region.

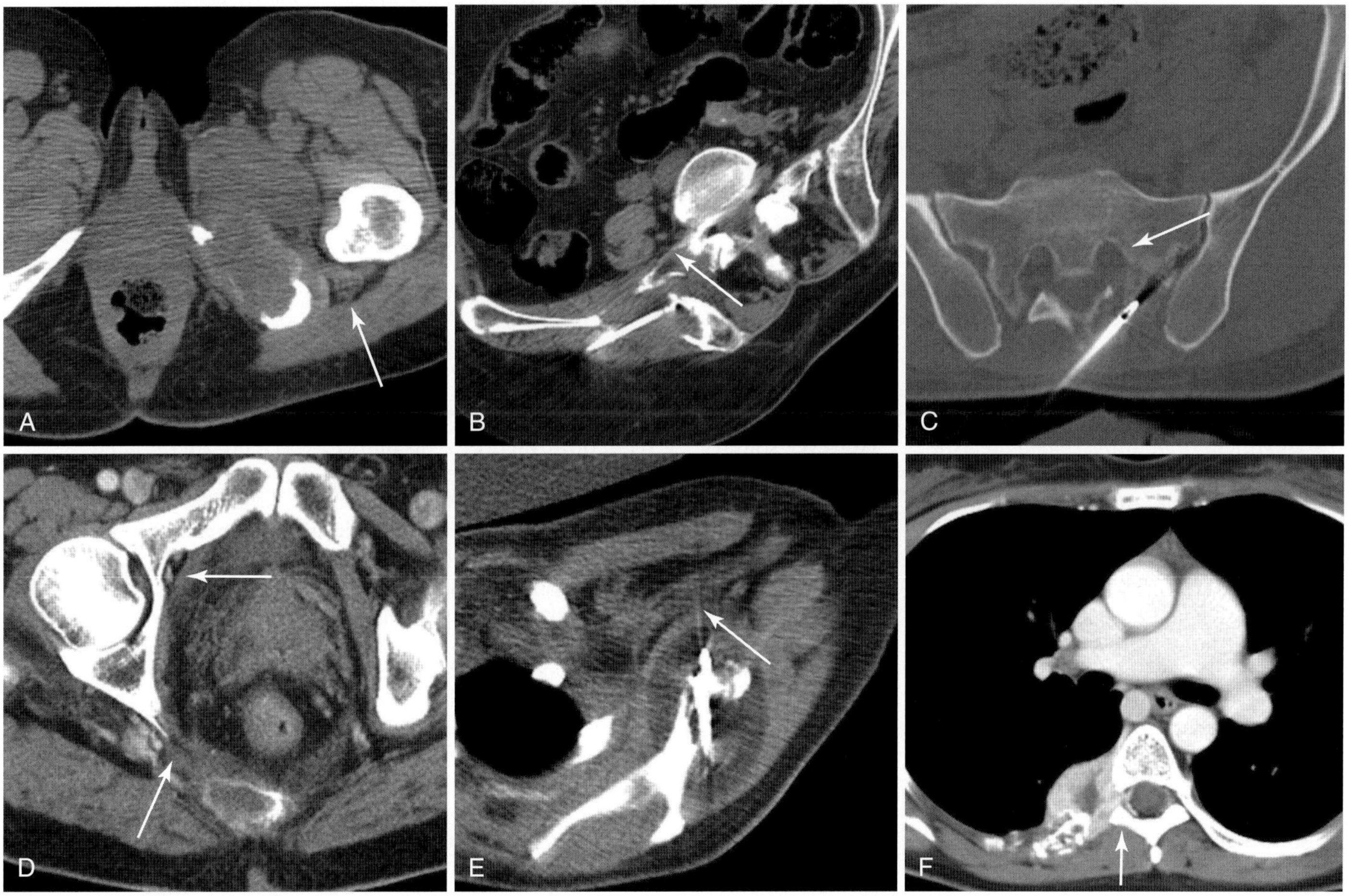

Figure 28-11 Common areas of concern for ablation of bone and soft tissue metastases. (A) A metastasis in the left inferior pubic ramus is in proximity to the sciatic nerve (*arrow*). (B) A cryoprobe is partially visualized in a metastasis in the right iliac bone with the lumbar plexus (*arrow*) along the anterior aspect of the sacrum. (C) A cryoprobe is in place in the posterior left sacrum. The S1 nerve root (*arrow*) is in close proximity. (D) An osteolytic metastasis is present in the inferior sacrum. The pudendal nerve (*long arrow*) is in close proximity. The obturator nerve (*short arrow*) is well separated from the tumor. (E) Two cryoprobes are partially imaged in a tumor involving the scapula, with a surrounding ice ball approaching the brachial plexus (*arrow*). (F) Paravertebral ablations that extend to the edge of the vertebral body and foramen should consider the potential adjacency of the artery of Adamkiewicz. This blood vessel, which provides blood supply to the ventral cord, originates from a segmental artery arising from the abdominal aorta. (*From Kurup AN, Callstrom MR: Ablation of skeletal metastases: current status,* J Vasc Interv Radiol *21(8 Suppl):S242-S250, 2010; Figure 1.)*

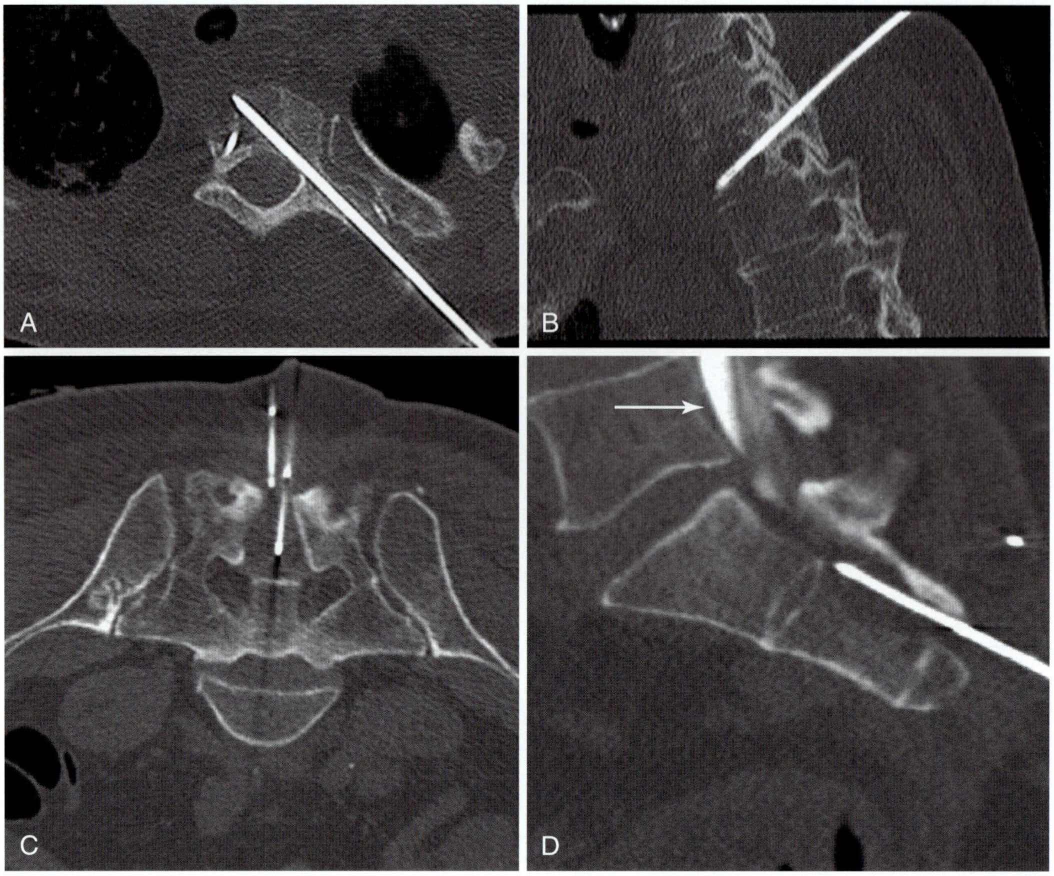

Figure 28-12 Special techniques to treat axial skeletal lesions. Tilting the CT gantry facilitates cryoprobe placement at an inferior angle along a transpedicular course to treat an osteolytic renal cell carcinoma metastasis in an upper thoracic vertebral body as shown on (A) axial and (B) sagittal reformatted CT images. (C) In a separate patient, the CT gantry was angulated to allow cryoprobes to be placed in a recurrent sacral chordoma as shown on an oblique axial CT image. (D) Sagittal reformatted CT image in the same patient shows the course of one of the cryoprobes. Note intrathecal contrast material (*arrow*) was administered prior to probe placement to allow identification of the thecal sac.

Additional local anatomic factors affect ablation technique. Targeting the bone–tumor interface may be sufficient for palliative treatment of painful skeletal metastases.[54] However, solitary or oligometastatic disease treated for local tumor control requires complete tumor coverage with the ablation zone, including a margin of normal tissue. Moreover, perfusion-mediated cooling or heating because of large blood vessels near ablated metastases may limit the temperatures reached locally to sublethal levels and thereby preserve adjacent tumor.[55,56] Presence of large vessels may make ablation a poor treatment option, require preablation embolization to maximize ablative effect, or lead to placement of additional applicators. Finally, the internal structure of tumors may influence applicator placement. Tumors with large necrotic regions may allow excessive, unintentional displacement of applicators during treatment and require additional applicators to be placed for complete tumor coverage.

In general, vertebral bodies are accessed via a transpedicular approach in the lumbar region, intercostopedicular approach at the thoracic level, and anteriorly in the cervical spine.[29] The sacrum is usually approached posteriorly. Access to the periacetabular region is typically from an anterolateral or posterolateral approach to avoid the femoral and sciatic nerves. However, any approach that safely avoids critical structures is acceptable.

ADJUNCTIVE PROCEDURES

Several adjunctive procedures may facilitate a tumor ablation treatment or further the goals of therapy (Figure 28-13, Table 28-5).

Tissue Displacement Of Adjacent Structures

Normal structures at risk for injury by the ablation energy may be displaced with fluid (hydrodisplacement or hydrodissection), angioplasty balloons, or gas (i.e., carbon dioxide). To prevent the theoretical extension of thermal energy through an ion-containing solution, sterile 5% dextrose in water should be used instead of normal saline for hydrodisplacement during RFA.[57] Hydrodisplacement and displacement using gas may be performed using any small-caliber needle or catheter.

Monitoring For Collateral Damage

Temperature monitoring may be performed by placing a thermocouple along a critical structure at the margin of an ablation zone. As nerve injury may occur with temperatures as low as 45°C for several minutes, ablations can be terminated as temperatures rise above this temperature.[51] Similarly, during cryoablation, neural injury may occur with temperatures below −10°C.[58,59] Electrophysiologic monitoring with somatosensory or motor evoked potentials provides immediate feedback regarding the functional status of vulnerable nerves.[60] Similarly, focused neurologic physical examination may provide information

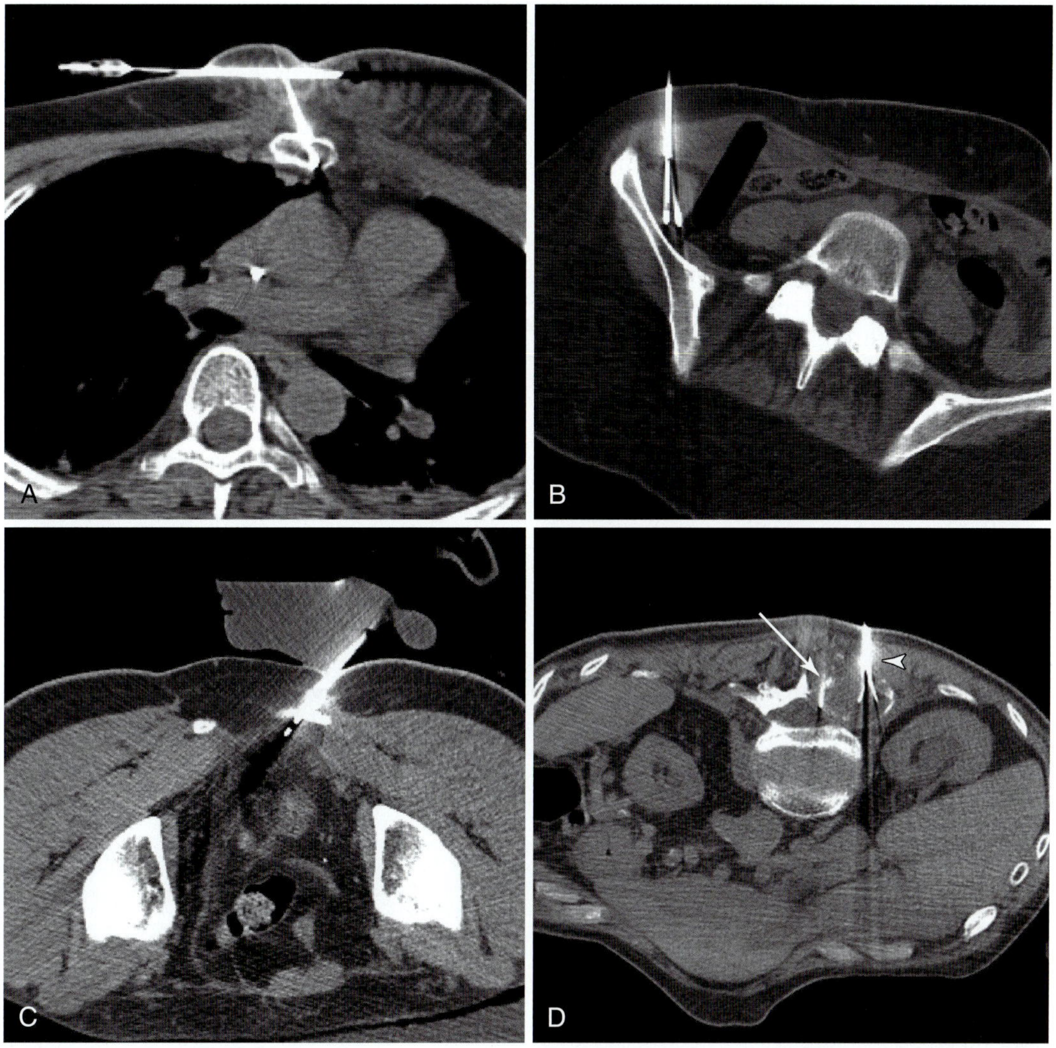

Figure 28-13 Adjunctive procedures during tumor ablation. (A) Hydrodisplacement performed to protect the skin during cryoablation of a breast carcinoma metastasis to the sternum. Axial CT image shows 5% dextrose in water instilled through a 5-French Yueh catheter. (B) Esophageal dilation balloon displacement of adjacent colon during cryoablation of an ovarian carcinoma metastasis in the pelvis. (C) Sterile glove containing tepid water placed for skin protection during cryoablation of a presacral mass (same case as Figure 28-2). (D) 3D volume-rendered CT image shows a thermocouple used to monitor temperature adjacent to the spinal canal during radiofrequency ablation of an osteolytic rectal carcinoma metastasis in an L1 transverse process. The thermocouple was placed medially compared to the multitined RFA electrode placed centrally within the tumor.

TABLE 28-5 Adjunctive Procedures Common to Percutaneous Ablation Procedures for Bone and Soft Tissue Metastases

Adjunctive Procedures for Bone and Soft Tissue Ablation
1. Displacement of adjacent structures
• Hydrodisplacement (Saline or D5W)
• Angioplasty balloon
• Gas (CO_2)
2. Monitoring for collateral damage
• Thermocouple
• Electrophysiologic monitoring (EMG)
• Limited neurologic exam
3. Skin protection
• Skin warmer (water in sterile glove)
4. Structural support
• Cementoplasty (or vertebroplasty)

regarding preserved nerve function in patients under minimal or no sedation.

Skin Protection

Skin overlying superficial tumors may be protected from thermal injury (burn or frostbite) using subcutaneous hydrodisplacement as well as placement of tepid water in a sterile glove on the skin surface.

Complications and Management

During tumor ablation or cementoplasty, adjacent normal structures may be injured directly during needle placement similar to other needle-based interventional procedures, albeit with larger-caliber bone access needles and drills. Thermal damage to normal structures may cause bowel or bladder perforation, infection, or fistula formation. These may require catheter drainage or surgical repair. Thermal-induced nerve dysfunction may present as weakness, paralysis, dysesthesia, paresthesias, or anesthesia. It may be managed expectantly, as it can resolve over weeks to months. Medications for neuropathic pain may be necessary. Skin burns may be produced when heat-based applicators are placed too close to the skin or as a result of excess heat generation at an RFA grounding pad. Similarly, frostbite may occur because of transgression of skin by the ice ball generated during cryoablation. These skin injuries can be managed with topical agents (e.g., silver sulfadiazine) as would skin injuries from other causes, depending on their severity. Injury to normal structures may be minimized through displacement, monitoring, and skin warming. In addition, pathologic fracture of an ablated bone may develop and may require surgical fixation. This complication may be minimized with adjunctive cementoplasty.

The main complications of cementoplasty result from cement leakage. Although this is typically asymptomatic, leaked cement which contacts neural tissue can lead to radiculopathy or neuropathy. Some authors have advocated immediately cooling freshly leaked cement close to nerve by injection of saline in the region.[61] Alternatively, perineural infiltration with steroids may minimize the injury.[29] Venous intravasation of cement may be asymptomatic if immediately recognized and limited to the basivertebral plexus. However, more extensive intravasation can lead to extension into the epidural space or pulmonary embolism (Figure 28-14).[62]

Outcomes and Results

Results from selected series and trials of treatment of painful bone metastases with the main ablation modalities are included in Table 28-6.

RADIOFREQUENCY ABLATION

RFA of painful bone metastases was first reported by Dupuy et al. in 1998 after treatment of 18 metastases in 16 patients.[41]

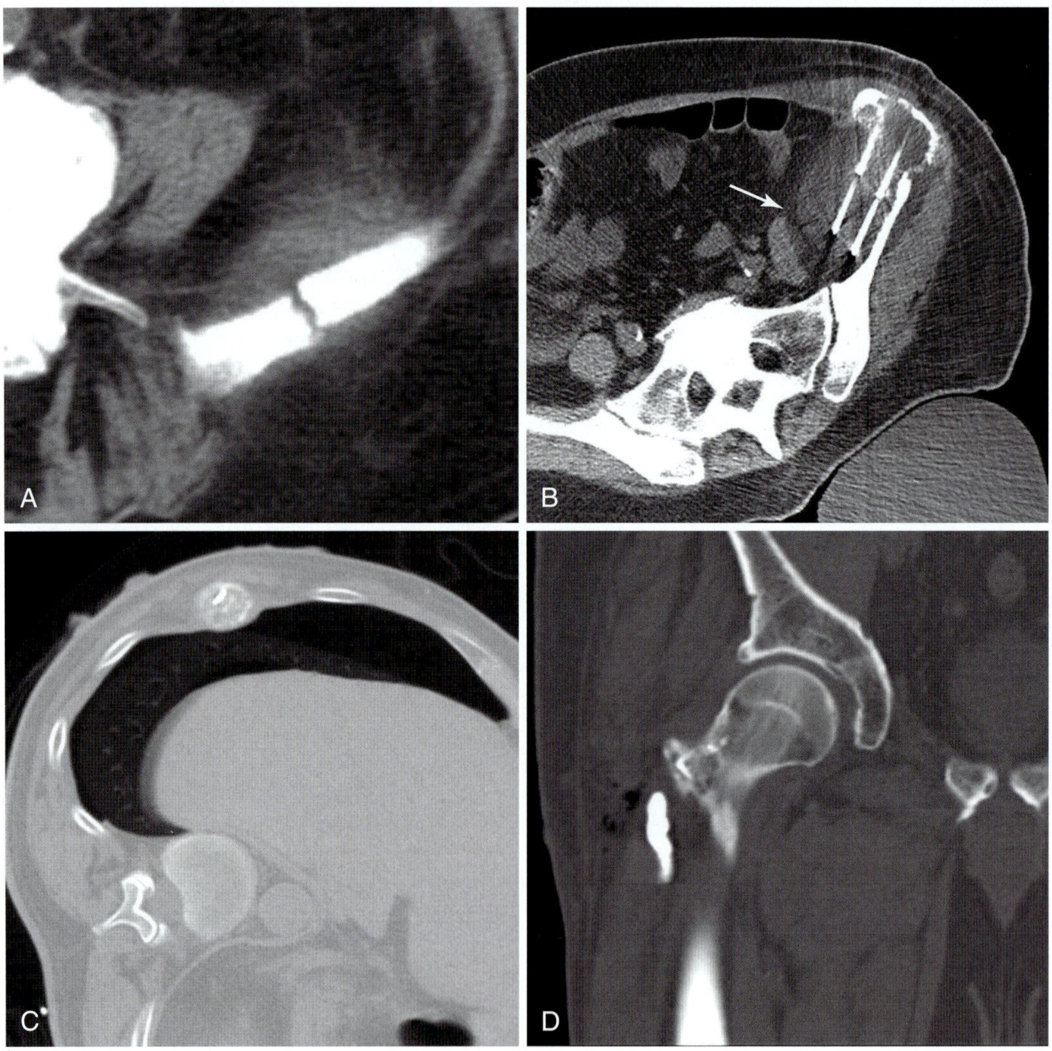

Figure 28-14 Complications following ablation and/or cementoplasty of musculoskeletal metastases. (A) Fracture of the iliac bone 1 week following cryoablation of a painful metastasis. (B) During cryoablation of a large, painful hepatocellular carcinoma metastasis to the left iliac bone in a 66-year-old woman, the ice ball encompassed the femoral nerve (*arrow* at expected location). The patient awoke with a severe femoral neuropathy, which slowly and incompletely recovered over several months. (C) Small pneumothorax during radiofrequency ablation of a right 8th rib metastasis from renal cell carcinoma in a 51-year-old man was immediately aspirated with a 5-French catheter. No chest tube was left in place. (D) Cement extravasation during combined ablation and cementoplasty of a painful proximal femoral metastasis from renal cell carcinoma in a 69-year-old man. Fortunately, the cement remained within the musculature and subcutaneous tissue of the lateral thigh, and the patient was asymptomatic.

TABLE 28-6 Selected Studies of Ablation of Painful Skeletal Metastases

Authors (et al.)	Year	Ablation Type (Manufacturer)	Patients (*n*)	Tumors (*n*)	Follow-up (months)	Pain Reduction* (No. of patients, Mean decrease)	Analgesic reduction (MED or % patients)	Complications (*n*, type)
Goetz[63]	2004	RFA (RITA)	43	43	6	41/43 points, 7.9–1.4	MED 99–93	3 (burn, incontinence, fracture)
Dupuy [64]	2009	RFA (Radionics)	55	55	3	14.2 points	NR	3 (local pain, neuro pain, foot drop)
Callstrom[73]	2006	Cryo (Endocare)	14	18	6	12/14 patients, 6.7–3.4 (2 m)	100% (8/8) dec opioids	None
Gangi[28]	1996	Ethanol	64	69	2–7	NR	73% dec opioids	1 (brachial plexus injury)
Liberman[76]	2009	FUS	31	32	3	18/25 patients, 5.9–1.8	67% (6/9) dec opioids	None
Gianfelice[77]	2008	FUS	11	12	3	6.0–0.5	100% (11/11) dec opioids	None
Anselmetti[78]	2008	Cementoplasty	50	70	3	9.1–2.1	94% (47/50) ceased opioids	2 (fractures)

Abbreviations: Cryo, cryoablation; dec, decreased; MED, morphine equivalent dose; NR, not reported; NSAIDs, nonsteroidal antiinflammatory drugs; RFA, radiofrequency ablation.

*Using an 11-point visual analog scale, except Dupuy et al. (which used a 100-point scale)

Since then, numerous case reports, series, and small trials of RFA of bone tumors have described RFA as effective and safe for the treatment of painful metastases.

Two major prospective, multicenter trials have evaluated the use of RFA in painful skeletal metastases. The first was a single-arm trial using the multitined RITA device (AngioDynamics, Lathum, NY) to treat 62 patients.[54,63] A clinically significant decrease (≥2 points on the BPI) in worst pain in a 24-hour period occurred in 59 of 62 patients (95%). A total of 6 patients (10%) experienced complications, including increase in tumor-cutaneous fistulae in 3 patients as well as solitary cases of transient bowel and bladder incontinence, second-degree skin burn at a grounding pad site, and pathologic fracture of an acetabular metastasis. In a second, single-arm, American College of Radiology Imaging Network (ACRIN) supported study, the Radionics Cool-tip device (Covidien, Boulder, CO) was used to treat 55 patients.[64] Using a 100-point pain scale, patients had decreased pain at 1 month (26.9 point decrease in pain intensity, 14.0 odds ratio for lower pain severity) and at 3 months (14.2 point decrease, 8.0 odds ratio). Major complications occurred in 3 patients (5%), including severe local pain, neuropathic pain, and foot drop.

MICROWAVE ABLATION

Fan et al. performed intraoperative microwave ablation to treat 62 patients with various bone tumors and achieved local tumor control in 57 of 62 patients.[65] Five patients experienced fracture complications. Multiple additional small series or case reports of percutaneous microwave ablation of skeletal metastases exist in the literature.[66-69]

LASER ABLATION

Laser ablation of osteoid osteoma has been reported in a large series.[70] Limited evaluation has been reported in the treatment of bone metastases. Groenmeyer et al. treated 3 patients with painful spine metastases with an Nd:YAG laser, resulting in 30%–45% pain reduction.[71] In a separate ongoing clinical trial of MRI-guided laser ablation, 7 patients with skeletal metastases have been successfully treated with no adverse event.[72]

CRYOABLATION

A prospective, single-institution, single-arm trial of cryoablation to treat 14 patients with painful bone metastases showed cryoablation to be safe and effective with durable results.[73] Mean BPI score for worst pain in a 24-hour period decreased from 6.7 to 3.8 over 4 weeks, and 80% of the patients who initially reported pain relief continued to report pain relief after 24 weeks. All 8 patients who were prescribed opioid analgesics prior to cryoablation decreased their dosage following the procedure. No serious complication occurred.

ETHANOL ABLATION

Gangi et al. treated 69 painful bone metastases in 64 patients with 1–3 doses of 3–30 mL of 95% ethanol and found reduction in opiate usage in 73% of patients.[28,74] Pain relief occurred within 1–2 days and lasted 2–7 months. The single serious complication observed was weakness after treatment of a spinal metastasis extending into the brachial plexus.

FOCUSED ULTRASOUND

FUS has been shown to produce effective palliation for painful skeletal metastases. In a prospective, multicenter trial involving 36 FUS treatments of 32 skeletal metastases in 31 patients, 18 of 25 patients (72%) with at least 3-month follow-up experienced a clinically significant pain reduction (≥2 points on the visual analog scale pain questionnaire, VAS).[75,76] In this trial, 9 patients experienced complete elimination of pain, 6 had no change, and 1 reported increased pain. Mean VAS score decreased from 5.9 to 1.8. A separate, single center trial included 11 patients with 12 bone tumors treated with MRI-guided FUS.[75-77] Mean VAS score decreased from 6.0 to 0.5 with 3-month follow-up. All patients decreased their analgesic usage, and 7 patients ceased using analgesic medications. No serious complication occurred.

CEMENTOPLASTY

In several studies, cementoplasty has been performed as solitary treatment or in combination with ablative therapy in the treatment of painful metastatic disease involving bone.[78-86] Anselmetti et al. reported on 50 patients with painful extraspinal osteolytic metastases treated with cementoplasty, including 7 patients who also had RFA for tumors greater than 7 cm.[78] Mean VAS scores decreased from 9.1/10 to 2.1/10 within 3 months, an effect that was durable for a 2-year period. Allowing for the small sample size, no significant difference in pain relief was identified between those treated with cementoplasty alone compared to combination therapy with RFA. Munk at al. used combined RFA and cementoplasty to treat 19 patients with 25 previously irradiated, painful metastatic lesions.[83] Mean pain scores decreased from 7.9/10 to 3.8/10 in 6 weeks, and 18 patients had increased mobility. A small study of cementoplasty alone in 5 patients with skeletal metastases by Hierholzer et al. found significant pain reduction.[86]

Summary

Percutaneous ablation of bone and soft tissue metastases may be performed for palliation of pain, prevention of complications due to progressive disease, and local disease control in nonsurgical patients. Patients treated for palliation of painful metastases should have at least moderate pain levels, pain referable to a limited number of metastatic lesions on imaging, and target lesions separated (or separable) from critical normal structures.

Preablation workup should include laboratory assessment and correction of coagulation parameters and platelets, pain and quality of life assessments using standardized scales, and focused physical examination to enable correlation of painful site(s) with imaging findings. Preablation imaging should guide safe percutaneous access to the bone or soft tissue metastasis and assessment of nearby vital structures, particularly nerves, to be avoided or monitored during treatment.

Radiofrequency ablation, cryoablation, laser ablation, microwave ablation, focused ultrasound, and ethanol ablation offer different advantages and disadvantages in the treatment of bone and soft tissue metastases. Cementoplasty provides structural support to ablated metastases at risk for fracture.

REFERENCES

The complete reference list is available online at www.expertconsult.com.

29

Vertebroplasty and Kyphoplasty in Malignant Vertebral Fracture

ALEXIS D. KELEKIS

KEY POINTS

- Vertebroplasty and kyphoplasty are mainly used for pain relief.
- Tumor dissemination is an unknown factor in these techniques.
- Locoregional tumor control can be effective when combined with other techniques.
- Excessive vertebral destruction might need additional support by other material.

Background

Most oncologic patients (~70%) eventually will develop a metastatic vertebral fracture/lesion because of their underlying disease.[1] Although these fractures/lesions can be located at any spine level, most commonly they are encountered in the thoracic and lumbar spine.[1] These fractures lead to augmented tumor load, vertebral body height reduction, and consequent spinal deformity along with intractable pain and mobility impairment. These symptoms lead to reduction of physical and social function, reduced lung capacity, negative influence on nutrition as well as on quality of life, and lead to hospitalization and an increase in mortality rates.

The therapeutic archer's quiver includes conservative therapy (bisphosphonates, bed rest and bracing, oral analgesics and opioids, etc.), chemotherapy, radiotherapy, and surgical options. In approximately one-third of these patients, these treatments do not result in significant pain reduction, increase in mobility, or improvement in quality of life.[2-4] In these patients, vertebral augmentation by means of vertebroplasty or kyphoplasty can be performed by aiming at vertebral body stabilization, with subsequent pain decrease and restoration of mobility.

Vertebroplasty was introduced to everyday clinical practice in 1987 when for the first time ever Galibert and Deramond performed the technique for the treatment of an aggressive hemangioma in the cervical spine.[5] The technique involves the image-guided, percutaneous needle placement in the vertebral body and the injection of a viscous implant (polymethyl methacrylate [PMMA]) for vertebral stabilization. Ever since along with the technological innovations, the indications of the technique expanded, including osteoporotic and traumatic vertebral fractures as well as metastatic lesions including lesions from multiple myeloma and lymphoma. In addition, the fact that the technique can be combined to other minimally invasive techniques for local tumor treatment plans further expands the indication list to include specific benign primary tumors (e.g., aneurysmal bone cyst, eosinophilic granuloma) and complex metastatic lesions (e.g., osteoblastic metastases).[6] More recent technologies provide vertebral augmentation combining PMMA injection to the assistance of specific devices such as radiofrequency electrodes, stents, and peek cages.

Kyphoplasty is another percutaneous, image-guided procedure used to treat symptomatic vertebral fractures and, in addition, aims in vertebral height restoration with subsequent reduction of the spine's biomechanical alterations.[7,8] The technique was introduced to everyday clinical practice in 1998 in the United States by an orthopedic surgeon. During kyphoplasty, cannulas are, bilaterally or unilaterally, introduced inside the vertebral body, a cavity is drilled, and inflatable balloon bone tabs are used to elevate the vertebral endplates, thus reducing the deformity and attempting to, at least temporarily, more or less restore the initial vertebral height. The intravertebral cavity created is subsequently filled with bone cement (PMMA). More recent technologies have reduced the size and diameter of the instruments used in kyphoplasty.

PMMA is a biocompatible and nonabsorbable implant that is injected in a viscous form and that rapidly solidifies, providing mechanical stability within a few hours postinjection.[9,10] Concerning interventional oncology, the use of PMMA as the viscous implant has proved useful, as it deters tumor growth.[11] The reason for this behavior of tumor cell in contact with PMMA is not yet clear, but the predominant hypothesis is that the exothermic reaction during polymerization creates a necrotic zone, which has an antimitotic effect on local tumor.[12] This energy release is directly proportional to the amount of cement injected and is limited by convective heat transfer due to blood perfusion. PMMA bone cement is suggested to be designed in a way that the maximum temperatures during this reaction are limited to 70°C.[12-15] Several studies have shown that the therapeutic temperatures raised during PMMA polymerization do not cause any damage in the spinal cord or surrounding nerve roots as long as the cement is confined to the boundaries of the vertebral body and does not come in direct contact (at large volumes) with the aforementioned nerve structures.[12-15] Another advantage of PMMA for interventional oncology is the fact that it does not undergo vascular invasion and bone or tumor ingrowth, resulting in resorption and remodeling.[12-15]

Concerning interventional oncology, both techniques constitute symptomatic (palliative) rather than curative treatments.[9,10] Although both techniques seem to be governed by excellent success rates (concerning pain reduction and mobility improvement) and low complication rates, it is beyond doubt that specifically for the application of percutaneous kyphoplasty in interventional oncology, more and extensive studies and meta-analyses are necessary. The same is true for all of the most recently developed vertebral augmentation techniques that combine cementoplasty to implantation of a specific biocompatible material (e.g., cage or stent).

Patient Selection

Proper patient selection is critical for a safe and efficacious technique. To begin with, one must consider the histology of the tumor, the general condition of the patient, the degree of bone destruction, and the potential of combining osteoplasty with other surgical or minimally invasive image-guided therapies. These considerations will assist to define whether the therapy will have curative intent (e.g., a case of solitary metastasis treated by a combination of chemoembolization, ablation, and cementoplasty), locoregional tumor control, or palliative intent (e.g., a case of multiple lesions treated with multilevel vertebroplasty or kyphoplasty aimed at pain reduction and mobility improvement).[16]

Biopsy of the lesion for histologic conformation is necessary and can be performed either prior to or at the same session with cementoplasty depending on treatment type. Indications for performing a biopsy include the possibility of lesions originating from unknown primary neoplasm, presence of more than one primary neoplasm coexisting and cases where imaging findings do not clearly attribute the lesions to the primary neoplasm.[17]

In general, the ideal candidate is a patient with symptomatic vertebral lesion of an osteolytic nature (metastasis, multiple myeloma, and lymphoma lesions) with pain, mobility impairment, and risk of compression fracture[18-25] (Figure 29-1). Osteoblastic lesions require a more complex technique during which, prior to cementoplasty, some osseous space must be created for PMMA to be injected (e.g., a cavity or osseous channels, formed by specific instruments) (Figure 29-2). Finally, in cases of aggressive benign vertebral tumors such as hemangioma, giant cell tumor (GCT), and aneurysmal bone cyst (ABC), the aim of vertebroplasty is to strengthen the vertebral body and devascularize the lesion, thus resulting in lowering of pain. In such cases, vertebroplasty can be combined to intralesional sclerotherapy.[16]

Disruption of the posterior wall is no longer considered a contraindication for both vertebroplasty and kyphoplasty. Retropulsed osseous fragment is a relative contraindication for kyphoplasty but not for vertebroplasty.[25,26] Other contraindications

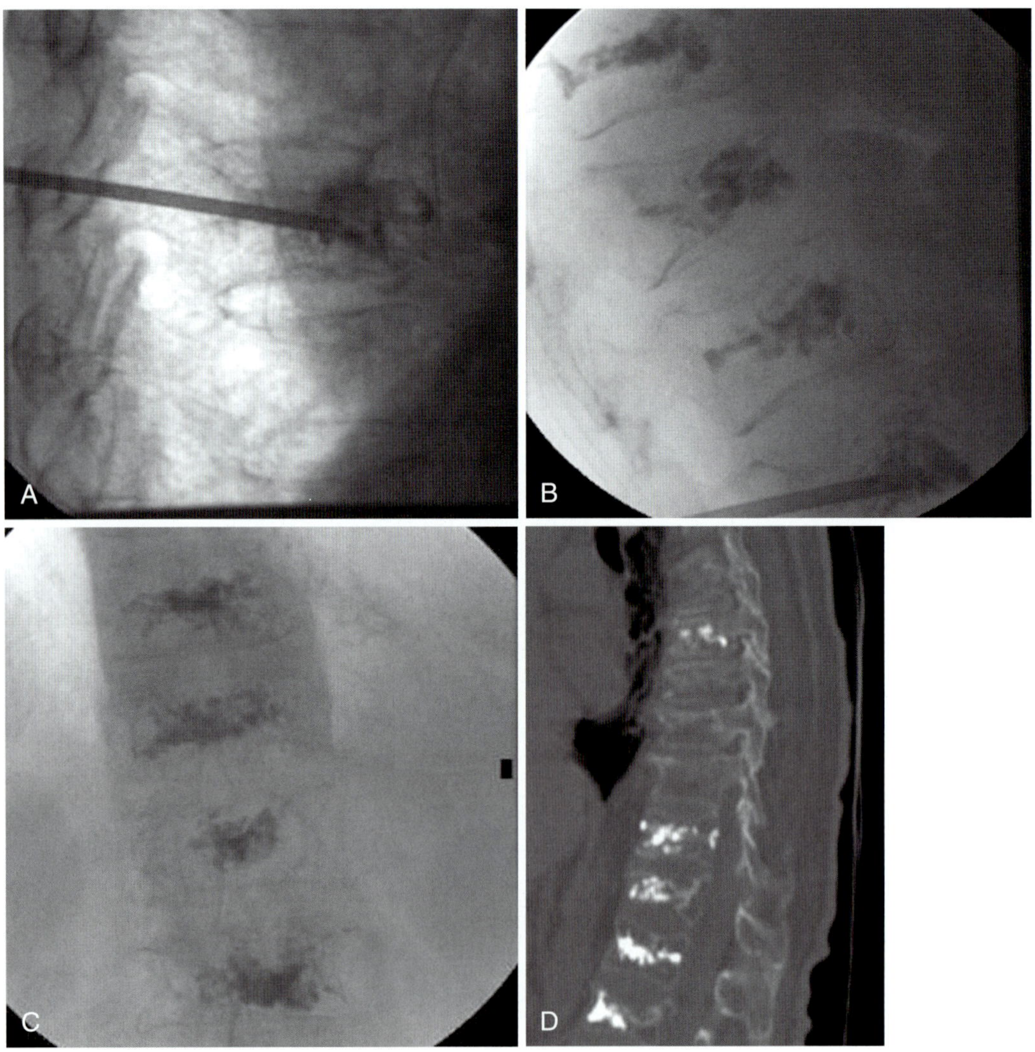

Figure 29-1 Female patient with multiple myeloma (A) Phlebography (intravertebral injection of small amount of contrast medium) prior to PMMA injection provides valuable information about the potential distribution of the cement (B) Lateral projection of the patient's spine post vertebroplasty. Cement is distributed within the vertebral bodies, creating a column from the upper to the lower end plate (C) AP projection of the patient's spine post vertebroplasty. Cement is centrally distributed within the vertebral bodies. (D) Sagittal reconstruction from the CT scan postvertebroplasty.

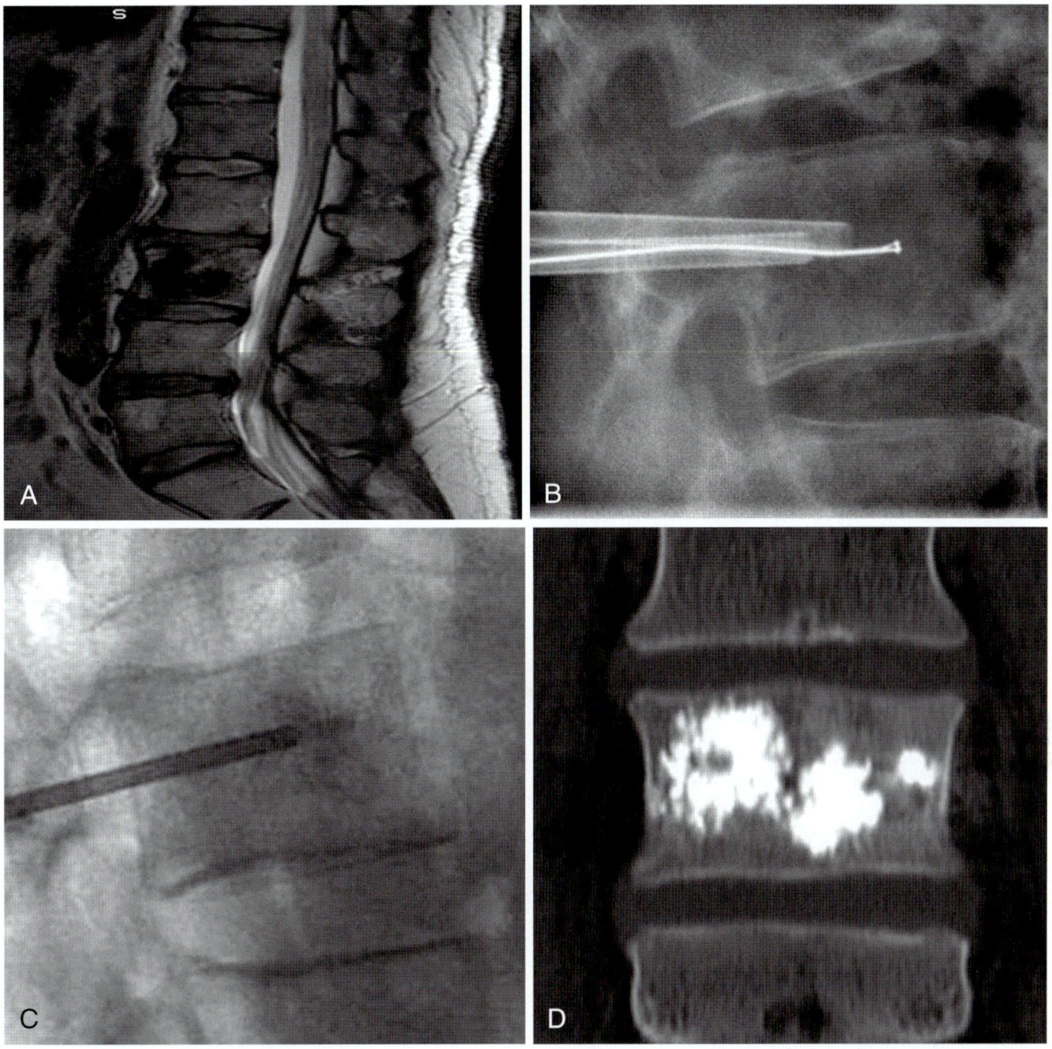

Figure 29-2 Patient with painful blastic metastasis at L3 vertebral body from prostate carcinoma (A) T2-weighted sagittal reconstruction illustrates the low signal lesion in the L3 vertebral body (B) Through the trocar a coblation electrode is introduced within the vertebral body, and the coblation session follows creating channels within the blastic lesion. (C) PMMA injection follows coblation. Cement fills in the created channels. (D) CT coronal multiplanar reconstruction post vertebroplasty illustrates the cement filling the lesion.

include a patient unwilling to consent, restricted span of life, local or systemic infection, allergy to any of the materials used (cement, opacifiers etc.), uncorrectable coagulopathy, and lesions that do not produce symptoms.

Preprocedural Care

Preprocedural imaging in oncologic patients should include magnetic resonance scans (including fat-saturated sequences prior to and after intravenous (IV) gadolinium chelate administration and short tau inversion recovery [STIR] sequence), bone scintigraphy exams, and computed tomography (CT) scans (extremely helpful in deferring osteolytic/osteoblastic lesions). Thorough medical record uptake and physical examination is combined to imaging and neurophysiologic studies. Correlation of physical examination findings to those of imaging and neurophysiology will provide most of the answers in clinical and diagnostic dilemmas.

Prior to the session, laboratory workup is necessary, including complete blood count and coagulation profile as well as electrocardiogram and cardiopulmonary control. Consultation with the anesthesiologist is performed after the aforementioned workup and prior to the therapeutic session.

Choice of anesthesia is left to the responsible anesthesiologist and varies from local anesthesia to general anesthesia (including epidural anesthesia with or without sedation). It is to be kept in mind that cement injection in neoplastic lesions can be quite painful; thus local anesthesia is usually not considered a choice.

Technique

VERTEBROPLASTY

Vertebroplasty is a minimally invasive, image-guided technique performed under fluoroscopy, CT (±CT fluoroscopy), cone beam CT, and magnetic resonance imaging (MRI). Preprocedural dose of prophylactic antibiotics is optional; however, it seems that it is a common practice in most centers throughout the globe. In any case, as far as immunocompromised patients are concerned, prophylactic antibiotics administration is mandatory. The technique is performed under vital signs monitoring and extended local sterility measures.

The patient is placed in prone position (whenever levels of interest are at thoracic or lumbar spine) or in supine position (whenever levels of interest are at cervical spine). Concerning thoracic and lumbar spine, the most common approach is the transpedicular one (either lateral or direct) performed unilaterally or bilaterally depending on the size and location of the lesion. On anteroposterior (AP) projection, the target point lies at 1–3 o' clock (or 9–11 o' clock, respectively) at the lateral pedicular wall (a breach of the upper-lateral pedicle poses less threat than a corresponding one in lower-medial part). AP and lateral projections verify the route of the needle within the pedicle until it reaches the posterior vertebral wall (a fact verified on lateral projections) (Figure 29-3). Once past the posterior wall, the needle is advanced toward the lesion. The use of beveled needles advocates easier guidance inside the bone (needle has the tendency to follow its tip); on the other hand, diamond-tip needles are better in cases where blastic bone has to be penetrated.

Intravertebral venography (i.e., intraosseous injection of 1–3 mL of iodinated contrast medium) is optional, because of the different viscosity properties between contrast and cement; however, it can provide valuable information concerning the lesion's vascularity and the potential distribution of the implant. Injection of PMMA is considered an act of embolization and should be performed under continuous imaging guidance (lateral projection is preferred because it allows early detection of epidural leakage and anterior body leakages; AP projections detect lateral leakages). In cases of solitary metastasis or primary lesion, the goal should be complete filling of the lesion. In cases of multiple lesions, stabilization of vertebral body is the target (ideally at least one-fourth of the vertebral body should be filled with PMMA that will create a column at midline extending from the upper to lower endplate). In any case where pain relief is the goal, even smaller cement amounts (1.5–2.5 mL) are enough. At room temperature (~20°C), most of the older cements were governed by an effective working time of 8–12 minutes. Nowadays, newer

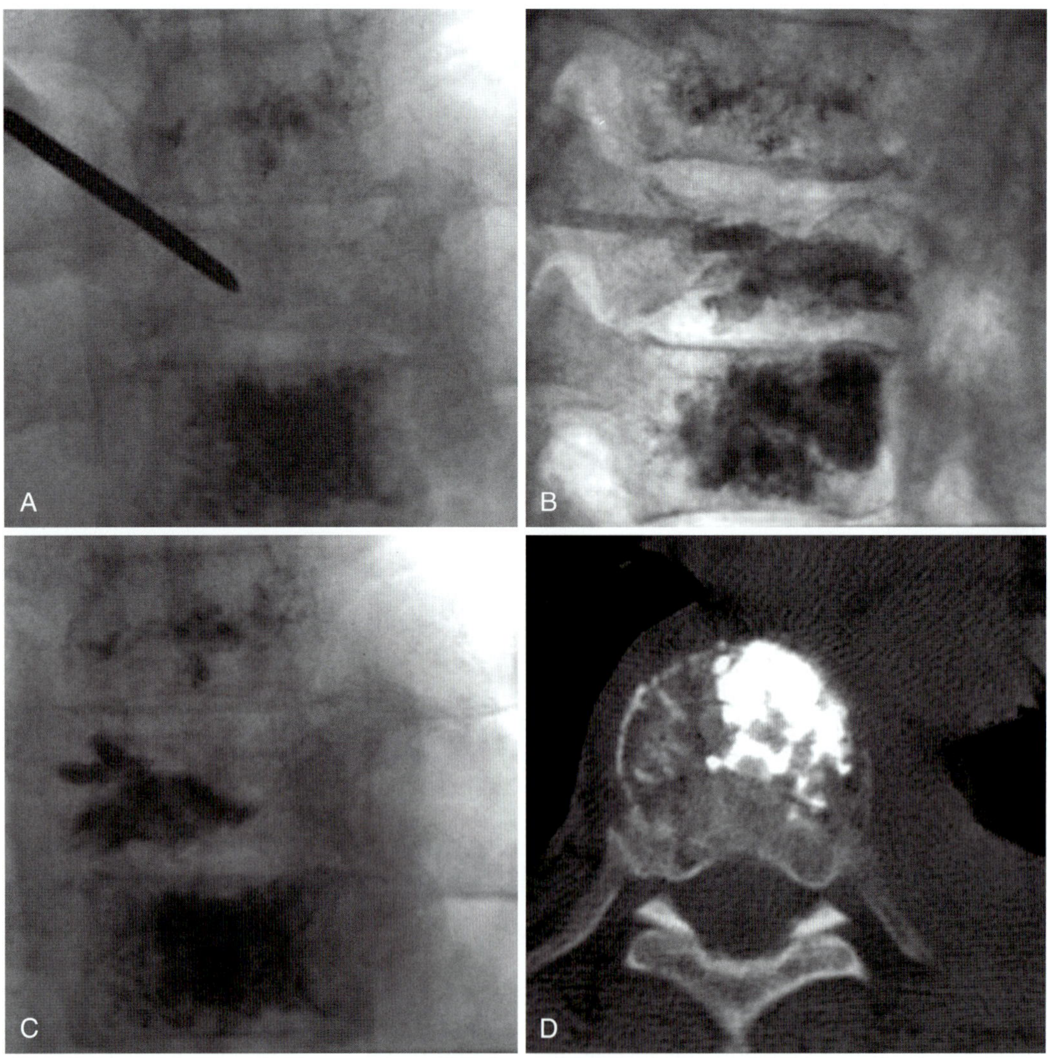

Figure 29-3 Female patient with vertebral metastasis from breast carcinoma (A) AP projection of the treated vertebral body. At its final position on this projection, the needle should be toward the midline (B) Lateral projection of the patient's spine post vertebroplasty. Cement is distributed within the vertebral bodies, creating a column from the upper to the lower end plate (C) AP projection of the patient's spine post vertebroplasty. Cement is centrally distributed within the vertebral bodies. (D) Axial CT scan post vertebroplasty illustrates the cement within the vertebral body without leakage.

cements provide up to 20 minutes of effective working time, or 10 minutes of working time at high viscosity.

Alternative approaches include the posterolateral (paravertebral) for the lumbar spine and the intercostovertebral route for the thoracic spine. Concerning cervical spine, an anterolateral approach is performed from C3 to C7 vertebrae (needle route should avoid the local major vessels) and a transoral approach at the C1 and C2 vertebral body. General anesthesia is required for performing vertebroplasty in the cervical spine.

KYPHOPLASTY

Prior to kyphoplasty, imaging studies (usually CT scan) are necessary for the evaluation of the vertebral posterior wall, fractured pedicles, and the possibility of retropulsed osseous fragment.

Kyphoplasty is performed only in lumbar or thoracic spine with the patient in prone position. The technique is usually performed under general anesthesia; extensive and strict local sterility measures are mandatory. Usually, a bilateral approach is chosen and a working cannula from each side is advanced through a transpedicular approach until the posterior third of the vertebral body, although a unipedicular approach has also been documented[27] (Figure 29-4). AP and lateral fluoroscopy images are used for screening the needle advancement inside the pedicle. By means of reaming tools, two working channels are created inside which the balloons are inserted. These balloons can measure 10, 15, or 20 mm in length and ideally are positioned in the anterior two-thirds of the vertebral bodies in the middle distance between the upper and lower endplates. Under visual field, the volume and pressure control balloons are inflated; end points of inflation include a pressure >400 psi, when the balloon comes in contact with the vertebral body endplate or cortical wall and when the balloon's maximum inflation volume is reached. Following injection, the balloons are deflated and removed. In the next step, the cement injector system is advanced through the working cannula until the cavity's anterior. Under continuous fluoroscopy, cement is slowly injected aiming to fill the cavity and the same procedure is repeated from the contralateral side as well. Use of highly viscous cement along with the created cavity minimizes the extravertebral leakage rate.

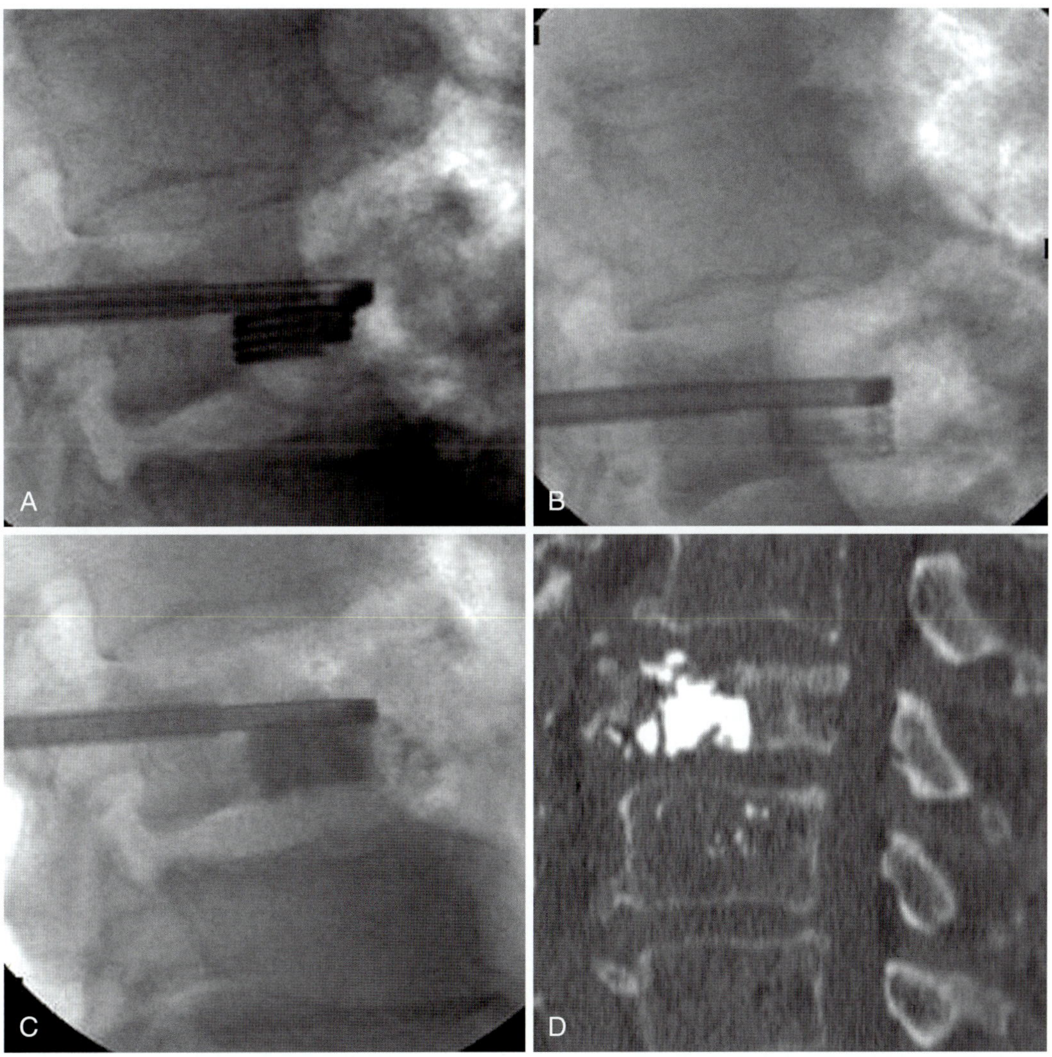

Figure 29-4 Patient with a medical record of renal cell carcinoma underwent kivoplasty due to a painful vertebral fracture. (A) Through the working cannulla, the Kiva coil is deployed within the vertebral body. (B) Over the Kiva coil, the peek polymer cage is deployed and the coil is subsequently retrieved. (C) The peek polymer cage is filled with PMMA. (D) Sagittal reconstruction from the CT scan the morning post kivoplasty.

Postprocedural Care

Patient remains on bed rest in supine position for approximately 4 hours (at that time period, most PMMA types have accessed ~90% of the desired stiffness and hardening).[9] Specifically for kyphoplasty, the patient is mobilized the morning after the session.[7,8] Vital signs are monitored every 15 minutes during the first hour. A responsible medical person is charged for assisting the patient to rise from the bed for the first time after the session. Clinical evaluation includes immediate study of patient's general condition and neurologic status. In case of any clinical or neurological deterioration, a CT scan is immediately performed; otherwise the scan is reserved for the morning after the session. Although many centers treat these lesions as an outpatient treatment, in our institution patients remain hospitalized overnight and exit the hospital the morning after. Analgesics and antiinflammatory drugs may be necessary because of small but painful hematomas at the puncture sites. Sometimes, a postembolic syndrome, associated with pain and fever, can occur because of tumor necrosis from the polymer.

Outcome

Vertebroplasty and kyphoplasty result in significant pain (>50% on the Numeric Visual Scale) and medication uptake (>50% decrease of narcotic analgesics) in 75%–85% of patients.[28-40] Combination of vertebroplasty to other local control ablative techniques is used for curative intent or locoregional tumor control. Such combinations include ablation and/or transarterial chemoembolization (TACE). They seem to be governed by higher success rates (especially when paravertebral tumor extension coexists to vertebral lesion).[28-40] In cases of triple combination (vertebroplasty, ablation, and TACE), embolization is performed on the first day and 24 hours later ablation and vertebroplasty are performed. Furthermore, it is mandatory to allow enough time between ablation and cement injection in order for vertebral body's temperature to normalize and thus avoid fast cement polymerization because of high temperature.

Controversies

1. Height restoration and kyphotic correction are not the prime goals in oncologic patients, where pain reduction and mobility enhancement are by far more important. Furthermore, it has been suggested that height restoration and kyphotic correction achieved by kyphoplasty are only temporary.
2. Kyphoplasty is less cost effective, lasting longer and requiring a higher level of anesthesia in many cases (many oncologic patients are not in a suitable physical condition for long-lasting sessions under general anesthesia).
3. Solitary metastatic intravertebral lesions can be treated curatively by a combination of thermal ablation and vertebroplasty (±TACE). Furthermore, studies have shown that combining these procedures results in higher pain reduction and mobility improvement levels. This combination is not so easily performed in cases of kyphoplasty.
4. Extravertebral leakages are more common in vertebroplasty than in kyphoplasty; however, the vast majority of them are not clinically significant. It has not been proved yet that clinically significant leakages rates are statistically different for the two therapies.
5. Displacement of tumor cells mainly by kyphoplasty and probably with vertebroplasty is an unknown factor in disease progression, although there are no studies showing worst Kaplan–Meier curves of survival of patients after vertebral augmentation.
6. Quite often, metastatic lesions can be located in the vertebral pedicles; in this case, vertebroplasty rather than kyphoplasty is the treatment of choice.[41]

Complications

The complication rate of vertebroplasty or kyphoplasty in malignant cases is <10%.[9,10] Generally, complications of these two minimally invasive techniques can be avoided by performing the technique in a state-of-the-art way and by using excellent imaging modalities for guidance, according to Interventional Society's standards.[9,10] Furthermore, although the use of specifically designed injectors for the implantation of PMMA and polymers inside the vertebral body increases the cost, it provides excellent control of the injection and contributes to minimizing the risk of leakages.

Cementoplasty's complications in the spine include leakage of the cement (38%–72.5%) beyond the vertebral borders (epidural–foraminal, intravascular, lateral, and inside the intervertebral disc), lung embolism, transient neurologic deficit lasting <30 days (~5%), permanent neurologic deficit (~2%), infection (<1%), iatrogenic fracture of the pedicle, endplate, or wall of the treated vertebra (<1%), fracture of adjacent vertebrae (or fracture of "sandwich" vertebrae), allergic reaction (hypotension and arrhythmias due to the cement), puncture site bleeding, and acute increased pain or new areas of pain (14%).[42-47]

Finally, an important issue especially in patients with multiple lesions treated in the same session is the potential of pulmonary fat embolism, the clinical significance of which probably increases in patients with compromised pulmonary function.

Technologic Advancements

During recent years, several new devices and instruments have been designed and released in the market aiming at further enhancement of vertebroplasty or kyphoplasty as well as at higher safety and efficacy levels. Regarding safety levels, new cements that are of higher viscosity or medium-viscosity cements with ideal radioopacity and optimal rheologic properties allowing longer injecting time (20 minutes) have been released in the market. Aiming at the same target, radiofrequency-assisted cement injection results in higher cement viscosity by means of an RF needle. Furthermore, covered self-expandable nitinol stents and decrease of the instrumental size used in kyphoplasty seem to enhance cementoplasty and increase safety levels.[48-51]

Nowadays, several different endovertebral prostheses can be used not only for achieving but also for reserving height restoration. Such devices include nitinol endovertebral cages, peek implant, or vertebral body stents.[48-51]

No doubt each one and all of these devices may be extremely helpful in enhancing the safety and efficacy of osteoplasty in the spine; however, further and more extended studies are necessary for proving their scientific importance. Most important of all, with all these new devices available nowadays, each case must be individualized and material selection should be performed based on the case requirements.

Conclusion

The improved survival of oncologic patients due to advancements in the fields of chemotherapy and radiotherapy has illustrated the importance of efficient pain control for these patients, because an extended life expectancy should be combined with life quality as well. Image-guided, percutaneous minimally invasive techniques such as vertebroplasty and balloon kyphoplasty are safe and efficacious therapies aiming at pain reduction and mobility improvement in patients with metastatic lesions or lesions from multiple myeloma or lymphoma. Obviously, these techniques work in an adjunctive way, along with radiation therapy and/or chemotherapy, for symptom regression and improvement of patients' condition.

REFERENCES

The complete reference list is available online at www.expertconsult.com.

30

Intraarterial Procedures for the Musculoskeletal System

MOHAMED ABDELSALEM | KATSUHIRO KOBAYASHI | RONY AVRISTCHER | SANJAY GUPTA | ALDA L. TAM

KEY POINTS

- Intraarterial procedures are useful for pain palliation, local disease control and as an adjunct to a planned surgical intervention.
- Meticulous angiographic technique and careful monitoring of the patient's neurologic status is essential for preventing complications during embolization of tumors in the spine.
- Specific strategies for embolization of tumors in the spine are discussed.

Background

The arterial system provides an extensive route of access to tumors of the musculoskeletal system, allowing for the precise delivery of embolic agents or antineoplastic chemotherapy. This chapter reviews how intraarterial procedures can be used as a tool for pain palliation, local disease control, and as an adjunct to support surgical interventions.

Patient Selection

Patients with primary or secondary musculoskeletal neoplasms often receive care from a multidisciplinary team of physicians, consisting of medical oncologists, orthopedic surgeons, radiation oncologists, and interventional radiologists, who make the collective decision to incorporate the use of intraarterial (IA) therapy. Evaluation of the patient in a clinic setting is essential for providing the patient with education regarding the potential risks and benefits of the procedure. A complete history and physical examination is necessary to document symptoms and their severity and to assess baseline physical function. The use of subjective pain assessment scales (Brief Pain Inventory or Memorial Pain Assessment Card) and the quantification of narcotic medications to a morphine-equivalent dose can be useful tools for determining treatment efficacy in follow-up. Patients with mild pain, <4 on a 10-point scale, usually do not experience significant pain relief following intervention and may not be appropriate candidates for arterial embolization. Patients who undergo a procedure for pain palliation should be counseled on the expected onset, degree, and duration of symptom relief. These patients require close clinical follow-up after the procedure to determine clinical effectiveness. Repeat embolizations may be indicated if pain symptoms recur or develop in a new location.

The diagnostic cross-sectional imaging must be reviewed for procedural planning. Routine laboratory values including coagulation studies and serum creatinine must be evaluated. Normal cardiac and renal function is required for the administration of chemotherapeutic agents.[1] Patients with uncorrectable coagulopathy, renal insufficiency, severe allergic reaction contrast media, or severe atherosclerotic disease may not be candidates for angiography.[2,3]

Technique

Intraarterial procedures are typically performed under monitored, moderate sedation using a combination of fentanyl and midazolam. Adequate hydration is recommended prior to angiography as the use of significant amounts of contrast media may be required. The placement of a urinary catheter may be helpful for monitoring urine output during the procedure and in the postoperative recovery period. Antibiotic prophylaxis is not routinely given.

INTRAARTERIAL INFUSION CATHETER PLACEMENT FOR LIMB INFUSION

After arterial access is achieved using Seldinger's technique, a guiding 4-F or 5-F catheter is directed into the main arterial trunk supplying the tumor. This is usually the common femoral artery for lower extremity lesions and the axillary artery for upper extremity lesions. Image acquisition during angiography should be performed in at least two different projections (anterior and lateral or oblique projections) to allow for the adequate evaluation of the arterial supply to the entire lesion.[1] Angiography should be performed using a power injector to deliver contrast at 3 to 5 mL per second for a total volume of 12–20 mL.[1] Image projections and contrast injection rates should be documented so that subsequent infusion sessions can use the same parameters, allowing for accurate assessment of tumor response during treatment.

Ideally, the catheter should be positioned to deliver the chemotherapy to the entire tumor while minimizing the exposure of uninvolved tissues. Once the catheter position has been optimized, an infusion wire (0.035 in. diameter, 145 cm length) with either a 6- or 12-cm working tip is inserted coaxially through the guide catheter. A longer working tip length is helpful in cases where the catheter must be placed to cross an arterial bifurcation point. For example, if a lesion derives supply from both the deep femoral and superficial femoral arteries, the working tip of the infusion wire should be placed in the deep femoral artery and extend back into the common femoral artery to ensure that chemotherapy is delivered through all arteries supplying the lesion. The infusion wire may be advanced through the guide catheter to the appropriate location in the artery; however, when feasible, a pull-back technique, where the guide catheter is retracted to uncover the infusion wire, should be used to minimize the risk of intimal injury.[1] Following infusion wire placement, contrast injection is performed to verify the appropriate placement.

BLAND ARTERIAL EMBOLIZATION

For embolization procedures, the arterial access can be secured with the placement of a 5-F sheath, which facilitates subsequent catheter exchanges and manipulations. A diagnostic angiogram is performed from the parent artery supplying the lesion using a 4-F or 5-F guide catheter to create a vascular map, defining the pathologic vessels that need to be targeted for embolization. Subselective catheterization of the vessels feeding the tumor is performed using a 3-F microcatheter, inserted coaxially through the guide catheter. Embolization of the tumor from a subselective location allows for tumor devascularization while minimizing the risk for nontarget embolization. Embolization is carried out until stasis of the vessel has been achieved. Postembolization angiography provides an assessment of the percentage reduction in tumor vascularity.

SPINAL ANGIOGRAPHY

The spine is a common location for bone metastases, and preoperative embolization of spinal tumors is routinely performed to reduce intraoperative blood loss. A comprehensive knowledge of the vascular anatomy of the spine and spinal cord is essential (Figure 30-1). There are three types of radicular arteries, classified according to their contribution to the spinal arteries. Simple radicular arteries supply the nerve roots and dura but do not supply the spinal cord; radiculopial arteries supply the posterior spinal arteries; and the radiculomedullary arteries supply the anterior spinal arteries, which provide the major blood supply to the spinal cord. Six to eight radiculomedullary arteries are present, each of which bifurcates near the midline into ascending and descending branches that form the anterior spinal artery.[4] The blood supply to the spine and spinal cord via the radiculomedullary arteries varies depending on the region of the spine. In the cervicothoracic (C1-T2) and thoracic regions, an average of three to four radiculomedullary arteries supply the spinal cord. In the lower thoracic and lumbar region, a single large radiculomedullary artery, called the artery of Adamkiewicz, supplies the spinal cord and its origin can be located anywhere between T8 and L3.[5,6]

A 5-F catheter is typically used to select the segmental artery. Digital subtraction angiography is performed using hand injections of 3–5 mL of noniodinated contrast.[7] The segmental arteries on both sides, two levels above and below the tumor site, should be interrogated to define the arterial supply to the tumor and the proximity of the origin of the anterior spinal artery, if present. Table 30-1 lists the arteries supplying the vertebral column that need to be investigated for tumor embolization in each spinal region. It is recommended that images be acquired with a large field of view at a high frame rate (6/second) until the draining veins are visualized.[8] These techniques are designed to maximize visualization of the feeding arteries of the spinal tumor and the radiculomedullary arteries. The radiculomedullary arteries have a classic hairpin turn as they join the anterior spinal artery, which appears as a midline vessel. In some cases, the use of cone-beam computed tomography (CBCT) with 3D soft tissue reconstructions has been helpful as a problem-solving tool for difficult cases[9-11] and can provide information about feeding arteries, tumor vascularity, and radiculomedullary arteries (Figure 30-2).

In spinal embolization, selective delivery of embolic agents to the tumor and protection of the radiculomedullary arteries are essential to reduce the risk of nontarget embolization, which may have catastrophic consequences. A coaxial microcatheter system permits safe, selective catheter position and minimizes nontarget embolization. Although small particles (100–300-μm) can be routinely used in embolization of peripheral bone tumors, medium-sized particles (250–500-μm) are recommended for embolization in the spine. Medium-sized particles will occlude tumor vessels proximal to or at the capillary bed[12] without blocking collateral arterial supply to the spinal cord, thus reducing the risk of cord ischemia and paralysis.[13] Table 30-2 lists some of the common embolic agents and their characteristics.

Strategies and techniques of spinal embolization depend on the angiographic findings: the size and number of feeding

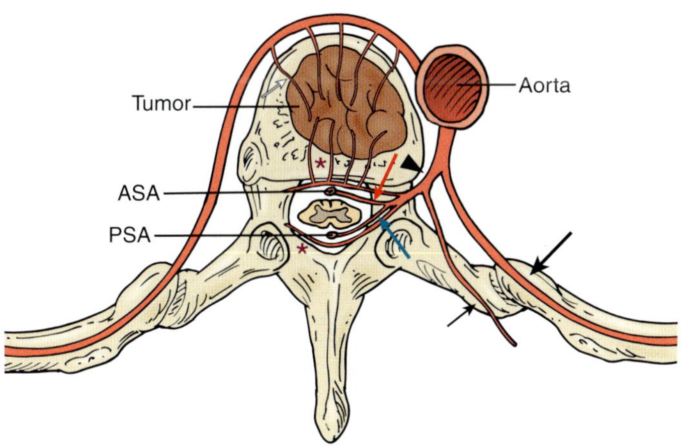

Figure 30-1 Vascular anatomy of the vertebral body and spinal cord. Branches supplying the vertebral body and spinal cord arise from the intercostal (or segmental) arteries at the midthoracic level. The intercostal artery divides into an anterior branch (*large black arrow*) that runs along the costal groove and a posterior branch to the spine (*black arrowhead*). The posterior branch gives off a radicular branch and a muscular branch (*small black arrow*). The radicular branch divides into the radiculomedullary artery (*red arrow*) and the radiculopial artery (*blue arrow*) which supply the anterior (ASA) and posterior (PSA) spinal arteries. The radicular artery also provides dorsal and ventral somatic branches to supply the anterior and posterior bony walls of the neural canal (*asterisk*). Small branches from the segmental artery perforate the anterior surface of the vertebral body (*white arrow*).

TABLE 30-1 Potential Sources of Arterial Supply to Tumors of the Spine

Cervicothoracic Spine	Thoracolumbar Spine	Sacrum
Vertebral arteries Ascending cervical trunk Deep cervical trunk Descending branches of thyrocervical trunk Supreme intercostal artery Intercostobrachial trunk	Segmental arteries (intercostal or lumbar) Iliolumbar arteries Median sacral artery	Iliolumbar arteries Internal iliac arteries Median sacral artery Lateral sacral arteries

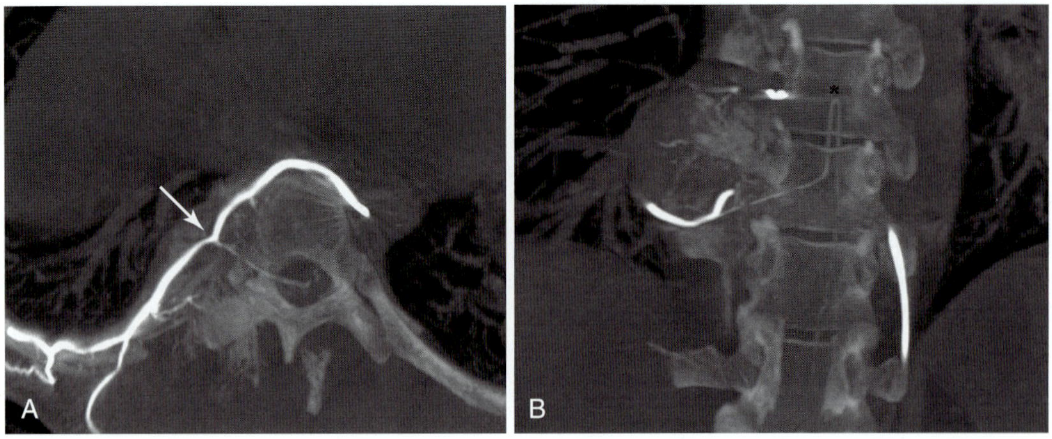

Figure 30-2 Use of cone beam CT (CBCT) as a problem-solving tool during angiography. In this case of metastatic sarcoma involving the T7 vertebral body, the origin of the radiculomedullary artery on the selective angiogram of the right T7 segmental artery was not clear (angiogram not shown). CBCT with soft tissue reconstruction images in the axial (A) and coronal (B) planes clearly demonstrates the origin of the radiculomedullary artery (*arrow*, A) and its subsequent connection to the anterior spinal artery, which is denoted by the hairpin configuration (*asterisk*, B).

TABLE 30-2 Characteristics of Common Embolic Agents

Embolic agents	Characteristics
Particles (PVA/Embosphere)	Inert, water-insoluble, nonabsorbable, defined sizes
Gel foam/sponge	No defined sizes, provides temporal occlusion, degraded by enzyme
Alcohol/*N*-butyl-cyanoacrylate	Liquid agents, high risk of nontarget embolization, increased rates of neurologic complications and skin/muscle necrosis; use should be limited to experienced operators
Metallic coils	Single use for proximal embolization is ineffective, frequently used in conjunction with particle embolization

TABLE 30-3 Embolization Strategies for Spine Tumors

Angiographic Pattern	Spinal Artery	Embolization Strategies/ Techniques	Category
Single or few feeding vessels that can be catheterized	Not visualized	Superselective catheterization of the feeding vessels followed by particulate embolization	A-1
Small feeding vessels that cannot be catheterized	Not visualized	Distal coil embolization of the segmental artery followed by particulate embolization	A-2
Origin of feeding vessels distal to that of the radiculomedullary artery	Visualized	Superselective catheterization distal to radiculomedullary artery followed by particulate embolization +/- distal coil embolization	B-1
Origin of feeding vessels close to that of radiculomedullary artery	Visualized	No embolization	B-2
Origin of feeding vessels proximal to that of radiculomedullary artery	Visualized	Unless superselective catheterization of the feeding arteries is possible, do not embolize	B-3

vessels to the tumor and the presence or absence of visualization of the spinal artery. Table 30-3 summarizes five common patterns of angiographic findings seen in hypervascular spinal tumors and proposes specific embolization strategies for each pattern (Figures 30-3 to 30-7). In addition to the five common angiographic patterns identified, other angiographic features warrant technical consideration. Arteriovenous shunting may be present on the segmental angiogram, and occlusion of the shunt can be attempted with large embolic agents or coils; however, if a large shunt persists, embolization is contraindicated because of the risk of pulmonary and systemic embolism. Occasionally, the radiculomedullary artery may only be visible following subselective catheterization or may be visible via an intersegmental anastomosis one level above or below the selected segmental artery. Embolization in both these cases is contraindicated if the feeding arteries are too close to the origin of the radiculomedullary artery. Lastly, the flow dynamics of the spinal tumor may change during the embolization procedure. The radiculomedullary artery may not be seen during preembolization subselective angiography because of diversion of contrast into the high-flow tumor but will become angiographically apparent once embolization has been initiated and flow to the tumor has been reduced.[14] Therefore, frequent angiographic investigation and careful monitoring of the patient's clinical status during the procedure are necessary to prevent nontarget embolization. If the patient reports altered sensation, onset of paresthesia, or muscle spasm during the embolization procedure, this may be a sign of nontarget embolization of a radiculomedullary artery and the procedure should be terminated.[15] In patients undergoing the procedure for preoperative purposes, if embolization of the spinal tumor was not feasible or if only a portion of the tumor could be embolized, this should be communicated to the surgeon so that additional precautions, if needed, can be taken during surgery.

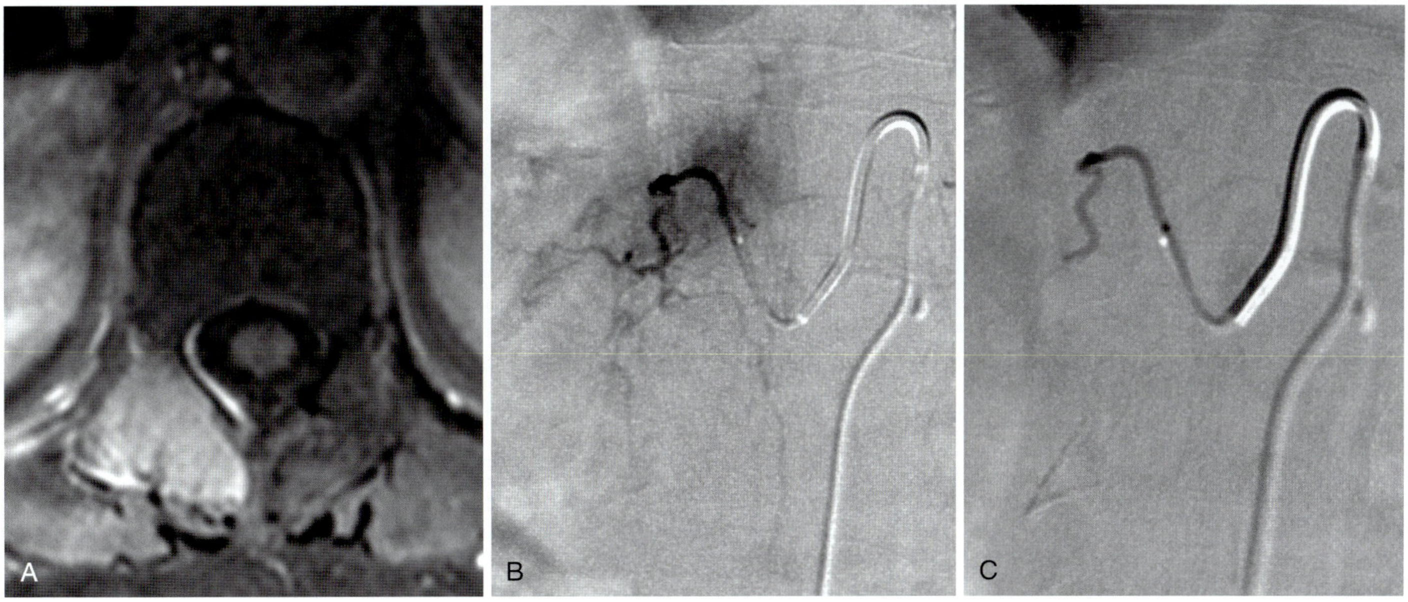

Figure 30-3 Embolization strategy for category A-1 lesions: superselective catheterization of the feeding arteries followed by particulate embolization. (A) Contrast-enhanced MRI of T12 shows metastatic thyroid cancer with an enhancing mass involving the posterior element of T12. (B) A selective right T12 segmental arteriogram performed from a microcatheter reveals a single feeding artery supplying the tumor. This artery was embolized using 300–500-μm particles. (C) A postembolization arteriogram shows successful embolization of the mass with significant reduction in tumor blush.

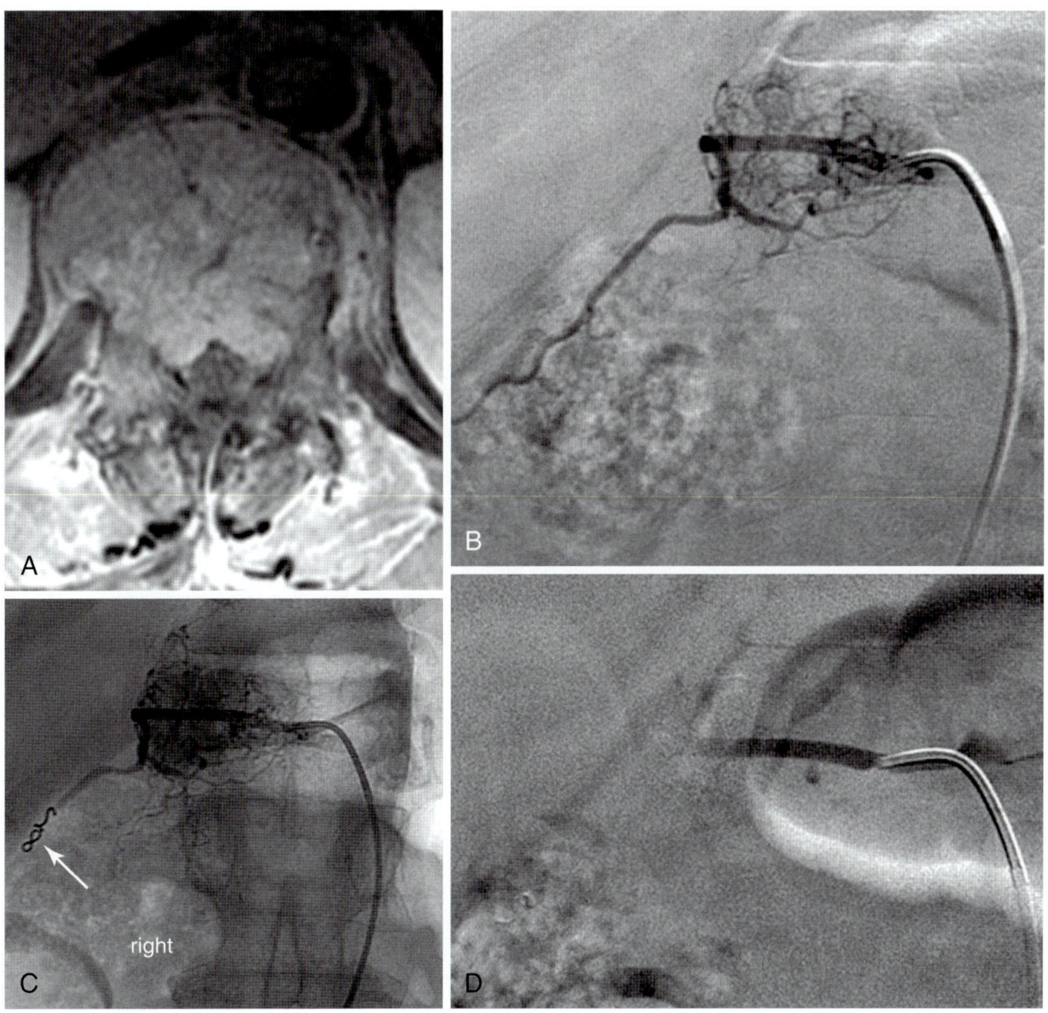

Figure 30-4 Embolization strategy for category A-2 lesions: distal coil embolization of the segmental artery followed by particulate embolization. (A) Contrast-enhanced MRI of T12 shows metastatic hepatocellular carcinoma involving the T12 body. (B) An arteriogram of the right T12 segmental artery reveals multiple, small feeding arteries that cannot be individually catheterized. The radiculomedullary artery is not seen. (C) Following distal segmental artery embolization with coils (*arrow*), these feeding arteries were embolized using 300–500-μm particles. (D) A postembolization arteriogram shows successful occlusion of the feeding arteries.

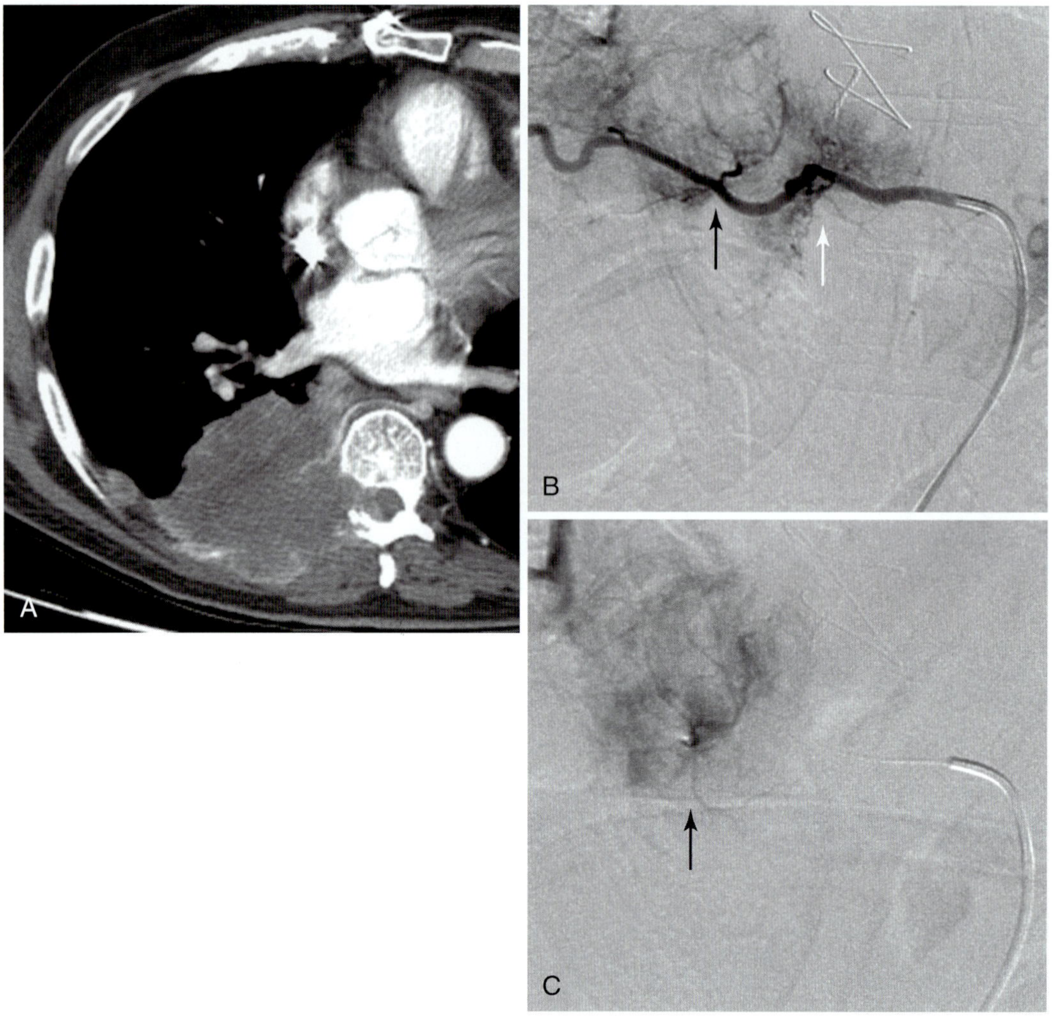

Figure 30-5 Embolization strategy for category B-1 lesions: superselective catheterization of feeders distal to radiculomedullary artery followed by particulate embolization. (A) Contrast-enhanced CT of T8 demonstrates a large metastatic lesion from renal cell carcinoma involving the paraspinal muscles and vertebra. (B) Selective arteriogram from the right T8 segmental artery shows the medial portion of the mass to be supplied by branches from the posterior division of the segmental artery, close to the origin of the radiculomedullary artery (*white arrow*). The lateral portion of the mass is supplied by branches from the anterior division of the segmental artery (*black arrow*). (C) Superselective catheterization of the artery feeding the lateral portion of the mass was achieved and the vessel was embolized using 300–500-μm particles. Because of the proximity of the origin of the radiculomedullary artery, only partial embolization of the mass could be performed and great care was taken to prevent the reflux of particles into the radiculomedullary artery.

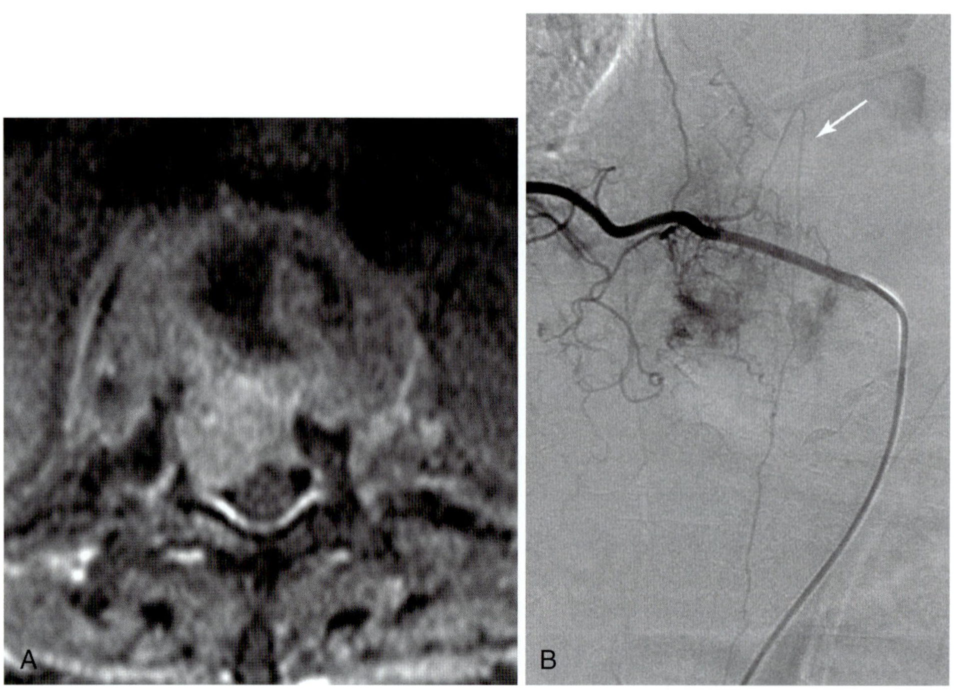

Figure 30-6 Embolization strategy for category B-2 lesions: embolization should not be performed unless the feeding arteries can be superselectively catheterized. (A) Contrast-enhanced MRI of T9 demonstrates a metastatic lesion from renal cell carcinoma involving the vertebral body with extension into the spinal canal and paraspinal spaces bilaterally. (B) Selective arteriogram of the right T9 segmental artery shows the mass to be supplied by branches from the posterior division, close the origin of the radiculomedullary artery (*white arrow*). Because of the proximity of the feeding arteries to the radiculomedullary artery, embolization cannot be performed. Evaluation of the contralateral segmental T9 and T10 arteries revealed additional feeding vessels that were successfully embolized (images not shown).

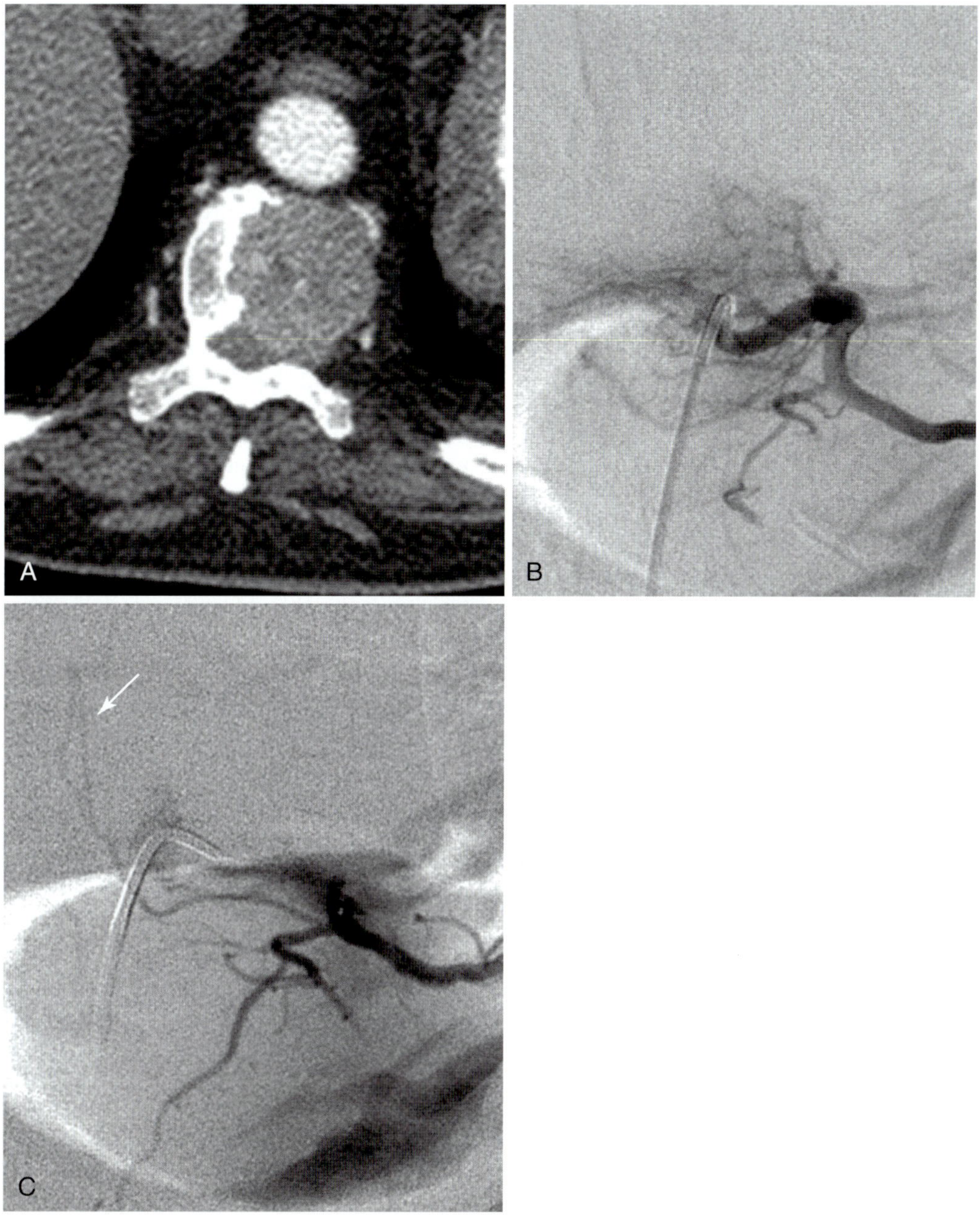

Figure 30-7 Embolization strategy for category B-3 lesions: embolization should not be performed unless the feeding arteries can be superselectively catheterized. (A) Contrast-enhanced CT demonstrates a metastatic lesion from renal cell carcinoma involving the T10 vertebral body and extending into the spinal canal and left neural foramen. (B) Selective arteriogram of the left T10 segmental artery demonstrates the mass is supplied by small branches from the segmental artery proximal to the bifurcation of the anterior and posterior branches. (C) Superselective arteriogram of the segmental artery demonstrates visualization of the radiculomedullary artery (*arrow*). Because of the inability to selectively catheterize the small feeding vessels, embolization was not performed.

Complications and Management

Placement of an IA catheter for chemotherapy infusion is a safe procedure. During chemotherapy infusion, the patient is restricted to bed rest and should be monitored for limb pain, edema, paresthesia, decreased pedal pulses, or hematoma formation at the arterial catheter insertion site.[1] The chemotherapy infusion should be stopped if a complication develops. There were no reported instances of death, limb loss, or other major complication in the combined results of four studies, consisting of over 450 infusion catheter placements.[16-19] Minor complications including transient arterial spasm and local hematoma have been reported.[16]

Postembolization syndrome is an expected occurrence following tumor embolization.[20,21] Signs and symptoms include local pain at the tumor site and low-grade fever, nausea, vomiting, all of which can be managed with over-the-counter medications and are expected to resolve within 3–5 days following the procedure. Nontarget embolization of tumors in the extremities, or the reflux of embolic material into the distal arteries of the hand or foot, may result in transient or permanent paresthesias, loss of sensation, or necrosis. Initial management includes conservative measures such as warm compresses, oral anticoagulation medications, and physical therapy. If portions of the distal extremity become nonviable, a surgical consult is warranted. Pathologic fracture is also a potential complication of tumor embolization in the extremities.

The most feared complication of embolization of spinal tumors is paralysis as a result of the inadvertent embolization of a radiculomedullary artery and subsequent spinal cord ischemia. This complication can be prevented by using meticulous angiographic technique, a coaxial microcatheter system during embolization, appropriately sized particles, and maintaining close monitoring of the patient's neurologic status.

Outcomes and Results

OSTEOSARCOMA

The use of IA chemotherapy with or without embolization before limb salvage surgery in osteosarcoma has been demonstrated to induce substantial tumor necrosis, reduce intraoperative blood loss, improve survival rates, and avoid limb amputation.[22-26] Delivering chemotherapy directly into the tumor via the IA route increases the concentration of the drug to the neoplastic tissue while limiting systemic toxicity,[27,28] may help prevent the development of micrometastases, and reduces the risk of tumor dissemination during surgery.[29]

At our institution, osteosarcoma patients usually receive four cycles of neoadjuvant chemotherapy, consisting of intravenous doxorubicin (30 mg/m^2) administered as a continuous infusion over 24 hours daily for 3 days and intraarterial cisplatin (120 mg/m^2) mixed in 300 mL of 3% (hypertonic) normal saline with 3000 units of heparin administered over 4 hours via an intraarterial infusion catheter, prior to surgical resection. The minimum time interval between treatment cycles is 21 days (Figure 30-8).

Others favor the use of intraarterial chemotherapy and embolization prior to osteosarcoma resection.[25,26] Zhang et al. compared a group of 47 patients who received intraarterial chemotherapy and embolization to a group of 65 patients who received no preoperative intervention and evaluated the effects of preoperative intervention on tumor necrosis and amount of blood loss during surgery.[25] The average amount of tumor necrosis induced by embolization was 83%, and the amount of blood loss and operative times were significantly less than that of the group who did not receive preoperative intervention. The authors also noted the formation of a "false capsule," a fibrous edematous band around the tumor, which facilitated tumor excision.[25] There were no major complications and all patients underwent successful limb salvage surgery.

BONE METASTASES

Bone metastases are the most common cause of cancer-related pain and a major contributor to patient morbidity, limiting mobility and affecting quality of life.[3,30] The etiology of the pain is multifactorial and related to the tumor exerting pressure on the periosteum and adjacent nerves, tumor-induced osteolysis and microfractures, and the production of growth factors and cytokines.[30,31] The goal of transarterial embolization is to devascularize and debulk the tumor, reducing the compression on the periosteum and pressure effects on surrounding structures and nerves, to provide symptomatic relief.[32,33]

The onset of symptomatic relief following transarterial embolization can be as early as 12 hours following the procedure and may last up to 3–9 months[20,34-40] for metastatic lesions and up to several years for nonmalignant bone tumors such as aneurysmal bone cysts (ABCs) and giant cell tumors (GCTs).[20,41] In one of the first series to report on the use of transarterial embolization for the palliation of bone metastases, Barton et al.[20] performed the procedure in 11 patients. All patients experienced pain relief within 12 hours of the procedure and were all successfully weaned from opiate analgesics. The duration of response was 2–8 months and 5 patients were pain free at the time of death. In a larger and more recent series, Rossi et al.[9] reported on a subset of more than 309 embolizations performed in 243 patients for pain palliation of bone metastases. A clinical response was achieved in 97% of procedures and associated with a greater than 50% reduction in pain score and analgesic use. The mean duration of pain relief was 8.1 months (range 1–12 months). Patients who experienced recurrent pain did so at a reduced intensity, and repeat embolizations were performed successfully with subsequent pain relief.[9] Although any hypervascular metastasis is amenable to transarterial embolization, patients with metastases secondary to renal cell and thyroid carcinomas have historically had better responses to therapy when compared to patients with bone metastases related to lung cancer[9,20,38,39](Figure 30-9).

Other authors have explored the use of transarterial chemoembolization of bone metastases for pain palliation. Chiras et al. evaluated the effect of chemoembolization on pain control and tumor growth in 25 patients with surgically unresectable metastatic bone tumors that were refractory to radiotherapy and chemotherapy.[42] These patients with analgesic-resistant bone pain from lytic metastases underwent superselective catheterization and chemoembolization of the lesions with pirarubicin and polyvinyl alcohol (PVA) foam followed by chemoinfusion with carboplatin. Eighty-three percent of patients experienced significant pain relief, with an associated decrease in analgesic use. The mean duration of response was 12 months (range 4–36 months). Measurement of tumor response was available for 65% of patients: 10 patients had stable disease, and partial and complete responses were observed in 4 and 2 patients, respectively. The authors concluded that chemoembolization is well tolerated and may be more effective and reliable as compared to bland embolization to provide pain relief.[42]

For select patients with oligometastatic disease to the bone, transarterial embolization can be used in conjunction with ablation or surgery for local disease control. In the case of hypervascular tumors, 3–4 cm in size, transarterial embolization prior to radiofrequency ablation is helpful to decrease the perfusion-mediated tissue cooling from the tumor and potentiate the effects of ablation.[43,44]

ANEURYSMAL BONE CYST AND GIANT CELL TUMOR

For benign tumors such as ABCs and GCTs, serial transarterial embolization may be used as the primary and definitive treatment, prior to surgical resection or for pain palliation in unresectable tumors.[41,45-50]

ABCs are benign lytic lesions of the bone that represent 1% of primary bone tumors.[51] As a result of rapid bone expansion, the lesion may cause pain and swelling and appear radiographically aggressive. The standard treatment for ABC

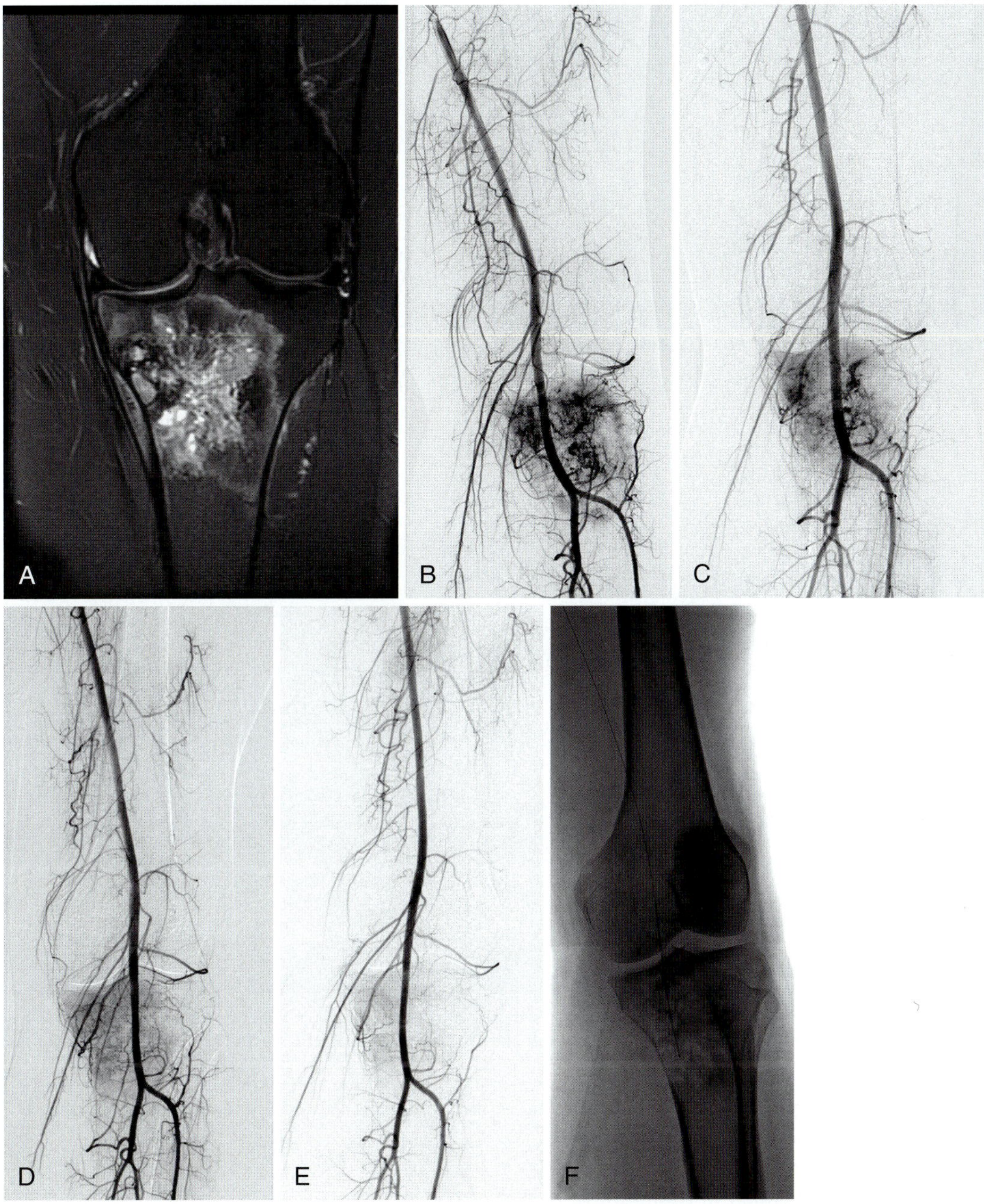

Figure 30-8 A 39-year-old woman with osteosarcoma of the left proximal tibia. (A) Coronal proton density MRI of the left knee before intervention demonstrates a large heterogeneous mass in the proximal tibia. (B–E) Digital subtraction angiography performed from the superficial femoral artery over a series of four infusion catheter placements, each 21 days apart, demonstrates a large hypervascular mass supplied by branches of the superficial femoral, popliteal, and anterior tibial arteries. There is progressive decrease in the vascularization of the mass over time. Arteriograms were performed in the frontal projection using an injection rate of 4 mL/second for a total of 12 mL of contrast administered. (F) Frontal projection radiograph demonstrates the position of a 6-cm working-length infusion wire positioned in the popliteal artery, just proximal to the trifurcation.

is surgical resection and curettage but local recurrence rates can be as high as 31%.[52] Embolization was initially introduced as a preoperative procedure to reduce intraoperative blood loss and for the treatment of ABCs located in areas such as the spine, sacrum, or pelvis that are not easily amenable to a surgical approach[51]; however, recent studies indicate that the tumor may respond to serial embolization without requiring further surgical intervention.[49-51,53] In the largest series, Rossi et al. reported on 55 embolization sessions performed in 36 patients with ABC.[51] Subselective embolization was performed in all patients using *N*-butyl-cyanoacrylate (NBCA). Twenty-four (67% of the total number of patients) were considered healed after no evidence of tumor recurrence at the 2-year follow-up mark (range 0.9–2 years).[51] Serial embolization was required in 39% of patients. The recurrence or persistence of disease rate was 21.2% in lesions less than 5 cm and 58.8% in lesions greater than 5 cm, for an overall recurrence rate of 39%[51] (Figure 30-10).

Although benign, GCTs are often locally aggressive, and when located in the sacrum, can be difficult to manage surgically, with local recurrence rates as high as 33%.[47,54] Three series, with a combined total of 33 patients with GCTs of the sacrum,

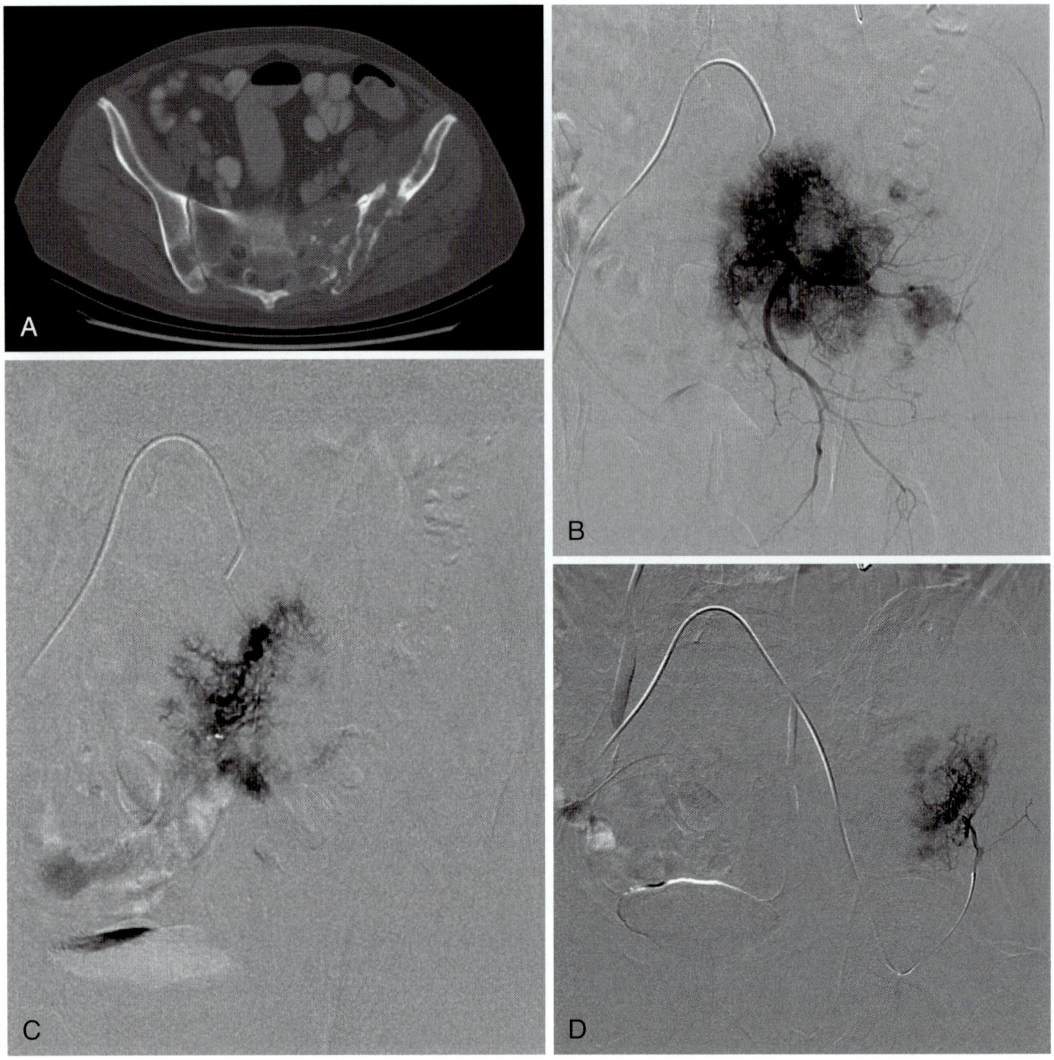

Figure 30-9 A 54-year-old man with metastatic renal cell carcinoma who presented with left buttock and pelvic pain. (A) Axial image from a contrast-enhanced CT scan demonstrates lytic bone metastases involving the left sacrum and iliac bone. (B) The patient presented for transarterial embolization for pain palliation and arteriogram from the left internal iliac artery demonstrates a corresponding hypervascular mass. (C and D) Arteriograms performed after subselective catheterization with a microcatheter demonstrate tumor blush from a branch of the posterior division of the internal iliac artery (C) and the deep circumflex iliac artery (D). Embolization with 300–500-μm particles was performed from these locations. The patient experienced pain relief for 8 months.

demonstrated serial embolization resulted in symptom resolution and tumor ossification.[46-48] Of the 33 patients, 25 demonstrated substantial pain relief with preservation of function and ossification or stabilization of tumor size. The follow-up in these patients ranged from 6 months to 21.2 years.[46-48] Recurrence rates were reported to be 31% at 10 years and 43% at 15 and 20 years in one series[47] (Figure 30-11).

HEMANGIOMA

Hemangiomas are benign vascular malformations that can be commonly found in the vertebrae. Although the treatment options for symptomatic or painful hemangiomas include sclerotherapy, vertebroplasty, radiation therapy or surgery, embolization has also been reported to be effective for pain palliation.[55-57] Additional case series have reported favorable results following hemangioma embolization,[58,59] and others have reported on the success of embolization as a definitive treatment for symptomatic hemangiomas, obviating the need for surgery.[9,56]

PREOPERATIVE EMBOLIZATION OF HYPERVASCULAR TUMORS IN THE SPINE

Preoperative embolization of bone tumors at any site (Figures 30-12 and 30-13) can be used to reduce intraoperative blood loss during surgical resection; however, the procedure is particularly useful as an adjunct to spine surgery. Spinal surgery of hypervascular tumors, most commonly metastatic renal cell carcinoma, is often complicated by intraoperative hemorrhage, which can prolong procedure time, obscure the surgical field, and lead to postoperative complications. Although there is a lack of prospective, randomized data on the benefits of preoperative spine embolization, enough evidence from retrospective studies, documenting that the intraoperative blood loss in patients who received preoperative spine embolization (550–4300 mL) is significantly lower than that in nonembolized patients (4700–8300 mL), exists to make preoperative embolization a prerequisite to surgery for most spine surgeons.[8,60-65] Preoperative embolization has also been associated with

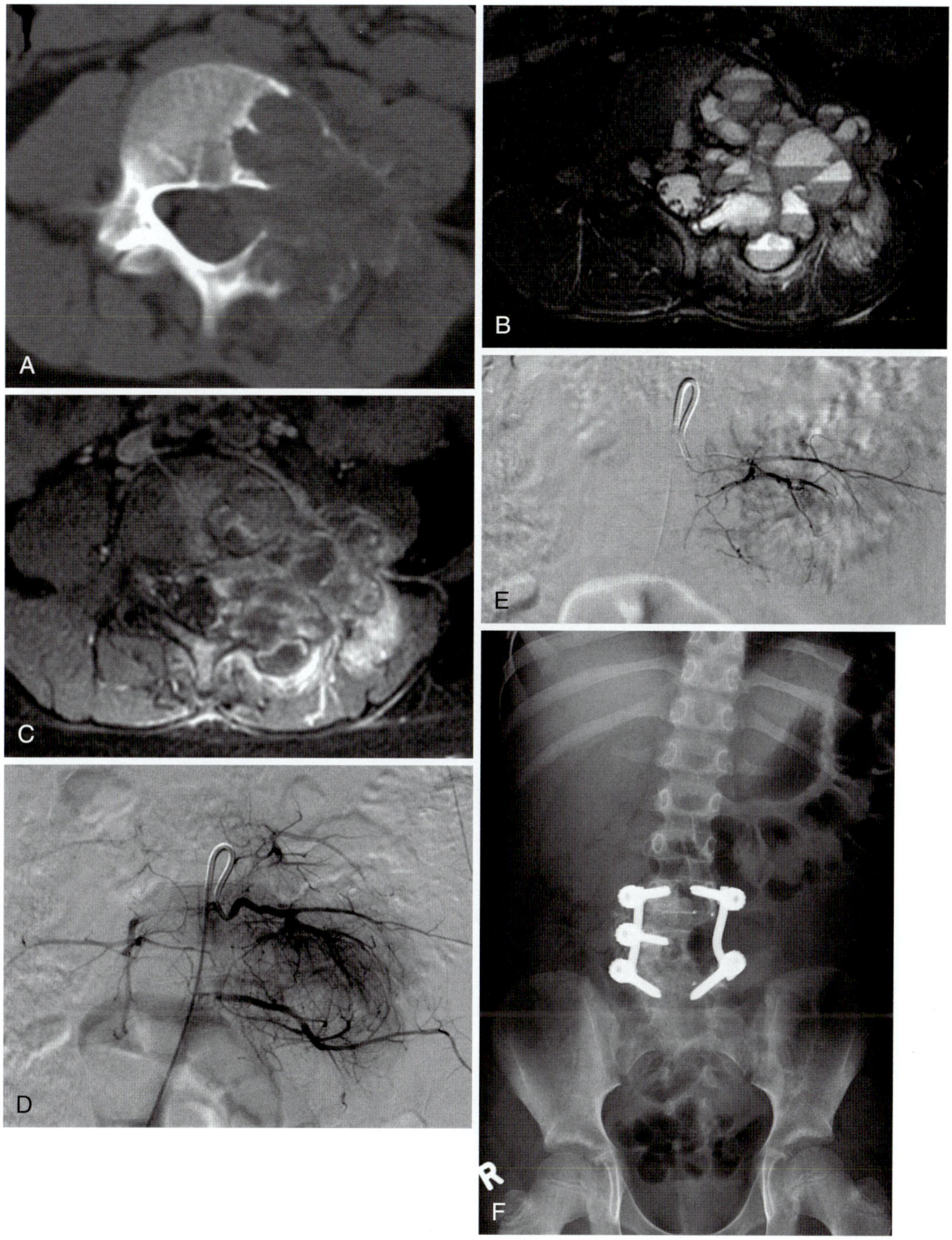

Figure 30-10 A 9-year-old boy who presented with low back pain. (A) Axial non-contrast-enhanced CT scan of the spine at L4 demonstrates an expansile lesion affecting the posterolateral vertebral body, pedicle, lateral elements, and lamina on the left side. This lesion was biopsy proven to be an aneurysmal bone cyst (ABC). Axial T2-weighted (B) and axial contrast-enhanced T1-weighted (C) MRI images of L4 demonstrate the cystic nature of this expansile lesion with multiple fluid–fluid levels. There is also a soft tissue component of the lesion that extends into the spinal canal, resulting in shifting of the thecal sac toward the right but without compression of its contents. (D) A SOS-2 (Cook, Inc., Bloomington, IN) catheter was used to select the left L3 lumbar artery. Arteriogram demonstrates hypervascular tumor blush of the ABC and no filling of the radiculomedullary artery. (E) Following selective catheterization of the L3 lumbar artery with a 3-F microcatheter, embolization was performed using 300–500-μm particles in preparation for surgery. The postembolization arteriogram demonstrates significant reduction in tumor hypervascularity. (F) Frontal radiograph demonstrates partial resection of L4 and posterior stabilization with pedicle screw and rod fixation at L3, L4, and L5. Although ABC can be managed with serial embolizations, the young age of this patient and risk of repeated radiation exposure made this option less ideal for this case. In addition, the lesion exhibited aggressive features with documented interval growth over a 2-month period and has a soft tissue component that abuts the thecal sac. Therefore, it was felt that a surgical resection would provide the best opportunity for disease control without compromising future growth. On the day after the embolization, the patient underwent partial L4 vertebrectomy, L3 and L4 laminectomy, L3 inferior facetectomy, and complete L4 facetectomy for radial resection of the tumor. Posterior arthrodesis from L3 to L5 was constructed using a mixture of allograft and demineralized bone matrix and posterior stabilization was performed from L3 to L5 using pedicle screw and rod fixation. The total estimated blood loss was 400 mL.

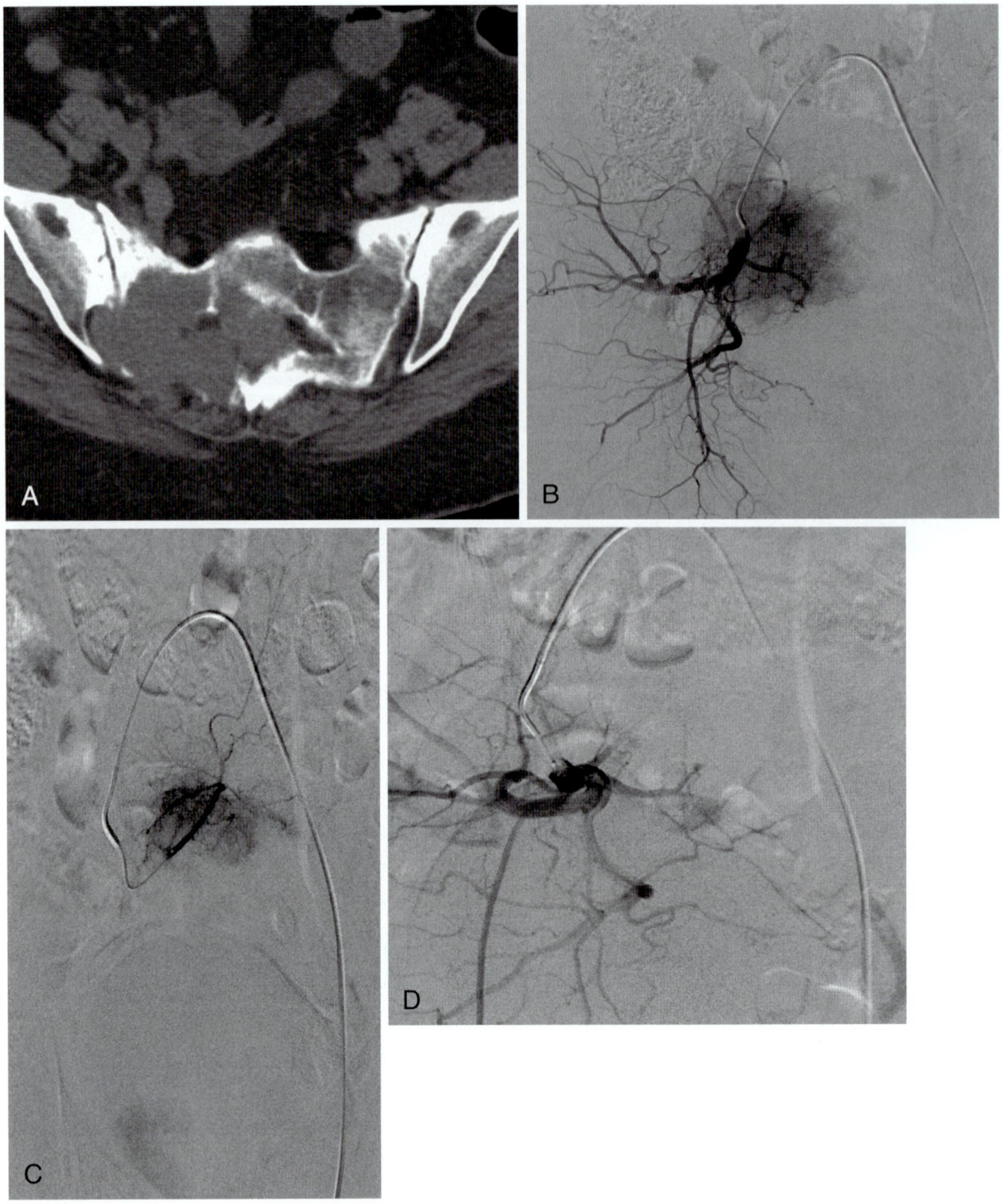

Figure 30-11 A 70-year-old woman with sacral pain. (A) Axial non-contrast-enhanced CT scan of the sacrum reveals a lytic lesion involving the right sacrum and iliac bone. This lesion was biopsied, and pathology revealed giant cell tumor. Although the tumor extends across midline to abut the S2 neural foramen, the patient denies neurologic dysfunction. Given the difficult surgical approach and likely requirement for extensive resection of the sacrum, the patient was referred for serial embolization. (B) Arteriogram from the right internal iliac artery demonstrates hypervascular tumor blush corresponding to the known lesion. (C) Following superselective catheterization with a 3-F microcatheter of a branch of the posterior division of the internal iliac artery, embolization was performed using 300–500-μm particles. (D) Postembolization arteriogram from the right internal iliac artery demonstrates near-total resolution of the tumor blush. The contralateral internal iliac artery was also interrogated and a branch from the posterior division, seen to supply the tumor, was successfully embolized (not shown).

shorter mean operating time, decreased need for transfusion, and decreased hospital stay.[8,66] Preoperative embolization should be performed 24–48 hours prior to surgical resection.

Summary

Intraarterial procedures provide versatility in the management of patients with either primary or secondary musculoskeletal lesions. These procedures can be used as a stand-alone therapy or in combination with ablative or surgical therapies to treat tumor pain, aid in local disease control, and as a preoperative adjunct to reduce intraoperative blood loss and reduce the incidence of postoperative complications.

REFERENCES

The complete reference list is available online at www.expertconsult.com.

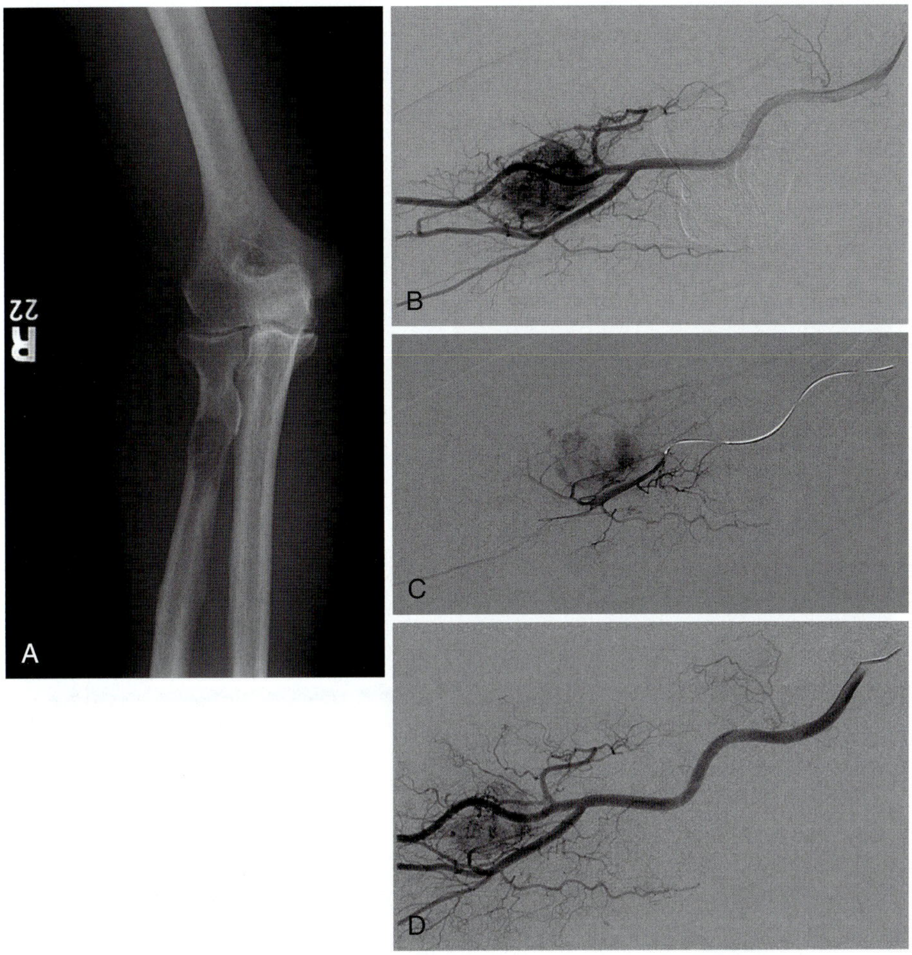

Figure 30-12 A 67-year-old man with metastatic renal cell carcinoma to the radius presented for preoperative embolization. (A) Frontal radiograph of the right elbow demonstrates a lytic, destructive lesion involving the proximal right radius. (B) Arteriogram from the axillary artery demonstrates a hypervascular lesion in the proximal radius. (C) Following subselective catheterization with a 3-F microcatheter, the recurrent radial artery that was noted to supply the lesion was embolized using 300–500-μm particles. (D) Postembolization arteriogram demonstrates an approximately 50% reduction in tumor vascularity. Other tumoral feeding branches were extremely small, could not be subselectively catheterized, and were therefore not embolized. The following day, the patient underwent curettage of the proximal radius lesion with reconstruction of the cavitary defect using polymethylmethacrylate and Steinmann pin. The estimated blood loss was minimal.

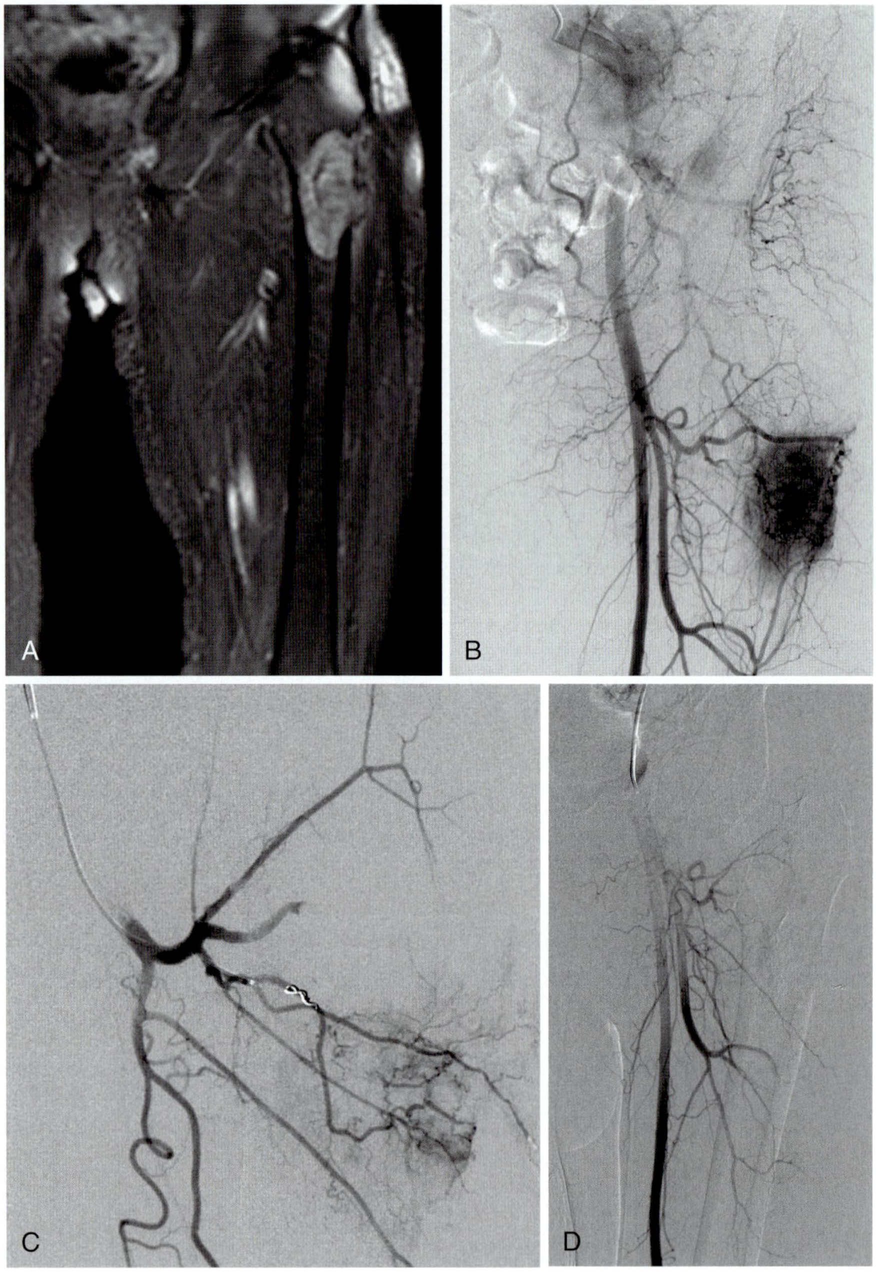

Figure 30-13 A 62-year-old man with metastatic renal cell carcinoma to the left femur presents for preoperative embolization. (A) Coronal T2-weighted MRI demonstrates a hyperintense lesion involving the proximal diaphysis of the left femur. (B) Arteriogram from the external iliac artery demonstrates the hypervascular tumor to be supplied by branches of the profunda femoris artery. (C) Following subselective catheterization with a 3-F microcatheter, a branch of the profunda femoris artery was embolized using 300–500-μm particles. (D) Postembolization arteriogram from the external iliac artery demonstrates near total resolution of the tumor blush. The patient underwent surgical resection of the femur with curettage of the lesion, reconstruction of the cavitary defect with polymethylmethacrylate and intramedullary rod fixation 48 hours after embolization. The estimated blood loss was 800 mL.

O

S